Marine Bioactive Peptides

Marine Bioactive Peptides: Structure, Function, and Therapeutic Potential

Special Issue Editor

Tatiana V. Ovchinnikova

MDPI • Basel • Beijing • Wuhan • Barcelona • Belgrade

MDPI

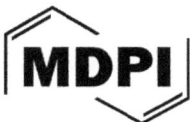

Special Issue Editor
Tatiana V. Ovchinnikova
Russian Academy of Sciences
Russia

Editorial Office
MDPI
St. Alban-Anlage 66
4052 Basel, Switzerland

This is a reprint of articles from the Special Issue published online in the open access journal *Marine Drugs* (ISSN 1660-3397) from 2018 to 2019 (available at: https://www.mdpi.com/journal/marinedrugs/special_issues/Marine_Bioactive_Peptides)

For citation purposes, cite each article independently as indicated on the article page online and as indicated below:

LastName, A.A.; LastName, B.B.; LastName, C.C. Article Title. *Journal Name* **Year**, *Article Number*, Page Range.

ISBN 978-3-03921-532-4 (Pbk)
ISBN 978-3-03921-533-1 (PDF)

Contents

About the Special Issue Editor

Tatiana V. Ovchinnikova, Head of the Science-Educational Centre, M.M. Shemyakin & Yu.A. Ovchinnikov Institute of Bioorganic Chemistry, Russian Academy of Sciences; Full Professor, Department of Bioorganic Chemistry, M.V. Lomonosov Moscow State University. She received her degree in Chemistry with Honors at the University of Kyiv (Ukraine) and then completed her Ph.D. in Bioorganic Chemistry at M.M. Shemyakin & Yu.A. Ovchinnikov Institute of Bioorganic Chemistry (Moscow, Russia). She obtained a Second Doctorate (Habilitation) degree in Bioorganic Chemistry and Biotechnology in 2011. Her research interests focus on discovery, isolation, structural elucidation, functional characterization, structure–function relationship analysis, and the evaluation of the therapeutic potential of novel antimicrobial and host defense peptides of animal and plant origin, investigation of their antimicrobial and anticancer activity, as well as mechanisms of their participation in innate immunity, screening of marine organisms for the discovery of novel peptides with high activities against microorganisms and transformed human cells, bioengineering of peptide molecules with improved therapeutic potency and efficacy for using in medicine and veterinary, design of innovative antibiotics and anticancer drugs. She has published over 450 scientific papers, reviews, book chapters, patents, and communications at national and international conferences, including over 150 peer-reviewed publications in international journals.

marine drugs

MDPI

Editorial

Structure, Function, and Therapeutic Potential of Marine Bioactive Peptides

Tatiana V. Ovchinnikova

M.M. Shemyakin & Yu.A. Ovchinnikov Institute of Bioorganic Chemistry, the Russian Academy of Sciences, Miklukho-Maklaya str. 16/10, 117997 Moscow, Russia; ovch@ibch.ru; Tel.: +7-495-336-44-44

Received: 14 August 2019; Accepted: 26 August 2019; Published: 28 August 2019

In recent years, bioactive peptides from marine organisms have gained increasing attention in the field of pharmaceutical, cosmeceutical, and nutraceutical product development owing to their interesting biological properties. They are involved in fundamental mechanisms that allow the survival of living organisms, including their defense, reproduction, growth, and homeostasis. Marine peptides that are diverse in structure and function have been found in various phyla, and their number has dynamically grown over the recent years. Some of them are evolutionary ancient molecular factors of innate immunity that play a key role in host defense [1]. Long-term evolution of marine organisms proceeded in continuous contact with pathogens, and efficient defense mechanisms were the necessary condition of their survival. Peptides with protective functions were isolated from tissues of many marine invertebrates and vertebrates. A plethora of biological activities, including antibacterial, antifungal, antiviral, cytotoxic, neurotoxic, anticoagulant, antidiabetic, antifreeze, endotoxin-binding, and immune-modulating, make marine peptides an attractive molecular basis for the design of innovative antibiotics, anticancer drugs, analgetics, medicines for neurological disorders, etc.

The Special Issue "Marine Bioactive Peptides: Structure, Function, and Therapeutic Potential" was aimed at collecting papers on up-to-date information regarding isolation, structural elucidation, functional characterization, and evaluation of the therapeutic potential of peptides from marine organisms. Chemical synthesis and biotechnological production of marine peptides and their mimetics were also a focus of this Special Issue. In total, 24 papers were accepted and included in the Special Issue, which are now published as a book. Getting started with this book, we planned to produce an interesting edition that would cover breakthroughs and recent trends in basic and applied research on marine peptides.

Bioactive peptides showing antihypertensive, antioxidative, and antidiabetic activities were isolated from seaweed [2]. Algae peptides have strong potential for use as therapeutic drugs, especially for treatment of cardiovascular diseases and diabetes, and as functional food formulations in health care. This Special Issue includes papers analyzing potential health impacts of bioactive peptides from the seaweed species *Pyropia yezoensis*, *Chlorella pyrenoidosa*, and *Gracilariopsis lemaneiformis*. In particular, the protective effects of the *P. yezoensis* peptide PYP15 against dexamethasone-induced myotube atrophy was revealed [3]. The effect of the *Chlorella pyrenoidosa* protein hydrolysate (CPPH) and *Chlorella pyrenoidosa* protein hydrolysate-calcium chelate (CPPH-Ca) on calcium absorption and gut microbiota composition was evaluated [4]. It was demonstrated that CPPH-Ca could promote calcium absorption partially through regulating specific gut microbiota and modulating expressions of the calcium absorption-related genes in kidney. Therefore, CPPH-Ca may be used to promote the calcium absorption and reduce the risk of calcium deficiency [4]. Two novel angiotensin-converting enzyme (ACE) inhibitory peptides were identified in the *Gracilariopsis lemaneiformis* protein hydrolysate. Both peptides were noncompetitive inhibitors of ACE and reduced systolic and diastolic blood pressure in spontaneously hypertensive rats [5].

All members of the phylum Cnidaria (sea anemones, corals, jellyfish, and hydra) are venomous [6]. Acid-sensing ion channel 3 (ASIC3) makes an important contribution to development and maintenance of inflammatory and acid-induced pain. An inhibition of ASIC3 was reported as an attractive approach to inducing analgesia. Different ASIC3 inhibitors including the peptides APETx2 and Ugr9-1 from the venom of the sea anemone *Urticina grebelnyi* and nonpeptide molecules sevanol and diclofenac were compared with a focus on their anti-inflammatory and analgesic effects [7]. All the tested compounds had distinct effects on pH-induced ASIC3 current. Comparison of the ASIC3-selective ligands in different animal pain models provides an opportunity to estimate their pharmacological potential and specify the properties of the most attractive compound for analgetics development [7]. The antitumor effect of the sea anemone *Anthopleura anjunae* peptide AAP-H in prostate cancer DU-145 cells was investigated in vitro and in vivo [8]. The obtained results indicated that AAP-H was nontoxic and exhibited the antitumor activity. The role of the phosphatidylinositol 3-kinase/protein kinase B/mammalian rapamycin target protein (PI3K/AKT/mTOR) signaling pathway in the antitumor mechanism of APP-H was investigated. It was shown that the antitumor mechanism of APP-H on DU-145 cells may involve regulation of the PI3K/AKT/mTOR signaling pathway, which eventually promotes apoptosis via mitochondrial and death receptor pathways [8].

Echinoderms are ancient marine invertebrates. The phylum Echinodermata contains about 7000 living species including sea stars (asteroids), sea urchins (echinoids), brittle stars (ophiuroids), sea lilies (crinoids), and sea cucumbers (holothurians). Previously, natural ACE-inhibitory peptides were obtained from the sea cucumber protein hydrolysates by a plastein reaction [9,10]. The aim of the published work was to prepare efficient ACE-inhibitory peptides from sea cucumber-modified hydrolysates by adding exogenous amino acids. Two novel efficient ACE-inhibitory peptides were purified and identified from the sea cucumber *Acaudina molpadioidea* which may be useful in the preparation of antihypertensive drugs [11].

Synthesis of bioactive peptides was detected in the neuroendocrine, immune, and gut system of mollusks [12]. A novel peptide, isolated from the abalone *Haliotis discus hannai* and designated as AATP, effectively inhibited matrix metalloproteinases (MMPs) by blocking MAPKs and NF-κB pathways, leading to the downregulation of metastasis of tumor cells [13]. Moreover, AATP significantly inhibited vasculogenic mimicry and pro-angiogenic factors, including vascular endothelial growth factor and MMPs by suppression of AKT/mTOR signaling. The anti-metastatic and anti-vascular effect of AATP in HT1080 cells revealed that AATP may be a potential anticancer lead compound [13]. Zinc-binding peptides were prepared from the oyster *Crassostrea gigas'* hydrolysates modified by the plastein reaction, and the zinc absorption mechanism of the peptide-zinc complex was examined [14]. The complex was shown to promote the intestinal absorption of zinc and have a great potential for zinc supplementation as a functional food ingredient [14]. Two novel multi-functional peptides were isolated from the marine snail *Neptunea arthritica cumingii*. Both peptides showed antioxidant, antidiabetic, and ACE-inhibitory activities [15]. The venom of each *Conus* species consists of a diverse array of neurophysiologically active peptides. Isolation and characterization of the first bioactive peptide from the venom of *Conus ateralbus*, named conotoxin AtVIA, was described [16]. AtVIA manifested an excitatory activity in mouse lumbar dorsal root ganglion neurons. AtVIA has homology with δ-conotoxins from other worm-hunters, including conserved elements in amino acid sequences of δ-conotoxins from fish-hunting *Conus*. The presence of δ-conotoxins that act on vertebrate Na$^+$-channels has thus been established in two divergent worm-hunting clades. The results are consistent with the hypothesis that certain worm-hunting *Conus* evolved δ-conotoxins that act to probably deter competitors in a defensive envenomation strategy [16]. To analyze putative conotoxin transcripts from the venom ducts of three vermivorous cone snails (*Conus caracteristicus*, *Conus generalis*, and *Conus quercinus*), high-throughput transcriptome sequencing was performed [17]. In total, 118, 61, and 48 putative conotoxins (across 22 superfamilies) were identified from the three *Conus* species, respectively [17]. Two comprehensive reviews included in this Special Issue deal with structural and functional analyses of cone snail toxins [18] and with computational studies on the conopeptides [19], providing a good overview of bioactive peptides from venoms of *Conus* species and their therapeutic potential.

Polychaeta is an almost uninvestigated class of invertebrates in the context of discovery of new host defense peptides. The large majority of polychaeta species are marine animals that inhabit all oceans and seas from the Arctic to the Antarctic. On the grounds of their morphology and physiology, polychaeta are considered as the most primitive annelids [20]. Papers included in this Special Issue deal with marine polychaeta, providing good examples of their biological potential. The peptides arenicins and nicomicins, isolated from *Arenicola marina* [21,22] and *Nicomache minor* [23], respectively, exhibited in vitro antimicrobial activity and possessed cytotoxicity against cancer cells. Arenicin was shown to modulate the human complement system [22]. At relatively low concentrations, the peptide stimulates complement activation and lysis of target erythrocytes, whereas at higher concentrations arenicin acts as a complement inhibitor [22]. The peptide PAP with anticancer activity was purified from the enzymatic hydrolysate of *Perinereis aibuhitensis* [24]. PAP inhibited proliferation and induced apoptosis of human lung cancer H1299 cells. The peptide may be used for prevention or treatment of human non-small cell lung cancer [24].

Crustaceans form a diverse arthropod taxon which contains about 67,000 described species including crabs, shrimps, lobsters, crayfish, prawns, krill, woodlice, and barnacles. Many crustaceans are free-living marine animals. A novel antimicrobial peptide polyphemusin III from the horseshoe crab *Limulus polyphemus* was examined against bacterial strains and human cancer, transformed, and normal cell cultures [25]. The peptide showed cytotoxic activity and caused fast permeabilization of the cytoplasmic membrane of human leukemia cells HL-60. In comparison to known polyphemusins and tachyplesins, polyphemusin III demonstrated a similar or lower antimicrobial effect, but significantly higher cytotoxicity against human cancer and transformed cells [25]. Anti-lipopolysaccharide factors (ALFs) are β-hairpin peptides with the ability to bind to microbial surface molecules. ALFs appear to be exclusive to marine chelicerates and crustaceans. The remarkable diversity of ALFs was demonstrated in the *Litopenaeus vannamei* shrimp [26]. At least seven members of the ALF family were found, all of which were encoded by different loci with conserved gene organization. The transcriptional profile of ALFs was compared in terms of tissue distribution, response to pathogens and shrimp development. ALFs were found to be constitutively expressed in hemocytes and to respond differently to tissue damage. ALFs form a family of shrimp peptides that has been the subject of intense diversification. These data suggest that multiple selection pressures have led to functional diversification of ALFs in shrimp [26].

Fish-derived bioactive peptides suggested to influence pathways involved in regulation of blood pressure, lipid and glucose metabolism, and body composition. Some of them could be developed as antihypertensive components in functional foods or nutraceuticals. The protective effects of the tilapia *Oreochromis niloticus* peptide against oxidative stress, inflammation, and endothelial injury were evaluated in angiotensin II (Ang II)-stimulated human umbilical vein endothelial cells [27]. The peptide moderated Ang II-stimulated oxidative stress and vascular endothelial dysfunction [27]. Another tilapia peptide with a high ACE-inhibitory activity was identified, and its antihypertensive effect was evaluated in vivo [28]. The obtained results showed that the tilapia peptide exerts an antihypertensive effect in spontaneously hypertensive rats, and the systolic and diastolic blood pressures of the rats remarkably decreased [28]. Thus, both tilapia peptides have potential for application in therapy of hypertensive disorders. Eight antioxidant peptides were purified from the hairtail *Trichiurus japonicas* [29]. The peptides might serve as potential antioxidants in pharmaceutical and health food industries. Several novel short antibacterial peptides were isolated from the half-fin anchovy *Setipinna taty* [30]. The peptides displayed antibacterial activity against *Escherichia coli* via inducing intracellular H_2O_2 production [30]. A novel peptide inhibiting the influenza A H1N1 virus neuraminidase was isolated from the skin hydrolysates of the cod *Gadus macrocephalus* [31]. The peptide acts as a neuraminidase blocker inhibiting influenza A virus in Madin–Darby canine kidney (MDCK) cells. Thus, the peptide has potential utility in treatment of the influenza virus infection.

As seen from the above overview, the papers included in this Special Issue deal with diverse marine organisms, providing an overall view of their biological potential. A range of new marine-derived peptides were isolated from evolutionarily distant species and characterized. Significantly, most of them displayed broad-spectrum biological activities and potential for use in clinical trials in humans. All the papers presented in this Special Issue underline the central role of bioactive peptides in innate immunity of marine organisms as well as their therapeutic potential for human health care.

In conclusion, the Guest Editor thanks all the authors who contributed to this Special Issue, all the reviewers for evaluating the submitted manuscripts, and the Editorial board of *Marine Drugs*, especially Orazio Taglialatela-Scafat, Editor-in-Chief of this journal, and Estelle Fan, Assistant Editor, for their kind help in bringing this book into reality.

References

1. Hancock, R.E.W.; Brown, K.L.; Mookherjee, N. Host defence peptides from invertebrates—Emerging antimicrobial strategies. *Immunobiology* **2006**, *211*, 315–322. [CrossRef] [PubMed]
2. Admassu, H.; Gasmalla, M.A.A.; Yang, R.; Zhao, W. Bioactive Peptides Derived from Seaweed Protein and Their Health Benefits: Antihypertensive, Antioxidant, and Antidiabetic Properties. *J. Food Sci.* **2018**, *83*, 6–16. [CrossRef] [PubMed]
3. Lee, M.-K.; Choi, J.-W.; Choi, Y.H.; Nam, T.-J. Protective Effect of *Pyropia yezoensis* Peptide on Dexamethasone-Induced Myotube Atrophy in C2C12 Myotubes. *Mar. Drugs* **2019**, *17*, 284. [CrossRef] [PubMed]
4. Hua, P.; Xiong, Y.; Yu, Z.; Liu, B.; Zhao, L. Effect of *Chlorella pyrenoidosa* Protein Hydrolysate-Calcium Chelate on Calcium Absorption Metabolism and Gut Microbiota Composition in Low-Calcium Diet-Fed Rats. *Mar. Drugs* **2019**, *17*, 348. [CrossRef] [PubMed]
5. Deng, Z.; Liu, Y.; Wang, J.; Wu, S.; Geng, L.; Sui, Z.; Zhang, Q. Antihypertensive Effects of Two Novel Angiotensin I-Converting Enzyme (ACE) Inhibitory Peptides from *Gracilariopsis lemaneiformis* (Rhodophyta) in Spontaneously Hypertensive Rats (SHRs). *Mar. Drugs* **2018**, *16*, 299. [CrossRef] [PubMed]
6. Turk, T.; Kem, W.R. The phylum Cnidaria and investigations of its toxins and venoms until 1990. *Toxicon* **2009**, *54*, 1031–1037. [CrossRef] [PubMed]
7. Andreev, Y.A.; Osmakov, D.I.; Koshelev, S.G.; Maleeva, E.E.; Logashina, Y.A.; Palikov, V.A.; Palikova, Y.A.; Dyachenko, I.A.; Kozlov, S.A. Analgesic Activity of Acid-Sensing Ion Channel 3 (ASIC3) Inhibitors: Sea Anemones Peptides Ugr9-1 and APETx2 versus Low Molecular Weight Compounds. *Mar. Drugs* **2018**, *16*, 500. [CrossRef]
8. Li, X.; Tang, Y.; Yu, F.; Sun, Y.; Huang, F.; Chen, Y.; Yang, Z.; Ding, G. Inhibition of Prostate Cancer DU-145 Cells Proliferation by *Anthopleura anjunae* Oligopeptide (YVPGP) via PI3K/AKT/mTOR Signaling Pathway. *Mar. Drugs* **2018**, *16*, 325. [CrossRef]
9. Zhao, Y.H.; Li, B.F.; Ma, J.J.; Dong, S.Y.; Liu, Z.Y.; Zeng, M.Y. Purification and synthesis of ACE-inhibitory peptide from *Acaudina molpadioidea* protein hydrolysate. *Chem. J. Chin. Univ.* **2012**, *33*, 308–312.
10. Shen, Q.; Zeng, M.; Zhao, Y. Modification of *Acaudina molpadioides* hydrolysates by plastein reaction and preparation of ACE-inhibitory peptides. *Chem. J. Chin. Univ.* **2014**, *35*, 965–970.
11. Li, J.; Liu, Z.; Zhao, Y.; Zhu, X.; Yu, R.; Dong, S.; Wu, H. Novel Natural Angiotensin Converting Enzyme (ACE)-Inhibitory Peptides Derived from Sea Cucumber-Modified Hydrolysates by Adding Exogenous Proline and a Study of Their Structure–Activity Relationship. *Mar. Drugs* **2018**, *16*, 271. [CrossRef] [PubMed]
12. Tascedda, F.; Ottaviani, E. Biologically active peptides in mollusks. *Invertebr. Surviv. J.* **2016**, *13*, 186–190.
13. Gong, F.; Chen, M.-F.; Zhang, Y.-Y.; Li, C.-Y.; Zhou, C.-X.; Hong, P.-Z.; Sun, S.-L.; Qian, Z.-J. A Novel Peptide from Abalone (*Haliotis discus hannai*) to Suppress Metastasis and Vasculogenic Mimicry of Tumor Cells and Enhance Anti-Tumor Effect In Vitro. *Mar. Drugs* **2019**, *17*, 244. [CrossRef] [PubMed]
14. Zhang, S.-S.; Han, L.-W.; Shi, Y.-P.; Li, X.-B.; Zhang, X.-M.; Hou, H.-R.; Lin, H.-W.; Liu, K.-C. Two Novel Multi-Functional Peptides from Meat and Visceral Mass of Marine Snail *Neptunea arthritica cumingii* and Their Activities In Vitro and In Vivo. *Mar. Drugs* **2018**, *16*, 473. [CrossRef] [PubMed]
15. Li, J.; Gong, C.; Wang, Z.; Gao, R.; Ren, J.; Zhou, X.; Wang, H.; Xu, H.; Xiao, F.; Cao, Y.; et al. Oyster-Derived Zinc-Binding Peptide Modified by Plastein Reaction via Zinc Chelation Promotes the Intestinal Absorption of Zinc. *Mar. Drugs* **2019**, *17*, 341. [CrossRef] [PubMed]

16. Neves, J.L.B.; Imperial, J.S.; Morgenstern, D.; Ueberheide, B.; Gajewiak, J.; Antunes, A.; Robinson, S.D.; Espino, S.; Watkins, M.; Vasconcelos, V.; et al. Characterization of the First Conotoxin from *Conus ateralbus*, a Vermivorous Cone Snail from the Cabo Verde Archipelago. *Mar. Drugs* **2019**, *17*, 432. [CrossRef] [PubMed]

17. Yao, G.; Peng, C.; Zhu, Y.; Fan, C.; Jiang, H.; Chen, J.; Cao, Y.; Shi, Q. High-Throughput Identification and Analysis of Novel Conotoxins from Three Vermivorous Cone Snails by Transcriptome Sequencing. *Mar. Drugs* **2019**, *17*, 193. [CrossRef] [PubMed]

18. Duque, H.M.; Dias, S.C.; Franco, O.L. Structural and Functional Analyses of Cone Snail Toxins. *Mar. Drugs* **2019**, *17*, 370. [CrossRef] [PubMed]

19. Mansbach, R.A.; Travers, T.; McMahon, B.H.; Fair, J.M.; Gnanakaran, S. Snails In Silico: A Review of Computational Studies on the Conopeptides. *Mar. Drugs* **2019**, *17*, 145. [CrossRef] [PubMed]

20. Tasiemski, A. Antimicrobial peptides in annelids. *Invertebr. Surviv. J.* **2008**, *5*, 75–82.

21. Orlov, D.S.; Shamova, O.V.; Eliseev, I.E.; Zharkova, M.S.; Chakchir, O.B.; Antcheva, N.; Zachariev, S.; Panteleev, P.V.; Kokryakov, V.N.; Ovchinnikova, T.V.; et al. Redesigning Arenicin-1, an Antimicrobial Peptide from the Marine Polychaeta *Arenicola marina*, by Strand Rearrangement or Branching, Substitution of Specific Residues, and Backbone Linearization or Cyclization. *Mar. Drugs* **2019**, *17*, 376. [CrossRef] [PubMed]

22. Umnyakova, E.S.; Gorbunov, N.P.; Zhakhov, A.V.; Krenev, I.A.; Ovchinnikova, T.V.; Kokryakov, V.N.; Berlov, M.N. Modulation of Human Complement System by Antimicrobial Peptide Arenicin-1 from *Arenicola marina*. *Mar. Drugs* **2018**, *16*, 480. [CrossRef] [PubMed]

23. Panteleev, P.V.; Tsarev, A.V.; Bolosov, I.A.; Paramonov, A.S.; Marggraf, M.B.; Sychev, S.V.; Shenkarev, Z.O.; Ovchinnikova, T.V. Novel Antimicrobial Peptides from the Arctic Polychaeta *Nicomache minor* Provide New Molecular Insight into Biological Role of the BRICHOS Domain. *Mar. Drugs* **2018**, *16*, 401. [CrossRef] [PubMed]

24. Jiang, S.; Jia, Y.; Tang, Y.; Zheng, D.; Han, X.; Yu, F.; Chen, Y.; Huang, F.; Yang, Z.; Ding, G. Anti-Proliferation Activity of a Decapeptide from *Perinereies aibuhitensis* toward Human Lung Cancer H1299 Cells. *Mar. Drugs* **2019**, *17*, 122. [CrossRef]

25. Marggraf, M.B.; Panteleev, P.V.; Emelianova, A.A.; Sorokin, M.I.; Bolosov, I.A.; Buzdin, A.A.; Kuzmin, D.V.; Ovchinnikova, T.V. Cytotoxic Potential of the Novel Horseshoe Crab Peptide Polyphemusin III. *Mar. Drugs* **2018**, *16*, 466. [CrossRef]

26. Matos, G.M.; Schmitt, P.; Barreto, C.; Farias, N.D.; Toledo-Silva, G.; Guzmán, F.; Destoumieux-Garzyn, D.; Perazzolo, L.M.; Rosa, R.D. Massive Gene Expansion and Sequence Diversification Is Associated with Diverse Tissue Distribution, Regulation and Antimicrobial Properties of Anti-Lipopolysaccharide Factors in Shrimp. *Mar. Drugs* **2018**, *16*, 381. [CrossRef]

27. Chen, J.; Gong, F.; Chen, M.-F.; Li, C.; Hong, P.; Sun, S.; Zhou, C.; Qian, Z.-J. In Vitro Vascular-Protective Effects of a Tilapia By-Product Oligopeptide on Angiotensin II-Induced Hypertensive Endothelial Injury in HUVEC by Nrf2/NF-κB Pathways. *Mar. Drugs* **2019**, *17*, 431. [CrossRef]

28. Sun, L.; Wu, B.; Yan, M.; Hou, H.; Zhuang, Y. Antihypertensive Effect in Vivo of QAGLSPVR and Its Transepithelial Transport Through the Caco-2 Cell Monolayer. *Mar. Drugs* **2019**, *17*, 288. [CrossRef]

29. Yang, X.-R.; Zhang, L.; Ding, D.-G.; Chi, C.-F.; Wang, B.; Huo, J.-C. Preparation, Identification, and Activity Evaluation of Eight Antioxidant Peptides from Protein Hydrolysate of Hairtail (*Trichiurus japonicas*) Muscle. *Mar. Drugs* **2019**, *17*, 23. [CrossRef]

30. Wang, J.; Wei, R.; Song, R. Novel Antibacterial Peptides Isolated from the Maillard Reaction Products of Half-Fin Anchovy (*Setipinna taty*) Hydrolysates/Glucose and Their Mode of Action in *Escherichia coli*. *Mar. Drugs* **2019**, *17*, 47. [CrossRef]

31. Li, J.; Chen, Y.; Yuan, N.; Zeng, M.; Zhao, Y.; Yu, R.; Liu, Z.; Wu, H.; Dong, S. A Novel Natural Influenza a H1N1 Virus Neuraminidase Inhibitory Peptide Derived from Cod Skin Hydrolysates and Its Antiviral Mechanism. *Mar. Drugs* **2018**, *16*, 377. [CrossRef] [PubMed]

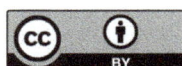

marine drugs

MDPI

Article

Protective Effect of *Pyropia yezoensis* Peptide on Dexamethasone-Induced Myotube Atrophy in C2C12 Myotubes

Min-Kyeong Lee [1], Jeong-Wook Choi [1], Youn Hee Choi [1,2,*] and Taek-Jeong Nam [1,3,*]

[1]   Institute of Fisheries Sciences, Pukyong National University, Busan 46041, Korea;
      3633234@hanmail.net (M.-K.L.); wook8309@naver.com (J.-W.C.)
[2]   Department of Marine Bio-Materials & Aquaculture, Pukyong National University, Busan 48513, Korea
[3]   Department of Food Science and Nutrition, Pukyong National University, Busan 48513, Korea
*   Correspondence: unichoi@pknu.ac.kr (Y.H.C.); namtj@pknu.ac.kr (T.-J.N.); Tel.: +82-51-629-5915 (Y.H.C.);
      +82-51-629-5846 (T.-J.N.)

Received: 11 April 2019; Accepted: 10 May 2019; Published: 11 May 2019

Abstract: Dexamethasone (DEX), a synthetic glucocorticoid, causes skeletal muscle atrophy. This study examined the protective effects of *Pyropia yezoensis* peptide (PYP15) against DEX-induced myotube atrophy and its association with insulin-like growth factor-I (IGF-I) and the Akt/mammalian target of rapamycin (mTOR)-forkhead box O (FoxO) signaling pathway. To elucidate the molecular mechanisms underlying the effects of PYP15 on DEX-induced myotube atrophy, C2C12 myotubes were treated for 24 h with 100 μM DEX in the presence or absence of 500 ng/mL PYP15. Cell viability assays revealed no PYP15 toxicity in C2C12 myotubes. PYP15 activated the insulin-like growth factor-I receptor (IGF-IR) and Akt-mTORC1 signaling pathway in DEX-induced myotube atrophy. In addition, PYP15 markedly downregulated the nuclear translocation of transcription factors FoxO1 and FoxO3a, and inhibited 20S proteasome activity. Furthermore, PYP15 inhibited the autophagy-lysosomal pathway in DEX-stimulated myotube atrophy. Our findings suggest that PYP15 treatment protected against myotube atrophy by regulating IGF-I and the Akt-mTORC1-FoxO signaling pathway in skeletal muscle. Therefore, PYP15 treatment appears to exert protective effects against skeletal muscle atrophy.

Keywords: dexamethasone; myotube atrophy; protein synthesis; proteolytic system; *Pyropia yezoensis* peptide; PYP15

1. Introduction

Bioactive peptides are generally composed of between three and 20 amino acid residues, and their activity is based on their amino acid composition and sequence [1]. The short chains of amino acids are in an inactive state within the sequence of the parent protein molecule, but can be liberated by proteolytic enzymes during gastrointestinal digestion or food processing and fermentation processes [2]. These peptides exhibit various physiological activities, such as anti-hypertensive [3], anti-oxidant [4–6], and anti-inflammatory effects [7,8] depending on their structural, sequential, and constitutive characteristics.

Pyropia yezoensis Ueda (Bangiaceae, Rhodophyta, Figure 1) is a commercially important red seaweed widely used as a food source in Korea, China, and Japan [9]. The protein content of *P. yezoensis* is higher than that of high protein foods such as soybeans, thus providing a rich source of biologically active peptides [10]. *P. yezoensis*-derived peptides are known to exert various biological effects, including antioxidant [11], antitumor [12], and anti-inflammatory activities [13]. Previous studies have reported that peptides synthesized from *P. yezoensis* reduced the inflammatory stress induced by lipopolysaccharides in RAW 264.7 cells, and cytotoxicity induced by acetaminophen in Chang cells [13,14]. Moreover, *P. yezoensis* peptides prevented the endoplasmic reticulum stress induced by perfluorooctane sulfonate in Chang cells [15]. A recent study also demonstrated that *P. yezoensis* peptide promoted collagen synthesis by activating the transforming growth factor-beta (TGF-β)/Smad signaling pathway in human dermal fibroblasts [16]. In addition, *P. yezoensis* peptides also protected against breast cancer by activating the mammalian target of rapamycin (mTOR) signaling pathway in MCF-7 cells [12]. Therefore, *P. yezoensis* is widely used as a health-promoting functional natural material due to its various physiological activities.

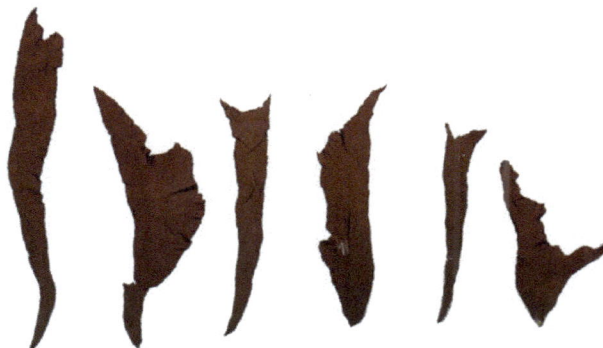

Figure 1. Image of *Pyropia yezoensis* Ueda (Bangiaceae, Rhodophyta).

Glucocorticoids (GCs) are steroid hormones widely administered for their anti-inflammatory and immunosuppressive activities [17]. However, sustained high-dose administration of GCs may lead to hyperglycemia, weight loss, osteoporosis, depression, hypertension, and skeletal muscle atrophy [18]. Many previous in vivo and in vitro experiments have suggested that synthetic GC dexamethasone (DEX) induces skeletal muscle atrophy by decreasing the protein synthesis rate and increasing the protein degradation rate [19,20].

The inhibitory effect on protein synthesis seen in GC-induced muscle atrophy occurs through multiple mechanisms. First, the catabolic effect of GCs inhibits the transport of amino acids within muscle, limiting protein synthesis [21]. Second, GCs inhibit the secretion of insulin-like growth factor I (IGF-I), which stimulates the phosphorylation of eIF4E-binding protein 4E-BP1 and p70 ribosomal S6 protein kinase (p70S6K), two factors that play key roles in protein synthesis by controlling the initiation of mRNA translation [20,22]. Third, GCs cause muscle atrophy by blocking myogenesis through the inhibition of myogenin, a transcription factor essential for the differentiation of satellite cells into muscle fibers [23]. It is well known that the inhibition of protein synthesis by GCs is mainly due to activation of the IGF-I-Akt-mTORC1 signaling pathway, which is involved in the phosphorylation of 4E-BP1 and p70S6K [24]. Previous studies have demonstrated that GCs in L6 myoblasts decrease the protein levels of insulin receptor substrate-1 (IRS-1), the first upstream component of the Akt-mTOR cascade [25,26]. In addition, GCs have been shown to inhibit the Akt-mTOR pathway by promoting the expression of microRNA miR1 [27]. These observations suggest that excess GCs may cause muscle atrophy by inhibiting the IGF-I-Akt-mTORC1 signaling pathway.

Akt also regulates the ubiquitin-proteasome system and autophagy-lysosomal system via the forkhead box O (FoxO) transcription factors, which are produced in muscle cell catabolism caused by GCs [28,29]. Mammalian cells express three FoxO isoforms, FoxO1, FoxO3, and FoxO4, which have been implicated in the regulation of genes involved in cell death, cell cycle arrest, and metabolism [30]. The absence of growth or survival signals inactivates Akt, thereby attenuating its inhibitory effects on FoxO transcription factors, which permits their translocation from the cytoplasm to the nucleus [31]. Nuclear translocation and activation of FoxO transcription factors are required to upregulate atrogenes, such as atrogin-1/muscle atrophy F-box (MAFbx), muscle RING finger 1 (MuRF1), and cathepsin-L. FoxO3 transfection of skeletal muscle cells was found to be sufficient for upregulating atrogin-1/MAFbx expression and muscle atrophy [32]. Moreover, previous studies employing inhibitors of the different proteolytic pathways have demonstrated that GCs stimulate not only ubiquitin-proteasome system-dependent proteolysis, but also autophagy-lysosomal system-dependent protein breakdown [30]. The role of the autophagy-lysosomal system in muscle atrophy induction by GCs is also demonstrated by the upregulation of muscle cathepsin-L expression [33–35] and by the upregulated conversion of LC3-I to LC3-II, an indicator of autophagy [36], in animals administered GCs. These findings suggest that activation of the ubiquitin-proteasome and autophagy-lysosomal systems in skeletal muscle atrophy induced by GC exposure may be mediated by the activation of FoxO through the inhibition of Akt expression.

Our previous study provided molecular evidence that the protective effects of the *P. yezoensis* peptide on DEX-induced muscle atrophy were due to downregulation of the muscle-specific E3 ubiquitin ligases atrogin-1/MAFbx and MuRF1 [37]. The present study was undertaken to investigate whether the protective effects of *P. yezoensis* peptide (PYP15) against DEX-induced myotube atrophy are associated with the proteolytic system, and whether this is regulated by the IGF-I-mediated Akt-mTOR and Akt-FoxO signaling pathways.

2. Results

2.1. Effects of DEX and PYP15 on C2C12 Myotube Viability

To evaluate the cytotoxic effects of PYP15 on C2C12 myotubes, MTS [(3-4,5-dimethylthiazol-2-yl)-5-(3-carboxymethoxyphenyl)-2-(4-sulfonyl)-2H-tetrazolium)] assays were carried out. C2C12 myotubes were incubated for 24 h with 100 μM DEX and PYP15 at concentrations ranging from 0 to 500 ng/mL. The DEX concentration (100 μM) was determined in a previous study [37]. As shown in Figure 2, PYP15 did not affect cell viability up to a concentration of 500 ng/mL. Thus, all subsequent experiments were performed 24 h after treatment with 500 ng/mL PYP15, which is the appropriate concentration that does not induce cytotoxicity, as described by Choi et al. [38].

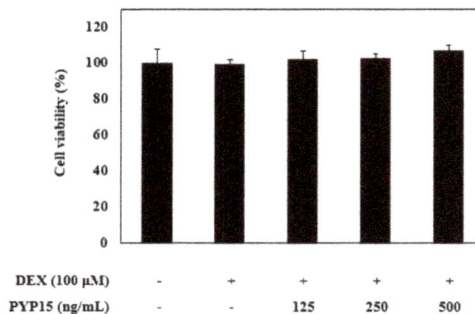

Figure 2. Effects of dexamethasone (DEX) and *Pyropia yezoensis* peptide (PYP15) on the cytotoxicity of C2C12 myotubes. C2C12 myoblasts were seeded in 96-well plates at a density of 1.5×10^4 cells/well and were allowed to attach for 24 h. After differentiation, the cells were treated with 100 μM DEX and 500 ng/mL PYP15 for 24 h. The viability of C2C12 myotubes was measured by MTS assay. The values are the mean ± SDs of three independent experiments.

2.2. PYP15 Treatment Attenuates the DEX-Induced Reduction in Insulin-Like Growth Factor I Receptor (IGF-IR) and IRS-1 Phosphorylation in C2C12 Myotubes

To determine whether PYP15 treatment led to changes in the IGF-I pathway in DEX-treated C2C12 myotubes, phosphorylation levels of insulin-like growth factor I receptor (IGF-IR) and insulin receptor substrate 1 (IRS-1) were examined using Western blot analysis. As shown in Figure 3, p-IGF-IR and p-IRS-1 protein expression levels was markedly decreased in DEX-stimulated C2C12 myotubes. However, the DEX-induced downregulation of p-IGF-IR and p-IRS-1 was attenuated by 500 ng/mL PYP15 treatment. Furthermore, C2C12 myotubes treated with PYP15 alone exhibited marked upregulation of the p-IGF-IR and p-IRS-1 protein expression levels compared with untreated control cells. These results suggest that PYP15 could induce muscle hypertrophy through activation of IGF-I signaling.

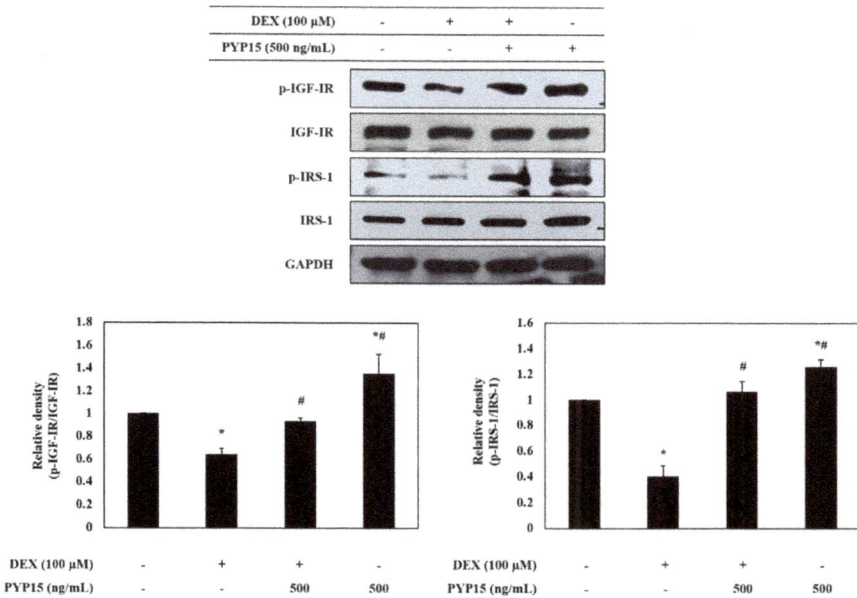

Figure 3. Effects of PYP15 on the phosphorylation of insulin-like growth factor I receptor (IGF-IR) and insulin receptor substrate 1 (IRS-1) in DEX-treated C2C12 myotubes. C2C12 myotubes were treated for 24 h with 100 μM DEX in the absence or presence of 500 ng/mL PYP15. The protein levels for p-IGF-IR, IGF-IR, p-IRS-1, and IRS-1 were assessed as described in Section 4. Glyceraldehyde-3-phosphate dehydrogenase (GAPDH) was the loading control. The values are the mean ± SD of three independent experiments. * $P < 0.05$ vs. corresponding control; # $P < 0.05$ vs. corresponding only DEX treatment.

2.3. PYP15 Treatment Attenuates the DEX-Induced Downregulation of the Akt-mTORC1 Signaling Pathway in C2C12 Myotubes

To further investigate the downstream signals regulated by activation of IGF-I signaling, the protein levels of Akt-mTORC1 pathway members were measured in C2C12 myotubes. As shown in Figure 4A, p-Akt and p-mTOR protein expression levels were markedly decreased in DEX-stimulated C2C12 myotubes. However, the DEX-induced downregulation of p-Akt and p-mTOR was attenuated by 500 ng/mL PYP15 treatment. In addition, to determine whether PYP15 induced changes in mTORC1 and mTORC2 protein levels in DEX-induced myotube atrophy, the protein and mRNA levels of Raptor, Rictor, REDD1, and KLF-15 were examined. As expected, Raptor protein expression levels was markedly decreased in DEX-stimulated C2C12 myotubes. However, the DEX-induced downregulation of Raptor was attenuated by 500 ng/mL PYP15 treatment (Figure 4A). The DEX-induced upregulation of REDD1 and KLF-15 was attenuated by 500 ng/mL PYP15 treatment (Figure 4B,C). However, no significant differences were observed in Rictor levels compared with the control group (Figure 4A).

These results demonstrate that PYP15 exerted protective effects against DEX-induced myotube atrophy via mTORC1 signaling activation.

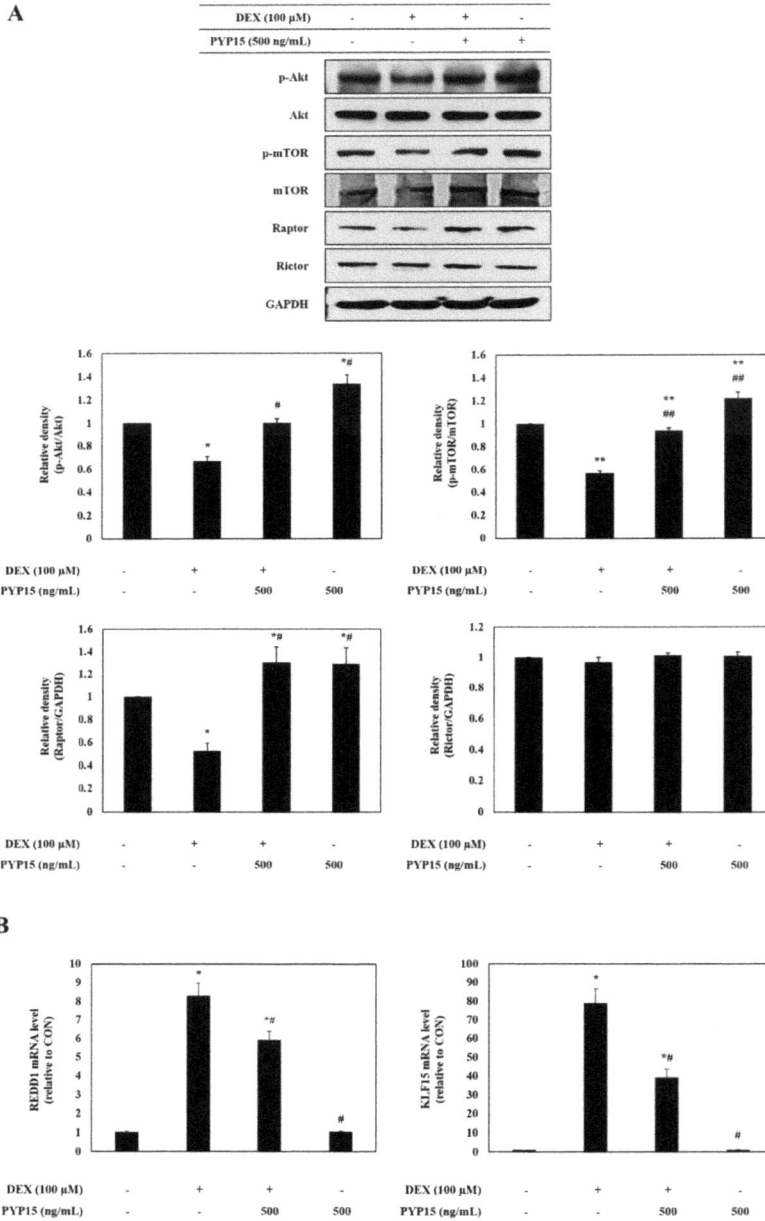

Figure 4. *Cont.*

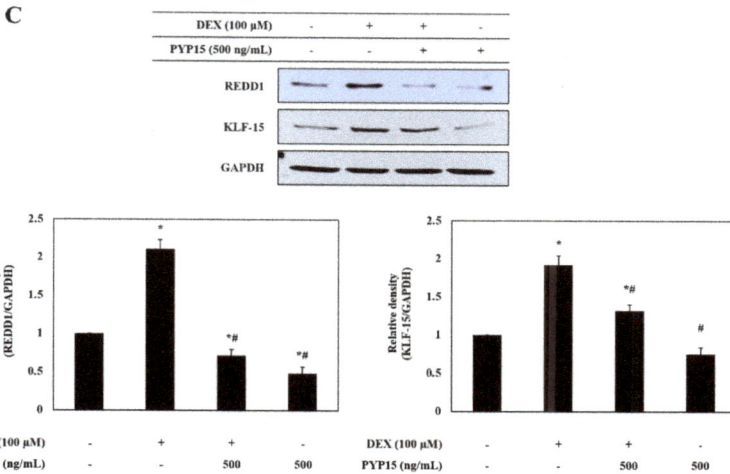

Figure 4. Effects of PYP15 on the Akt/mammalian target of rapamycin (mTOR) signaling pathway in DEX-stimulated C2C12 myotubes. C2C12 myotubes were treated for 24 h with 100 μM DEX in the absence or presence of 500 ng/mL PYP15. (**A**) The protein levels for p-Akt, Akt, p-mTOR, mTOR, Raptor, and Rictor were assessed as described in Section 4. (**B**) The mRNA levels for REDD1 and KLF15 were assessed as described in Section 4. (**C**) The protein levels for REDD1 and KLF15 were assessed as described in Section 4. GAPDH was the loading control. The values are the mean ± SD of three independent experiments. * $P < 0.05$ vs. corresponding control; # $P < 0.05$ vs. corresponding only DEX treatment.

2.4. PYP15 Treatment Attenuates the DEX-Induced Decreases in p70S6K and 4E-BP1 Phosphorylation in C2C12 Myotubes

To further determine the downstream signals regulated by mTORC1 activation, the protein levels of p70S6K and 4E-BP1 signaling members were measured in C2C12 myotubes. As shown in Figure 5A, Rheb protein expression levels were markedly decreased in DEX-stimulated C2C12 myotubes. However, the DEX-induced downregulation of Rheb was attenuated by 500 ng/mL PYP15 treatment. In addition, the DEX-induced downregulation of p-p70S6K, p-S6, p-4E-BP1, and eIF4E was attenuated by 500 ng/mL PYP15 treatment (Figure 5A,B).

A

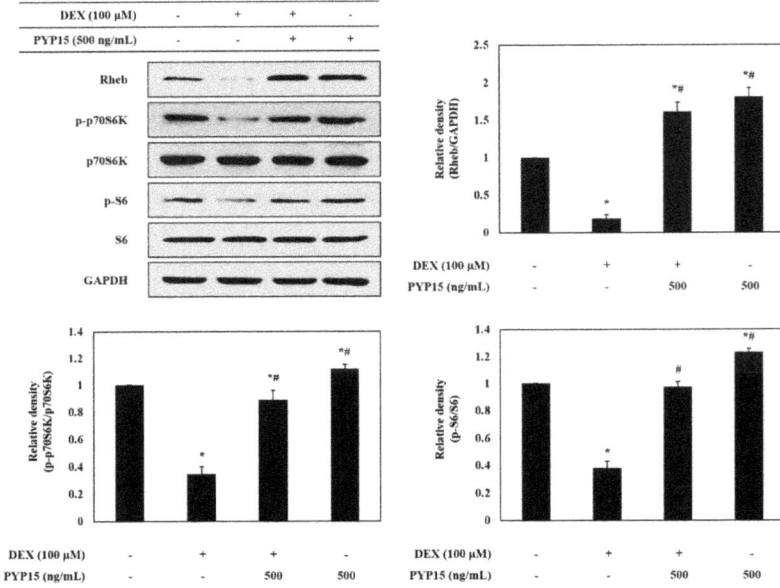

B

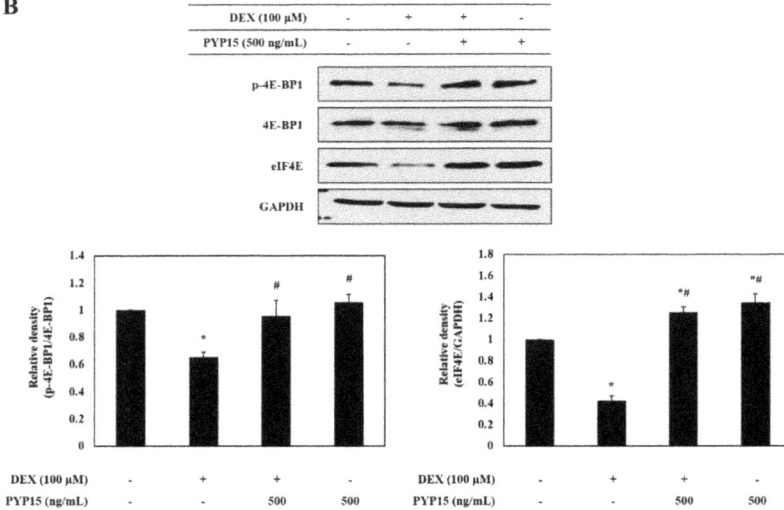

Figure 5. Effects of PYP15 on the mTORC1 downstream signaling components in DEX-stimulated C2C12 myotubes. C2C12 myotubes were treated for 24 h with 100 μM DEX in the absence or presence of 500 ng/mL PYP15. (**A**) The protein levels for Rheb, p-p70S6K, p70S6K, p-S6, and S6 were assessed as described in Section 4. (**B**) The protein levels for p-4EBP1, 4E-BP1, and eIF4E were assessed as described in Section 4. GAPDH was the loading control. The values are the mean ± SD of three independent experiments. * $P < 0.05$ vs. corresponding control; # $P < 0.05$ vs. corresponding only DEX treatment.

2.5. PYP15 Treatment Downregulates the DEX-Induced Increase in Nuclear Translocation of FoxO1 and FoxO3a in C2C12 Myotubes

To further determine the mechanism underlying transcriptional control by PYP15, the effects of PYP15 on the transcriptional activation of FoxO1 and FoxO3a were measured in DEX-stimulated C2C12 myotubes. As shown in Figure 6A, FoxO1 and FoxO3a protein expression levels were significantly increased in DEX-stimulated C2C12 myotubes ($P < 0.05$). However, the DEX-induced upregulation of total FoxO1 and FoxO3a was attenuated by 500 ng/mL PYP15 treatment. In addition, the DEX-induced reduction in p-FoxO1 and p-FoxO3a was attenuated by 500 ng/mL PYP15 treatment. The dephosphorylation of FoxO1 and FoxO3a accelerated their nuclear translocation. The levels of nuclear FoxO1 and FoxO3a were significantly increased by DEX treatment, but were significantly decreased by PYP15 treatment ($P < 0.05$, Figure 6B).

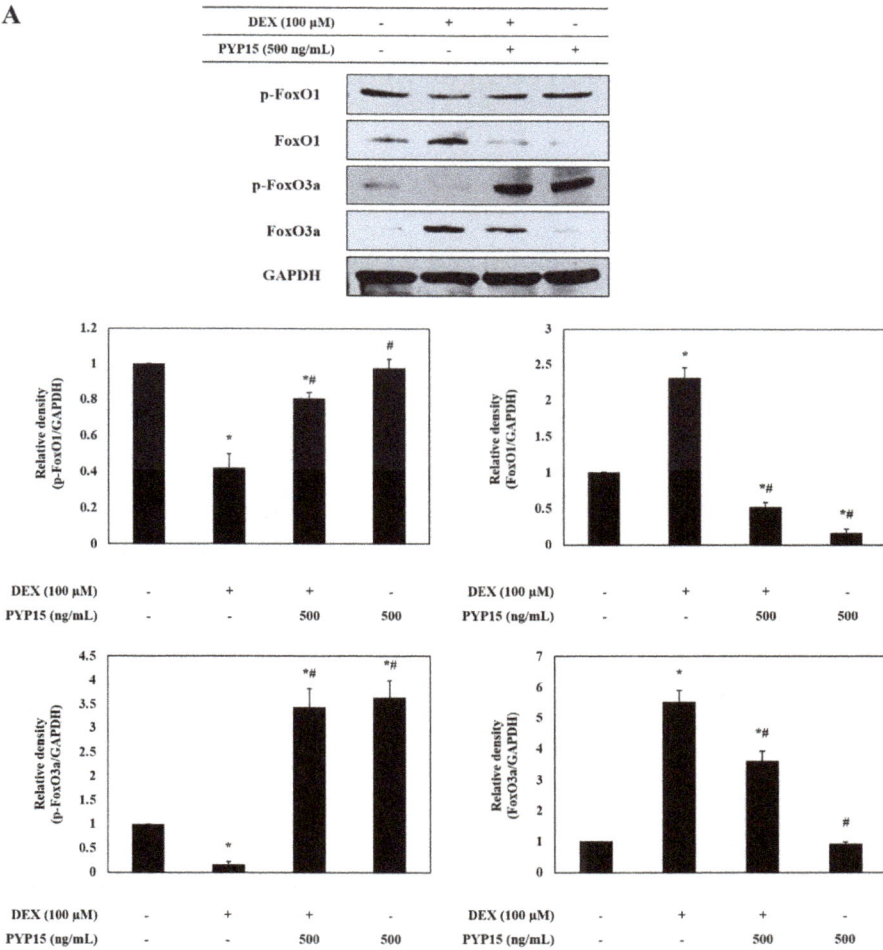

Figure 6. *Cont.*

B

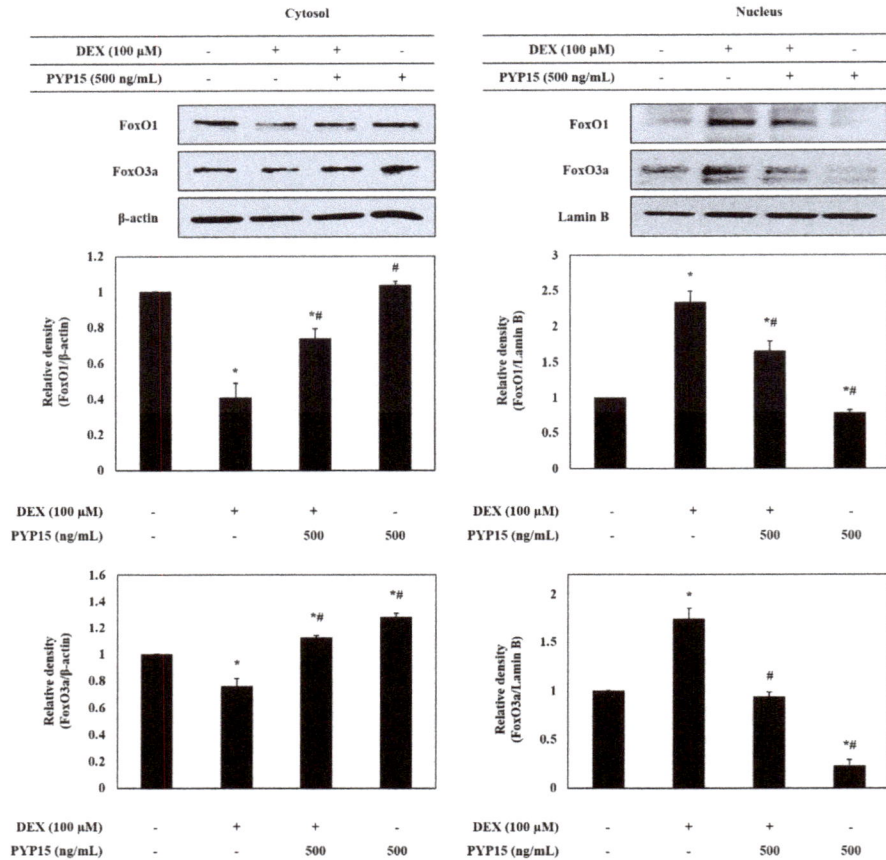

Figure 6. Effects of PYP15 on the activation and translocation of forkhead box O (FoxO) transcription factors FoxO1 and FoxO3a in DEX-stimulated C2C12 myotubes. C2C12 myotubes were treated for 24 h with 100 μM DEX in the absence or presence of 500 ng/mL PYP15. (**A**) The protein levels for total p-FoxO1, FoxO1, p-FoxO3a, and FoxO3a were assessed as described in Section 4. (**B**) The protein levels for cytosolic and nucleus fractions were assessed as described in Section 4. GAPDH, β-actin, and lamin B were the loading control. The values are the mean ± SD of three independent experiments. * $P < 0.05$ vs. corresponding control; # $P < 0.05$ vs. corresponding only DEX treatment.

2.6. PYP15 Treatment Inhibits DEX-Induced 20S Proteasome Activity in C2C12 Myotubes

To identify the ubiquitin-proteasome system regulated by FoxO transcription factors, 20S proteasome activity in C2C12 myotubes was measured using an ELISA kit. As shown in Figure 7, DEX treatment significantly increased 20S proteasome activity ($P < 0.05$). However, treatment with PYP15 attenuated the DEX-induced increase in 20S proteasome activity.

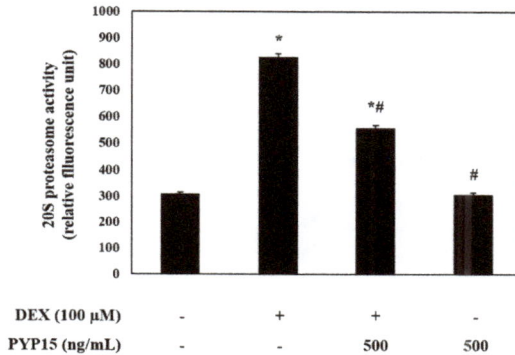

Figure 7. Effects of PYP15 on 20S proteasome activity in DEX-stimulated C2C12 myotubes. 20S proteasome activity was assessed as described in Section 4. The values are the mean ± SD of three independent experiments. * $P < 0.05$ vs. corresponding control; # $P < 0.05$ vs. corresponding only DEX treatment.

2.7. PYP15 Treatment Downregulates the DEX-Induced Activation of the Autophagy-Lysosomal System in C2C12 Myotubes

The effects of PYP15 on the expression of cathepsin-L and autophagy-related genes in DEX-treated C2C12 myotubes were assessed by real-time polymerase chain reaction (PCR) and Western blot analysis. As shown in Figure 8A,B, the mRNA and protein expression levels of cathepsin-L were significantly increased in DEX-stimulated C2C12 myotubes ($P < 0.05$). However, the DEX-induced upregulation of cathepsin-L was attenuated by 500 ng/mL PYP15 treatment. In addition, DEX treatment increased the conversion of LC3-I to LC3-II, which was attenuated by PYP15 treatment (Figure 8C).

A

DEX (100 µM)	-	+	+	-
PYP15 (ng/mL)	-	-	500	500

B

DEX (100 µM)	-	+	+	-
PYP15 (ng/mL)	-	-	500	500

C

DEX (100 µM)	-	+	+	-
PYP15 (ng/mL)	-	-	500	500

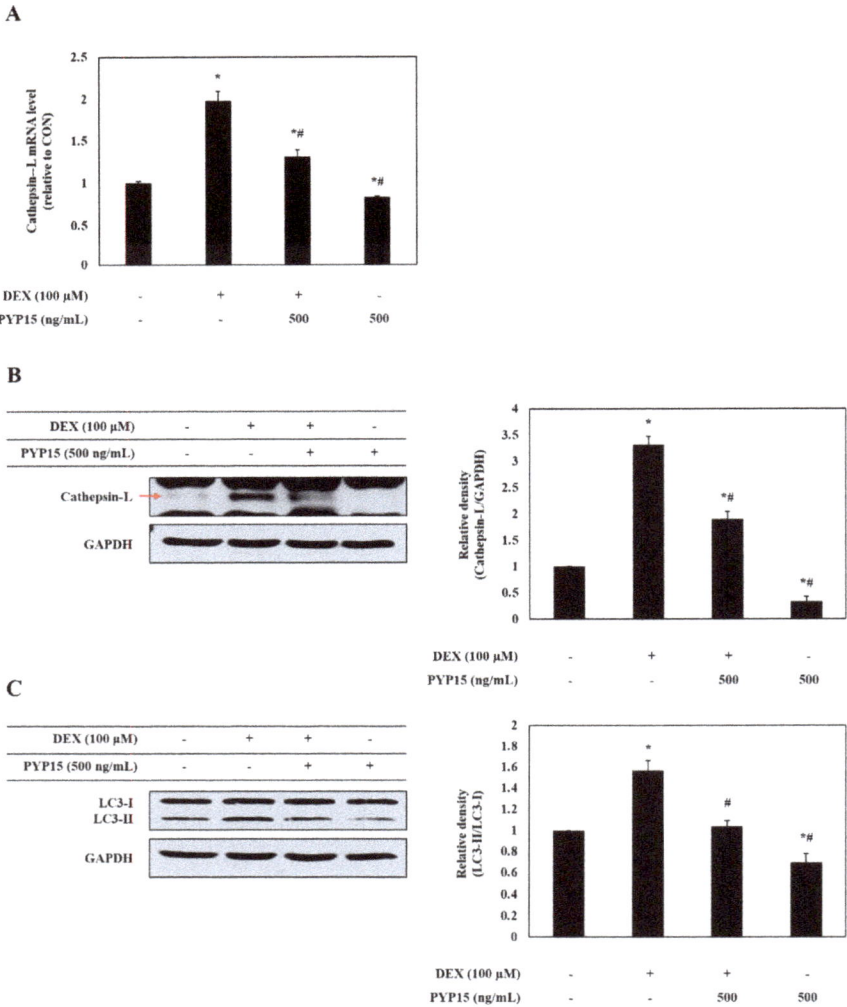

Figure 8. Effects of PYP15 on cathepsin-L and LC3-I/II levels in DEX-stimulated C2C12 myotubes. C2C12 myotubes were treated for 24 h with 100 µM DEX in the absence or presence of 500 ng/mL PYP15. (**A**) The mRNA levels for cathepsin-L were assessed as described in Section 4. (**B**) The protein levels for cathepsin-L and (**C**) LC3-I/II were assessed as described in Section 4. GAPDH was the loading control. The values are the mean ± SD of three independent experiments. * $P < 0.05$ vs. corresponding control; # $P < 0.05$ vs. corresponding only DEX treatment.

2.8. Analysis of Myotube Atrophy Marker Genes after Akt siRNA Transfection

We investigated the expression of E3 ubiquitin ligases after knocking down Akt gene expression to clarify whether Akt plays a role in the PYP15-mediated inhibition of E3 ubiquitin ligases in C2C12 myotubes. As shown in Figure 9A, the protein level of Akt was markedly reduced after treatment with Akt siRNA2, in comparison with the universal negative control siRNA. These results confirmed that C2C12 myotubes were successfully transfected with Akt siRNA2. Therefore, Akt siRNA2 was used in subsequent experiments. Following this, we transfected cultured myotubes with Akt siRNA2 to test whether the effects of PYP15 on the DEX-induced upregulation of atrogin-1/MAFbx, MuRF1, and cathepsin-L expression are inhibited after Akt knockdown. Transfection of C2C12 myotubes with Akt siRNA2 significantly increased the mRNA and protein levels of atrogin-1/MAFbx, MuRF1, and cathepsin-L, and these increases in expression were attenuated by PYP15 treatment (Figure 9B,C). These results demonstrate that PYP15 prevents myotube atrophy by blocking proteolytic systems through Akt activation.

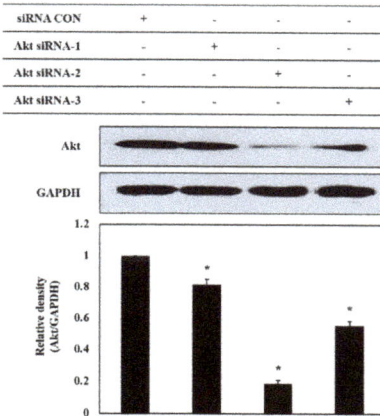

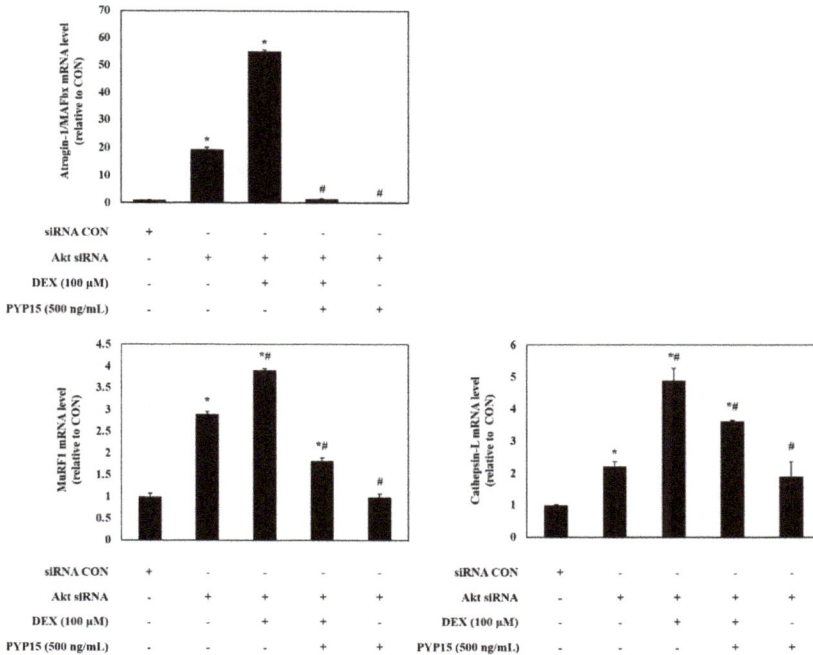

Figure 9. *Cont.*

C

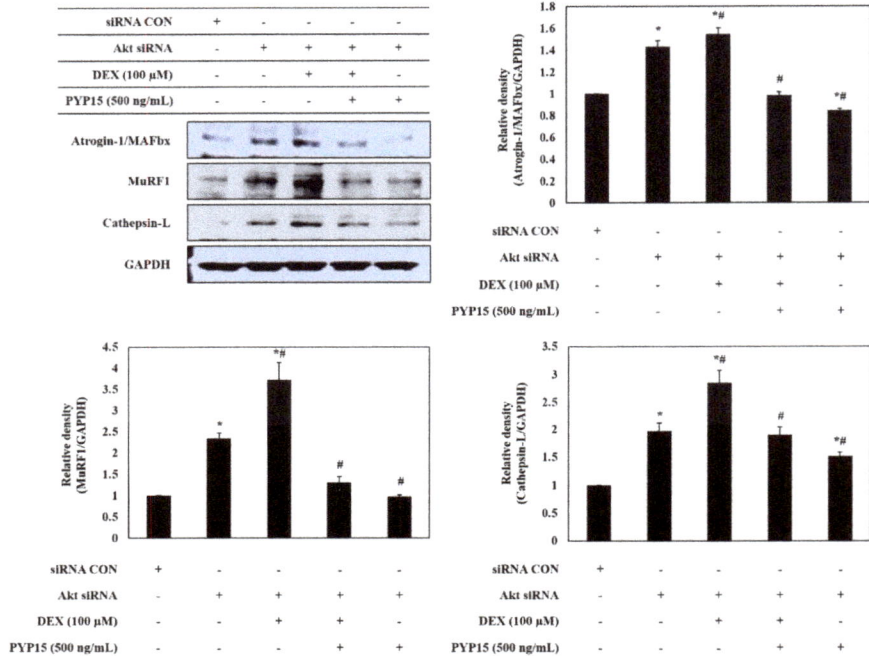

Figure 9. Effects of PYP15 on the levels of ubiquitin-E3 ligases following DEX-induced myotube atrophy in transfected C2C12 myotubes. (**A**) Changes in Akt protein levels by Akt knockdown were measured as described in Section 4. (**B,C**) The mRNA and protein levels of atrogin-1/MAFbx, MuRF1, and cathepsin-L in the five treatment groups were measured as described in Section 4. GAPDH was the loading control. The values are the mean ± SD of three independent experiments. * $P < 0.05$ vs. corresponding control; # $P < 0.05$ vs. corresponding only Akt siRNA treatment.

3. Discussion

In this study, we used an in vitro model to investigate the protective role of PYP15, and the mechanisms of its anti-atrophic effects, against DEX-induced muscle atrophy. DEX induces atrophy in skeletal muscle by decreasing the protein synthesis rate and increasing the protein degradation rate [39]. The inhibitory effect of DEX on muscle protein synthesis is mainly induced by inhibition of the IGF-I signaling pathway, which is an anabolic growth factor [40]. Previous studies have demonstrated that IGF-I is sufficient to induce skeletal muscle hypertrophy [41,42]. The inverse of muscle atrophy is muscle hypertrophy, defined as an increase in muscle mass resulting from an increase in size, as opposed to by an increase in the number of muscle fibers [28,43]. The effects of IGF-I are mainly mediated by IGF-IR, which exhibits tyrosine kinase activity and signals via adaptor proteins, such as IRS-1 [44]. In this study, the DEX-induced reductions in IGF-IR and IRS-1 phosphorylation were ameliorated by treatment with PYP15 (Figure 3). These results suggest that PYP15 could protect C2C12 myotubes from DEX-induced myotube atrophy through the activation of IGF-I signaling. The downstream signaling mechanisms induced by IGF-I required for muscle hypertrophy remain controversial, but many studies have focused on the Akt-mTOR pathway downstream of IGF-I, demonstrating that Akt is activated by IGF-I [28,45]. In our results, DEX inhibited the phosphorylation of Akt and mTOR, but treatment with PYP15 increased this phosphorylation (Figure 4A). mTOR interacts with several proteins to form two distinct multiprotein complexes, mTORC1 and mTORC2. The inhibition of protein synthesis by

DEX is known to be mainly due to inhibition of mTORC1 [40]. This inhibition of mTORC1-signaling by DEX is induced by the transcriptional stimulation of REDD1 and KLF-15, which are inhibitors of mTORC1 signaling [40]. PYP15 treatment activated Raptor expression in DEX-induced C2C12 myotubes and reduced the DEX-induced expression of REDD1 and KLF15 (Figure 4). These results suggest that PYP15 inhibits muscle atrophy through activation of the mTORC1 signaling pathway in DEX-stimulated C2C12 myotubes. Activation of the Akt-mTORC1 signaling pathway stimulates protein synthesis by increasing protein translation through the activation of p70S6K and inhibition of 4E-BP1 [28]. In our study, PYP15 treatment increased the phosphorylation of p70S6K, S6, and 4E-BP1 as well as the expression of eIF4E (Figure 5). Interestingly, C2C12 myotubes treated with PYP15 alone exhibited marked upregulation of the IGF-I-Akt-mTORC1 signaling pathway compared with untreated control cells. Taken together, these results demonstrate that PYP15 could protect C2C12 myotubes from DEX-induced myotube atrophy by inducing muscle hypertrophy through the activation of Akt-mTORC1 pathway via the activation of IGF-I signaling.

DEX-induced myotube atrophy is mediated by FoxO transcription factors [18]. In addition to stimulating protein synthesis pathways, Akt activation inhibits proteolytic systems by inducing phosphorylation of the downstream target FoxO transcription factors, thus blocking nuclear translocation [17]. Previous studies have shown that the reduced activity of the Akt pathway observed in the muscle atrophy model markedly increases the levels of phosphorylated FoxO in the cytoplasm as well as the nuclear expression of FoxO [46]. In addition, FoxO transgenic mice reportedly exhibit markedly reduced muscle mass, further supporting that FoxO is sufficient to stimulate muscle atrophy [47,48]. Our results demonstrate that the phosphorylation of FoxO is activated by treatment with PYP15, resulting in decreased nuclear translocation (Figure 6). These results indicate that PYP15 effectively blocks the nuclear translocation and activation of FoxO1 and FoxO3a by promoting the phosphorylation of FoxO1 and FoxO3a.

The increased expression of FoxO contributes to the activation of muscle proteolysis through the ubiquitin-proteasome system and lysosomal system [30]. The ubiquitin-proteasome system functions in processing and degrading cellular proteins, which is essential for basic cellular processes, such as differentiation, proliferation, and immune and inflammatory responses [49,50]. The degradation of a target protein by the ubiquitin-proteasome system is labeled by the covalent bonds of multiple ubiquitin molecules, comprising 76 amino acids; the proteins are then degraded by proteolytic enzymes [51]. Previous studies have shown that the ubiquitin-proteasome pathway is downregulated by the IGF-I-mediated Akt-FoxO signaling pathway [31] and that the inhibition of proteasomal activity markedly inhibits muscle proteolysis in muscle atrophy [52]. Our study showed that the DEX-stimulated expression of atrogin-1/MAFbx and MuRF1 and the activity of the 20S proteasome were downregulated by PYP15 treatment (Figure 7). In addition to the ubiquitin-proteasome system, the proteolytic system found to be regulated by the Akt-FoxO signaling pathway is the autophagy-lysosomal system [53]. Previous studies have demonstrated the downregulation of the autophagy-lysosomal pathway by the Akt-FoxO signaling pathway [54]. DEX exerts its atrophic effects by activating the autophagy-lysosomal system through increased cathepsin-L muscle expression and increased conversion of LC3-I to LC3-II, which is an indicator of autophagy [34–36]. In this study, the DEX-induced increased expression of cathepsin-L and autophagy-related genes were downregulated by PYP15 treatment (Figure 8). We also confirmed that Akt knockdown induced the upregulation of atrogin-1/MAFbx, MuRF1, and cathepsin-L, effects that were reduced by PYP15 treatment (Figure 9). These results suggest that PYP15 protects DEX-induced myotube atrophy by blocking the ubiquitin-proteasome and autophagy-lysosomal pathways through downregulation of atrogenes activated by nuclear translocation of FoxO. Our results also suggest that the activation of IGF-I-mediated Akt signaling is essential for the regulation of muscle atrophy in proteolytic systems by PYP15.

In summary, these data provide molecular evidence that the anti-muscle atrophy effects of PYP15 are at least partially regulated by the Akt-mTORC1 and Akt-FoxO signaling pathways and reflect inhibited upregulation of the ubiquitin-proteasome and autophagy-lysosomal pathways.

4. Materials and Methods

4.1. Preparation of PYP15

PYP15 (D-P-K-G-K-Q-Q-A-I-H-V-A-P-S-F) was synthesized by Peptron (Daejeon, Korea). PYP15 was purified using the Shimadzu Prominence HPLC system (Shimadzu Corporation, Kyoto, Japan) and a Capcell Pak C18 column (column dimensions, 150 × 4.6 mm; particle size, 2.7 μM; Shiseido Corporation, Tokyo, Japan), with a gradient of 10% to 70% ACN (0% to 20% ACN for 2 min, 20% to 50% ACN for 10 min, 50% to 80% ACN for 2 min) in 0.1% trifluoroacetic acid (TFA; v/v in water), a flow rate of 1.0 mL/min, and UV detection at 220 nm, controlled via the software package Class-VP (ver. 6.14; Shimadzu Corporation, Kyoto, Japan). The molecular weight of PYP15 was determined to be 1622 Da using an HP 110 Series liquid chromatography/mass spectrometric detector (LC/MSD) [ionization mode, positive; nitrogen flow, 7 L/min; high vacuum, 1.3×10^{-5} torr; neb press, 40 psi; quadrupole temperature, 100 °C; flow rate, 0.4 mL/min (isocratic ACN: DW = 8:2, 0.1% (v/v) TFA/water); Agilent Technologies, Santa Clara, CA, USA)] [37].

4.2. Cell Culture and Differentiation

C2C12 mouse skeletal muscle cells were obtained from the American Type Culture Collection (CRL-1722; ATCC, Manassas, VA, USA). Cells were maintained in a humidified 5% CO_2 incubator at 37 °C in Dulbecco's modified Eagle's medium (DMEM; Gibco, Thermo Fisher Scientific, Waltham, MA, USA) supplemented with 10% fetal bovine serum (FBS; Gibco, Thermo Fisher Scientific, Waltham, MA, USA), 100 U/mL penicillin (Gibco, Thermo Fisher Scientific, Waltham, MA, USA), and 100 mg/mL streptomycin (Gibco, Thermo Fisher Scientific, Waltham, MA, USA). C2C12 myoblasts were grown to 70% to 80% confluence in culture dishes (100 mm) at 37 °C, then trypsinized and seeded (4×10^4 cells/well) into six-well culture plates for experiments. Cells were grown to 70% to 80% confluence in DMEM supplemented with 10% FBS at 37 °C for 24 h, at which time the medium was replaced with DMEM containing 2% FBS to induce differentiation into myotubes; the medium was replaced every 2 days. Cells were allowed to differentiate for 6 days, at which point 90% of the cells had fused into myotubes [37].

4.3. Treatment with DEX and PYP15

Following 6 days of differentiation, C2C12 myotubes were subdivided into four groups: The control group, in which cells were incubated in serum-free medium (SFM; DMEM containing 100 U/mL penicillin and 100 mg/mL streptomycin); the DEX group, in which cells were treated with 100 μM DEX (Sigma-Aldrich, St. Louis, MO, USA); the DEX + PYP15 group, in which cells were treated with 100 μM DEX and 500 ng/mL PYP15; and the PYP15 group, in which cells were treated with 500 ng/mL PYP15. All groups were incubated in SFM at 37 °C for 24 h prior to harvesting cells for experiments. The concentrations of DEX and PYP15 used here were based on previous studies [37].

4.4. MTS Assay

Cell viability was measured using the CellTiter 96 Aqueous Non-Radioactive Cell Proliferation Assay (Promega Corporation, Madison, WI, USA), which is based on the formation of a formazan product from tetrazolium compound MTS [(3-4,5-dimethylthiazol-2-yl)-5-(3-carboxymethoxyphenyl)-2-(4-sulfonyl)-2H-tetrazolium)]. Briefly, cells (1.5×10^4 cells/well) were seeded into 96-well plates in 100 μL DMEM supplemented with 10% FBS and were allowed to attach at 37 °C for 24 h. After differentiation, the cells were incubated with 100 μM DEX and 500 ng/mL PYP15 for 24 h at 37 °C. MTS solution (10 μL) was added and the cells were incubated at 37 °C for 30 min. The absorbance at 490 nm was measured using a Gen5 ELISA (Bio-Tek, Houston, TX, USA) [37]. Experiments were performed in triplicate.

4.5. Real-Time PCR

The mRNA expression levels of specific genes were evaluated using real-time PCR. Total RNA was isolated from C2C12 myotubes using TRIzol reagent (Invitrogen Life Technologies, Carlsbad, CA, USA). The resulting RNA was evaluated by measuring the absorbance at 260 and 280 nm to determine the RNA concentration and purity, respectively. A RevoScript Reverse Transcriptase PreMix Kit (Intron Biotechnology Co., Ltd., Seongnam, Korea) was used to prepare cDNA according to the manufacturer's instructions, and the samples were stored at −50 °C. Real-time PCR was conducted in 20-μL reactions using the TOPreal qPCR 2X preMIX (Enzynomics, Inc., Daejeon, Korea) and the Illumina Eco real-time PCR system (Illumina, Inc., Hayward, CA, USA). All mRNA levels were normalized using glyceraldehyde-3-phosphate dehydrogenase (GAPDH) as an internal control [37]. The primers used for amplification are shown in Table 1.

Table 1. Oligonucleotide primer sequences used in real-time PCR.

Gene	Accession No.	Sequence (5′–3′)	Amplicon Size (bp)
Atrogin-1/MAFbx	NM_026346.3	F: ATGCACACTGGTGCAGAGAG R: TGTAAGCACACAGGCAGGTC	168
Cathepsin-L	M20495.1	F: GACCGGGACAACCACTGTG R: CCCATCAATTCACGACAGGAT	61
GAPDH	NM_008084.3	F: ACTCCACTCACGGCAAATTCA R: CGCTCCTGGAAGATGGTGAT	91
KLF-15	NM_001355668.1	F: CGAGAAGCCCTTTGCCTGCA R: ATCGCCGGTGCCTTGACAAC	70
MuRF1	DQ_229108.1	F: CGAGAAGCCCTTTGCCTGCA R: GTGCCGGTCCATGATCACTT	59
REDD1	NM_029083.2	F: TGGTGCCCACCTTTCAGTTG R: GTCAGGGACTGGCTGTAACC	121

4.6. Preparation of Total Cell Lysates

Cell were allowed to differentiate for 6 days at 37 °C, followed by incubation at 37 °C for 24 h in either SFM (control group) or SFM containing 100 μM DEX (DEX group), 100 μM DEX + 500 ng/mL PYP15 (DEX + PYP15 group), or 500 ng/mL PYP15 (PYP15 group). Cells were washed twice with PBS (Gibco, Thermo Fisher Scientific) and lysed with extraction buffer [1% NP-40, 0.25% sodium deoxycholate, 1 mM ethylene glycol-bis (β-aminoethyl ether)-N,N,N′N′-tetraacetic acid, 150 mM NaCl, and 50 mM Tris-HCl, pH 7.5] containing protease inhibitors (1 mg/mL aprotinin, 1 mg/mL leupeptin, 1 mg/mL pepstatin A, 200 mM Na_3VO_4, 500 mM NaF, and 100 mM PMSF) on ice. After incubation for 30 min at 4 °C, the extracts were centrifuged at $16,000 \times g$ for 10 min at 4 °C, and protein levels were quantified using a bicinchoninic acid (BCA) protein assay kit (Pierce, Thermo Fisher Scientific) according to the manufacturer's instructions. The supernatant was then used in Western blot analysis [37].

4.7. Preparation of Cytosolic and Nuclear Extracts

Cells were treated and harvested as described above, lysed with hypotonic lysis buffer (25 mM HEPES, pH 7.5, 5 mM EDTA, 5 mM $MgCl_2$, and 5 mM DTT) containing protease inhibitors (1 mg/mL aprotinin, 1 mg/mL leupeptin, 1 mg/mL pepstatin A, 200 mM Na_3VO_4, 500 mM NaF, and 100 mM PMSF), and incubated for 15 min on ice. Cells were further lysed by adding 2.5% NP-40. After 10 min, nuclei were collected by centrifugation at $7500 \times g$ for 15 min at 4 °C. The supernatant (cytosolic fraction) was immediately transferred to clean pre-chilled tubes. The insoluble (pellet) fraction is the nuclear fraction. The nuclear fraction was resuspended in cell extraction buffer (10 mM HEPES pH 7.9, 100 mM NaCl, 1.5 mM $MgCl_2$, 0.1 mM EDTA, and 0.2 mM DTT) containing protease inhibitors (1 mg/mL aprotinin, 1 mg/mL leupeptin, 1 mg/mL pepstatin A, 200 mM Na_3VO_4, 500 mM NaF, and 100 mM PMSF). The samples were placed on ice and vortexed for 15 s every 10 min for a total of 40 min. Extracts were centrifuged at 16,000 × *g* for 10 min, and protein levels were determined using a BCA protein assay kit (Pierce, Thermo Fisher Scientific, Waltham, MA, USA) according to the manufacturer's instructions. Both fractions were then used in Western blot analysis [37].

4.8. Western Blot Analysis

Equal amounts of proteins (40 µg) were separated by 6% to 12.5% sodium dodecyl sulfate-polyacrylamide gel electrophoresis (SDS-PAGE) and transferred to a polyvinylidene fluoride membrane (Millipore, Bedford, MA, USA). The membrane was blocked at room temperature with 1% bovine serum albumin (BSA) in TBS-T (10 mM Tris-HCl, 150 mM NaCl, and 0.1% Tween-20) and then incubated with primary antibodies (Table 2). The secondary antibodies (diluted 1:10,000 to 1:20,000) were horseradish peroxidase-conjugated anti-rabbit IgG (7074S; Cell Signaling Technology, Inc., Beverly, MA, USA), donkey anti-goat IgG (A50-101P; Bethyl Laboratories, Inc., Montgomery, TX, USA), or goat anti-mouse IgG (sc-2031; Santa Cruz Biotechnology, Inc., Santa Cruz, CA, USA). Signals were detected using an enhanced chemiluminescence Western blot analysis kit (Thermo Fisher Scientific). Experiments were performed in triplicate and densitometry analysis was performed using Multi-Gauge software version 3.0 (Fujifilm Life Science, Tokyo, Japan) [37].

Table 2. Primary antibodies used in Western blot analysis.

Antibody	Manufacturer and Catalog No.	Species of Origin	Dilution Rate
4E-BP1	Santa Cruz Biotechnology: sc-9977	Mouse	1:1000
Akt	Santa Cruz Biotechnology: sc-8312	Rabbit	1:1000
Atrogin-1/MAFbx	Santa Cruz Biotechnology: sc-27645	Goat	1:2000
β-actin	Santa Cruz Biotechnology: sc-47778	Mouse	1:1000
Cathepsin-L	Santa Cruz Biotechnology: sc-6498	Goat	1:1000
eIF4E	Santa Cruz Biotechnology: sc-514875	Mouse	1:1000
FoxO1	Santa Cruz Biotechnology: sc-374427	Mouse	1:500
FoxO3a	Santa Cruz Biotechnology: sc-9813	Goat	1:1000
GAPDH	Santa Cruz Biotechnology: sc-25778	Rabbit	1:1000
IGF-IR	Santa Cruz Biotechnology: sc-713	Rabbit	1:1000
IRS-1	Santa Cruz Biotechnology: sc-560	Rabbit	1:1000
KLF-15	Santa Cruz Biotechnology: sc-27165	Mouse	1:1000
Lamin B	Santa Cruz Biotechnology: sc-377000	Mouse	1:1000
LC3-I/II	Cell Signaling: #4108S	Rabbit	1:1000
mTOR	Santa Cruz Biotechnology: sc-8319	Rabbit	1:1000
MuRF1	Santa Cruz Biotechnology: sc-27642	Goat	1:2000
p-4E-BP1	Santa Cruz Biotechnology: sc-293124	Mouse	1:1000
p70S6K	Santa Cruz Biotechnology: sc-8418	Mouse	1:1000
p-Akt	Santa Cruz Biotechnology: sc-135650	Mouse	1:500
p-FoxO1	Cell Signaling: #9461S	Rabbit	1:500
p-FoxO3a	Cell Signaling: #9466S	Rabbit	1:1000
p-IGF-IR	Santa Cruz Biotechnology: sc-101703	Rabbit	1:1000
p-IRS-1	Santa Cruz Biotechnology: sc-17200	Goat	1:1000
p-mTOR	Santa Cruz Biotechnology: sc-293132	Mouse	1:1000
p-p70S6K	Santa Cruz Biotechnology: sc-8416	Mouse	1:1000
p-S6	Santa Cruz Biotechnology: sc-293144	Mouse	1:1000
Raptor	Santa Cruz Biotechnology: sc-81537	Mouse	1:1000
REDD1	Santa Cruz Biotechnology: sc-376671	Mouse	1:1000
Rheb	Santa Cruz Biotechnology: sc-271509	Mouse	1:1000
Rictor	Santa Cruz Biotechnology: sc-81538	Mouse	1:1000
S6	Santa Cruz Biotechnology: sc-74459	Mouse	1:1000

4.9. Akt Small Interfering RNA (siRNA) Transfection

For gene silencing, three different siRNA oligonucleotides (predesigned and synthesized by Bioneer, Daejeon, Korea) targeting Akt (GenBank accession No. NM_009652.2) were transfected into differentiated C2C12 myotubes using Lipofectamine RNAiMAX transfection reagent (Invitrogen Life Technologies) according to the manufacturer's instructions. The siRNA sequences are listed in Table 3. Negative controls were employed to evaluate siRNA specificity and for siRNA optimization. Briefly, siRNA (50 µM) and Lipofectamine RNAiMAX were separately diluted in Opti-MEM (Invitrogen Life Technologies) and then combined. The mixture was incubated for 20 min at room temperature and added to the cells for 24 h at 37 °C. After 24 h, 4% FBS and antibiotic/antimycotic-free DMEM were added to the cells, resulting in a final FBS concentration of 2%. The cells were further incubated for 24 h in a CO_2 incubator to silence Akt expression. The efficiency of Akt siRNA silencing was assessed by measuring Akt protein levels by Western blotting. After siRNA transfection, myotubes were exposed to 100 µM DEX and 500 ng/mL PYP15 for 24 h.

Table 3. Small interfering RNA (siRNA) sequences used for Akt knockdown.

Gene	Accession No.	Sequence (5'–3')
Akt siRNA1	NM_009652.2	F: CUCAAGUGAGGUUGACAGA
		R: UCUGUCAACCUCACUUGAG
Akt siRNA2	NM_009652.2	F: CCACGGAUACCAUGAACGA
		R: UCGUUCAUGGUAUCCGUGG
Akt siRNA3	NM_009652.2	F: GACGAUGGACUUCCGAUCA
		R: UGAUCGGAAGUCCAUCGUC

4.10. 20S Proteasome Activity Assay

The chymotrypsin-like activity of the 20S proteasome was measured as changes in the fluorescence of 7-amino-4-methylcoumarin (AMC) conjugated to the chymotrypsin peptide substrate LLVY, using a 20S proteasome activity assay kit (Chemicon, Temecula, CA, USA). Briefly, cells were suspended in RIPA lysis buffer (50 mM Tris-HCl, pH 7.5, 150 mM sodium chloride, 0.5% sodium deoxycholate, 1% Triton X-100, 0.1% SDS, and 2 mM EDTA) containing protease inhibitors (1 mg/mL aprotinin, 1 mg/mL leupeptin, 1 mg/mL pepstatin A, 200 mM Na_3VO_4, 500 mM NaF, and 100 mM PMSF) and centrifuged at $16,000 \times g$ for 10 min at 4 °C. The protein concentration in supernatants was determined using the BCA protein assay kit (Pierce). The cell lysates were incubated for 90 min at 37 °C with a labeled substrate, Leu-Leu-Val-Tyr (LLVY)-AMC, and the cleavage activity was monitored by detecting the free fluorophore AMC using a fluorescence plate reader (Gen5 ELISA, Bio-Tek, Winooski, VT, USA).

4.11. Statistical Analysis

Mean values were compared by analysis of variance using SPSS software (ver. 10.0; SPSS Inc., Chicago, IL, USA). The values are presented as the mean ± SD. Different letters indicate significant differences among groups according to Duncan's multiple-range test [37].

Author Contributions: Conceptualization, T.-J.N.; Formal analysis, M.-K.L.; Funding acquisition, T-J.N.; Investigation, M.-K.L. and J.-W.C.; Methodology, M.-K.L.; Resources, T.-J.N.; Supervision, T.-J.N.; Validation, T.-J.N.; Visualization, M.-K.L.; Writing-original draft, M.-K.L.; Writing-review and editing, Y.H.C.

Funding: This study was supported by the Basic Science Research Program through the National Research Foundation of Korea (NRF), funded by the Ministry of Education (grant No. 2012R1A6A1028677).

Conflicts of Interest: The authors declare no conflict of interest.

References

1. Qian, Z.-J.; Jung, W.K.; Kim, S.K. Free radical scavenging activity of a novel antioxidative peptide purified from hydrolysate of bullfrog skin, Rana catesbeiana Shaw. *Bioresour. Technol.* **2008**, *99*, 1690–1698. [CrossRef]
2. Korhonen, H.; Pihlanto, A. Bioactive peptides: Production and functionality. *Int. Dairy J.* **2006**, *16*, 945–960. [CrossRef]
3. Suetsuna, K.; Maekawa, K.; Chen, J. Antihypertensive effects of Undaria pinnatifida (wakame) peptide on blood pressure in spontaneously hypertensive rats. *J. Nutr. Biochem.* **2004**, *15*, 267–272. [CrossRef]

4. Jung, W.K.; Rajapakse, N.; Kim, S.K. Antioxidative activity of low molecular peptide derived from the sauce of fermented blue mussel, Mytilus edulis. *Eur. Food Res. Technol.* **2005**, *220*, 535–539. [CrossRef]

5. Kim, S.K.; Kim, Y.T.; Byun, H.G.; Park, P.J.; Ito, H. Purification and characterization of antioxidative peptides from bovine skin. *BMB Rep.* **2001**, *34*, 219–224.

6. Rajapakse, N.; Mendis, E.; Jung, W.K.; Je, J.Y.; Kim, S.K. Purification of radical scavenging peptide from fermented mussel sauce and its anti-oxidant properties. *Food Res. Int.* **2005**, *38*, 175–182. [CrossRef]

7. Chen, J.; Suetsuna, K.; Yamauchi, F. Isolation and characterization of immunostimulative peptides from soybean. *J. Nutr. Biochem.* **1995**, *6*, 310–313. [CrossRef]

8. Tsuruki, T.; Kishi, K.; Takahashi, M.; Tanaka, M.; Matsukawa, T.; Yoshikawa, M. Soymetide, an immunostimulating peptide derived from soybean β-conglycinin, is an Fmlp agonist. *FEBS Lett.* **2003**, *540*, 206–210. [CrossRef]

9. Lee, M.K.; Kim, I.H.; Choi, Y.H.; Choi, J.W.; Kim, Y.M.; Nam, T.J. The proliferative effects of *Pyropia yezoensis* peptide on IEC-6 cells are mediated through the epidermal growth factor receptor signaling pathway. *Int. J. Mol. Med.* **2015**, *35*, 909–914. [CrossRef] [PubMed]

10. Fleurence, J.; Morancais, M.; Dumay, J. Seaweed proteins. In *Protein in Food Processing*; Yada, R.Y., Ed.; Woodhead Publishing Limited: Cambridge, UK, 2014; pp. 197–213.

11. Kim, E.Y.; Choi, Y.H.; Nam, T.J. Identification and antioxidant activity of synthetic peptides from phycobiliproteins of *Pyropia yezoensis*. *Int. J. Mol. Med.* **2018**, *42*, 789–798. [CrossRef]

12. Park, S.J.; Ryu, J.; Kim, I.H.; Choi, Y.H.; Nam, T.J. Activation of the mTOR signaling pathway in breast cancer MCF-7 cells by a peptide derived from *Porphyra yezoensis*. *Oncol. Rep.* **2015**, *33*, 19–24. [CrossRef] [PubMed]

13. Lee, H.A.; Kim, I.H.; Nam, T.J. Bioactive peptide from *Pyropia yezoensis* and its anti-inflammatory activities. *Int. J. Mol. Med.* **2015**, *36*, 1701–1706. [CrossRef] [PubMed]

14. Choi, Y.H.; Kim, E.Y.; Mikami, K.; Nam, T.J. Chemoprotective effects of a recombinant protein from *Pyropia yezoensis* and synthetic peptide against acetaminophen-induced change liver cell death. *Int. J. Mol. Med.* **2015**, *36*, 369–376. [CrossRef]

15. Oh, J.H.; Kim, E.Y.; Choi, Y.H.; Nam, T.J. Negative regulation of ERK1/2 by PI3K is required for the protective effects of *Pyropia yezoensis* peptide against perfluorooctane sulfonate-induced endoplasmic reticulum stress. *Mol. Med. Rep.* **2017**, *15*, 2583–2587. [CrossRef]

16. Kim, C.R.; Kim, Y.M.; Lee, M.K.; Kim, I.H.; Choi, Y.H.; Nam, T.J. *Pyropia yezoensis* peptide promotes collagen synthesis by activating the TGF-β/Smad signaling pathway in the human dermal fibroblast cell line Hs27. *Int. J. Mol. Med.* **2017**, *39*, 31–38. [CrossRef] [PubMed]

17. Zhang, P.; Chen, X.; Fan, M. Signaling mechanisms involved in disuse muscle atrophy. *Med. Hypotheses* **2007**, *69*, 310–321. [CrossRef] [PubMed]

18. Schakman, O.; Gilson, H.; Thissen, J.P. Mechanisms of glucocorticoid-induced myopathy. *J. Endocrinol.* **2008**, *197*, 1–10. [CrossRef]

19. Auclair, D.; Garrel, D.R.; Chaouki Zerouala, A.; Ferland, L.H. Activation of the ubiquitin pathway in rat skeletal muscle by catabolic doses of glucocorticoids. *Am. J. Physiol. Cell Physiol.* **1997**, *272*, C1007–C1016. [CrossRef]

20. Shah, O.J.; Kimball, S.R.; Jefferson, L.S. Acute attenuation of translation initiation and protein synthesis by glucocorticoids in skeletal muscle. *Am. J. Physiol. Endocrinol. Metab.* **2000**, *278*, E76–E82. [CrossRef]

21. Kostyo, J.L.; Redmond, A.F. Role of protein synthesis in the inhibitory action of adrenal steroid hormones on amino acid transport by muscle. *Endocrinology* **1966**, *79*, 531–540. [CrossRef]

22. Shah, O.J.; Kimball, S.R.; Jefferson, L.S. Among translational effectors, p70S6K is uniquely sensitive to inhibition by glucocorticoids. *Biochem. J.* **2000**, *347*, 389–397. [CrossRef] [PubMed]

23. Te Pas, M.F.; de Jeong, P.R.; Verburg, F.J. Glucocorticoid inhibition of C2C12 proliferation rate and differentiation capacity in relation to mRNA levels of the MRF gene family. *Mol. Biol. Rep.* **2000**, *27*, 87–98. [CrossRef]

24. Jellyman, J.K.; Martin-Gronert, M.S.; Cripps, R.L.; Giusseni, D.A.; Ozanne, S.E.; Shen, Q.W.; Du, M.; Fowden, A.L.; Forhead, A.J. Effects of cortisol and dexamethasone on insulin signaling pathways in skeletal muscle of the ovine fetus during late gestation. *PLoS ONE* **2012**, *7*, e52363. [CrossRef]

25. Nakao, R.; Hirasaka, K.; Goto, J.; Ishidoh, K.; Yamada, C.; Ohno, A.; Okumura, Y.; Nonaka, I.; Yasuromo, K.; Baldwin, K.M.; et al. Ubiquitin ligase Cb1-b is a negative regulator for insulin-like growth factor 1 signaling during muscle atrophy caused by unloading. *Mol. Cell. Biol.* **2009**, *29*, 4798–4811. [CrossRef] [PubMed]

26. Zheng, B.; Ohkawa, S.; Li, H.; Roberts-Wilson, T.K.; Price, S.R. FoxO3a mediates signaling crosstalk that coordinates ubiquitin and atrogin-1/MAFbx expression during glucocorticoid-induced skeletal muscle atrophy. *FASEB J.* **2010**, *24*, 2660–2669. [CrossRef]

27. Kukreti, H.; Amuthavalli, K.; Harikumar, A.; Sathiyamoorthy, S.; Feng, P.Z.; Anantharaj, R. Muscle-specific microRNA1 (miR1) targets heat shock protein 70 (HSP70) during dexamethasone mediated atrophy. *J. Biol. Chem.* **2013**, *288*, 6663–6678. [CrossRef] [PubMed]

28. Stitt, T.N.; Drujan, D.; Clarke, B.A.; Panaro, F.; Timofeyva, Y.; Kline, W.O.; Gonzalez, M.; Yancopoulos, G.D.; Glass, D.J. The IGF-I/PI3K/Akt pathway prevents expression of muscle atrophy-induced ubiquitin ligases by inhibiting FOXO transcription factors. *Mol. Cell* **2004**, *14*, 395–403. [CrossRef]

29. Mammucari, C.; Milan, G.; Romanello, V.; Masiero, E.; Rudolf, R.; Del Piccolo, P.; Buren, S.J.; Di Lisi, R.; Sandri, C.; Zhao, J.; et al. FoxO3 controls autophagy in skeletal muscle in vivo. *Cell Metab.* **2007**, *6*, 458–471. [CrossRef]

30. Hasselgren, P.O. Glucocorticoids and muscle catabolism. *Curr. Opin. Clin. Nutr. Metab. Care* **1999**, *2*, 201–205. [CrossRef]

31. Leger, B.; Cartoni, R.; Praz, M.; Lamon, S.; Deriaz, O.; Crettenand, A.; Gobelet, C.; Rohmer, P.; Konzelmann, M.; Luthi, F.; et al. Akt signaling through GSK-3β, mTOR and FoxO1 is involved in human skeletal muscle hypertrophy and atrophy. *J. Physiol.* **2006**, *576*, 923–933. [CrossRef]

32. Sandri, M.; Sandri, C.; Gilbert, A.; Skurk, C.; Calabria, E.; Picard, A.; Kenneth, W.; Schiaffino, S.; Lecker, S.H.; Goldberg, A.L. FoxO transcription factors induce the atrophy-related ubiquitin ligase atrogin-1 and cause skeletal muscle atrophy. *Cell* **2004**, *117*, 399–412. [CrossRef]

33. Deval, C.; Mordier, S.; Obled, C.; Bechet, D.; Combaret, L.; Attaix, D.; Ferrara, M. Identification of cathepsin-L as a differentially expressed message associated with skeletal muscle wasting. *Biochem. J.* **2001**, *360*, 143–150. [CrossRef]

34. Komamura, K.; Shirotani-Ikejima, H.; Tatsumi, R.; Tsujita-Kuroda, Y.; Kitakaze, M.; Miyatake, K.; Sunagawa, K.; Miyata, T. Differential gene expression in the rat skeletal and heart muscle in glucocorticoid-induced myopathy: Analysis by microarray. *Cardiovasc. Drugs Ther.* **2003**, *17*, 303–310. [CrossRef]

35. Sacheck, J.M.; Ohtsuka, A.; Mclary, S.C.; Goldberg, A.L. IGF-I stimulates muscle growth by suppressing protein breakdown and expression of atrophy-related ubiquitin ligases, atrogin-1 and MuRF1. *Am. J. Physiol. Endocrinol. Metab.* **2004**, *287*, E591–E601. [CrossRef]

36. Yamamoto, D.; Maki, T.; Herningtyas, E.H.; Ikeshita, N.; Shibahara, H.; Sugiyama, Y.; Nakanishi, S.; Iida, K.; Iguchi, G.; Takahashi, Y.; et al. Branched-chain amino acids protect against dexamethasone-induced soleus muscle atrophy in rats. *Muscle Nerve* **2010**, *41*, 819–827. [CrossRef]

37. Lee, M.K.; Kim, Y.M.; Kim, I.H.; Choi, Y.H.; Nam, T.J. *Pyropia yezoensis* peptide PYP15 protects against dexamethasone-induced muscle atrophy through the downregulation of atrogin1/MAFbx and MuRF1 in mouse C2C12 myotubes. *Mol. Med. Rep.* **2017**, *15*, 3507–3514. [CrossRef] [PubMed]

38. Choi, Y.H.; Yamaguchi, K.; Oda, T.; Nam, T.J. Chemical and mass spectrometry characterization of the red alga *Pyropia yezoensis* chemoprotective protein (PYP): Protective activity of the N-terminal fragment of PYP1 against acetaminophen-induced cell death in Chang liver cells. *Int. J. Mol. Med.* **2015**, *35*, 271–276. [CrossRef]

39. Desler, M.M.; Jones, S.J.; Smith, C.W.; Woods, T.L. Effects of dexamethasone and anabolic agents on proliferation and protein synthesis and degradation in C2C12 myogenic cells. *J. Anim. Sci.* **1996**, *74*, 1265–1273. [CrossRef] [PubMed]

40. Schakman, O.; Kalista, S.; Barbe, C.; Loumaye, A.; Thissen, J.P. Glucocorticoid-induced skeletal muscle atrophy. *Int. J. Biochem. Cell Biol.* **2013**, *45*, 2163–2172. [CrossRef]

41. Adams, G.R.; Mccue, S.A. Localized infusion of IGF-I results in skeletal muscle hypertrophy in rats. *J. Appl. Physiol.* **1998**, *84*, 1716–1722. [CrossRef]

42. Lee, S.H.; Barton, E.R.; Sweeney, H.L.; Farrar, R.P. Viral expression of insulin-like growth factor-I enhances muscle hypertrophy in resistance-trained rats. *J. Appl. Physiol.* **2004**, *96*, 1097–1104. [CrossRef]

43. Glass, D.J. Skeletal muscle hypertrophy and atrophy signaling pathways. *Int. J. Biochem. Cell Biol.* **2005**, *37*, 1974–1984. [CrossRef] [PubMed]

44. Clemmons, D.R. Role of IGF-I in skeletal muscle mass maintenance. *Trends Endocrinol. Metab.* **2009**, *20*, 349–356. [CrossRef]

45. Latres, E.; Amini, A.R.; Amini, A.A.; Griffiths, J.; Martin, F.J.; Lin, H.C.; Yancopoulos, G.D.; Glass, D.J. Insulin-like growth factor-1 (IGF-1) inversely regulates atrophy-induced genes via the phosphatidylinositol 3-kinase/Akt/mammalian target of rapamycin (PI3K/Akt/mTOR) pathway. *J. Biol. Chem.* **2005**, *280*, 2737–2744. [CrossRef]

46. Calnan, D.R.; Brunet, A. The FoxO code. *Oncogene* **2008**, *27*, 2276–2288. [CrossRef]

47. Kamei, Y.; Miura, S.; Suzuki, M.; Kai, Y.; Mizukami, J.; Taniguchi, T.; Mochida, K.; Hata, T.; Matsuda, J.; Aburatani, H.; et al. Skeletal muscle FOXO1 (FKHR) transgenic mice have less skeletal muscle mass, down-regulated type I (slow twitch/red muscle) fiber genes, and impaired glycemic control. *J. Biol. Chem.* **2004**, *279*, 41114–41123. [CrossRef] [PubMed]

48. Southgate, R.J.; Neill, B.; Prelovsek, O.; El-Osta, A.; Kamei, Y.; Miura, S.; Exaki, O.; McLoughlin, T.J.; Zhang, W.; Unterman, T.G.; et al. FoxO1 regulates the expression of 4E-BP1 and inhibits mTOR signaling in mammalian skeletal muscle. *J. Biol. Chem.* **2007**, *282*, 21176–21186. [CrossRef] [PubMed]

49. Naujokat, C.; Hoffmann, S. Role and function of the 26S proteasome in proliferation and apoptosis. *Lab. Investig.* **2002**, *82*, 965–980. [CrossRef] [PubMed]

50. Wolf, D.H.; Hilt, W. The proteasome: A proteolytic nanomachine of cell regulation and waste disposal. *Biochim. Biophys. Acta* **2004**, *1695*, 19–31. [CrossRef] [PubMed]

51. Lecker, S.H.; Goldberg, A.L.; Mitch, W.E. Protein degradation by the ubiquitin-proteasome pathway in normal and disease states. *J. Am. Soc. Nephrol.* **2006**, *17*, 1807–1819. [CrossRef]

52. Jagoe, R.T.; Goldberg, A.L. What do we really know about the ubiquitin-proteasome pathway in muscle atrophy? *Curr. Opin. Clin. Nutr. Metab. Care* **2001**, *4*, 183–190. [CrossRef] [PubMed]

53. Mammucari, C.; Schiaffino, S.; Sandri, M. Downstream of Akt: FoxO3 and mTOR in the regulation of autophagy in skeletal muscle. *Autophagy* **2008**, *4*, 524–526. [CrossRef] [PubMed]

54. Zaho, J.; Brault, J.J.; Schild, A.; Cao, P.; Sandri, M.; Schiaffino, S.; Lecker, S.H.; Goldberg, A.L. FoxO3 coordinately activates protein degradation by the autophagic/lysosomal and proteasomal pathways in atrophying muscle cells. *Cell Metab.* **2007**, *6*, 472–483. [CrossRef] [PubMed]

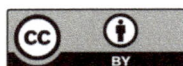

marine drugs

MDPI

Article

Effect of *Chlorella Pyrenoidosa* Protein Hydrolysate-Calcium Chelate on Calcium Absorption Metabolism and Gut Microbiota Composition in Low-Calcium Diet-Fed Rats

Pengpeng Hua [1,2], **Yu Xiong** [1], **Zhiying Yu** [1], **Bin Liu** [1,2,*] and **Lina Zhao** [1,*]

[1] National Engineering Research Center of JUNCAO Technology, Fujian Agriculture and Forestry University, Fuzhou 350002, China; huapengpeng_flower@163.com (P.H.); aindxiong@163.com (Y.X.); 18838018055@163.com (Z.Y.)

[2] College of Food Sciences, Fujian Agriculture and Forestry University, Fuzhou 350002, China

* Correspondence: liubin618@hotmail.com (B.L.); zln20002000@163.com (L.Z.); Tel.: +86-591-8353-0197 (B.L. & L.Z.)

Received: 30 April 2019; Accepted: 3 June 2019; Published: 11 June 2019

Abstract: In our current investigation, we evaluated the effect of *Chlorella pyrenoidosa* protein hydrolysate (CPPH) and *Chlorella pyrenoidosa* protein hydrolysate-calcium chelate (CPPH-Ca) on calcium absorption and gut microbiota composition, as well as their in vivo regulatory mechanism in SD rats fed low-calcium diets. Potent major compounds in CPPH were characterized by HPLC-MS/MS, and the calcium-binding mechanism was investigated through ultraviolet and infrared spectroscopy. Using high-throughput next-generation 16S rRNA gene sequencing, we analyzed the composition of gut microbiota in rats. Our study showed that HCPPH-Ca increased the levels of body weight gain, serum Ca, bone activity, bone mineral density (BMD) and bone mineral content (BMC), while decreased serum alkaline phosphatase (ALP) and inhibited the morphological changes of bone. HCPPH-Ca up-regulated the gene expressions of transient receptor potential cation V5 (TRPV5), TRPV6, calcium-binding protein-D9k (CaBP-D9k) and a calcium pump (plasma membrane Ca-ATPase, PMCA1b). It also improved the abundances of *Firmicutes* and *Lactobacillus*. *Bifidobacterium* and *Sutterella* were both positively correlated with calcium absorption. Collectively, these findings illustrate the potential of HCPPH-Ca as an effective calcium supplement.

Keywords: *Chlorella pyrenoidosa* protein hydrolysate (CPPH); *Chlorella pyrenoidosa* protein hydrolysate-calcium chelate (CPPH-Ca); calcium absorption; gene expression; gut microbiota

---

1. Introduction

As one of the most abundant mineral elements in human body, calcium plays a critical role in human bone health, especially for children [1] and the elderly [2]. A low intake and bioavailability of calcium may cause calcium deficiency [3], which is characterized by low levels of calcium and alkaline phosphatase (ALP) in serum, as well as low bone mass. Calcium deficiency causes microarchitectural deterioration of bone tissue, leading to increased bone fragility and risk of fracture [4–6]. Considerable efforts have been devoted to developing appropriate treatments because of the medical importance of calcium deficiency. Although many calcium supplements are available on the market, their efficacies are often low and side effects are common [7]. Calcium gluconate (HGCa), inorganic calcium (CaCO$_3$) and calcium lactate are the main forms of ionized calcium in the intestinal environment, which have the disadvantage of easily forming calcium phosphate deposition [7]. As a result, the bioavailability and the absorption of dietary calcium is severely lowered [8]. Therefore, a well-tolerated treatment with minimal side effects for calcium absorption is urgently required. Many calcium-containing complexes and commercial products are currently available to prevent calcium deficiency in humans [9]. Previous studies have shown that substances such as casein phosphopeptides (CPPs) and phosvitin phosphopeptides (PPPs) can improve calcium absorption [10–12]. In addition, soybean, fish bone, hen egg white peptides (EPs), shrimp processing by-products and whey protein have also been shown to facilitate the in vivo calcium absorption, while their in vivo effect remains largely unclear [13–20].

Chlorella pyrenoidosa is a genus of unicellular green algae which contains many substances that could be beneficial for human health, such as proteins, β-carotene and amino acids [21–23]. It is a good material for biotechnology research, and is also a source of high-quality single-cell protein [24–27]. At present, active peptides derived from *Chlorella pyrenoidosa* proteins are research hotspots worldwide. Most studies focus on the development of functional peptides, such as *Chlorella pyrenoidosa* protein (CCP), which has antioxidant, antimicrobial, blood pressure-reducing, lipid-lowering and immune regulatory properties [28–33]. However, there is almost no research on the activity of *Chlorella pyrenoidosa* calcium-chelating peptide.

At the molecular level, transient receptor potential cation V5 (TRPV5) [34–36], TRPV6 [37,38], calcium-binding protein-D9k (CaBP-D9k) and a calcium pump (plasma membrane Ca-ATPase, PMCA1b) [39–46] can modulate calcium re-absorption in the renal tubules [47,48]. It is widely accepted that gut microbiota has beneficial effects on calcium absorption and bone health. Some bacterial genera, such as *Bifidobacterium* and *L. reuteri*, are positively correlated with levels of serum Ca, ALP, bone mineral content (BMC) and bone mineral density (BMD) [49]. Moreover, Marine algae can regulate the composition of microbiota [50] and have a beneficial effect on the improvement the Ca absorption [51]. However, the calcium-promoting mechanism of *Chlorella pyrenoidosa* protein hydrolysate-calcium chelate (CPPH-Ca) has not been well studied. Therefore, in the present study, we aimed to assess the potential calcium absorption of HCPPH-Ca in rats fed low-calcium diets. Furthermore, we also determined the specific gene expression and the composition of gut microbiota.

2. Results

2.1. Characterization of Potent Major Compounds of CPPH and Structural Characterization of CPPH-Ca

Table S1 illustrates the identified peptide sequences of CPPH. A total of 43 peptide sequences were detected from CPPH. Retention times ranged from 4.21 min to 8.37 min. Figure S1 shows that the ultraviolet absorption spectrum of CPPH and CPPH-Ca demonstrated obvious band shifts. When the CPPH and Ca ions chelated, the UV absorption spectra of CPPH obviously shifted/changed both in band and intensity in the area of 223 to 274 nm. The absorption peak of WPH shifted from 230 to 265 nm. The CPPH-Ca presented distinct UV absorption spectra compared with CPPH, suggesting that the new substance was formed when CPPH interacted with calcium ions. Figure S2 shows that the FT-IR spectrum curve of CPPH-Ca was different from CPPH. CPPH-Ca had obvious fluctuations at 3410 cm^{-1}, 1650 cm^{-1} and 1400 cm^{-1}, while CPPH exhibited obvious absorption peak at around 3350 cm^{-1}, 1642 cm^{-1} and 1476 cm^{-1}. Meanwhile, the spectra of the CPPH showed two strong bands at 1642 cm^{-1} and 1625 cm^{-1}(amide-I). After binding with calcium, two peaks appeared at 1650 cm^{-1} and 1400 cm^{-1}, with that at 1400 cm^{-1} showing the symmetric stretching vibration of -COO. The results indicate that the interaction site between calcium and CPPH is carboxyl oxygen.

2.2. Body Weight and Biochemical Parameters in Serum

Table 1 lists the changes in the body weights of rats in different groups. During the experimental period, no rats died. At week 0, no significant difference in terms of initial body weight was observed among the 10 groups. After 4 weeks, the body weight of low calcium diet-fed (model) was obviously lower compared with the normal diet-fed (control) group. In addition, after 8 weeks, the rats fed with HCPPH-Ca in the high dose group gained body weight more rapidly compared with the model group and HCaCO3 ($p < 0.05$). However, there was no significant difference between the HCPPH-Ca group and control group. After 8 weeks, the final body weight gain of the MCPPH + MCaCO3, HCPPH +

HCaCO$_3$, MCPPH-Ca and HCPPH-Ca groups was significantly higher than that of the model group (p < 0.05). These results indicated that CPPH-Ca could effective improve body weight to a normal level, even in the middle dose group, that HCPPH-Ca was better than HCaCO$_3$, even in HGCa, and that calcium in CPPH-Ca was more easily to be absorbed.

Table 1. Changes in the body weight of rats in the different groups during the experimental period.

Groups	Weight (g)			
	0 Weeks	4 Weeks	8 Weeks	Weight Gain
Control	120.04 ± 4.66[a]	303.62 ± 10.43[a]	371.21 ± 14.01[a]	245.13 ± 9.00[a]
Model	125.19 ± 4.79[a]	267.32 ± 5.62[b]	308.56 ± 4.58[e]	189.36 ± 8.33[f]
HCaCO$_3$	120.39 ± 9.22[a]	269.63 ± 14.27[b]	326.33 ± 19.47[bcd]	211.42 ± 9.63[bcd]
HGCa	122.70 ± 2.19[a]	271.54 ± 13.35[b]	331.92 ± 11.43[bc]	221.79 ± 10.96[bc]
LCPPH + LCaCO$_3$	122.443 ± 4.75[a]	266.95 ± 11.27[b]	320.97 ± 14.36[cde]	196.53 ± 11.53[ef]
MCPPH + MCaCO$_3$	119.72 ± 5.43[a]	271.54 ± 17.60[b]	328.01 ± 24.35[bcd]	208.23 ± 21.50[cde]
HCPPH + HCaCO$_3$	123.94 ± 4.76[a]	269.85 ± 12.52[b]	333.47 ± 17.22[bc]	214.70 ± 11.34[bcd]
LCPPH-Ca	123.34 ± 4.49[a]	267.35 ± 9.50[b]	325.72 ± 20.89[bcd]	202.38 ± 17.97[def]
MCPPH-Ca	121.65 ± 4.63[a]	269.20 ± 6.67[b]	332.21 ± 11.45[bc]	204.33 ± 15.22[de]
HCPPH-Ca	121.85 ± 7.19[a]	270.62 ± 13.87[b]	340.02 ± 20.01[a]	223.41 ± 13.03[b]

Note: control, normal group; model, low calcium group; HCaCO$_3$, high dosage of CaCO$_3$ group; HGCa, high dosage of calcium gluconate group; LCPPH + LCaCO$_3$, low dosage of CPPH supplemented with low dosage of CaCO$_3$ group; MCPPH + MCaCO$_3$, model dosage of CPPH supplemented with model dosage of CaCO$_3$ group; HCPPH + HCaCO$_3$, high dosage of CPPH supplemented with high dosage of CaCO$_3$ group; LCPPH-Ca, low dosage of CPPH-Ca group; MCPPH-Ca, model dosage of CPPH-Ca group; HCPPH-Ca, high dosage of CPPH-Ca group. Data are expressed as the mean ± SD (n = 10). One-way ANOVA with Tukey's test. Different letters indicate significant effect with p < 0.05.

Figure 1 summarizes the changes about the biochemical parameters in the serum. After 8 weeks, the serum phosphorus (p) level was not significantly changed under different treatments (p < 0.05) (Figure 1B). However, rats fed with the serum Ca level increased significantly in control group compared with the model group (p < 0.05) (Figure 1A), the serum ALP activity were decreased significantly in control group compared with the model group (p < 0.05) (Figure 1C). Particularly, rats fed with supplements at low, medium or high dose of CPPH-Ca and high dose of CPPH + CaCO$_3$ showed a significant increase of serum Ca level compared with the model group even CaCO$_3$ group (p < 0.05), while those groups were no different significantly from control group and HGCa group. The ALP activity in the serum showed no significant difference between the HCPPH-Ca and control groups (Figure 1C), while those groups showed a significant decrease in ALP compared with the model group (p < 0.05). A high dosage of CPPH + CaCO$_3$ and CPPH-Ca deduced a greater ALP activity compared with low dosages of CPPH + CaCO$_3$ and CPPH-Ca. Therefore, these results reveal that CPPH-Ca, even in the low dose group, was more easily absorbed and calcified.

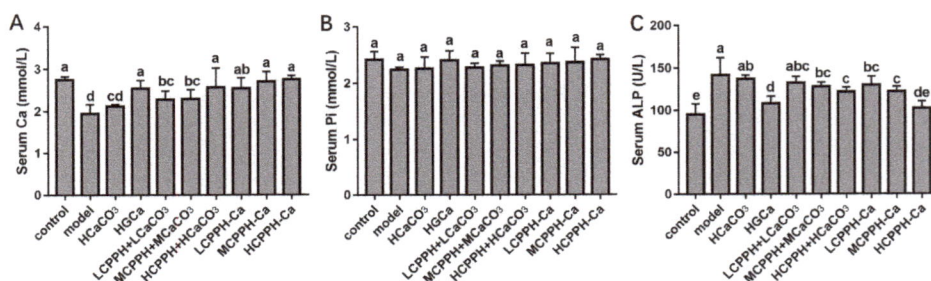

Figure 1. Biochemical parameters in the serum of Ca-deficient rats after oral gavage with different Ca. Serum Ca (**A**), Serum P (**B**), Serum alkaline phosphatase (Serum ALP) (**C**). Note: control, normal group; model, low calcium group; HCaCO$_3$, high dosage of CaCO$_3$ group; HGCa, high dosage of calcium gluconate group; LCPPH + LCaCO$_3$, low dosage of CPPH supplemented with low dosage of CaCO$_3$ group; MCPPH + MCaCO$_3$, model dosage of CPPH supplemented with model dosage of CaCO$_3$ group; HCPPH + HCaCO$_3$, high dosage of CPPH supplemented with high dosage of CaCO$_3$ group; LCPPH-Ca, low dosage of CPPH-Ca group; MCPPH-Ca, model dosage of CPPH-Ca group; HCPPH-Ca, high dosage of CPPH-Ca group. Data are expressed as the mean ± SD ($n = 10$). One-way ANOVA with Tukey's test. Different letters indicate significant effect with $p < 0.05$.

2.3. Bone Biomechanical Parameters and Histomorphometry

To measure the assimilation and metabolism of calcium, femur properties were monitored in the experiment. Figure 2 presents the dry weight (DW) index, length and diameter of femurs and tibias of all rats. At the end of 8 weeks, no significant differences in tibial diameter were observed in any group (Figure 2F) ($p < 0.05$). The femur weight index, femur length, femur diameter, tibial weight index and tibial length of the high dose of CPPH-Ca and HGCa groups were significantly increased compared to the model group (Figure 2A–E) ($p < 0.05$). Meanwhile, there was no statistically significant difference between the HCPPH-Ca group or HGCa group and control group in the femur weight index, femur length, femur diameter, tibial weight index and tibial length ($p < 0.05$). The femur weight and the length of high dose of CaCO$_3$, HGCa and the medium and high dose of CPPH-Ca groups were significantly higher compared with the model group ($p < 0.05$), while no significant differences among HCaCO$_3$, HGCa and HCPPH-Ca groups were observed (Figure 2A,B,D,E). Particularly, the bone biomechanical parameters of rats in the low, medium and high dose CPPH-Ca groups were higher than those in the CPPH + CaCO$_3$ group. Figure 3 indicates that the levels of BMD and BMC at the proximal, central, and distal ends of the femur at the end of 8 weeks were significantly increased in the high dose of CPPH-Ca, HGCa and control groups compared with the model and HCaCO$_3$ groups ($p < 0.05$). However, the femur BMD and BMC were significantly different between the high dose of CPPH-Ca and HGCa groups, and the high dose of CPPH-Ca group exhibited a greater effect compared with the HGCa group. The administration of high doses of CPPH-Ca significantly increased the levels of BMD and BMC compared with the high dose of CPPH + CaCO$_3$ group at the end of the experiment (8 weeks) ($p < 0.05$) (Figure 3A–F). There was no significant difference in the levels of BMD and BMC of low and medium doses of CPPH + CaCO$_3$, while the level of distial BMD reached that of the control group when fed with high doses of CPPH-Ca. H&E staining exhibited the effect of CPPH-Ca on pathological profiles in the femur (Figure 4). According to microarchitectural of femoral necks analysis, the sections of femur tissues in the control group showed normal level (Figure 4A). However, the model group showed abnormal (Figure 4B) bone volume per tissue volume (BV/TV), trabecular thickness (Tb.Th), trabecular number (Tb.No). In the rats fed with CPPH-Ca, we found that the bone volume compared to the tissue volume (BV/TV), trabecular thickness (Tb.Th), trabecular number (Tb.No) was significantly increased, whereas trabecular separation (Tb.Sp) was dramatically decreased. The aforementioned results indicate the beneficial effects of HCPPH-Ca and HCPPH + HCaCO$_3$ treatments on the femoral pathology in calcium-deficient rats (Figure 4G,J).

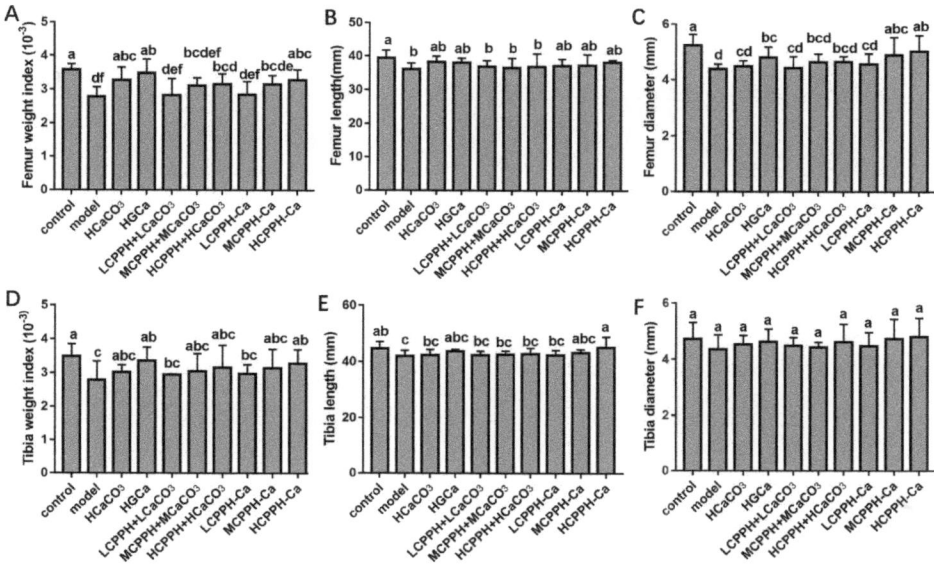

Figure 2. Weight index, length and diameter of femurs and tibias of Ca-deficient rats after treatment with different Ca. Femur weight index (**A**), Femur length (**B**), Femur diameter (**C**), Tibia weight index (**D**), Tibia length (**E**), Tibia diameter (**F**). Note: control, normal group; model, low calcium group; HCaCO$_3$, high dosage of CaCO$_3$ group; HGCa, high dosage of calcium gluconate group; LCPPH + LCaCO$_3$, low dosage of CPPH supplemented with low dosage of CaCO$_3$ group; MCPPH + MCaCO$_3$, model dosage of CPPH supplemented with model dosage of CaCO$_3$ group; HCPPH + HCaCO$_3$, high dosage of CPPH supplemented with high dosage of CaCO$_3$ group; LCPPH-Ca, low dosage of CPPH-Ca group; MCPPH-Ca, model dosage of CPPH-Ca group; HCPPH-Ca, high dosage of CPPH-Ca group. Data are expressed as the mean ± SD (*n* = 10). One-way ANOVA with Tukey's test. Different letters indicate significant effect with *p* < 0.05.

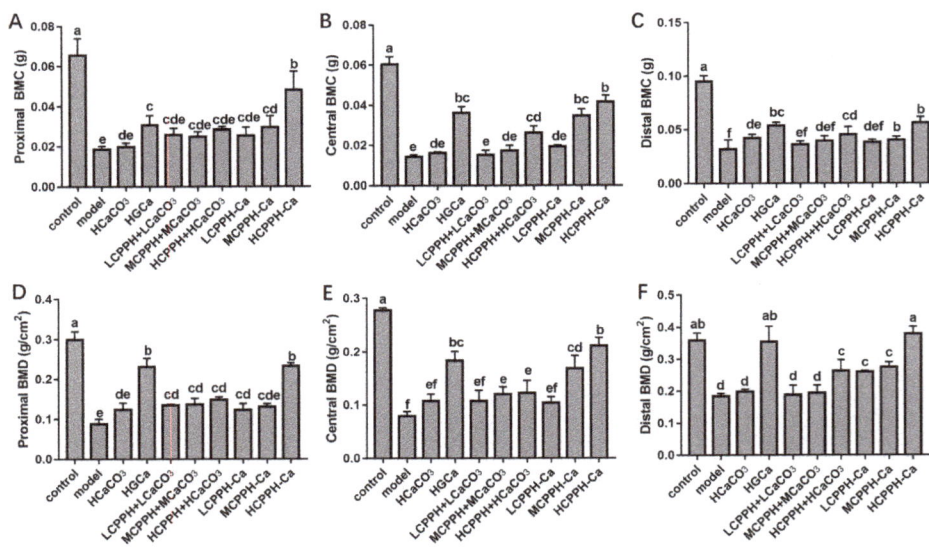

Figure 3. Femurs bone mineral content (BMC) and bone mineral density (BMD) of Ca-deficient rats after oral gavage with different Ca in the experimental period. Proximal BMC (**A**), Central BMC (**B**), Distal BMC (**C**), Proximal BMD (**D**), Centrality BMD (**E**), Distal BMD (**F**). Note: control, normal group; model, low calcium group; HCaCO$_3$, high dosage of CaCO$_3$ group; HGCa, high dosage of calcium gluconate group; LCPPH + LCaCO$_3$, low dosage of CPPH supplemented with low dosage of CaCO$_3$ group; MCPPH + MCaCO$_3$, model dosage of CPPH supplemented with model dosage of CaCO$_3$ group; HCPPH + HCaCO$_3$, high dosage of CPPH supplemented with high dosage of CaCO$_3$ group; LCPPH-Ca, low dosage of CPPH-Ca group; MCPPH-Ca, model dosage of CPPH-Ca group; HCPPH-Ca, high dosage of CPPH-Ca group. Data are expressed as the mean ± SD ($n = 10$). One-way ANOVA with Tukey's test. Different letters indicate significant effect with $p < 0.05$.

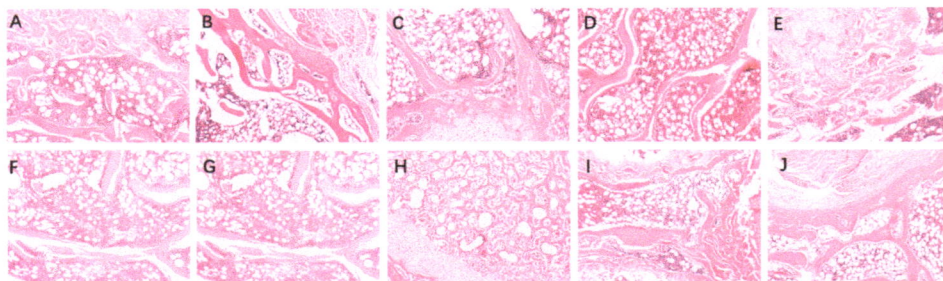

Figure 4. Histopathological analysis of rat kidney tissues in different groups at 100× magnification. control (**A**), model (**B**), HCaCO$_3$ (**C**), HGCa (**D**), LCPPH + LCaCO$_3$ (**E**), MCPPH + MCaCO$_3$ (**F**), HCPPH + HCaCO$_3$ (**G**), LCPPH-Ca (**H**), MCPPH-Ca (**I**), HCPPH-Ca (**J**).

2.4. Calcium Balance

Figure 5 shows that the oral administration of low, medium and high doses of CPPH-Ca remarkably improved the apparent calcium absorption (ACAR) of rats compared with CaCO$_3$ ($p < 0.05$) (Figure 5A), and that these groups had no significant difference in ACAR between the control and HGCa group. Meanwhile, the administration of the low, middle and high doses of CPPH-Ca significantly increased the calcium accumulation rate (CAR) ($p < 0.05$), indicating the beneficial effects of CPPH-Ca treatment on calcium absorption in calcium-deficient rats. Moreover, the CAR in the low, medium and high doses CPPH-Ca groups were significantly higher compared with the $HCaCO_3$ group ($p < 0.05$). Rats in the HCPPH-Ca group showed significantly higher ACAR and CAR compared with the HCPPH + $HCaCO_3$ group ($p < 0.05$). The ACAR and CAR of the CPPH + $CaCO_3$ group at different doses were not significantly different from those of the corresponding CPPH-Ca groups ($p < 0.05$).

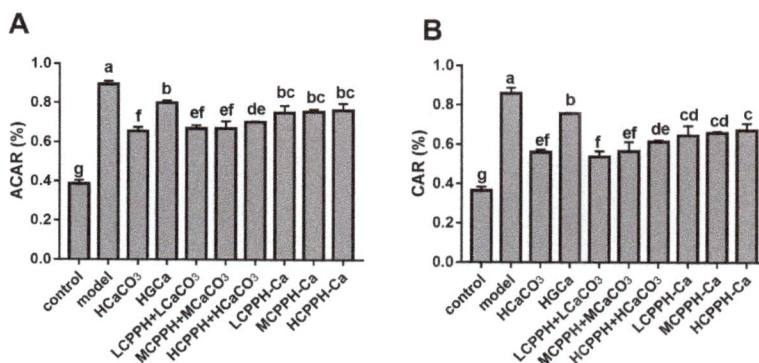

Figure 5. Apparent calcium absorption rate (ACAR) and calcium accumulation rate (CAR) of Ca-deficient rats after oral gavage with different Ca. ACAR (**A**), CAR (**B**). Note: control, normal group; model, low calcium group; $HCaCO_3$, high dosage of $CaCO_3$ group; HGCa, high dosage of calcium gluconate group; LCPPH + $LCaCO_3$, low dosage of CPPH supplemented with low dosage of $CaCO_3$ group; MCPPH + $MCaCO_3$, model dosage of CPPH supplemented with model dosage of $CaCO_3$ group; HCPPH + $HCaCO_3$, high dosage of CPPH supplemented with high dosage of $CaCO_3$ group; LCPPH-Ca, low dosage of CPPH-Ca group; MCPPH-Ca, model dosage of CPPH-Ca group; HCPPH-Ca, high dosage of CPPH-Ca group. Data are expressed as the mean ± SD ($n = 10$). One-way ANOVA with Tukey's test. Different letters indicate significant effect with $p < 0.05$.

2.5. Gene Expression of Corresponding Receptors in the Kidney of the Rats

We examined the expressions of genes involved in calcium absorption in the kidney to assess the molecular mechanisms of CPPH-Ca in regulating the calcium absorption mechanism (Figure 6). Our data revealed that there was a significant increase in most genes at the mRNA level responsible for calcium absorption in kidney of CaBP-D9k, TRPV6 and TRPV5 by the HGCa and the high dose of CPPH-Ca treatment when compared with the model group ($p < 0.05$) (Figure 6A,B,D). PMCA1b is located on the basolateral membrane and plays a role in the extrusion of calcium. We found that the PMCA1b expression was significantly elevated in the HCPPH-Ca group compared with the control group ($p < 0.05$) (Figure 6C). Collectively, these results indicated that HCPPH-Ca promoted calcium absorption in the kidney of calcium-deficient rats, suggesting that calcium supplementation of HCPPH-Ca enhanced calcium absorption, activated calcium transport channels and up-regulated intracellular calcium buffering genes.

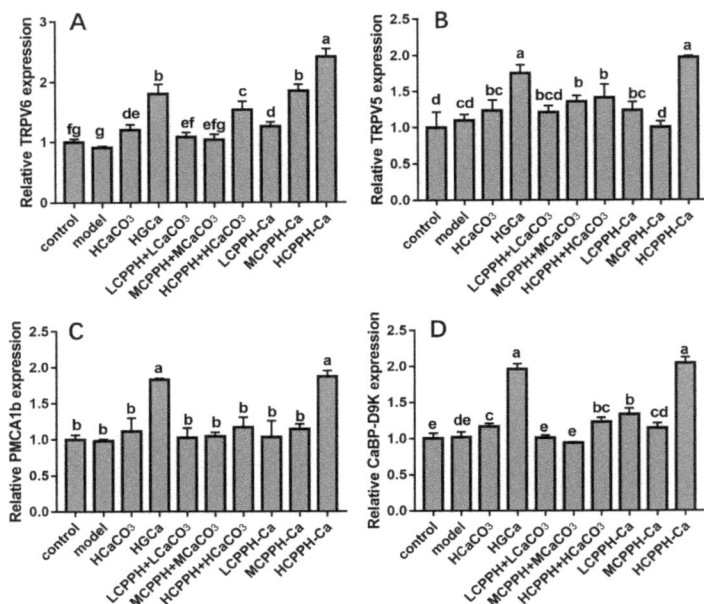

Figure 6. mRNA expression levels of genes involved in calcium-promoting mechanism as determined using real-time PCR. Transient receptor potential cation V6 (TRPV6) (**A**), Transient receptor potential cation V5 (TRPV5) (**B**), calcium-binding protein-D9k (CaBP-D9K) (**C**), plasma membrane Ca-ATPase (PMCA1b) (**D**). Note: control, normal group; model, low calcium group; HCaCO$_3$, high dosage of CaCO$_3$ group; HGCa, high dosage of calcium gluconate group; LCPPH + LCaCO$_3$, low dosage of CPPH supplemented with low dosage of CaCO$_3$ group; MCPPH + MCaCO$_3$, model dosage of CPPH supplemented with model dosage of CaCO$_3$ group; HCPPH + HCaCO3, high dosage of CPPH supplemented with high dosage of CaCO$_3$ group; LCPPH-Ca, low dosage of CPPH-Ca group; MCPPH-Ca, model dosage of CPPH-Ca group; HCPPH-Ca, high dosage of CPPH-Ca group. Data are expressed as the mean ± SD (n = 10). One-way ANOVA with Tukey's test. Different letters indicate significant effect with $p < 0.05$.

2.6. CPPH-Ca Modulates Caecal Microbiota Composition of Calcium-Deficient Rats

To identify the effects of HCPPH-Ca on the compositional distribution of caecal microbiota, we investigated the dominant microbial populations in the other groups (Figure 7) using high-throughput sequencing (HTS) technology. Additionally, the V3–V4 regions of the 16S rRNA gene from fecal samples were sequenced using the Illumina MiSeq platform. At the genus level of metagenomic analysis, the calcium deficiency induced by low calcium diet changed the composition of the intestinal microbiota when compared with the control group. However, the gut microbiota populations of the HCPPH-Ca group recovered. In this study, *Allobaculum, Lactobacillus, Oscillospira, Desulfovibrio, Coprococcus, Oscillospira, Akkermansia, Adlercreutzia, Dorea, Blautia, Ruminococcus, Bifidobacterrium* and *Clostridium* were the prevailing genera in different groups. Through 8 weeks of HCPPH-Ca treatment, the relative abundances of these bacteria were significantly altered, and *Allobaculum, Lactobacillus* and *Ruminococcus* were the most prominently enriched ones after HCPPH-Ca treatment at the genus level. In addition, the abundance of *Coprococcus* was reduced in the HCPPH-Ca group compared with the model group. These results suggested that low-calcium diets could dysregulate the distribution of gut microbiota, while HGCa treatment might have the ability to restore the ecological imbalance of the intestinal flora, maintaining its healthy composition.

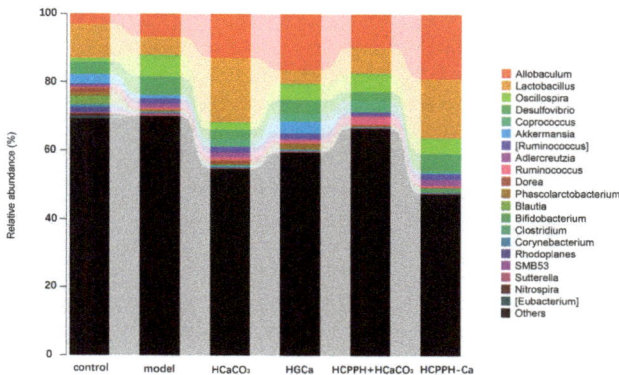

Figure 7. Changes in the bacterial composition of rat intestinal contents according to different genera. Composition of gut microbiota at the genus level. Note: control, normal group; model, low calcium group; HCaCO₃, high dosage of CaCO₃ group; HGCa, high dosage of calcium gluconate group; LCPPH + LCaCO₃, low dosage of CPPH supplemented with low dosage of CaCO₃ group; MCPPH + MCaCO₃, model dosage of CPPH supplemented with model dosage of CaCO₃ group; HCPPH + HCaCO₃, high dosage of CPPH supplemented with high dosage of CaCO₃ group; LCPPH-Ca, low dosage of CPPH-Ca group; MCPPH-Ca, model dosage of CPPH-Ca group; HCPPH-Ca, high dosage of CPPH-Ca group. T-test was used to calculate significant differences between group.

2.7. Correlations of Biochemical Data and Key Phylotypes of Caecal Microbiota

In the present study, we explored the interactive features between the calcium absorption and gut microbiota during the calcium deficiency-induced development. The correlation between the composition of gut microbiota and biochemical indicators induced by HCPPH-Ca was also assessed by Spearman's algorithm (Figure 8). The microbes, including *Lactobacillus*, *Rothia*, *Streptococcus* and *Turicibacter*, showed a positive correlation with abnormal parameters, such as serum Ca and body weight, while *Sutterella* was negatively correlated with the serum Ca and body weight. Interestingly, *D-75-a5*, *Akkeruansia*, *Rothia* and Streptococcus were positively correlated with serum P, serum Ca levels and body weight. These results indicated that these bacteria played an important role in the beneficial effects of HCPPH-Ca.

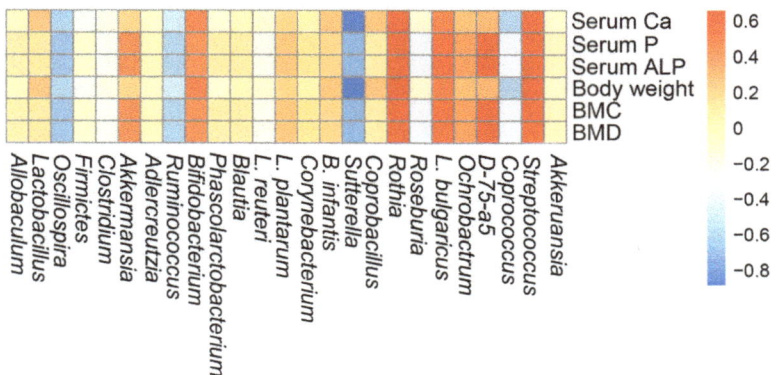

Figure 8. Heatmap of Spearman's correlation between caecal microbiota of significant differences and biochemical indexes. The depth of the color corresponds the extent of relevance between caecal microbiota and biochemical indexes. (FDR adjusted $p < 0.05$).

3. Discussion

To provide more information on the binding of metal ions with organic ligand groups of peptide, the FTIR spectra are shown (Figure S2).The specific FTIR absorption peak of amide-A stretching vibration had significant fluctuations at 3410 cm^{-1}, which might be attributed to the substitution of N-OH bonds (hydrogen bonds) with Ca-N bonds after calcium chelation [51,52]. The amide-I vibration and amide-II vibration were important vibrational modes of amides. The amide-I vibration is primarily caused by the stretching of C=O bonds and amide-II vibration is assigned to deformation of N-H bonds and stretching of C–N bonds [13,14]. The absorption band of FY at 1642 cm^{-1} for the amide I band shifted to a higher frequency (1650 cm^{-1}) when chelating with calcium, showing that the -COO- group participated in the covalent combining reaction with the metal cations [13]. After chelation, the spectrum shifted towards high-frequency wavenumbers (3500–2800 cm^{-1}), indicating that the dipole field effect or induced effect led to the electron cloud density and frequency increase. Strong absorption peaks at 1600 cm^{-1} and 1300 cm^{-1} for the amide I band showed that the -COO- group participated in the covalent combination reaction with the metal cations [53]. The maximum absorption peak of the CPPH was at around 230 nm, and the maximum absorption peak of the CPPH-Ca was transferred at around 223 nm. This showed that the chromophore groups (C=O, -COOH) and auxochrome groups (-OH, -NH$_2$) induced intensity changes and red shift in the ultraviolet spectrum when the CPPH was combined with calcium ions to form a chiral spatial structure [54]. Therefore, structural characterization of CPPH-Ca showed that CPPH and Ca^{2+} were combined to form a new substance.

Low-calcium diets may cause a significant reduction in body weight and changes in the serum parameters, gut microbiota disturbance and intestinal barrier dysfunction as well as osteoporosis, hypertension and rickets [55,56]. Therefore, various types of calcium-fortified medicines and foods have come onto the market. However, calcium deficiency is still widespread due to insufficient absorption of the intake calcium and low bioavailability [57–60]. Currently, organic calcium (especially the peptide-calcium complex) as a new type of calcium supplement has become a hot research topic, due to its good therapeutic effects in clinical practice [61,62]. In the present study, we investigated whether CPPH + CaCO$_3$ and CPPH-Ca promoted calcium absorption and how such an effect might impair kidney gene expression and gut microbiota. Rats fed with high doses of CPPH-Ca increased serum Ca and P concentration, and decreased serum ALP level. The results indicated that high doses of CPPH-Ca increased serum Ca and P concentrations, which rose to values comparable to those of the control group [4]; this was consistent with previously reported studies [63,64]. Meanwhile, CPPH-Ca may influence organism growth. These results of this observation could be the ability of a high dose of CPPH-Ca to increase the calcium retention and prevent mineral loss [4]. ALP play an important role in the process of bone calcification; it will increase when calcification is abnormal [64]. High serum ALP level may interfere with calcium absorption [65–68]. The results illustrated that the high dose of CPPH-Ca treatment could restore calcification to a normal level, and that calcium in HCPPH-Ca was more easily absorbed, calcified and its effect was better compared with inorganic calcium, even in the HGCa.

Femoral properties are the ideal monitoring indicators in the calcium supplementation experiment because they are sensitive to Ca assimilation and metabolism [63]. The consumption of low calcium (model) obviously decreased the dry weight (DW) index, length and diameter of femurs and tibias, indicating that calcium deficiency resulted in calcification of rat bone, which were consistent with a previous study [63]. In our study, the high dose of CPPH-Ca supplementation significantly alleviated the levels of femoral and tibial weight index, length and diameter in low-calcium diet-fed rats during eight-weeks, suggesting that HCPPH-Ca had positive effects on calcium absorption and bone calcification. Bone content (BMC) and bone mineral density (BMD) are used to assess the bone strength and quality of bone [62]. The loss of bone mass is accompanied by increased bone remodeling, evidenced by elevated serum ALP activity. Interestingly, our results illustrated that HCPPH-Ca treatment could effectively improve bone index parameters, and more effective absorption and utilization of calcium were found in rats fed HCPPH-Ca compared with inorganic calcium and even HGCa [67]. BMD and

BMC are the gold standards for the evaluation of low-calcium deficiency risk [66]. In addition, the BMD of femur and tibia were markedly reduced in the model and $HCaCO_3$ groups compared with the HCPs-Ca, HGCa and control groups. The 8-week treatment of HCPPH-Ca improved BMD and BMC and prevented the bone loss induced by calcium deficiency. As previously described, calcium deficiency is a metabolic bone disease characterized by reduced BMD and BMC. BMC and BMD in rats can be improved by supplementation of bovine and caprine cheese [68]. In addition, these changes of calcium deficiency phenotypes might be associated with femoral mineralization. In this study, low-calcium diets could cause morphological changes of trabecular bone and femoral mineralization of rats [68]. Histopathological analyses revealed visible differences of femur tissue structure in these ten groups. The histopathological femur was improved by HCPPH-Ca supplementation, for which the result was similar to previous research [66]. Meanwhile, the calcium bioavailability of a body is usually increased in cases of severe calcium deficiency. A previous study showed that effective calcium supplementation can improve the ACAR and CAR [57]. In our experiment, after 8 weeks, HCPPH-Ca treatment significantly elevated ACAR and CAR compared with the HCPPH + $HCaCO_3$ and $HCaCO_3$ groups ($p < 0.05$). With long-term low-calcium intake or bioavailability, the calcium level in the circulation decreases to below normal levels. Therefore, in order to maintain the blood calcium level, calcium is taken from the bone into the blood. These findings confirmed that HCPPH-Ca could be used as an effective calcium supplement in ameliorating the low-calcium diet-induced effects.

To further understand the molecular mechanism of HCPPH-Ca underlying the calcium re-absorption, we examined the expressions of the genes involved in kidney at the mRNA level, including CaBP-D9k [37], TRPV6 [36] and TRPV5 [35], as well as the expression of PMCA1b [69]. In the kidney, TRPV5, TRPV6, PMCA1 and CaBP-9k were principally expressed in the basolateral layer of the distal and proximal convoluted tubules. Several calcium transporters (CaBP-D9k, and PMCA1) have already been shown to express in the convoluted tubules [64], as has the function of calcium transporters transport active calcium in the kidney. When the body is deficient in calcium, calcium ions are removed from kidneys through calcium transport genes such as TRPV5, TRPV6, CaBP-D9k, and PMCA1 [70]. Calcium supplementation can help to prevent serious disorders such as hypercalcemia and hypocalcemia [64]. TRPV6 is an apical calcium entry channel in the kidney in general and particularly is to renal transcellular Ca^{2+} re-absorption, which regulates two separate active transcellular pathways for Ca^{2+} absorption [70] Importantly, co-localization of TRPV5 and TRPV6 in the kidney may have significant functional relevance, because it was recently shown that TRPV5 and TRPV6 can form heterotetrameric Ca^{2+} channels with distinct functionality [70]. The pathway regulated by TRPV6 is dependent on CaBP-D9k and PMCA1 for Ca^{2+} absorption [36]. In addition, TPPV6 is activated when the hyperpolarization of apical membrane occurs. Moreover, TPPV6 can be modulated by vitamin D3 along with CaBP-D9k and PMCA1b [47,48], indirectly indicating that HCPPH-Ca is the active ingredient responsible for calcium absorption. This process is possibly regulated by interacting with these calcium transporters and enzymes involved in intestinal calcium absorption and increasing parathyroid hormone [35–38].

The gut microbial community plays an important role in maintaining the normal physiological functions of the human body [71]. Therefore, we compared the caecal microbiota of rats in different groups to elucidate the precise underlying mechanism of improved calcium absorption by HCPPH-Ca. Our results showed that HCPPH-Ca treatment significantly changed the relative abundances of gut microbiota induced by low-calcium diets, including *L. reuteri*, *L. plantarum*, *Firmicutes*, *L. bulgaricus*, *Streptococcus thermophilus* and *Lactobacillus* ($p < 0.05$). *Bifidobacterium* and *L. reuteri* showed a positive correlation with the levels of serum Ca, ALP, BMC and BMD. Previous work has demonstrated that the beneficial effect of *L. reuteri* on bone health is dependent on immunomodulation of key pathways involved in osteoclastogenesis, estrogen signaling [71–73] and BMD [74–79]. Different strains of *Lactobacillus* and *Bifidobacterium* possess anti-inflammatory effects, which can improve vitamin D absorption and diminish osteoclast differentiation, thereby preventing the ovariectomy-induced bone loss in mice [80–82]. Treatment of either *Lactobacillus rhamnosus GG* (LGG) or the commercially available probiotic supplement reduces gut permeability in mice, inhibits the intestinal and bone marrow inflammation, and completely prevents bone loss after sex steroid deprivation, leading to both down-regulation of bone resorption markers and up-regulation of bone formation markers [83–85]. *Lactobacillus* salivarius significantly increases cellular calcium uptake [86,87]. Several studies have shown that administration of probiotics, such as *Lactobacillus (L) reuteri, L. plantarum, Bifidobacterium (B) longum*, or mixtures of several species, can exert a protective effect against bone loss in ovariectomized mice. Moreover, HCPPH-Ca reduced the abundance of *Firmicutes* and enhanced the abundance of Bacteroidetes in caecal contents. UTOHERE It is necessary to determine whether other gut microbiome play a causal role in bone calcium absorption in CPPH-Ca [88]. Taken together, we offered convincing evidence for the potential use of CPPH-Ca in calcium deficiency and showed that the gut microbiota played a potent regulatory role in attenuating metabolic abnormalities. Figure S3 illustrates the mechanism by which HCPPH-Ca promoted calcium absorption. HCPPH-Ca could promote calcium absorption partially through regulating specific gut microbiota and modulating the expressions of the calcium absorption-related genes in the kidney. Therefore, HCPPH-Ca could be beneficially used to promote the calcium absorption and reduce the risk of calcium deficiency.

4. Materials and Methods

4.1. Preparation of CPPH, CPPH-Ca and HPLC-MS/MS Analysis

Chlorella pyrenoidosa powder was purchased from King Dnarmsa *Spirulina* Co., Ltd. (Fuqing, China). In order to get the CPPH and CPPH-Ca, CPP was first prepared. Briefly, *Chlorella pyrenoidosa* powder was dissolved in 0.2 M NaOH solution at a concentration of 3.3%. CPP was extracted at 60 °C for 60 min. The extract was centrifuged at 4500 rpm for 10 min, and then the pH of supernatant was adjusted to 3.0 by 4 M HCl solution and allowed to stand for 30 min. The precipitate was collected by centrifugation at 5000 rpm for 10 min and freeze-dried for further enzymatic hydrolysis. The mixture of CPP powder and ultra-pure water (powder: water, 1:30; W/W) was hydrolyzed by neutral protease (3%, neutral protease: substrate, protein basis) at pH 7.5 for 6 h at 40 °C. and the hydrolyzed solution was incubated in boiling water for 10 min to inactivate the enzyme. The pH of the mixture was adjusted to neutral, followed by centrifugation at 5000 rpm for 10 min. The supernatant was freeze-dried, and CPPH was yielded. CPPH-Ca was obtained by mixing 4% CPP solution with $CaCl_2$ (4.5 g/100 g peptide) at pH 9, followed by incubation at 50 °C for 30 min. Thereafter, the free calcium was removed with a semi-permeable membrane with a cut-off of 100 Da (Thermo Fisher Scientific Inc., Waltham, UK). Subsequently, 95% ethanol was added, and the mixture was allowed to stand at 25 °C for 24 h, followed by centrifugation at 4500 rpm for 10 min. The supernatant was discarded, and the precipitate was collected and washed with 70% ethanol for three times to remove the superfluous Ca^{2+}. Finally, the precipitate was freeze-dried and labeled as CPPH-Ca. The obtained CPPH-Ca was stored in a desiccator for further analysis. Peptide contents of CPPH and CPPH-Ca were determined by Testing Center of Fuzhou University. The calcium concentration of CPPH-Ca was determined with an atomic absorption spectrophotometer (AA-6300C, Shimadzu, Kyoto, Japan). The components of CPPH were determined on an HPLC-MS/MS, and the analytical column was a Waters BEH C18 column (1.7 µm, 2.1 × 50 mm) (Macherey-Nagel, Düren, Germany) as previously described [89].

4.2. Structural Characterization of Peptide-Calcium Chelate by Ultraviolet Spectroscopy and FTIR Analysis

The ultraviolet spectra of CPPH and CPPH-Ca were monitored by an ultraviolet spectrophotometer (UV-2600, UNICO Instrument Co. Ltd., Shanghai, China) in the wavelength range of 190–400 nm. The mixture of lyophilized sample (1 mg) and dried KBr (100 mg) were loaded onto a Fourier transform infrared spectrometer. Infrared spectral scans of wavelengths from 4000 cm^{-1} to 400 cm^{-1} were recorded by FTIR spectroscopy infrared spectrophotometer (360 Intelligent, Thermo Nicolet Co., Madison, WI, USA).

4.3. Animals

Male SD rats (3 weeks old) were purchased from Wu's Experimental Animal Company (Fuzhou, China). The animals were bred in stainless steel wire-bottomed cages under hygienic standard environmental conditions (23 ± 1 °C; humidity of 60 ± 5%; 12 h dark/light cycle). The rats were given free access to commercial food, which was prepared according to the AIN-93 (normal diet: 5000 mg Ca/kg; low-calcium diet: 1000 mg Ca/kg), and tap water. The AIN-93 diet was provided by Trophic Animal Feed High-Tech Co., Ltd. (Nantong, China). All animal-related protocols were in accordance with laboratory animal welfare ethics and daily animal care guidelines, and approved by the Ethics Review Committee of the College of Food Science, Fujian Agriculture and Forestry University (No. FS-2018-008). After animals were acclimatized for 1 week, 100 rats were randomly and evenly divided into 10 groups (Table 2). The rats in the control group were fed with the normal diet. Remaining rats were fed with a low-Ca diet, which were randomly assigned into 9 groups of 10 rats each, 9 groups as follows: model group, HCaCO$_3$ group, LCPPH + LCaCO$_3$ group, MCPPH + MCaCO$_3$ group, HCPPH + HCaCO$_3$ group, or LCPPH-Ca group, MCPPH-Ca group and HCPPH-Ca group.

Table 2. Oral administration dosages of peptides and Ca for each group.

No.	Group	n	Given Dosage of N Content and Ca, mg/kg bw
1	Control	10	Deionized water
2	Model	10	Deionized water
3	HCaCO$_3$	10	Ca 119.97
4	HGCa	10	Ca 119.97
5	LCPPH + LCaCO$_3$	10	CPPH 465 + Ca 39.99
6	MCPPPH + MCaCO$_3$	10	CPPH 930 + Ca 79.98
7	HCPPH + HCaCO$_3$	10	CPPH1395 + Ca 119.97
8	LCPPH-Ca	10	Ca 39.99
9	MCPPH-Ca	10	Ca 79.98
10	HCPPH-Ca	10	Ca 119.97

Note: Control, normal group; model, low-calcium group; HCaCO$_3$, high dosage of CaCO$_3$ group; HGCa, high dosage of calcium gluconate group; LCPPH + LCaCO$_3$, low dosage of CPPH and low dosage of CaCO$_3$ group; MCPPH + MCaCO$_3$, middle dosage of CPPH and middle dosage of CaCO$_3$ group; HCPPH + HCaCO$_3$, high dosage of CPPH and high dosage of CaCO$_3$ group; LCPPH-Ca, low dosage of CPPH-Ca group; MCPPH-Ca, middle dosage of CPPH-Ca group; HCPPH-Ca, high dosage of CPPH-Ca group.

4.4. Sample Collection

During a 4-week experimental period, body weight, food intake, the amounts of feces and urine were recorded daily. After the 8-week experiment, all rats were starved for 12 h, anesthetized (1 mg kg^{-1} pentobarbital sodium) and dissected to obtain blood specimens. Blood was collected from the heart, centrifuged at 3000 rpm for 10 min at 4 °C and then stored at −80 °C until further analysis. Kidneys were weighed and cut into several sections. One part of kidney was stained by haematoxylin and eosin (H&E) for histopathological analysis. Another part of kidney was stored at −80 °C until further analysis of the mRNA expressions involved in calcium absorption metabolism. The samples of fresh caecal contents were also immediately collected before snap-freezing in liquid nitrogen and stored at −80 °C. Finally, the left and right femurs and tibias of each rat were dissected and cleaned of soft tissues. The left femur was stored in 4% paraformaldehyde for histopathological analysis.

4.5. Serum Calcium, Phosphorus Content and ALP Activity

Levels of serum calcium, phosphorus and ALP were determined using the corresponding assay kits (Nanjing Jiancheng Bioengineering Institute, Nanjing, China).

4.6. Bone Index Parameter and Histomorphometry Analysis

The left femurs of all rats were measured with a digital caliper (Exploit, Beijing, China). Then, femurs were dried in an oven at 105 °C overnight and weighed on an analytical balance (ML204, METTLER TOLEDO, Zurich, Switzerland). Dry weight index (DW index) was calculated according to the equation: DW index (10^{-3}) = Dry weight × 1000/Body weight. Bone mineral content (BMC) and bone mineral density (BMD) were assayed by the PIXImus dual energy X-ray absorptiometry method (LUNAR Corporation, Mississauga, ON, Canada) as described by Fonseca and Ward [90]. The femurs tissues were removed from each mice and samples were subsequently fixed in 4% 128 (v/v) paraformaldehyde/PBS then treated with ethanol solution. After that, all femur samples were decalcified in 10% EDTA (pH 7.4) for 3 weeks and were embedded in paraffin, the slices of distal femur were sectioned at 5 mm then were stained with H&E to observe the morphological changes under the high magnification of an optical microscope with high magnification (Nikon Eclipse TE2000-U, Nikon, Japan) [91].

4.7. Calcium Balance Study

Food consumption was recorded, and the urine and feces were measured and collected daily. The calcium balance experiment was conducted. After sample collection, the urine was immediately centrifuged at 3000× g for 10 min, and the supernatant was obtained. Fresh fecal samples were collected immediately after defecation and freeze-dried. The calcium contents of urine and feces were determined by a flame atomic absorption spectrometer (AA-6300C, Shimadzu). The ACAR and CAR were calculated as follows:

$$ACAR\ (\%) = (Ca\ intake - feces\ Ca) \times 100/Ca\ intake \tag{1}$$

$$CAR\ (\%) = (Ca\ intake - feces\ Ca - urine\ Ca) \times 100/Ca\ intake \tag{2}$$

4.8. RT-qPCR Analysis

Total RNA was extracted from the frozen kidney tissues by using TRIzol reagent (Invitrogen, Carlsbad, CA, USA). Purified RNA was reversely transcribed into cDNA using PrimeScript™ RT reagent Kit with gDNA Eraser (Takara, Kusatsu, Japan). The expressions of TRPV6, TRPV5 and CaBP-D9K were assessed by RT-qPCR using the SYBR® Premix Ex Taq™ II (Takara, Kusatsu, Japan) on an AB7300 Real-Time PCR system (Applied Biosystems, Foster City, CA, USA). GAPDH was selected as the housekeeping gene. The primer sequences were as follows: TRPV6, F: 5′-GCACCTTCGAGCTGTTCC-3′, R: 5′-CAGTGAGTGTCGCCCATC-3′; TRPV5, F: 5′-CGAGGATTCCAGATGC-3′, R: 5′-GACCATAGCCATTAGCC-3′; PMCA1b, F: 5′-TTCAGGTACTCATGTGATGGAAGG-3′, R: 5′-CAGCCCCAAGCAAGGTAAA-3′; CaBP-D9K, F: 5′-GACCTCACCTGTTCCTGTCTG-3′, R: 5′- GCTCCTTCTTCTGGCTTCATT-3′; GAPDH, F: 5′-TGACTTCAACAGCGACACCCA -3′, R: 5′-CACCCTGTTGCTGTAGCCAAA-3′. Briefly, after an initial denaturation step at 95 °C for 30 s, the amplifications were carried out with 40 cycles at a melting temperature of 95 °C for 5 s, an annealing temperature of 60 °C for 30 s, and an extension temperature of 72 °C for 30 s. The data were analyzed using Rotor-gene Q software ver. 1.7 (Qiagen). Relative gene expressions were calculated by the comparative $2^{-\Delta\Delta Ct}$ method.

4.9. Extraction of Caecal Genomic DNA for High Throughput Sequencing

Gut microbiota analysis was performed on ten samples per group. Metagenomic DNA was extracted from the caecal contents of the rats using a PowerSoil DNA Isolation Kit (MO BIO Laboratory Inc., Carlsbad, CA) according to the manufacturer's instructions. The 16S rRNA gene (V3-V4 hypervariable regions) from the caecal microbiota was amplified using specific primers (forward primer 5′-CCTACGGRRBGCASCAGKVRVGAAT-3′ and reverse primer 5′-GGACTACNVGGGTWTCTAATCC-3′) [92]. Sequencing was performed using a 2 × 300 paired-end

(PE) configuration, and the amplification bias caused by a non-official barcode was avoided. Finally, the image analysis and base calling were conducted on the MiSeq reagent kit v2 (300 cycles) by the MiSeq platform (Illumina, Inc., San Diego, CA, USA). The initial taxonomy analysis was performed on Illumina's BaseSpace cloud computing platform.

4.10. Bioinformatics Analysis

High-quality sequences were assigned to samples according to barcodes. The valid sequences were denoised in order to assess the species diversity. Results were generated using Usearch (Version 7.1, http://drive5.com/uparse/) with a disagreement of 3% [93].

4.11. Statistical Analysis

Data for each group were expressed as mean ± SD (*n* = 10). Statistical significance was measured using one-way analysis of variance (ANOVA) with Tukey's test. Statistical significance was expressed by a p-value of less than 0.05. Spearman's rank correlation coefficient was used to assess the correlation between gut microbiota and lipid metabolic parameters.

5. Conclusions

Collectively, the structural characterization of CPPH-Ca showed that CPPH and Ca^{2+} were combined to form a new substance. This study indicated that the HCPPH-Ca exerted its promotive effects on calcium absorption in the kidney by influencing relational gene expressions, enhancing bone tissues in rapidly growing rats, improving calcium absorption utilization and regulating gut microbiota. Additionally, HCPPH-Ca could improve femoral morphological abnormalities. Moreover, HCPPH-Ca treatment exerted promotive effects on calcium absorption by up-regulating TRPV6, TRPV5, CaBP-D9K and CMBP1b signaling pathways in kidney and affecting the composition of gut microbiome induced by low-calcium diets. Meanwhile, HCPPH-Ca also had beneficial effects on bone tissues in rats compared with the inorganic calcium. Taken together, our study, for the first time, clarified the new potential therapeutic role of HCPPH-Ca. However, in the study, bacterial 16S rRNA gene sequencing could not be fully characterized to assign accurate classification information beyond the genus level due to the limited read length of the Illumina MiSeq platform. Therefore, future studies should further explore changes in gut flora at the species level.

Supplementary Materials: The following are available online at http://www.mdpi.com/1660-3397/17/6/348/s1, Figure S1: UV spectra of CPPH and CPPH-Ca over the wavelength range from 190 to 400 nm, Figure S2: Fourier transform infrared (FTIR) spectra of CPPH and CPPH-Ca chelate in the regions from 4000 to 400 cm^{-1}, Figure S3: summary of the mechanism underlying the preventive effects of CPPH-Ca on calcium absorption, Table S1: peptide profile of CPPH identified by HPLC-MS/MS.

Author Contributions: P.H. and Z.Y. had performed the research work, Y.X. interpreted the results, P.H. critically analyzed the important data and drafted the paper; B.L. contributed to design the research protocol, L.Z. reviewed the manuscript, B.L. and L.Z. provided useful suggestion to improve the manuscript.

Funding: This research was funded by the Fujian Science and Technology Plan project (No. 2017N5003), the Science Foundations of Fujian Agriculture and Forestry University (XJQ201608), the National Natural Science Foundation of China (31501432), the National Science Foundation for Post-doctoral Scientists of China (2017M612117), Fujian Agriculture and Forestry University International Cooperation Project (No. KXG15001A), the 13th Five-year Plan on Fuzhou Marine Economic Innovation and Development Demonstration Project.

Conflicts of Interest: The authors declare no conflict of interest.

References

1.   Nicklas, T.A. Calcium intake trends and health consequences from childhood through adulthood. *J. Am. Coll. Nutr.* **2003**, *22*, 340–356. [CrossRef] [PubMed]

2.   Zemel, M.B.; Miller, S.L. Dietary calcium and dairy modulation of adiposity and obesity risk. *Nutr. Rev.* **2004**, *62*, 125–131. [CrossRef] [PubMed]

3. Cashman, K.D. Calcium intake, calcium bioavailability and bone health. *Br. J. Nutr.* **2002**, *87*, 169–177. [CrossRef]
4. Chen, D.; Mu, X.M.; Huang, H.; Nie, R.Y.; Liu, Z.Y.; Zeng, M.Y. Isolation of a calcium-binding peptide from tilapia scale protein hydrolysate and its calcium bioavailability in rats. *J. Func. Foods* **2014**, *6*, 575–584. [CrossRef]
5. Benzvi, L.; Gershon, A.; Lavi, I.; Wollstein, R. Secondary prevention of osteoporosis following fragility fractures of the distal radius in a large health maintenance organization. *Arch. Osteoporos.* **2016**, *11*, 20–25. [CrossRef] [PubMed]
6. Harvey, N.C.; Curtis, E.M.; Velde, R. On epidemiology of fractures and variation with age and ethnicity. *Bone* **2016**, *93*, 230–231. [CrossRef] [PubMed]
7. Aeberli, D.; Eser, P.; Bonel, H.; Widmer, J.; Caliezi, G.; Varisco, P.A.; Möller, B.; Villiger, P.M. Reduced trabecular bone mineral density and cortical thickness accompanied by increased outer bone circumference in metacarpal bone of rheumatoid arthritis patients: A cross-sectional study. *Arthritis Res. Ther.* **2010**, *12*, 45–57. [CrossRef] [PubMed]
8. Zhou, J.; Wang, X.; Ai, T.; Cheng, R.X.; Guo, H.Y.; Teng, G.X.; Mao, X.Y. Preparation and characterization of b-lactoglobulin hydrolysate-iron complexes. *J. Dairy Sci.* **2012**, *95*, 4230–4236. [CrossRef] [PubMed]
9. Harvey, J.A.; Kenny, P.; Poindexter, J.; Pak, C.Y. Superior calcium absorption from calcium citrate than calcium carbonate using external forearm counting. *J. Am. Coll. Nutr.* **1990**, *9*, 583–587. [CrossRef]
10. Cosentino, S.; Donida, B.M.; Marasco, E.; Favero, E.D.; Cantu, L.; Lombardi, G.; Colmbini, A.; Lametti, S.; Valaperta, S.; Fiorilli, A.; et al. Calcium ions enclosed in casein phosphopeptide aggregates are directly involved in the mineral uptake by differentiated HT-29 cells. *Int. Dairy J.* **2010**, *20*, 770–776. [CrossRef]
11. Holt, C.; Timmins, P.A.; Errington, N.; Leaver, J. A core-shell model of calcium phosphate nanoclusters stabilized by β-casein phosphopeptides, derived from sedimentation equilibrium and small-angle X-ray and neutron-scattering measurements. *Eur. J. Biochem.* **1998**, *252*, 73–78. [CrossRef] [PubMed]
12. Lee, Y.S.; Noguchi, T.; Naito, H. An enhanced intestinal absorption of calcium in the rat directly attributed to dietary casein. *Agric. Biol. Chem.* **1979**, *43*, 2009–2011.
13. Zhao, L.N.; Cai, X.X.; Huang, S.L.; Wang, S.Y.; Huang, Y.F.; Hong, J.; Rao, P.F. Isolation and identification of a whey protein-sourced calcium-binding tripeptide Tyr-Asp-Thr. *Inter. Dairy J.* **2015**, *40*, 16–23. [CrossRef]
14. Bao, X.L.; Lv, Y.; Yang, B.C.; Ren, C.G.; Guo, S.T. A study of the soluble complexes formed during calcium binding bysoybean protein hydrolysates. *J. Food Sci.* **2008**, *73*, 117–121. [CrossRef] [PubMed]
15. Jung, W.K.; Kim, S.K. Calcium-binding peptide derived from pepsinolytic hydrolysates of hoki (*Johnius belengerii*) frame. *Eur. Food Res. Technol.* **2007**, *224*, 763–767. [CrossRef]
16. Huang, G.G.; Ren, L.; Jiang, J.X. Purification of a histidine-containing peptide with calcium binding activity from shrimp processing byproducts hydrolysate. *Eur. Food Res. Technol.* **2011**, *232*, 281–287. [CrossRef]
17. Pan, D.D.; Lu, H.Q.; Zeng, X.Q. A newly isolated Ca binding peptide from whey protein. *Int. J. Food Prop.* **2013**, *16*, 1127–1134. [CrossRef]
18. Han, Y.; He, H.; Zhao, N.N.; Li, J.T.; Wang, Z.Z.; Nie, Z.K. Effect of egg white peptide binding with calcium on promotion of calcium absorption in vivo. *Food Sci.* **2012**, *33*, 262–265.
19. Ferraretto, A.; Signorile, A.; Gravaghi, C.; Tettamanti, G. Casein phosphopeptides influence calcium uptake by cultured human intestinal HT-29 tumor cells. *J. Nutr.* **2001**, *131*, 1655–1661. [CrossRef]
20. Zhen, D.; Liu, L.; Guan, C.; Zhao, N.; Tang, X. High prevalence of vitamin D defciency among middle-aged and elderly individuals in northwestern China: Its relationship to osteoporosis and lifestyle factors. *Bone* **2015**, *71*, 1–6. [CrossRef]
21. Guzman, S.; Gato, A.; Calleja, J.M. Antiinflammatory, analgesic and free radical scavenging activities of the marine microalgae *Chlorella stigmatophora* and *Phaeodactylum tricornutum*. *Phytother. Res.* **2001**, *15*, 224–230. [CrossRef] [PubMed]
22. Yamagishi, S.; Nakamura, K.; Inoue, H. Therapeutic potentials of unicellular green alga *Chlorella* in advanced glycation end product (AGE)-related disorders. *Med. Hypotheses* **2005**, *65*, 953–955. [CrossRef] [PubMed]
23. Jeong, H.; Kwon, H.J.; Kim, M.K. Hypoglycemic effect of *Chlorella vulgaris* intake in type 2 diabetic Goto-Kakizaki and normal Wistar rats. *Nutr. Res. Pract.* **2009**, *3*, 23–30. [CrossRef] [PubMed]
24. Gouveia, L.; Batista, A.P.; Sousa, I.; Raymundo, A.; Bandarra, N.M. Microalgae in novel food products. *Food Chem. Res. Dev.* **2008**, *3*, 1–37.

25. Queiroz, M.L.; Da Rocha, M.C.; Torello, C.; Souza Queiroz, J.; Bincoletto, C.; Morgano, M.A. *Chlorella Vulgaris* restores bone marrow cellularity and cytokine production in lead-exposed mice. *Food. Chem. Toxicol.* **2011**, *49*, 2934–2941. [CrossRef] [PubMed]

26. Yun, H.; Kim, I.; Kwon, S.H.; Kang, J.S.; Om, A.S. Protective effect of *Chlorella Vulgaris* against lead-induced oxidative stress in rat brains. *J. Health. Sci.* **2011**, *57*, 245–454. [CrossRef]

27. Aizzat, O.; Yap, S.W.; Sopiah, H.; Madiha, M.M.; Hazreen, M.; Shailah, A.; Wan, J.W.; Nur, S.A.; Srijit, D.; Musalmah, M.; et al. Modulation of oxidative stress by *Chlorella vulgaris* in streptozotocin (STZ) induced diabetic Sprague-Dawley rats. *Adv. Med. Sci.* **2010**, *55*, 281–288. [CrossRef]

28. Shibata, S.; Hayakawa, K.; Egashira, Y.; Sanada, H. Hypocholesterolemic mechanism of *Chlorella*: *Chlorella* and its indigestible fraction enhance hepatic cholesterol catabolism through up-regulation of cholesterol 7alpha-hydroxylase in rats. *Biosci. Biotechnol. Biochem.* **2007**, *71*, 916–925. [CrossRef]

29. Vijayavel, K.; Anbuselvam, C.; Balasubramanian, M.P. Antioxidant effect of the marine algae *Chlorella vulgaris* against naphthalene-induced oxidative stress in the albino rats. *Mol. Cell. Biochem.* **2007**, *303*, 39–44. [CrossRef]

30. Sibi, G.; Rabina, S. Inhibition of Pro-inflammatory mediators and cytokines by *Chlorella Vulgaris* extracts. *Pharmacognosy Res.* **2016**, *8*, 118–122. [CrossRef]

31. Shih, M.F.; Chen, L.C.; Cherng, J.Y. *Chlorella* 11-peptide inhibits the production of macrophage-induced adhesion molecules and reduces endothelin-1 expression and endothelial permeability. *Mar. Drugs* **2013**, *11*, 3861–3877. [CrossRef] [PubMed]

32. Renju, G.L.; Muraleedhara Kurup, G.; Saritha Kumari, C.H. Effect of lycopene from *Chlorella marina* on high cholesterol induced oxidative damage and inflammation in rats. *Inflammopharmacology* **2014**, *22*, 45–54. [CrossRef] [PubMed]

33. Shrafi, A.; Ebrahimi Mamaghani, S.; Kakaei, F.; Javadzadeh, Y.; Asghari Jafarabadi, M. The Effect of complex *Chlorella Vulgaris* microlevel on inflammatory factors in patients with non-alcoholic fatty liver: A double-sided clinical trial. *J. Mazandaran Univ. Med. Sci.* **2014**, *24*, 113–121.

34. Suzuki, Y.; Kovacs, C.S.; Takanaga, H.; Peng, J.B.; Landowski, C.P.; Hediger, M.A. Calcium channel TRPV6 is involved in murine maternal-fetal calcium transport. *J. Bone Miner. Res.* **2008**, *23*, 1249–1256. [CrossRef] [PubMed]

35. Yang, H.; Lee, G.S.; Yoo, Y.M.; Choi, K.C.; Jeung, E.B. Sodium/potassium/calcium exchanger 3 is regulated by the steroid hormones estrogen and progesterone in the uterus of mice during the estrous cycle. *Biochem. Biophys. Res. Commun.* **2009**, *385*, 279–283. [CrossRef] [PubMed]

36. Nijenhuis, T.; Hoenderop, J.G.; van der Kemp, A.W.; Bindels, R.J. Localization and regulation of the epithelial Ca^{2+} channel TRPV6 in the kidney. *J. Am. Soc. Nephrol.* **2003**, *14*, 2731–2740. [CrossRef] [PubMed]

37. Zhang, Y.; Dong, X.L.; Leung, P.C.; Che, C.T.; Wong, M.S. Fructus ligustri lucidi extract improves calcium balance and modulates the calciotropic hormone level and vitamin D-dependent gene expression in aged ovariectomized rats. *Menopause* **2008**, *15*, 558–565. [CrossRef] [PubMed]

38. Shin, N.R.; Whon, T.W.; Bae, J.W. Proteobacteria: Microbial signature of dysbiosis in gut microbiota. *Trends Biotechnol. Sep.* **2015**, *33*, 496–503. [CrossRef]

39. Busse, B.; Djonic, D.; Milovanovic, P.; Hahn, M.; Püschel, K.; Ritchie, R.O.; Djuric, M.; Amling, M. Decrease in the osteocyte lacunar density accompanied by hypermineralized lacunar occlusion reveals failure and delay of remodeling in aged human bone. *Aging Cell* **2010**, *9*, 1065–1075. [CrossRef]

40. Currey, J.D.; Shahar, R. Cavities in the compact bone in tetrapods and fish and their effect on mechanical properties. *J. Struct. Biol.* **2013**, *183*, 107–122. [CrossRef]

41. Gourion-Arsiquaud, S.; Burket, J.C.; Havill, L.M.; DiCarlo, E.; Doty, S.B.; Mendelsohn, R.; Van Der Meulen, M.C.H.; Boskey, A.L. Spatial variation in osteonal bone properties relative to tissue and animal age. *J. Bone Miner. Res.* **2009**, *24*, 1271–1281. [CrossRef] [PubMed]

42. Hannah, K.M.; Thomas, C.D.L.; Clement, J.G.; De Carlo, F.; Peele, A.G. Bimodal distribution of osteocyte lacunar size in the human femoral cortex as revealed by micro-CT. *Bone* **2010**, *47*, 866–871. [CrossRef] [PubMed]

43. Nalla, R.K.; Kruzic, J.J.; Kinney, J.H.; Balooch, M.; Ager, J.W.; Ritchie, R.O. Role of microstructure in the aging-related deterioration of the toughness of human cortical bone. *Mater. Sci. Eng.* **2006**, *C 26*, 1251–1260. [CrossRef]

44. Pfeiffer, S.; Crowder, C.; Harrington, L.; Brown, M. Secondary osteon and Haversian canal dimensions as behavioral indicators. *Am. J. Phys. Anthropol.* **2006**, *131*, 460–468. [CrossRef] [PubMed]
45. Seeman, E.; Delmas, P.D. Bone quality—The material and structural basis of bone strength and fragility. *N. Engl. J. Med.* **2006**, *354*, 2250–2261. [CrossRef] [PubMed]
46. Van Oers, R.F.M.; Ruimerman, R.; Tanck, E.; Hilbers, P.A.J.; Huiskes, R. A unified theory for osteonal and hemi-osteonal remodeling. *Bone* **2008**, *42*, 250–259. [CrossRef] [PubMed]
47. Bronner, F. Mechanisms and functional aspects of intestional calcium absorption. *J. Exp. Zool. A Comp. Exp. Biol.* **2003**, *300A*, 47–52. [CrossRef] [PubMed]
48. Asagiri, M.; Takayanagi, H. The molecular understanding of osteoclast differentiation. *Bone* **2007**, *40*, 251–264. [CrossRef]
49. Whisner, C.M.; Martin, B.R.; Nakatsu, C.H.; McCabe, G.P.; McCabe, L.D.; Peacock, M.; Weaver, C.M. Soluble maize fibre affects short-term calcium absorption in adolescent boys and girls: A randomised controlled trial using dual stable isotopic tracers. *Br. J. Nutr.* **2014**, *112*, 446–456. [CrossRef]
50. Zhao, C.; Yang, C.F.; Chen, M.J.; Lv, X.C.; Liu, B.; Yi, L.Z.; Cornara, L.; Wei, M.C.; Yang, Y.C.; Tundis, R.; et al. Regulatory efficacy of brown seaweed lessonia nigrescens extract on the gene expression profile and intestinal microflora in type 2 diabetic mice. *Mol. Nutr. Food Res.* **2018**, *62*, 1700730. [CrossRef]
51. Cai, X.X.; Lin, J.P.; Wang, S.Y. Novel peptide with specific calcium-binding capacity from *Schizochytrium* sp. protein hydrolysates and calcium bioavailability in Caco-2 Cells. *Mar. Drugs* **2017**, *15*, 3. [CrossRef] [PubMed]
52. Hua, P.P.; Yu, Z.Y.; Xiong, Y.; Liu, B.; Zhao, L.N. Regulatory efficacy of *Spirulina platensis* protease hydrolyzate on lipid metabolism and gut microbiota in high-fat diet-fed rats. *J. Mol. Sci.* **2018**, *19*, 4023. [CrossRef] [PubMed]
53. Siping, X.; Xiao, Y.; Xiaofei, Y. Immunization with Na+/K+ ATPase DR peptide prevents bone loss in an ovariectomized rat osteoporosis mode. *Biochem. Pharmacol.* **2018**, *23*, 223–225.
54. Lozupone, C.A.; Hamady, M.; Kelley, S.T.; Knight, R. Quantitative and qualitative beta diversity measures lead to different insights into factors that structure microbial communities. *Appl. Environ. Microbiol.* **2007**, *73*, 1576–1585. [CrossRef] [PubMed]
55. Wan, X.Z.; Li, T.T.; Liu, D.; Chen, Y.H.; Liu, Y.Y.; Liu, B.; Zhang, H.Y.; Zhao, C. Effect of marine microalga *Chlorella pyrenoidosa* ethanol extract on lipid metabolism and gut microbiota composition in high-fat diet-fed rats. *Mar. Drugs* **2018**, *16*, 498. [CrossRef] [PubMed]
56. Huang, S.L.; Zhao, L.N.; Cai, X.X.; Wang, S.Y.; Huang, Y.F.; Hong, J.; Rao, P.F. Purification and characterisation of a glutamic acid-containing peptide with calcium-binding capacity from whey protein hydrolysate. *J. Dairy Res.* **2015**, *82*, 29–35. [CrossRef]
57. Liu, F.R.; Wang, L.; Wang, R.; Chen, Z.X. Calcium-binding capacity of wheat germ protein hydrolysate and characterization of peptide-calcium complex. *J. Agric. Food Chem.* **2013**, *61*, 7537–7544. [CrossRef]
58. Wang, X.L.; Li, K.; Yang, X.D.; Wang, L.L.; Shen, R.F. Complexation of Al(III) with reduced glutathione in acidic aqueous solutions. *J. Inorg. Biochem.* **2009**, *103*, 657–665. [CrossRef]
59. Centeno, V.; Diaz de Barboza, G.; Marchionatti, A.; Rodriguez, V.; Tolosa de Talamoni, N. Molecular mechanisms triggered by low-calcium diets. *Nutr. Res. Rev.* **2009**, *22*, 163–174. [CrossRef]
60. Lv, Y.; Yang, B.C.; Guo, S.T. Aggregation of hydrophobic soybean protein hydrolysates: Changes in molecular weight distribution during storage. *LWT Food Sci. Techonol.* **2009**, *42*, 914–917. [CrossRef]
61. Liu, H.; Xu, J.; Guo, S.T. Soybean peptide aggregates improved calcium binding capacity. *LWT Food Sci. Techonol.* **2016**, *3*, 174–180. [CrossRef]
62. Yang, H.; Ahn, C.; Jeung, E.B. Differential expression of calcium transport genes caused by COMT inhibition in the duodenum, kidney and placenta of pregnant mice. *Mol. Cell. Endocrinol.* **2015**, *401*, 45–55. [CrossRef] [PubMed]
63. Shapiro, R.; Heaney, R.P. Co-dependence of calcium and phosphorus for growth and bone development under conditions of varying deficiency. *Bone* **2003**, *32*, 532–540. [CrossRef]
64. Robison, R.; Macleod, M.; Rosenheim, A.H. The possible significance of hexosephosphoric esters in ossification. *Biochem. J.* **1923**, *17*, 286–293. [CrossRef] [PubMed]
65. Wang, L.C.; Chen, S.Y.; Liu, R.; Wu, H. A novel hydrolytic product from flesh of mactra veneriformis and its bioactivities in calcium supplement. *J. Ocean Uni. China* **2012**, *11*, 389–396. [CrossRef]

66. Zhang, Y.; Wang, Z.Y.; Ding, L.; Damaolar, A.; Li, Z.Q.; Qiu, Y.S.; Yin, Z.H. Lentivirus-TAZ administration alleviates osteoporotic phenotypes in the femoral neck of ovariectomized rats. *Cell. Physiol. Biochem.* **2016**, *38*, 283–294.

67. Applegate, T.J.; Lilburn, M.S. Growth of the femur and tibia of a commercial broiler line. *Poul. Sci.* **2002**, *81*, 1289–1294. [CrossRef]

68. Mora-Gutierrez, A.; Farrell, H.M.J.; Attaie, R. Effects of bovine and caprine Monterey Jack cheeses fortified with milk calcium on bone mineralization in rats. *Int. Dairy J.* **2007**, *17*, 255–267. [CrossRef]

69. Stewart, A.F.; Cain, R.L.; Burr, D.B.; Jacob, D.; Turner, C.H.; Hock, J.M. Six-month daily administration of parathyroid hormone and parathyroid hormone-related protein peptides to adult ovariectomized rats markedly enhances bone mass and biomechanical properties: A comparison of human parathyroid hormon 1-34, parathyroid hormone-related protein 1-36, and SDZ-parathyroid hormone 893. *J. Bone Miner Res.* **2000**, *15*, 1517–1525.

70. Lieben, L.; Benn, B.S.; Ajibade, D.; Stockmans, I.; Moermans, K.; Hediger, M.A. Trpv6 mediates intestinal calcium absorption during calcium restrictionn and contributes to bone homeostasis. *Bone* **2010**, *47*, 301–308. [CrossRef]

71. Hanzlik, R.P.; Fowler, S.C.; Fisher, D.H. Relative bioavailability of calcium from calcium formate, calcium citrate, and calcium carbonate. *J. Pharmacol. Exp. Ther.* **2005**, *313*, 1217–1222. [CrossRef] [PubMed]

72. Titi, L.; Zemin, X.; Fei, C. Theabrownin suppresses, in vitro, osteoclastogenesis and prevents bone loss in ovariectomized rats. *Biomed. Pharmacother.* **2018**, *106*, 1339–1347.

73. Mentaverri, R.; Yano, S.; Chattopadhyay, N.; Petit, L.; Kifor, O.; Kamel, S.; Terwilliger, E.F.; Brazier, M.; Brown, E.M. The calcium sensing receptor is directly involved in both osteoclast differentiation and apoptosis. *Faseb J.* **2006**, *20*, 2562–2564. [CrossRef] [PubMed]

74. Kellett, G.L. Alternative perspective on intestinal calcium absorption: Proposed complementary actions of Ca(v)1.3 and TRPV6. *Nutr. Rev.* **2011**, *69*, 347–370. [CrossRef] [PubMed]

75. Lee, S.J.; Kim, Y.S.; Hwang, J.W.; Kim, E.K.; Moon, S.H.; Jeon, B.T.; Jeon, Y.J.; Kim, J.M.; Park, P.J. Purification and characterization of a novel antioxidative peptide from duck skin byproducts that protects liver against oxidative damage. *Food Res. Int.* **2012**, *49*, 285–295. [CrossRef]

76. Wang, G.; Wang, J.; Sun, D. Short-term hypoxia accelerates bone loss in ovariectomized rats by suppressing osteoblastogenesis but enhancing osteoclastogenesis. *Med. Sci. Monit.* **2016**, *22*, 2962–2971. [CrossRef] [PubMed]

77. Zhang, J.; Lazarenko, O.P.; Kang, J. Feeding blueberry diets to young rats dose-dependently inhibits bone resorption through suppression of RANKL in stromal cells. *PLoS ONE* **2013**, *8*, 78–89. [CrossRef]

78. Nilsson, A.G.; Sundh, D.; Bäckhed, F.; Lorentzon, M. *Lactobacillus reuteri* reduces bone loss in older women with low bone mineral density: A randomized, placebo-controlled, double-blind, clinical trial. *J. Intern. Med.* **2018**, *284*, 307–317. [CrossRef]

79. Parvaneh, K.; Ebrahimi, M.; Sabran, M.R. Probiotics (*Bifidobacterium longum*) increase bone mass density and upregulate Sparc and Bmp-2 genes in rats with bone loss resulting from ovariectomy. *Bio. Med. Res. Int.* **2015**, *2015*, 1–10.

80. Britton, R.A.; Irwin, R.; Quach, D. Probiotic *L. reuteri* treatment prevents bone loss in a menopausal ovariectomized mouse model. *J. Cell. Physiol.* **2014**, *229*, 1822–1830. [CrossRef]

81. Ohlsson, C.; Engdahl, C.; Fåk, F. Probiotics protect mice from ovariectomyinduced cortical bone loss. *PLoS ONE* **2014**, *9*, 21–24. [CrossRef] [PubMed]

82. Amdekar, S.; Singh, V.; Singh, R. *Lactobacillus casei* reduces the inflammatory joint damage associated with collagen-induced arthritis (CIA) by reducing the pro-inflammatory cytokines: *Lactobacillus casei*: COX-2 inhibitor. *J. Clin. Immunol.* **2011**, *31*, 147–156. [CrossRef] [PubMed]

83. Zhou, X.; Wu, L.F.; Wang, W.Y.; Lu, X.; Jiang, Z.H.; Zhang, Y.H.; Jiang, D.H.; Jiang, J.N.; Gao, H.Q.; Lei, S.F.; et al. Anxa2 attenuates osteoblast growth and is associated with hip BMD and osteoporotic fracture in Chinese elderly. *PLoS ONE* **2018**, *13*, e0194781. [CrossRef] [PubMed]

84. Nishide, Y.; Tadaishi, M.; Kobori, M. Possible role of S-equol on bone loss via amelioration of inflammatory indices in ovariectomized mice. *J. Clin. Biochem. Nutr.* **2013**, *53*, 41–48. [CrossRef] [PubMed]

85. Nima, M.N.; Younes, G.; Hossein, D.M. Supportive role of probiotic strains in protecting rats from ovariectomy-induced cortical bone loss. *Probiotics Antimicrob. Proteins* **2018**, *65*, 34–38.

86. Saltzman, J.R.; Russell, R.M. The aging gut. Nutritional issues. *Gastroenterol Clin. North Am.* **1998**, *27*, 309–324. [CrossRef]

87. Schwarzer, M.; Makki, K.; Storelli, G.; Machuca-Gayet, I.; Srutkova, D.; Hermanova, P.; Martino, M.E.; Balmand, S.; Hudcovic, T.; Heddi, A.; et al. Lactobacillus plantarum strain maintains growth of infant mice during chronic undernutrition. *Science* **2016**, *351*, 854–857. [CrossRef]

88. Yan, J.; Herzog, J.W.; Tsang, K.; Brennan, C.A.; Bower, M.A.; Garrett, W.S.; Sartor, B.R.; Aliprantis, A.O.; Charles, J.F. Gut microbiota induce IGF-1 and promote bone formation and growth. *Proc. Natl. Acad. Sci. USA* **2016**, *113*, E7554–E7563. [CrossRef]

89. Bryk, G.; Coronel, M.Z.; Pellegrini, G. Effect of a combination GOS/FOS prebiotic mixture and interaction with calcium intake on mineral absorption and bone parameters in growing rats. *Eur. J. Nutr.* **2015**, *54*, 913–923. [CrossRef]

90. Fonseca, D.; Ward, W.E. Daidzein together with high calcium preserve bone mass and biomechanical strength at multiple sites in ovariectomized mice. *Bone* **2004**, *35*, 489–497. [CrossRef]

91. Rodrigues, F.C.; Castro, A.S.B.; Rodrigues, V.C. Yacon flour and *Bifidobacterium longum* modulate bone health in rats. *J. Med. Food.* **2012**, *15*, 664–670. [CrossRef] [PubMed]

92. Pérez-Conesa, D.; López, G.; Abellán, P.; Ros, G. Bioavailability of calcium, magnesium and phosphorus in rats fed probiotic, prebiotic and synbiotic powder follow-up infant formulas and their effect on physiological and nutritional parameters. *J. Sci. Food Agric.* **2006**, *86*, 2327–2336. [CrossRef]

93. Gilman, J.; Cashman, K.D. The effect of probiotic bacteria on transepithelial calcium transport and calcium uptake in human intestinal-like Caco-2 cells. *Curr. Issues Intest. Microbiol.* **2006**, *7*, 1–5. [PubMed]

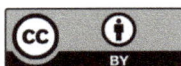

marine drugs

MDPI

Article

Antihypertensive Effects of Two Novel Angiotensin I-Converting Enzyme (ACE) Inhibitory Peptides from *Gracilariopsis lemaneiformis* (Rhodophyta) in Spontaneously Hypertensive Rats (SHRs)

Zhenzhen Deng [1,2,3,4,†], **Yingjuan Liu** [1,2,3,4,†], **Jing Wang** [1,2,3,4], **Suhuang Wu** [1,2,3,4], **Lihua Geng** [1,2,3,4], **Zhenghong Sui** [5,*] **and Quanbin Zhang** [1,2,3,4,*]

[1] CAS Key Laboratory of Experimental Marine Biology, Institute of Oceanology, Chinese Academy of Sciences, Qingdao 266071, China; dengzhenzhen16@mails.ucas.ac.cn (Z.D.); liuyingjuan829@163.com (Y.L.); jingwang@qdio.ac.cn (J.W.); wusuhuang16@mails.ucas.ac.cn (S.W.); genglihua13@mails.ucas.ac.cn (L.G.)
[2] Lab for Marine Biology and Biotechnology, Qingdao National Lab for Marine Sci. & Tech, Qingdao 266071, China
[3] University of Chinese Academy of Sciences, Beijing 100049, China
[4] Center for Ocean Mega-Science, Chinese Academy of Sciences, 7 Nanhai Road, Qingdao 266071, China
[5] College of Marine Life Sciences, Ocean University of China, Qingdao 266071, China
* Correspondence: suizhengh@ouc.edu.cn (Z.S.); qbzhang@qdio.ac.cn (Q.Z.);
  Tel./Fax: +86-532-8203-1128 (Z.S.); +86-532-8289-8703 (Q.Z.)
† These authors contributed equally to this work.

Received: 23 July 2018; Accepted: 21 August 2018; Published: 27 August 2018

Abstract: A variety of biologically active products have been isolated from *Gracilariopsis lemaneiformis*. In the present study, two novel angiotensin-converting enzyme (ACE) inhibitory peptides, FQIN [M(O)] CILR, and TGAPCR, were screened and identified from *G. lemaneiformis* protein hydrolysates by LC-MS/MS. The IC50 values of FQIN [M(O)] CILR and TGAPCR were 9.64 ± 0.36 μM and 23.94 ± 0.82 μM, respectively. In the stability study, both peptides showed stabilities of pH, temperature, simulated gastrointestinal digestion, and ACE hydrolysis. The Lineweaver–Burk plot showed that the two peptides were noncompetitive inhibitors of ACE. Molecular docking simulated the intermolecular interactions of two peptides and ACE, and the two peptides formed hydrogen bonds with the active pockets of ACE. However, FQIN [M(O)] CILR was more closely linked to the active pockets of ACE, thereby exerting better ACE inhibition. Spontaneously hypertensive rats (SHRs) were studied with an oral dose of 10 mg/kg body weight. Both peptides reduced systolic blood pressure (SBP) and diastolic blood pressure (DBP) in SHRs, of which FQIN [M(O)] CILR was able to reduce the systolic blood pressure by 34 mmHg (SBP) ($p < 0.05$). Therefore, FQIN [M(O)] CILR was an excellent ACE inhibitory peptide.

Keywords: *Gracilariopsis lemaneiformis*; ACE-inhibitory activity; peptide; molecular docking; SHRs

---

1. Introduction

Hypertension (high blood pressure) refers to the main feature of increased body circulation arterial blood pressure (systolic blood pressure ≥ 140 mmHg and diastolic blood pressure ≥ 90 mmHg), which is associated with increased mortality of cardiovascular disease and diabetes [1]. The WHO reported that more than 17.5 million people have died each year as a result of cardiovascular disease. Hypertension has become the leading global cause of death [2]. Human blood pressure is mainly regulated by the systemic renin-angiotensin system (RAS) and the kallikrein-bradykinin system (KKS). The role of the renin-angiotensin system in regulating blood pressure relies on the proteolytic cascade of two enzymes: renin (EC 3.4.23.15), an aspartyl protease secreted into the blood from the liver, and angiotensin I-converting enzyme (ACE; EC 3.4.15.1), a carboxypeptidase present on the external surface of endothelial cells of the lung [3]. Renin hydrolyzes the angiotensinogen (α-globulin) secreted by the liver to the inactive angiotensin I. Next, angiotensin I is hydrolyzed by ACE to angiotensin II, which then binds to angiotensin receptors and causes vasoconstriction [4]. In addition, ACE can inactivate bradykinin, a nonapeptide with cardiac protection. When bradykinin binds to β-receptor, a series of reactions are generated and causes the intracellular Ca^{2+} levels to increase significantly. Ca^{2+} stimulates the nitric oxide synthase (eNOS) reaction to produce NO, which results in vasodilation and reduced blood pressure [5]. Angiotensin I-converting enzyme is a ubiquitous Zn^{2+}-dependent carboxydiopeptidase in mammalian tissues that regulates the renin-angiotensin system (RAS) and the kallikrein-bradykinin system (KKS) and is considered useful therapeutic target for treating hypertension [6–8]. The common ACE inhibitors on the market are mostly "Prils", such as captopril, enalapril, lisinopril, fosinopril and the like. While these drugs can produce a strong antihypertensive effect, they may also cause a series of side effects such as cough, rash, nausea, acute renal failure, and proteinuria. These drugs are believed to reduce patients' compliance, leading eventually to exacerbated disease conditions, and increased health care costs [9]. For this reason, researchers are increasingly interested in developing natural ACE inhibitory peptides with low-toxicity that could replace or complement antihypertensive drugs [10]. Food-derived active peptides not only produce the same activity as ACE inhibitor drugs but are also safer in terms of having low toxicity due to their natural source. Components of proteins in food are containing sequences of bioactive peptides, which could exert a physiological effect in the body. These short chains of amino acids are inactive within the sequence of the parent protein, but can be released during gastrointestinal digestion, food processing, or fermentation [11]. It has been reported that ACE inhibitory peptides obtained from enzymatic, fermentative, or gastrointestinal digestion of foods exert significant antihypertensive effects in clinical and preclinical studies [12]. This demonstrates the significance and prospect of finding active ACE inhibitory peptides from healthy foods.

Gracilariopsis lemaneiformis is a red algae that is widely distributed in the marine environment and has important economic value [13]. *Gracilariopsis lemaneiformis* belongs to the family *Gracilariopsisceae* (Rhodophyta), in which a majority of the members are utilized as the main sources of the manufacture of agar [14]. *Gracilariopsis lemaneiformis* is rich in polysaccharides, protein, vitamins, and multiple minerals such as phosphorus, calcium, iodine, iron, zinc and magnesium [15]. Polysaccharides, phycoerythrin, agar and other active substances isolated from *G. lemaneiformis* have proven to show a range of biological activities such as antioxidation, antitumor, immune regulation and alcoholic liver injury protection [16–19]. There are few studies, however, investigating active peptides of *G. lemaneiformis*, particularly ACE inhibitory peptides. To date, ACE inhibitory peptides have been extracted from various types of marine algae, such as *Saccharina longicruris* [20], *Palmaria palmate* [21], *Pyropia columbina* [22], *Enteromorpha clathrata* [23], *Ulva rigida* C. [24], *Chlorella vulgaris* [25], and *Porphyra yezoensis* [26]. This demonstrates that marine algae are an important source of active peptides.

In this study, ACE inhibitory peptides were screened from *G. lemaneiformis* enzymatic hydrolyte. By searching the online database, the physicochemical properties of the peptides were investigated. The stabilities of such peptides against pH, temperature, gastrointestinal digestion and ACE hydrolysis were then assessed. Molecular docking was used to simulate the intermolecular interactions of peptides with ACE. Finally, the antihypertensive activities of the peptides were tested in vivo in spontaneously hypertensive rats (SHRs).

2. Results

2.1. Screening of the Active ACE Inhibitory Peptides.

Two ACE inhibitory peptides were screened and identified by LC-MS/MS; the sequences are FQIN [M(O)] CILR and TGAPCR. The result shows that the peptides are two novel ACE inhibitors with the IC50 value of 9.64 ± 0.36 µM and 23.94 ± 0.82 µM, respectively.

2.2. Properties of Peptides

The physicochemical properties of the peptide were obtained by online database search. Table 1 shows that the isoelectric points (PI) of FQIN [M(O)] CILR and TGAPCR are 8.61 and 8.55, respectively. Both peptides are non-toxic and can be used for animal studies. FQIN [M(O)] CILR has poor water solubility.

Table 1. Physicochemical characteristics of the two peptides.

Peptides	Number of Residues	Molecular Weight (Da)	ToxiPed	Solubility in Water	Iso-Electric Point (PI)
FQIN [M(O)] CILR	9	1153.43	non-toxin	poor	8.61
TGAPCR	6	603.69	non-toxin	good	8.55

2.3. Stability Study for ACE Inhibitory Activity

The pH and thermal stability of the peptides were measured. The results show that the peptides could maintain their ACE inhibitory activity after pH and heat treatment (Figure 1a,b). Both peptides show pH and thermal stability.

The stability of the peptides in the simulated gastric juice and intestinal fluid is shown in Figure 2. After digestion in simulated gastric juice and intestinal fluid containing the corresponding enzymes, the ACE inhibitory activity of the peptides did not display any significant changes. The results demonstrate that these peptides have gastrointestinal stability, and they may also produce antihypertensive effects in vivo.

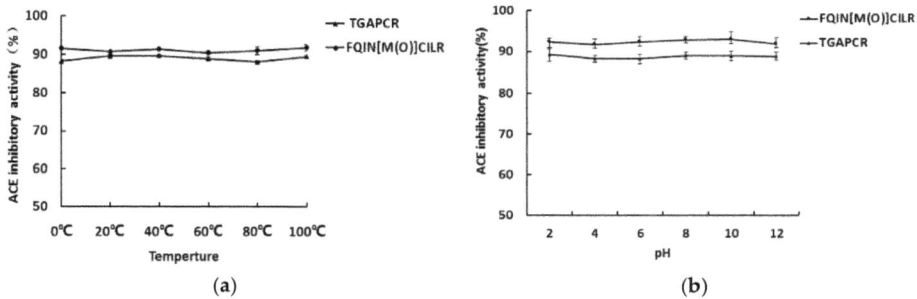

Figure 1. Temperature (**a**) and pH (**b**) stability of peptides FQIN [M(O)] CILR and TGAPCR. The concentration of peptides was 0.5 mg/mL; values represent mean ± SD ($n = 3$).

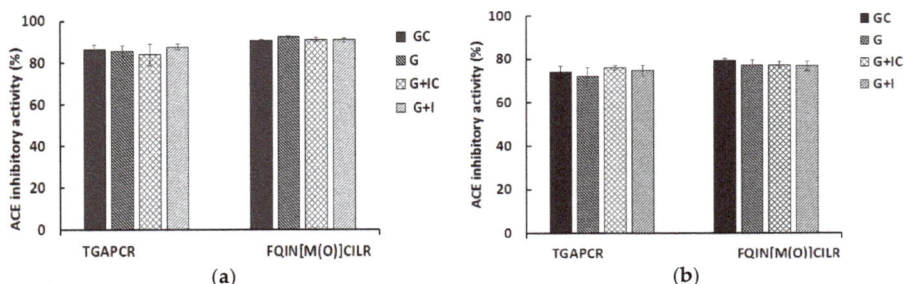

Figure 2. Stability of FQIN [M(O)] CILR and TGAPCR under simulated gastrointestinal digestion. The final concentrations of peptides were 0.5 mg/mL (**a**) and 0.1 mg/mL (**b**), respectively. GC, peptide sample and simulated gastric fluid without pepsin; G, peptide sample with gastric fluid with pepsin; G + IC, peptide sample and simulated gastrointestinal fluid without pepsin and pancreatin; G + I, peptide sample with gastrointestinal fluid with pepsin and pancreatin. Values represent mean ± SD (*n* = 3).

2.4. Stability of Peptides against ACE

Figure 3 shows no significant changes of ACE inhibitory activity within incubation of ACE for 24 h. The peptides maintained stable ACE inhibitory activity, suggesting that they were not hydrolyzed by ACE.

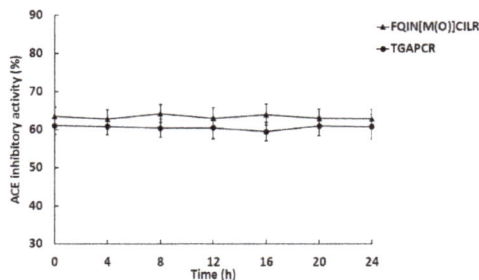

Figure 3. Stability of peptides against ACE. The concentration of peptides was 0.1 mg/mL; values represent mean ± SD (*n* = 3).

2.5. Characterization of the Inhibition Pattern on ACE

Based on the results of the Lineweaver–Burk plots, both FQIN [M(O)] CILR and TGAPCR are noncompetitive inhibitors of ACE. Table 2 shows the kinetic parameters of the two peptides binding to ACE. Combined with the results shown in Figure 4, the value of Km (2.26 ± 0.21 mM) is constant, which is an important characteristic of noncompetitive inhibition. In the noncompetitive inhibition pattern, the substrate and the inhibitory peptide bind to different parts of the enzyme. Thus, the apparent affinity of the substrate and the enzyme is a constant [27]. The Vmax (2.23 ± 0.67 $mg^{-1} \cdot mL \cdot min$) decreases as the concentration of inhibitory peptide increases. This is due to the reduction of the apparent catalytic efficiency of ACE, which leads to the decrease of the enzymatic reaction efficiency [23]. At the same concentration, the Vmax of FQIN [M(O)] CILR is smaller than TGAPCR, indicating that FQIN [M(O)] CILR produce a better inhibitory activity than TGAPCR.

The Ki of FQIN [M(O)] CILR and TGAPCR are 0.71 ± 0.04 mM and 0.86 ± 0.06 mM, respectively. The Ki value indicates the affinity of ACE inhibitory peptide to ACE. The lower the inhibition constant

(Ki), the higher the affinity of the inhibitors to ACE. The results show that FQIN [M(O)] CILR can produce better inhibitory activity than TGAPCR.

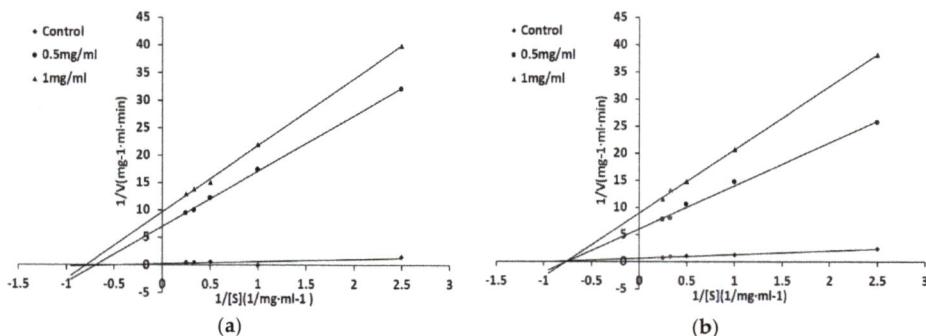

(a)

(b)

Figure 4. Lineweaver–Burk plots of ACE inhibited by the peptides. $1/V$ and $1/S$ represents the reciprocal of reaction velocity and substrate concentration, respectively. (a) FQIN [M(O)] CILR; (b) TGAPCR.

Table 2. Kinetics parameters of ACE-catalyzed reactions in different peptide concentrations.

Kinetics Parameters	Control	FQIN [M(O)] CILR		TGAPCR	
		1 mg/mL	0.5 mg/mL	1 mg/mL	0.5 mg/mL
Km (mM)	2.66 ± 0.21	2.66 ± 0.21		2.66 ± 021	
Vmax $(mg^{-1} \cdot mL \cdot min)$	2.23 ± 0.67	0.10 ± 0.05	0.14 ± 0.02	0.11 ± 0.03	0.17 ± 0.02
Ki (mM)		0.71 ± 0.04		0.86 ± 0.06	

2.6. Molecular Docking

CDOCKER was used to discover the ligand–receptor interaction mechanism. The -CDOCKER ENERGY and -CDOCKER INTERACTION ENERGY of FQIN [M(O)] CILR are 158.117 kcal·mol^{-1} and 105.509 kcal·mol^{-1}, respectively. The -CDOCKER ENERGY and -CDOCKER INTERACTION ENERGY of TGAPCR are 90.4226 kcal·mol^{-1} and 105.509 kcal·mol^{-1}, respectively (Table 3). Both peptides have a stable docking structure with ACE. The 2D and 3D structures of the peptide-ACE complexes are displayed in Figure 5a–d.

There are three main active site pockets in the ACE molecule. S1 pocket has three residues, Ala354, Glu384, and Tyr523. S2 pocket comprises of Gln281, His353, Lys511, His513, and Tyr520. S1'pocket includes residue Glu162 [28,29]. Inhibitory peptides interact with the active pockets of ACE through a variety of forces: electrostatic forces, hydrogen bonds, van der Waals forces, and hydrophobic interactions (Figure 5b,d). Of these forces, hydrogen bonds play a major role. Table 4 shows that FQIN [M(O)] CILR forms twelve hydrogen bonds with ACE residues Asn277, Gln281, Lys511, Tyr523, Ser517, Ser516, Glu123, His353, Glu376. Specifically, FQIN [M(O)] CILR constructs one hydrogen bond with S1 pocket (Tyr523), four bonds with S2 pocket (His353, Lys511, Gln281, His353). TGAPCR forms seven hydrogen bonds with ACE residues Lys511, Gln281, Glu376, Glu384, His353, Tyr394, Arg402. Specifically, Lys511, Gln281 and His353 belong to S2 pocket, link with TGAPCR through three hydrogen bonds and Glu384 belongs to S1 pocket. We speculate that FQIN [M(O)] CILR has a lower IC50 than TGAPCR because FQIN [M(O)] CILR forms a tighter bond with ACE.

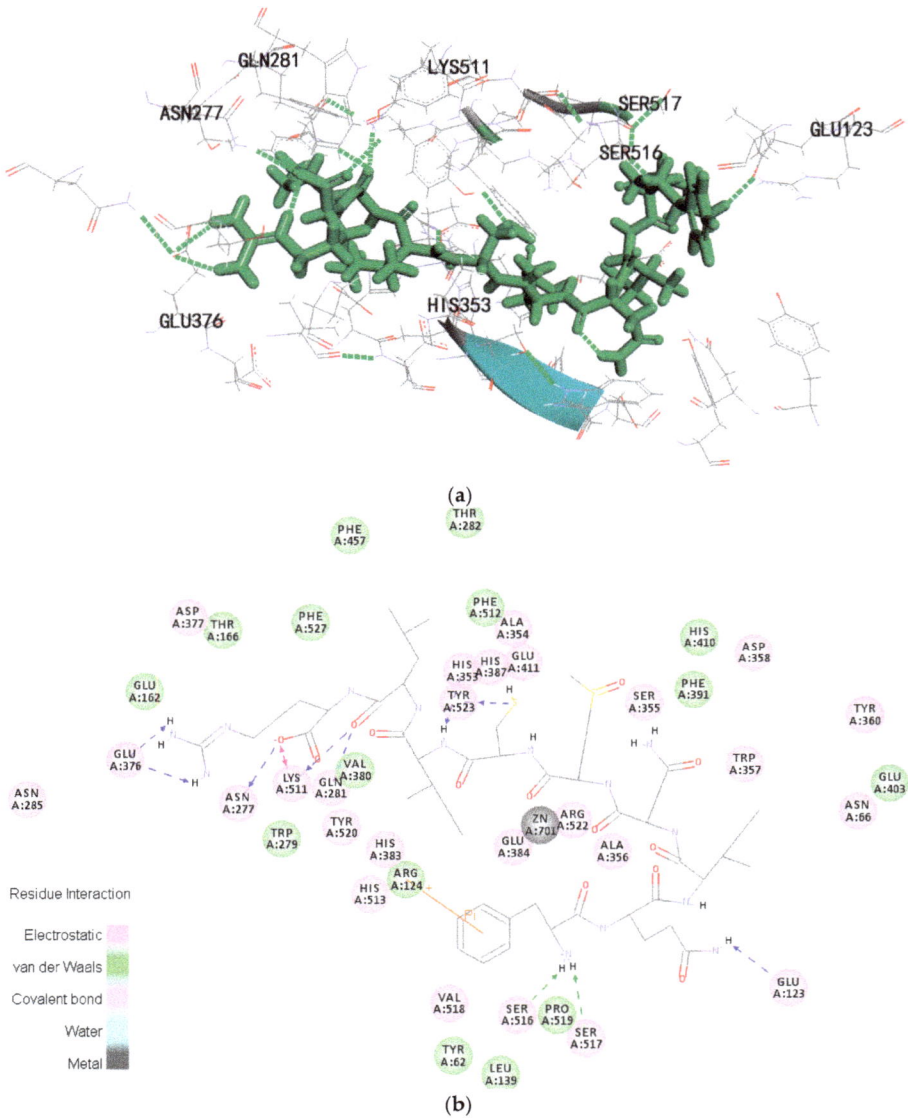

(a)

(b)

Figure 5. *Cont.*

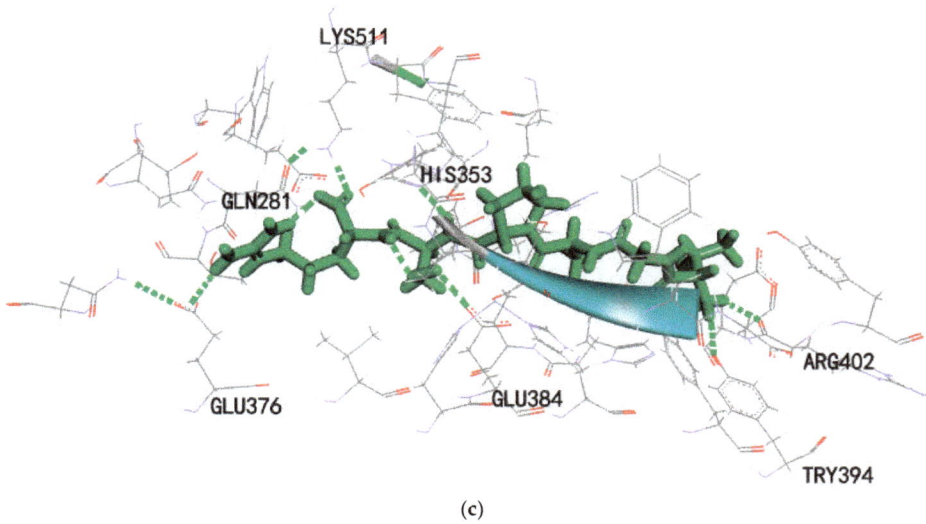

(c)

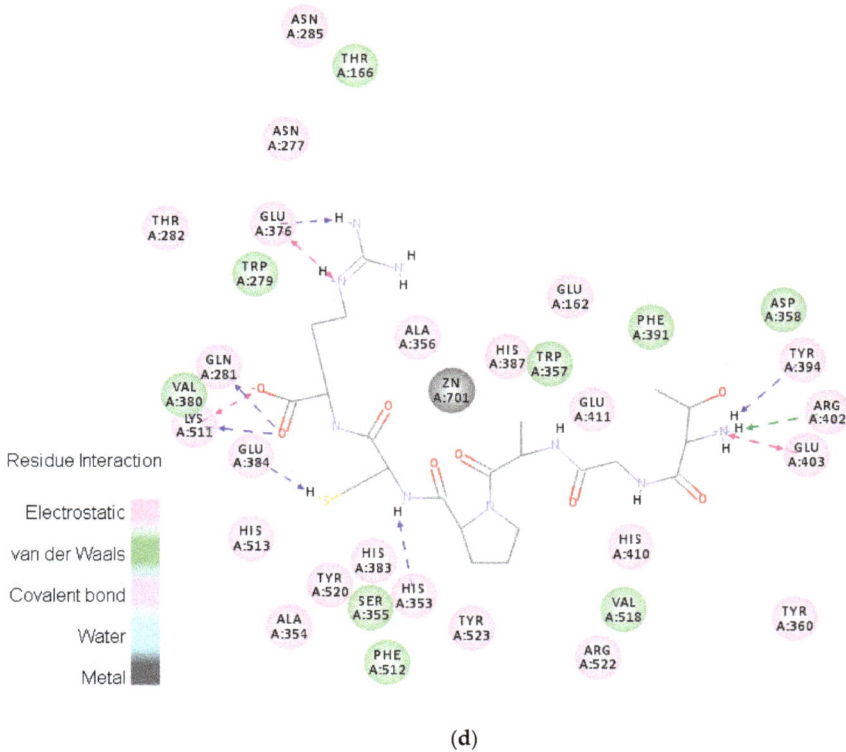

(d)

Figure 5. Molecular docking simulation of the peptides. (**a,b**) are local overview and two-dimensional (2D) diagram of FQIN [M(O)] CILR; (**c,d**) are local overview and two-dimensional (2D) diagram of TGAPCR.

Table 3. Docking energies for optimal conformation of two ACE inhibit peptides and ACE.

Peptides	-CDOCKER ENERGY (kcal·mol^{-1})	-CDOCKER INTERACTION ENERGY (kcal·mol^{-1})
FQIN [M(O)] CILR	158.117	145.01
TGAPCR	90.4226	105.509

Table 4. Hydrogen bonds formed between two ACE inhibitory peptides and ACE.

Peptides	Donor Atom	Acceptor Atom	Distance (Å)	Active Pocket
FQIN [M(O)] CILR	A: ASN277: HD22	F: O125	2.39	
	A: GLN281: HE22	F: O89	1.97	S2
	A: LYS511: HZ1	F: O89	2.02	S2
	A: LYS511: HZ3	F: O126	2.31	S2
	A: TYR523: HH	F: S63	2.24	S1
	F: H145	A: SER517: O	1.95	
	F: H146	A: SER516: O	1.98	
	F: H148	A: GLU123: OE1	2.14	
	F: H158	A: HIS353: NE2	2.33	S2
	F: H161	A: GLU376: OE1	2.44	
	F: H161	A: GLU: 376: OE2	2.03	
	F: H163	A: GLU: 376: OE1	2.32	
TGAPCR	A: GLN281: HE22	T: O2	2.06	S2
	A: LYS511: HZ1	T: O2	1.78	S2
	T: H71	A: GLU376: OE2	2.16	
	T: H75	A: GLU384: OE2	2.26	S1
	T: H76	A: HIS353: NE2	2.24	S2
	T: H78	A: TYR394: OH	2.32	
	T: H79	A: ARG402: O	2.41	

F is an abbreviation of FQIN [M(O)] CILR; T is an abbreviation of TGAPCR.

2.7. Antihypertensive Activity of the Two Peptides on SHRs

The in vivo antihypertensive activity of peptides was assessed by SHRs with a gavage dose of 10 mg/mL. Both FQIN [M(O)] CILR and TGAPCR decreased the SBP of SHRs. FQIN [M(O)] CILR significantly decreased the SBP between 2 to 4 h ($p < 0.05$), with the largest decrease of SBP from 204 to 170 mmHg occurring at 2 h. The SBP then began to recover and maintained a level of 200 mmHg at 8 h (Figure 6a). It was notable that the FQIN [M(O)] CILR reduced the SBP of SHRs by 34 mmHg to the maximum extent. TGAPCR reduced SBP to the lowest point at 2 h. The greatest decline observed was approximately 28 mmHg of SBP from 205 mmHg to 178 mmHg.

In addition, both FQIN [M(O)] CILR and TGAPCR could also affect DBP (Figure 6b). FQIN [M(O)] CILR could significantly reduce the DBP of SHRs from 145 mmHg to 118 mmHg at 2 h ($p < 0.05$), then restore to its original level at 8 h. TGAPCR could decrease DPH to 120 mmHg at 1 h and maintain the DPH until 4 h. TGAPCR can maintain low DBP for a longer period of time compared to FQIN [M(O)] CILR. In general, FQIN [M(O)] CILR has a better antihypertensive effect in SHRs than TGAPCR.

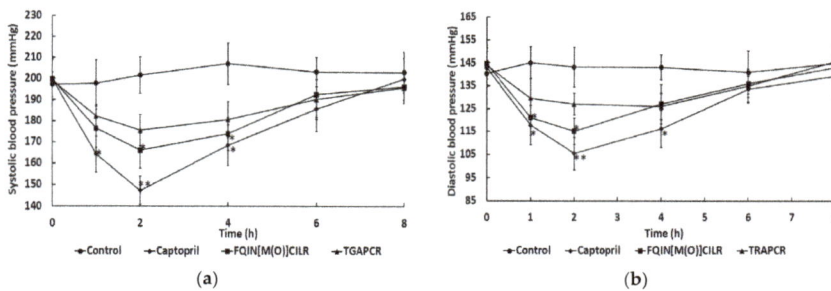

Figure 6. Changes of spontaneously hypertensive rats' systolic blood pressure (SBP) and diastolic blood pressure (DBP) after oral administration of the two peptides. Saline and Captopril were used as the control and positive control, respectively. Single oral administration was performed with a dose of 10 mg/kg body weight. Blood pressures were measured prior to and 1, 2, 4, 6, 8 h after oral administration. The difference with a value of $p < 0.05$ was considered to be significant. (**a**) SBP changes; (**b**) DBP changes.

3. Discussion

Natural products and derivate are considered relatively safe with limited side effects and thus will become an important source for clinical medications of hypertension in the future [30]. An increasing number of researchers have been investigating natural antihypertensive peptides, in which a variety of antihypertensive peptides with specific sequences and limited side effects have been extracted from animals and plants [10]. Algae accounts for 50% of marine living resources. Thus, marine algae can be used as an important source for extracting active peptides. Researchers have extracted antihypertensive peptides from *Saccharina longicruris* [20], *Palmaria palmate* [21], *Pyropia columbina* [22], and other types of marine algae. However, there are few reports of extracting antihypertensive peptides from *G. lemaneiformis*. Here, we reported that two peptides extracted from *G. lemaneiformis* have the activity to inhibit ACE.

D.Q. Cao et al. have reported that a peptide (QVEY, IC50 = 474.36 µM) isolated from trypsin hydrolyzate of *G. lemaneiformis* had ACE inhibitory activity [31]. FQIN [M(O)] CILR (IC50 = 9.64 ± 0.36 µM) and TGAPCR (IC50 = 23.94 ± 0.82 µM) were also screened from trypsin hydrolyzate of *G. lemaneiformis*, but the two peptides have lower IC50 values than the ACE inhibitory peptide reported above. The two peptides isolated from *G. lemaneiformis* showed higher activity than some reported C-terminal arginine ACE inhibitory peptides YIPIQYVLSR (IC50 = 132.5 µM), YASGR (IC50 = 184 µM) and GNGSGYVSR (IC50 = 29 µM) [32,33]. According to earlier studies, C-terminal arginine plays an important role in inhibiting the activity of ACE. The interaction between C-terminal arginine and ACE can be further analyzed in the molecular docking results.

The properties and stabilities of peptides are prerequisites for the preparation of "functional peptides". According to the information in the Innovagen server, FQIN [M(O)] CILR has poor water solubility. However, in our study, we found that the FQIN [M(O)] CILR had good water solubility when the concentration was lower than 10 mg/mL. The solubility gradually decreased when the concentration was above 10 mg/mL. The hydrophobicity of FQIN [M(O)] CILR is related to the presence of hydrophobic amino acids, such as Phe, Leu, Ile, and Met. The hydrophobicity of FQIN [M(O)] CILR may facilitate the binding of peptides to the hydrophobic active center of ACE, in turn, produce better inhibitory activity.

Small molecule peptides can cross the intestinal wall and enter the blood circulation. Prior to this, peptides must resist the gastrointestinal digestion and maintain their integrity, otherwise their biological activity may be activated or inactivated [34]. Our results suggested that the peptides can maintain the inhibitory activity after being absorbed into the blood.

Angiotensin I-converting enzyme is a carboxypeptidase with very broad substrate specificity [35]. Some ACE inhibitory peptides may become substrates of ACE, which are cleaved into smaller fragments. As a result, the activity of the peptides is altered [34]. For example, ACE hydrolyzed FFGRCVSP isolated from dried bonito to four fragments FF, GR, GV, SP, while the IC50 value increased from 0.4 μM to 4.6 μM [7]. LKPNM (IC50 = 2.4 μM) isolated from dried bonito was hydrolyzed into LKP and NM, and the IC50 value of LKPNM became 1/3 after the pre-incubation with ACE [7]. In view of this, the stability of peptide binding to ACE must be taken into account. Our results proved that FQIN [M(O)] CILR and TGAPCR are stable ACE inhibitors but not substrates of ACE.

There are multiple inhibition patterns of ACE inhibitory peptides: competitive inhibition, noncompetitive inhibition, and mixed-competitive inhibition [36]. The results suggested that both peptides are noncompetitive inhibitors of ACE. Some peptides isolated from food stuffs have also been observed working in noncompetitive inhibition, for example, IFL from fermented soybean food [37], AVKVL from hazelnut [38], and VELWP from cuttlefish [39].

Molecular docking has become an important tool for elucidating the mechanisms of action between ligands and receptors [40]. The results of molecular docking suggested that the two peptides were linked to several pivotal amino acids that are important for ACE. His353, Ala354, and His513 were reported as important residues interacting with Lisinopril which formed six hydrogen bonds with ACE in the absence of the H_2O molecule [3,28,41]. FQIN [M(O)] CILR and TGAPCR also formed hydrogen bonds with one of the three important residues (His353). Glu384 is the one formed coordination effect with Zn^{2+} [3]. Therefore, TGAPCR may also interfere ACE from combining with Zn^{2+}, which in turn may contribute to ACE inhibitory activity. The results also highlighted the important role of arginine in the ACE inhibitory activity of the peptides [32]. The arginine of FQIN [M(O)] CILR formed five hydrogen bonds with the ACE residues Glu376, Asn277, Lys511. ACE residues Glu376, Lys511 and Gln281 formed three hydrogen bonds with the arginine of TGAPCR. Arginine enabled the peptides to form a tight bond with ACE, which facilitated the peptides' inhibitory activity against ACE.

Antihypertensive activity of peptides were further evaluated using spontaneously hypertensive rats (SHRs). The results indicated that captopril resulted in maximal antihypertensive effect on SHRs. Overall, drugs can exert better antihypertensive effects than hydrolysates and antihypertensive peptides derived from foods [2,42]. This may be because antihypertensive drugs have a more stable conformation and a more stringent structure. Both FQIN [M(O)] CILR and TGAPCR decreased the SBP of SHRs. FQIN [M(O)] CILR and TGAPCR reduced the SBP of SHRs by 34 mmHg and 28 mmHg to the maximum extent, respectively. FQIN [M(O)] CILR also decreased the DBP of SHRs significantly ($p < 0.05$). HLFGPPGKKDPV (IC50 = 125 μM), separated from fertilized eggs, had the greatest SBP drop of 30 mmHg, following an oral dose of 10 mg/kg [43]. QPGPT (IC50 = 80.67 μM) and GDIGY (IC50 = 32.56 μM), isolated from jellyfish, reduced the SBP by 13.75 mmHg and 20.67 mmHg, respectively [44]. In comparison to the aforementioned peptides, FQIN [M(O)] CILR (IC50 = 9.64 ± 0.36 μM) may have a strong antihypertensive effect, suggesting that it has considerable potential in the control of blood pressure.

FQIN [M(O)] CILR and TGAPCR are two novel ACE inhibitory peptides, isolated from the trypsin hydrolysate of *G. lemaneiformis*. The results demonstrated that FQIN [M(O)] CILR and TGAPCR not only showed strong ACE inhibitory activity in vitro but also showed strong antihypertensive effects in SHRs. This study suggested that these two natural peptides have the potential to be developed for both antihypertensive drugs and health care products.

4. Materials and Methods

4.1. Chemicals

ACE (from rabbit lung), hippuryl-histidyl-leucine (HHL), high-performance liquid chromatography (HPLC)-grade acetonitrile (ACN), trifluoroaceticacid (TFA) and porcine pancreatin (8× USP) were purchased from Sigma-Aldrich Co. (St. Louis, MO, USA). Trypsin (EC 3.4.23.4, ≥250. N.F.U/mg solid), pepsin (EC 3.4.23.1, ≥250 U/mg solid), and captopril (>99% purity) were obtained from Solarbio (Beijing, China). All other chemical reagents were of analytical grade.

4.2. Preparation of G. Lemaneiformis Hydrolysates

G. lemaneiformis was hydrolyzed with 2% trypsin (EC 3.4.23.4, ≥250. N. F. U./mg solid) for 2 h. The 80% alcohol was used to precipitate the impurities in the hydrolysates. The supernatant was concentrated to remove ethanol. Next, the concentrated supernatant was fractionated by ultrafiltration (LNG-UF-101, Laungy Membrane Filtration Technology Co. Ltd., Shanghai, China) and the fraction (<3 KDa) was collected and freeze-dried before storage at −80 °C.

4.3. Identification of Peptides by LC-MS/MS

Peptide sequences were determined according to Kai Lin [45]. Identification of peptides in 3 KDa permeates was performed using a Q-Exactive mass spectrometer (Thermo Fisher Scientific, Waltham, MA, USA) coupled with a Thermo Scientific EASY-nLC 1000 System (Thermo Fisher Scientific, Waltham, MA, USA). Samples were loaded in a reverse-phase trap column (2 cm × 100 μm, 5 μm-C18), which was connected to a reverse-phase analytical column (75 μm × 100 μm, 3 μm-C18). The purified sample was injected into the trapping column at a flow rate of 300 nL/min. The mass spectrometer (MS) was operated in positive-ion detection mode, and the most abundant precursor ions from the scanning range of 300−1800 m/z were selected to obtain MS data. Peptide sequences were determined based on the MS/MS spectra and Mascot 2.2 (Matrix Science Inc., Boston, MA, USA) searches of dataset of *G. lemaneiformis* (Accession: SRX258772, download from SRA database of NCBI).

4.4. Synthesis of ACE Inhibitory Peptides

The inhibitory peptides were chemically synthesized in Shanghai Qiangyao Biotechnology Co., Ltd. (Shanghai, China). The peptides were synthesized using the Fmoc solid-phase method. To increase the stability of FQINMCILR, Methionine is selectively modified to methionine sulfoxide (FQIN [M(O)] CILR). The purity of the two peptides is 97.85% and 97.59%.

4.5. Measurement of ACE Inhibition Activity

ACE inhibition activity was assayed according to Cushman and Cheung, with some modification [27]. ACE was dissolved in sodium borate buffer (pH 8.3, containing 0.3 M sodium chloride) to 0.1 U/mL for the assay. Synthetic peptides were dissolved in distilled water to seven concentration levels. Then, 20 μL of a certain concentration of peptide was mixed with 10 μL ACE solution. The mixture was incubated at 37 °C for 5 min, and then 50 μL of 5 mM HHL (sodium borate buffer pH 8.3, containing 0.3 M sodium chloride) was added to the above mixture to start the reaction. The reaction was maintained at 37 °C for 60 min, and then 150 μL of 1 M HCl was added to stop the reaction. The solution was filtered through a 0.22 micron membrane. Next, 20 μL of reaction solution was injected into a RP-HPLC (Shimadzu, Kyoto, Japan) fixed with Eclipse XDB-C18 column (4.6 mm × 150 mm × 5 μm, Agilent Technologies Inc., St. Clara, CA, USA) to measure the concentration of hippuric acid (HA). The absorbance was detected at 228 nm. All determinations were triplicate. The activity of ACE inhibition was calculated as followed:

$$\text{ACE inhibitory activity } (\%) = (A_{control} - A_{inhibitor})/A_{control} \times 100$$

where $A_{inhibitor}$ is the relative area of the hippuric acid (HA) peak obtained from the reaction of ACE and HHL with inhibitor. $A_{control}$ is the relative area of the hippuric acid (HA) peak obtained from the reaction of ACE and HHL without inhibitor. IC50 is defined as the concentration of peptides that can inhibit half of the ACE activity.

4.6. Properties of Peptides

The properties of ACE inhibitory peptides are important for future research. These parameters can be retrieved from the online database. The ToxinPred server can analyze toxicity of the peptides (http://crdd.osdd.net/raghava/toxinpred/). The online Innovagen server was used to evaluate the solubility of the peptide (www.innovagen.com/proteomics-tools).

4.7. Stability Study for ACE Inhibitory Activity

4.7.1. Thermal Stability for Peptides

The synthetic peptide solutions (0.5 mg/mL) were incubated at different temperatures (0 °C, 20 °C, 40 °C, 60 °C, 80 °C, 100 °C) for 2 h. Next, 20 μL of peptide was used to assay the ACE inhibitory activity using the above method [39].

4.7.2. pH Stability for Peptides

The synthetic peptide solutions (0.5 mg/mL) were incubated at different pH levels (2, 4, 6, 8, 10, 12) for 2 h, and then solutions were neutralized to pH 7.0 [39]. Then, 20 μL of peptide was used to assay the ACE inhibitory activity using the above method.

4.7.3. Gastrointestinal Stability of Peptides

Gastrointestinal stability of peptides was evaluated in vitro [46,47]. Peptides were dissolved in a 0.1 M KCl-HCl buffer (pH 2.0) to the concentration of 0.1 mg/mL and 0.5 mg/mL. Pepsin ($\geq$250 U/mg) was added to a peptide solution to the final concentration 0.8 mg/mL. The solution was then incubated at 37 °C for 4 h. The pepsin was inactivated through boiling the solution for 10 min. The pH of the solution was adjusted to 7.0 with 1 M NaOH. The solution was centrifuged at 12,000 rpm for 5 min and the supernatant (20 μL) was taken out to determine the ACE inhibitory activity. The remaining supernatant was further incubated with pancreatin (10 mg/mL, 8× USP) at 37 °C for 4 h. The reaction was stopped by boiling the solution for 10 min. The solution was centrifuged at 12,000 rpm for 10 min, and then the supernatant (20 μL) was used to detect ACE inhibitory activity.

4.8. Stability of Peptides against ACE

The stability of peptides against ACE was assayed according to Salampessy. J and Fujita. H [48,49]. 30 μL of peptides (0.1 mg/mL) reacted with 30 μL 0.1 U/mL ACE solution at 37 °C for 24 h. The ACE was then inactivated through boiling the solution for 10 min. Then, 20 μL of peptides were used to detect ACE inhibitory activity in the above method.

4.9. Determination of Inhibitory Pattern

Peptides were dissolved in distilled water to the concentration of 1 mg/mL and 0.5 mg/mL, and HHL was dissolved to the concentration of 4 mg/mL, 2 mg/mL, 1 mg/mL and 0.5 mg/mL. Different concentrations of the peptide were reacted at different concentrations of HHL. Then, 20 μL of peptide solution was used to determine the ACE inhibitory activity using the above method. Lineweaver—Burk plots were applied to confirm the ACE inhibitory pattern of peptide. The inhibitory constant (Ki) was the intercept of the *X*-axis of the plot, of which the *Y*-axis displayed the slopes of Lineweaver-Burk line and the *X*-axis indicted peptides concentrations [25].

4.10. Molecular Docking

The affinity of peptides to inhibit ACE was simulated and evaluated by Discovery Studio 3.5 (DS 3.5, Accelrys, San Diego, CA, USA), according to the reported method with some modification [32]. In the docking experiments, the crystal structure of human tACE (PDB ID: 1O8A, http://www.rcsb.org/pdb/explore/explore.do?structureId=1O8A) was as receptor. The 3D structure of the peptides was designed by Discovery Studio 3.5 (DS 3.5, Accelrys, San Diego, CA, USA). Then the peptide was protonated at pH 7.0 and energetically minimized by the CHARMm force field. The structure of ACE was removed water, cleaned protein and added hydrogen. The CDOCKER was selected to simulate the docking of receptors and peptide ligands. The binding site sphere was x: 40.302, y: 37.243 and z: 48.948. Rigid residues were residues within the sphere with a 20 Å radius and with zinc as the center. CDOCKER module uses a CHARMm-based molecular dynamics (MD) scheme to dock ligands into a receptor binding site. Random ligand conformations are generated using high-temperature MD. The conformations are then translated into the binding site. Candidate poses are then created using random rigid-body rotations followed by simulated annealing. A final minimization is used to refine the ligand poses. -CDOCKER ENERGY and -CDCKER INTERACTION ENERGY are two criteria for evaluating CDOCKER results. -CDOCKER ENERGY indicates the negative of the total energy. -CDOCKER INTERACTION ENERGY indicates the negative of the interaction energy. The optimal conformation of peptide-ACE complex has the highest values of -CDOCKER ENERGY and -CDOCKER INTERACTION ENERGY.

4.11. Antihypertensive Effect on SHRs

Spontaneously hypertensive rats (SHRs) (male, 10-week-old, 250–300 g body weight, specific, pathogen-free) were bought from Vital River Laboratory Animal Co., Ltd. (Beijing, China). Animals used in this study were maintained in accordance with the guidelines of the Institutional Research Council's Guide for the Care and Use of Laboratory Animals. SHRs were housed under 12 h day/night cycle at 22 ± 2 °C and fed with tap water and a standard diet ad libitum. The SHRs were randomly separated into a positive group, control group, and two experiment groups. There were six SHRs in each group. Before the formal start of the test, SHRs had to adapt to measuring the environment in advance. Once the tail systolic blood pressure (SBP) rates were above 180 mmHg, the gavage administration could start.

Normal saline was the solvent to dissolve peptides and control reagent. Captopril (99% purity, Solarbio Technology Co., Ltd., Beijing, China) was the positive group. The same volume of normal saline was the control group. Tail-cuff method was performed for systolic blood pressure (SBP) and diastolic blood pressure (DBP) measurements with a non-invasive CODA device (Kent Scientific Co., Torrington, CT, USA). The blood pressure was measured in 0, 1, 2, 4, 6, 8 h after gavage administration. Measurements were repeated three times at each time point.

4.12. Statistical Analysis

Data analysis was performed using SPSS Version 17.0 (SPSS Inc., Chicago, IL, USA). To compare the mean differences among the groups, one-way analysis of variance was used. The results are shown as the mean $\pm$ SD, and $p < 0.05$ was considered to be statistically significant.

5. Conclusions

Two ACE inhibitory peptides, identified as FQIN [M(O)] CILR and TGAPCR from *G. lemaneiformis*, inhibit ACE in a noncompetitive pattern. Molecular docking results showed that the peptides were mainly linked to ACE via hydrogen bonds and produce inhibitory activity. Animal experiment has shown that FQIN [M(O)] CILR and TGAPCR can reduce blood pressure of SHRs. Therefore, these peptides have the potential to treat hypertension, while *G. lemaneiformis* can be developed as an antihypertensive food.

Author Contributions: Z.D. conceived, designed, and performed the experiments; Y.L. performed the experiments; J.W., S.W. and L.G. analyzed the data; Q.Z. conceive the experiments.

Funding: This research was funded by the Fujian STS project of Chinese Academy of Sciences, the Science and Technology project of Fujian Province (No. 2017T3015, 2017T3013), the Key Research and Development Project of Shandong Province (grant number 2016YYSP002), the Youth Innovation Promotion Association of CAS (grant number 2016190) and K.C. Wong Education Foundation, CAS.

Acknowledgments: We thank Elservier (https://www.elsevier.com/) for its linguistic assistance during the preparation of this manuscript. We thanks professor Zhenghong Sui provided us with the database. Finally, I am grateful to my teacher Quanbin Zhang for his guidance and support for my work.

Conflicts of Interest: The authors declare no conflict of interest.

References

1. Cornélissen, G.; Delcourt, A.; Toussaint, G.; Otsuka, K.; Watanabe, Y.; Siegelova, J.; Fiser, B.; Dusek, J.; Homolka, P.; Singh, R.B.; et al. Opportunity of detecting pre-hypertension: worldwide data on blood pressure overswinging. *Biomed. Pharmacother.* **2005**, *59*, S152–S157. [CrossRef]

2. Faria, M.; Costa, E.L.; Gontijo, J.A.; Netto, F.M. Evaluation of the hypotensive potential of bovine and porcine collagen hydrolysates. *J. Méd. Food* **2008**, *11*, 560–567. [CrossRef] [PubMed]

3. Natesh, R.; Schwager, S.L.U.; Sturrock, E.D.; Acharya, K.R. Crystal structure of the human angiotensin-converting enzyme–lisinopril complex. *Nature* **2003**, *421*, 551. [CrossRef] [PubMed]

4. Pacurari, M.; Kafoury, R.; Tchounwou, P.B.; Ndebele, K. The Renin-Angiotensin-aldosterone system in vascular inflammation and remodeling. *Int. J. Inflamm.* **2014**, *2014*, 689360. [CrossRef] [PubMed]

5. Chen, C.C.; Ke, W.H.; Ceng, L.H.; Hsieh, C.W.; Wung, B.S. Calcium- and phosphatidylinositol 3-kinase/Akt-dependent activation of endothelial nitric oxide synthase by apigenin. *Life Sci.* **2010**, *87*, 743–749. [CrossRef] [PubMed]

6. Martin, J.; Hartl, F.U. Molecular chaperones in cellular protein folding. *Bioessays* **1994**, *16*, 689–692. [CrossRef] [PubMed]

7. Fujita, H.; Yokoyama, K.; Yoshikawa, M. Classification and antihypertensive activity of angiotensin I-converting enzyme inhibitory peptides derived from food proteins. *J. Food Sci.* **2000**, *65*, 564–569.

8. Alemán, A.; Giménez, B.; Pérez-Santin, E.; Gómez-Guillén, M.C.; Montero, P. Contribution of Leu and Hyp residues to antioxidant and ACE-inhibitory activities of peptide sequences isolated from squid gelatin hydrolysate. *Food Chem.* **2011**, *125*, 334–341. [CrossRef]

9. García-Mora, P.; Martín-Martinez, M.; Bonache, M.A.; Gonzalez-Muniz, M.; Peñas, E.; Frias, J.; Martínez-Villaluenga, C. Identification, functional gastrointestinal stability and molecular docking studies of lentil peptides with dual antioxidant and angiotensin I converting enzyme inhibitory activities. *Food Chem.* **2017**, *221*, 464–472. [CrossRef] [PubMed]

10. Aluko, R.E. Structure and function of plant protein-derived antihypertensive peptides. *Curr. Opin. Food Sci.* **2015**, *4*, 44–50. [CrossRef]

11. Wijesekara, I.; Kim, S. Angiotensin-I-converting enzyme (ACE) inhibitors from marine resources: Prospects in the pharmaceutical industry. *Mar. Drugs* **2010**, *8*, 1080–1093. [CrossRef] [PubMed]

12. Aluko, R.E. Antihypertensive peptides from food proteins. *Annu. Rev. Food Sci. Technol.* **2015**, *6*, 235–262. [CrossRef] [PubMed]

13. Chen, B.; Zou, D.; Zhu, M.; Yang, Y. Effects of CO_2 levels and light intensities on growth and amino acid contents in red seaweed Gracilaria lemaneiformis. *Aquac. Res.* **2016**, *48*, 2683–2690. [CrossRef]

14. Fan, Y.; Wang, W.; Song, W.; Chen, H.; Teng, A.; Liu, A. Partial characterization and anti-tumor activity of an acidic polysaccharide from Gracilaria lemaneiformis. *Carbohydr. Polym.* **2012**, *88*, 1313–1318. [CrossRef]

15. Li, P.; Ying, J.; Chang, Q.; Zhu, W.; Yang, G.; Xu, T.; Yi, H.; Pan, R.; Zhang, E.; Zeng, X.; et al. Effects of phycoerythrin from Gracilaria lemaneiformis in proliferation and apoptosis of SW480 cells. *Oncol. Rep.* **2016**, *36*, 3536–3544. [CrossRef] [PubMed]

16. Jin, M.; Liu, H.; Hou, Y.; Chan, Z.; Di, W.; Li, L.; Zeng, R. Preparation, characterization and alcoholic liver injury protective effects of algal oligosaccharides from Gracilaria lemaneiformis. *Food Res. Int.* **2017**, *100*, 186–195. [CrossRef] [PubMed]

17. Ren, Y.; Zheng, G.; You, L.; Wen, L.; Li, C.; Fu, X.; Zhou, L. Structural characterization and macrophage immunomodulatory activity of a polysaccharide isolated from Gracilaria lemaneiformis. *J. Funct. Foods* **2017**, *33*, 286–296. [CrossRef]

18. Wen, L.; Zhang, Y.; Sun-Waterhouse, D.; You, L.; Fu, X. Advantages of the polysaccharides from Gracilaria lemaneiformis over metformin in antidiabetic effects on streptozotocin-induced diabetic mice. *RSC Adv.* **2017**, *7*, 9141–9151. [CrossRef]

19. Yuan, S.; Duan, Z.; Lu, Y.; Ma, X.; Wang, S. Optimization of decolorization process in agar production from Gracilaria lemaneiformis and evaluation of antioxidant activities of the extract rich in natural pigments. *Biotech.* **2018**, *8*, 8. [CrossRef] [PubMed]

20. Beaulieu, L.; Bondu, S.; Doiron, K.; Rioux, L.; Turgeon, S.L. Characterization of antibacterial activity from protein hydrolysates of the macroalga Saccharina longicruris and identification of peptides implied in bioactivity. *J. Funct. Foods* **2015**, *17*, 685–697. [CrossRef]

21. Beaulieu, L.; Sirois, M.; Tamigneaux, É. Evaluation of the in vitro biological activity of protein hydrolysates of the edible red alga, Palmaria palmata (dulse) harvested from the Gaspe coast and cultivated in tanks. *J. Appl. Phycol.* **2016**, *28*, 3101–3115. [CrossRef]

22. Cian, R.E.; Garzón, A.G.; Ancona, D.B.; Guerrero, L.C.; Drago, S.R. Hydrolyzates from Pyropia columbina seaweed have antiplatelet aggregation, antioxidant and ACE I inhibitory peptides which maintain bioactivity after simulated gastrointestinal digestion. *LWT Food Sci. Technol.* **2015**, *64*, 881–888. [CrossRef]

23. Pan, S.; Wang, S.; Jing, L.; Yao, D. Purification and characterisation of a novel angiotensin-I converting enzyme (ACE)-inhibitory peptide derived from the enzymatic hydrolysate of Enteromorpha clathrata protein. *Food Chem.* **2016**, *211*, 423–430. [CrossRef] [PubMed]

24. Paiva, L.; Lima, E.; Neto, A.I.; Baptista, J. Isolation and characterization of angiotensin I-converting enzyme (ACE) inhibitory peptides from *Ulva rigida* C. Agardh protein hydrolysate. *J. Funct. Foods* **2016**, *26*, 65–76. [CrossRef]

25. Xie, J.; Chen, X.; Wu, J.; Zhang, Y.; Zhou, Y.; Zhang, L.; Tang, Y.; Wei, D. Antihypertensive Effects, Molecular Docking Study, and Isothermal Titration Calorimetry Assay of Angiotensin I-Converting Enzyme Inhibitory Peptides from Chlorella vulgaris. *J. Agric. Food Chem.* **2018**, *66*, 1359–1368. [CrossRef] [PubMed]

26. Qu, W.; Ma, H.; Li, W.; Pan, Z.; Owusu, J.; Venkitasamy, C. Performance of coupled enzymatic hydrolysis and membrane separation bioreactor for antihypertensive peptides production from Porphyra yezoensis protein. *Process Biochem.* **2015**, *50*, 245–252. [CrossRef]

27. Li, H.; Aluko, R.E. Kinetics of the inhibition of calcium/calmodulin-dependent protein kinase II by pea protein-derived peptides. *J. Nutr. Biochem.* **2005**, *16*, 656–662. [CrossRef] [PubMed]

28. Wu, Q.; Jia, J.; Yan, H.; Du, J.; Gui, Z. A novel angiotensin-capital I, Ukrainian converting enzyme (ACE) inhibitory peptide from gastrointestinal protease hydrolysate of silkworm pupa (Bombyx mori) protein: Biochemical characterization and molecular docking study. *Peptides* **2015**, *68*, 17–24. [CrossRef] [PubMed]

29. Rohit, A.C.; Sathisha, K.; Aparna, H.S. A variant peptide of buffalo colostrum beta-lactoglobulin inhibits angiotensin I-converting enzyme activity. *Eur. J. Med. Chem.* **2012**, *53*, 211–219. [CrossRef] [PubMed]

30. Furuta, T.; Miyabe, Y.; Yasui, H.; Kinoshita, Y.; Kishimura, H. Angiotensin I Converting Enzyme Inhibitory Peptides Derived from Phycobiliproteins of Dulse Palmaria palmata. *Mar. Drugs* **2016**, *14*, 32. [CrossRef] [PubMed]

31. Cao, D.; Lv, X.; Xu, X.; Yu, H.; Sun, X.; Xu, N. Purification and identification of a novel ACE inhibitory peptide from marine alga Gracilariopsis lemaneiformis protein hydrolysate. *Eur. Food Res. Technol.* **2017**, *243*, 1829–1837. [CrossRef]

32. Guo, M.; Chen, X.; Wu, Y.; Zhang, L.; Huang, W.; Yuan, Y.; Fang, M.; Xie, J.; Wei, D. Angiotensin I-converting enzyme inhibitory peptides from Sipuncula (*Phascolosoma esculenta*): Purification, identification, molecular docking and antihypertensive effects on spontaneously hypertensive rats. *Process Biochem.* **2017**, *63*, 84–95. [CrossRef]

33. Maruyama, S.; Mitachi, H.; Awaya, J.; Kurono, M.; Tomizuka, N.; Suzuki, H. Angiotensin I-Converting Enzyme Inhibitory Activity of the C-Terminal Hexapeptide of αs1-Casein. *Agric. Biol. Chem. Tokyo* **1987**, *51*, 2557–2561. [CrossRef]

34. Escudero, E.; Mora, L.; Toldrá, F. Stability of ACE inhibitory ham peptides against heat treatment and in vitro digestion. *Food Chem.* **2014**, *161*, 305–311. [CrossRef] [PubMed]

35. Tagliazucchi, D.; Martini, S.; Shamsia, S.; Helal, A.; Conte, A. Biological activities and peptidomic profile of invitro-digested cow, camel, goat and sheep milk. *Int. Dairy J.* **2018**, *81*, 19–27. [CrossRef]

36. Maeno, M.; Yamamoto, N.; Takano, T. Identification of an antihypertensive peptide from casein hydrolysate produced by a proteinase from Lactobacillus helveticus CP790. *J. Dairy Sci.* **1996**, *79*, 1316–1321. [CrossRef]

37. Kuba, M.; Tanaka, K.; Tawata, S.; Takeda, Y.; Yasuda, M. Angiotensin I-converting enzyme inhibitory peptides isolated from tofuyo fermented soybean food. *Biosci. Biotechnol. Biochem.* **2003**, *67*, 1278–1283. [CrossRef] [PubMed]

38. Liu, C.; Fang, L.; Min, W.; Liu, J.; Li, H. Exploration of the molecular interactions between angiotensin-I-converting enzyme (ACE) and the inhibitory peptides derived from hazelnut (*Corylus heterophylla* Fisch.). *Food Chem.* **2018**, *245*, 471–480. [CrossRef] [PubMed]
39. Balti, R.; Bougatef, A.; Sila, A.; Guillochon, D.; Dhulster, P.; Nedjar-Arroume, N. Nine novel angiotensin I-converting enzyme (ACE) inhibitory peptides from cuttlefish (Sepia officinalis) muscle protein hydrolysates and antihypertensive effect of the potent active peptide in spontaneously hypertensive rats. *Food Chem.* **2015**, *170*, 519–525. [CrossRef] [PubMed]
40. Khan, M.T.H.; Dedachi, K.; Matsui, T.; Kurita, N.; Borgatti, M.; Gambari, R.; Sylte, I. Dipeptide Inhibitors of Thermolysin and Angiotensin I-Converting Enzyme. *Curr. Top. Med. Chem.* **2012**, *12*, 1748–1762. [CrossRef] [PubMed]
41. Wu, Q.; Du, J.; Jia, J.; Kuang, C. Production of ACE inhibitory peptides from sweet sorghum grain protein using alcalase: Hydrolysis kinetic, purification and molecular docking study. *Food Chem.* **2016**, *199*, 140–149. [CrossRef] [PubMed]
42. Kuramoto, S.; Kaneyoshi, G.; Morinaga, Y.; Matsue, H.; Iwai, K. Angiotensin-Converting enzyme-Inhibitory peptides isolated from pepsin hydrolyzate of apios americana tuber and their hypotensive effects in spontaneously hypertensive rats. *Food Sci. Technol. Res.* **2013**, *19*, 399–407. [CrossRef]
43. Duan, X.; Wu, F.; Li, M.; Yang, N.; Wu, C.; Jin, Y.; Yang, J.; Jin, Z.; Xu, X. Naturally occurring angiotensin I-Converting enzyme inhibitory peptide from a fertilized egg and its inhibitory mechanism. *J. Agric. Food Chem.* **2014**, *62*, 5500–5506. [CrossRef] [PubMed]
44. Liu, X.; Zhang, M.; Jia, A.; Zhang, Y.; Zhu, H.; Zhang, C.; Sun, Z.; Liu, C. Purification and characterization of angiotensin I converting enzyme inhibitory peptides from jellyfish Rhopilema esculentum. *Food Res. Int.* **2013**, *50*, 339–343. [CrossRef]
45. Lin, K.; Zhang, L.; Han, X.; Meng, Z.; Wu, Y.; Zhang, J.; Cheng, D. Quantitative Structure-Activity Relationship Modeling Coupled with Molecular Docking Analysis in Screening of Angiotensin I-Converting Enzyme Inhibitory Peptides from Qula Casein Hydrolysates Obtained by Two-Enzyme Combination Hydrolysis. *J. Agric. Food Chem.* **2018**, *66*, 3221–3228. [CrossRef] [PubMed]
46. Wu, H.; He, H.; Chen, X.; Sun, C.; Zhang, Y.; Zhou, B. Purification and identification of novel angiotensin-I-converting enzyme inhibitory peptides from shark meat hydrolysate. *Process Biochem.* **2008**, *43*, 457–461. [CrossRef]
47. Marambe, H.K.; Shand, P.J.; Wanasundara, J.P.D. Release of angiotensin I-converting enzyme inhibitory peptides from flaxseed (*Linum usitatissimum* L.) protein under simulated gastrointestinal digestion. *J. Agric. Food Chem.* **2011**, *57*, 9596–9604. [CrossRef] [PubMed]
48. Salampessy, J.; Reddy, N.; Phillips, M.; Kailasapathy, K. Isolation and characterization of nutraceutically potential ACE-Inhibitory peptides from leatherjacket (Meuchenia sp.) protein hydrolysates. *LWT-Food. Sci. Technol.* **2017**, *80*, 430–436. [CrossRef]
49. Fujita, H.; Yoshikawa, M. LKPNM: A prodrug-type ACE-inhibitory peptide derived from fish protein. *Immunopharmacology* **1999**, *44*, 123–127. [CrossRef]

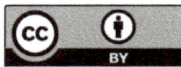

marine drugs

MDPI

Article

Analgesic Activity of Acid-Sensing Ion Channel 3 (ASIC3) Inhibitors: Sea Anemones Peptides Ugr9-1 and APETx2 versus Low Molecular Weight Compounds

Yaroslav A. Andreev [1,2,†], **Dmitry I. Osmakov** [1,2,†], **Sergey G. Koshelev** [1], **Ekaterina E. Maleeva** [1], **Yulia A. Logashina** [1,2], **Victor A. Palikov** [3], **Yulia A. Palikova** [3], **Igor A. Dyachenko** [3] and **Sergey A. Kozlov** [1,*]

[1] Shemyakin-Ovchinnikov Institute of Bioorganic Chemistry, Russian Academy of Sciences, ul. Miklukho-Maklaya 16/10, 117997 Moscow, Russia; yaroslav.andreev@yahoo.com (Y.A.A.); osmadim@gmail.com (D.I.O.); sknew@yandex.ru (S.G.K.); katerina@1ns.ru (E.E.M.); yulia.logashina@gmail.com (Y.A.L.)

[2] Institute of Molecular Medicine, Sechenov First Moscow State Medical University, Trubetskaya str. 8, bld. 2, Moscow 119991, Russia

[3] Branch of the Shemyakin-Ovchinnikov Institute of Bioorganic Chemistry, Russian Academy of Sciences, 6 Nauki Avenue, 142290 Pushchino, Russia; viktorpalikov@mail.ru (V.A.P.); ulia2791@rambler.ru (Y.A.P.); dyachenko@bibch.ru (I.A.D.)

* Correspondence: serg@ibch.ru; Tel.: +7-495-336-40-22

† These authors contributed equally to this work.

Received: 28 September 2018; Accepted: 10 December 2018; Published: 12 December 2018

Abstract: Acid-sensing ion channel 3 (ASIC3) makes an important contribution to the development and maintenance of inflammatory and acid-induced pain. We compared different ASIC3 inhibitors (peptides from sea anemones (APETx2 and Ugr9-1) and nonpeptide molecules (sevanol and diclofenac)) in anti-inflammatory action and analgesic effects. All tested compounds had distinct effects on pH-induced ASIC3 current. APETx2 inhibited only transient current, whereas Ugr9-1 and sevanol decreased transient and sustained components of the current. The effect on mice was evaluated after administering an intramuscular injection in the acetic acid writhing pain model and the complete Freund's adjuvant-induced thermal hyperalgesia/inflammation test. The bell-shaped dependence of the analgesic effect was observed for APETx2 in the acetic acid-induced writhing test, as well as for sevanol and peptide Ugr9-1 in the thermal hyperalgesia test. This dependence could be evidence of the nonspecific action of compounds in high doses. Compounds reducing both components of ASIC3 current produced more significant pain relief than APETx2, which is an effective inhibitor of a transient current only. Therefore, the comparison of the efficacy of ASIC3 inhibitors revealed the importance of ASIC3-sustained currents' inhibition for promotion of acidosis-related pain relief.

Keywords: acid-sensing ion channel; animal models; pain relief; toxin; Ugr 9-1; APETx2

---

1. Introduction

Different types of cells use special molecular sensors on the membrane to detect extracellular pH. The most specialized sensors of the concentration of protons are members of the degenerin-epithelial Na^+-channel family called acid-sensing ion channels (ASICs) [1]. Four genes (ACCN1-4) encode at least six splice variants of ASIC subunits: ASIC1a, $-1b$, $-2a$, 2b, -3, and -4 [2]. In the central nervous system (CNS), they are involved in monitoring of extracellular pH levels during normal neuronal activity and in the development of pathological processes upon stressful conditions. For example, hypoxia of the brain results in increased glycolysis following an accumulation of lactic acid and acidosis that leads to neuronal cell death. The ASIC1a inhibitors produce a neuroprotective effect in the ischemia model caused by hypoxia in mice [3]. During peripheral inflammation, expression levels of ASIC1a and −2a isoforms were increased in the rat spinal dorsal horn [4]. The potential role for ASICs in the pathogenesis of Parkinson's disease was shown on the 1-methyl-4-phenyl-1, 2, 3, 6-tetrahydropyridine mouse model [5] but further this data were controverted [6].

In the peripheral nervous system and in the tissues of internal organs, ASICs are responsible for the sensitivity to tissue acidosis, cardiac ischemia, corneal damage, inflammation, and local infections [7,8]. ASIC3 channels are mainly represented in the peripheral nervous system, especially in dorsal root ganglion (DRG) neurons [9–11], and inhibition of activity of these channels by the selective ligands is considered to be a promising tool for pain relief [12].

An inhibition of ASIC3 was reported to be an attractive approach to producing analgesia. A diuretic agent amiloride, a nonspecific blocker of sodium channels, is one of the most well-known molecules possessing a nonspecific inhibitory effect on ASICs [13]. Other nonspecific substances can also influence ASIC3 activity. Nonsteroidal anti-inflammatory drugs, salicylic acid, and diclofenac were found to inhibit ASICs currents directly on sensory neurons and heterologous-expressed ASIC3 channels [14]. The local anaesthetic tetracaine was found to inhibit the transient ASIC3 currents in a concentration-dependent manner with dependence arising from the extracellular pH value. In addition to ASIC3, tetracaine inhibited the ASIC1a and ASIC1b currents [15]. A small-molecule inhibitor, A-317567, blocked ASIC3's sustained and transient currents and produced an analgesic effect in an inflammatory thermal hyperalgesia model induced by complete Freund's adjuvant (CFA) in rats [16].

Natural ASIC3 inhibitors were found to produce analgesia in different animal models of pain. Levo-tetrahydropalmatine (l-THP), a bioactive compound from Chinese herbs of the genera *Stephania* and *Corydalis*, decreased the amplitude of proton-gated currents in DRG neurons and inhibited the nociceptive response to intraplantar acetic acid injections in rats [17]. A natural coumarin derivative osthol was reported to block voltage-gated Na^+-channels and inhibit ASIC3 [18]. Sevanol from thyme inhibited the amplitude of transient and sustained ASIC3 currents and exhibited pronounced analgesic and anti-inflammatory activity in mice at doses of 1–10 mg/kg [19].

Peptide antagonists of ASIC3 channels were isolated from the venom of sea anemones; that is, the toxin APETx2, its close structural homologue Hcr1b-1, and peptide Ugr9-1 [20–22]. APETx2 was shown to inhibit the transient component of ASIC3 current and produce potent analgesic effects in several models of pain on rats (acid-induced muscle pain, peripheral inflammatory pain, and postoperative pain) [23–25]. Ugr9-1 was shown to inhibit both components of the ASIC3 current and demonstrated a significant analgesic effect in vivo at 0.1–0.5 mg/kg doses [22,26].

To date, many reports support the direct correlation between ASIC3 activation and inflammatory pain. Here, for the first time, we compare the activity of ASIC3 inhibitors in vitro and in vivo under the same conditions. For this purpose, we selected four compounds that act differently on ASIC3 channels: peptide APETx2 inhibiting only a transient component of the current; peptide Ugr9-1 acting on both components of the current; low-molecular weight compound sevanol, which inhibits two components of the current; and diclofenac, a potent nonsteroidal anti-inflammatory drug, as a positive control of analgesic effects and an inhibitor of the sustained component of the current. The comparison of ASIC3-selective ligands in different animal pain models provides an opportunity to estimate their pharmacological potential and specify the properties of the most attractive compound for drug development.

2. Results

2.1. Whole Cell Electrophysiology

The activity of ligands was checked on human ASIC3 (hASIC3) channels expressed in *Xenopus laevis* oocytes. Sevanol, diclofenac, and two recombinant analogues of peptides (APETx2 and Ugr9-1) were analysed. Two different protocols were used to reveal the effects of ligands on sustained and transient components of acid-induced hASIC3 currents. The influence of the compounds on the transient current amplitude was estimated after preincubation for 15 s before the activation in a low alkali bath solution (pH 7.8), which ensured an absence of steady-state desensitization for the transient current [27] (Figure 1A). The compounds' inhibition effectiveness was calculated using the value of maximal amplitudes. As expected from previous reports, the APETx2 toxin was the most effective inhibitor of the transient current (Figure 1C). The peptide Ugr9-1 also completely blocked the transient current of ASIC3, but in 30-times greater concentration. Nonpeptide ligand sevanol had much less potency and inhibited transient currents in submillimolar concentrations. Thus, both peptides and sevanol inhibited dose-dependent transient currents at pH 7.8, and the complete inhibition was observed for all of them. The inhibitory effect was concentration-dependent and fit well using a logistic equation. The estimated IC_{50} and Hill coefficient (n_H) values are summarized in Table 1. The inhibition of transient current by diclofenac was not detected.

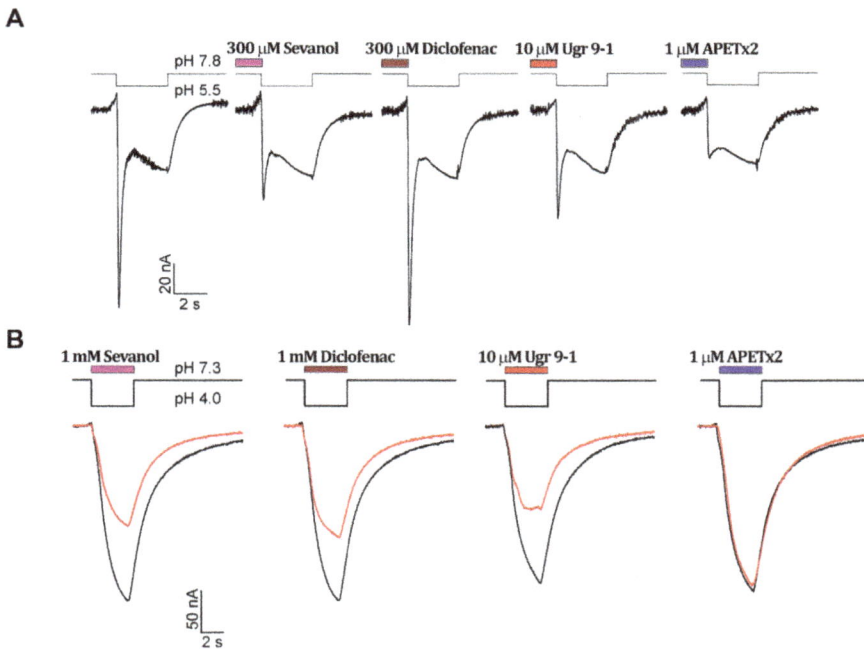

Figure 1. *Cont.*

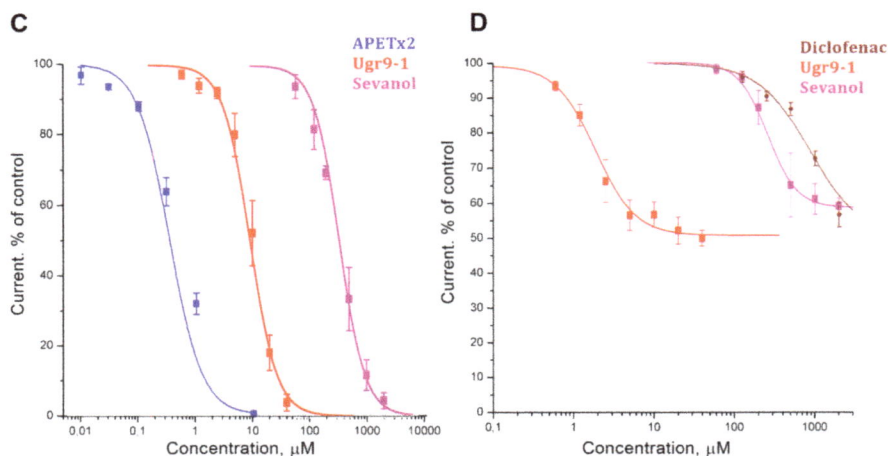

Figure 1. Comparison of ligands' antagonistic effects on hASIC3 channels. Whole-cell currents were induced by pH drops and recorded at the holding potential −50 mV. (**A**) Effect of ligands on the transient component of current at conditioning pH 7.8. The control trace is shown first; (**B**) Effect of ligands on the sustained component at conditioning pH 7.3. The black line is the control trace, and the red line is the trace of activation in the presence of a ligand. Dose-response curves for transient (**C**) and sustained (**D**) currents' inhibitions are shown. Data are shown as mean ± SEM (n = 4–6) and fitted with the logistic equation (solid lines).

Table 1. Inhibition potency of hASIC3 antagonists.

Antagonist	Transient Currents		Sustained Currents	
	IC$_{50}$ (µM)	Hill Coefficient	IC$_{50}$ (µM)	Hill Coefficient
APETx2	0.344 ± 0.080	1.5 ± 0.2	-	-
Ugr 9-1	9.1 ± 0.9	1.86 ± 0.16	1.88 ± 0.36	1.74 ± 0.51
sevanol	331 ± 21	1.98 ± 0.24	259 ± 39	2.4 ± 0.4
diclofenac	-	-	856 ± 106	1.35 ± 0.21

The analysis of a sustained component of the current was carried out in a bath solution (pH 7.3) where the transient component of the current was completely desensitized by protons [27]. The pH activation stimulus (3.5 s) was applied in the presence of the testing compound (Figure 1B). APETx2 did not inhibit the sustained current as reported earlier [20]. Sevanol and diclofenac were significantly weaker in their inhibitory potency when compared to peptide toxin Ugr9-1 (Figure 1D, Table 1). The sustained current amplitude was not completely blocked by any of the applied antagonists. The saturation concentrations of ligands (about 3 mM for sevanol and diclofenac and 50 µM for Ugr9-1) inhibited approximately 50% of the sustained current amplitude. The inhibitory effect was concentration-dependent, and the calculated IC$_{50}$ and n_H values are summarized in Table 1.

Thus, we evaluated and generally confirmed the pharmacological properties of the compounds inhibiting ASIC3. Tested compounds differ in their abilities to inhibit transient and sustained current components and have activity in broad ranges of concentrations (IC$_{50}$ range 0.3–300 µM for a transient current and 1–800 µM for a sustained current).

2.2. Open Field Test

An open field test was carried out on mice to estimate the possible sedative effects of compounds administration. No statistically significant changes were detected between ASIC3 antagonist-treated groups and the control animals group in 5-min observations of 12 parameters. Animals treated with APETx2, Ugr9-1, and sevanol had a greater travelled distance, a less percentage of time spent freezing (Figure 2A,B) and less travelling distance in the central area, but each of these differences was nonsignificant. Thus, the compounds did not impair locomotion, and the CNS-mediated behaviour and, most likely, their analgesic effects are the result of direct action on peripheral nociceptors.

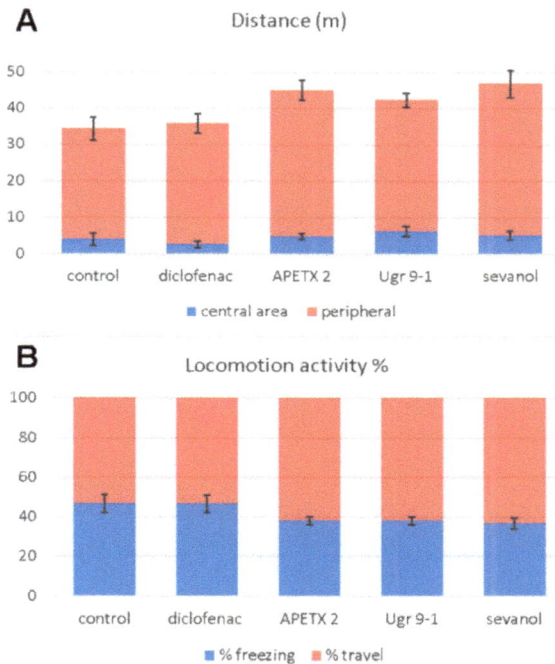

Figure 2. Open field experiments on mice. Administration of compounds at a 1 mg/kg dose intramuscularly was done 4 h before of the measurements. (**A**) Travelling distance and (**B**) locomotion activity presented as mean ± SEM for 5-min recording period ($n = 6$–7).

2.3. Acetic Acid-Induced Writhing

Acetic acid-induced writhing is based on irritation of tissues and organs of the abdomen by low pH and could be considered the most appropriate test for influence on acid-induced pain. The dose of 1 mg/kg of all testing compounds was able to reduce the number of writhes significantly and had no influence on the latency time of the first response (Figure 3A). A dose-dependent analysis revealed a bell-shaped profile of APETx2 activity. The APETx2 toxin was surprisingly much less effective at 1 mg/kg than at 0.2 mg/kg dose (19% vs. 76%). The maximal effect was registered for Ugr9-1 at a 0.02 mg/kg dose (74% inhibition) and for APETx2 at a 0.2 mg/kg dose (76% inhibition) (Figure 3B,D). The plant lignan sevanol showed a linear dose dependence with a maximal effect at a 10 mg/kg dose (76% inhibition). It is interesting that the effects of sevanol and Ugr9-1 plateaued at a wide range of doses (0.01–1mg/kg for sevanol and 0.02–1 mg/kg Ugr9-1) (Figure 3C,D).

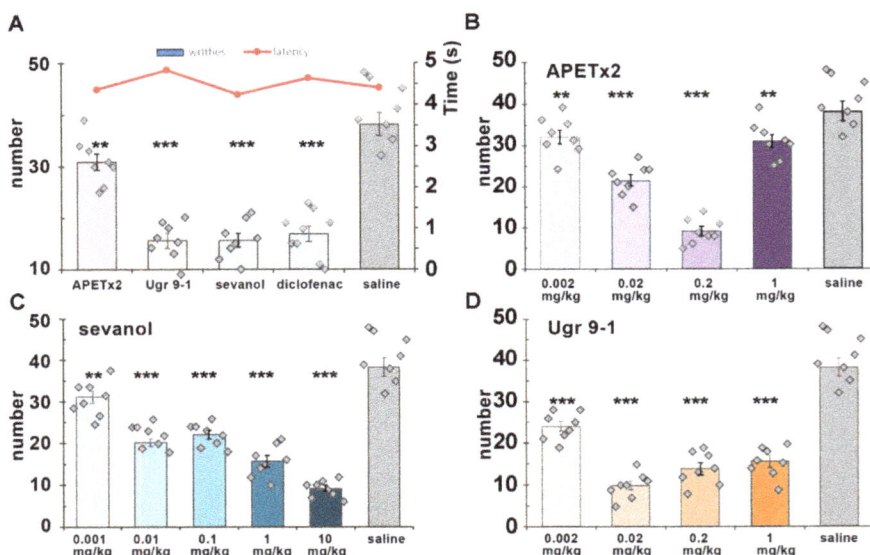

Figure 3. Effects of ligands in an acetic acid-induced writhing test. Pretreatment of mice with APETx2, sevanol, and Ugr9-1 (2 h before testing) attenuated the response to the intraperitoneal administration of acetic acid. (**A**) Efficacy of ASIC3 antagonists at a dose of 1 mg/kg. (**B–D**) Dose-dependent chart of ligands' effects: APETx2 (**B**), sevanol (**C**), and Ugr9-1 (**D**). Results are presented as mean $\pm$ SEM ($n = 8$). ** $p < 0.01$, *** $p < 0.001$ versus saline group (ANOVA followed by a Tukey's test).

2.4. CFA-Induced Inflammation

CFA-induced thermal hyperalgesia is a result of different inflammatory pathways' action on thermal sensitivity of the paw. Injection of CFA into the hind paw provokes increased sensitivity to noxious mechanical and thermal stimuli together with swelling of the paw due to the inflammatory process. Diclofenac and APETx2 at 1 mg/kg doses showed equal potency in the reversal of thermal hyperalgesia, which exceeded the analgesic potency of sevanol and Ugr9-1 at the same dosage (Figure 4A). For APETx2 (Figure 4B), sevanol (Figure 4C), and Ugr9-1 (Figure 4D), the dose dependency of the analgesic effect was evaluated. The effect of APETx2 was dose-dependent with a minimal active dose of 0.02 mg/kg (47% of reversal), and the complete reversal of thermal hyperalgesia was reached at doses of more than 0.2 mg/kg. The effects of sevanol and Ugr9-1 were bell-shaped, so the reversal of thermal hyperalgesia for 1 mg/kg and 0.001–0.002 mg/kg doses did not differ significantly (Figure 4C,D). The maximal effect value for both samples was observed in doses of 0.01–0.02 mg/kg. Additionally, the effect of sevanol at 0.01 mg/kg and Ugr9-1 at 0.02 mg/kg was confirmed in the independent experiment (data not shown).

To reveal the anti-inflammatory effects of ASIC3 antagonists, paw oedema changes were also evaluated (Figure 5). Diclofenac, sevanol, and Ugr9-1 did not produce significant anti-inflammatory effects within 4 h after administration. APETx2 in a dose of 1 mg/kg reduced paw oedema by 16%, 24%, and 44% compared to the control group at 2, 4, and 24 h after administration, respectively. APETx2 at 0.2 mg/kg reduced inflammation by approximately 20% only 24 h after administration. Peptide Ugr9-1 (0.02 mg/kg) and sevanol (2.5 mg/kg) also reduced the inflammation process within 24 h by 31% and 22%, respectively.

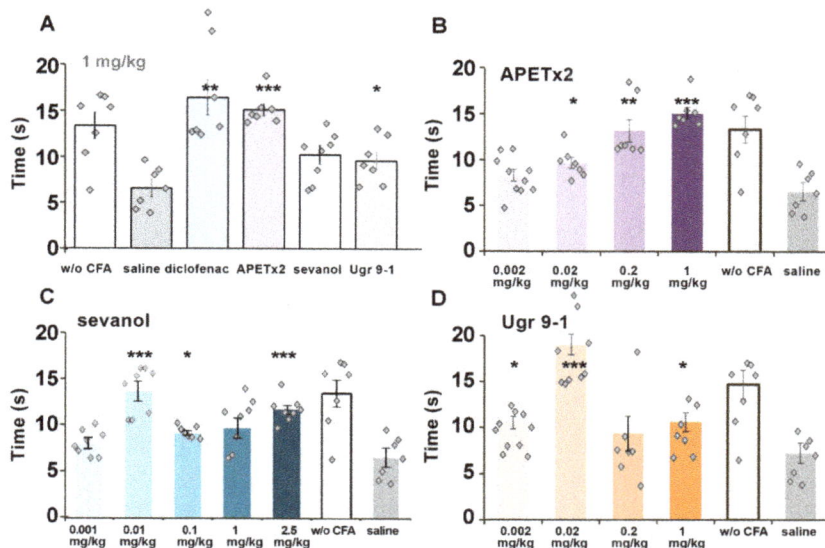

Figure 4. Effect of ligands on the CFA-induced thermal hyperalgesia test. Test was performed 2 h after intramuscular administration of ASIC3 antagonists. (**A**) Comparison between ligands at the dose of 1 mg/kg; (**B–D**) Dose-dependent chart of ligands' effect. APETx2 (**B**), sevanol (**C**), and Ugr9-1 (**D**) reversed CFA-induced thermal hyperalgesia and prolonging withdrawal latency of the inflamed hind paw on a hot plate. Results are presented as mean ± SEM (*n* = 7–8). * *p* < 0.05, ** *p* < 0.01, *** *p* < 0.001 versus saline group (ANOVA followed by a Tukey's test).

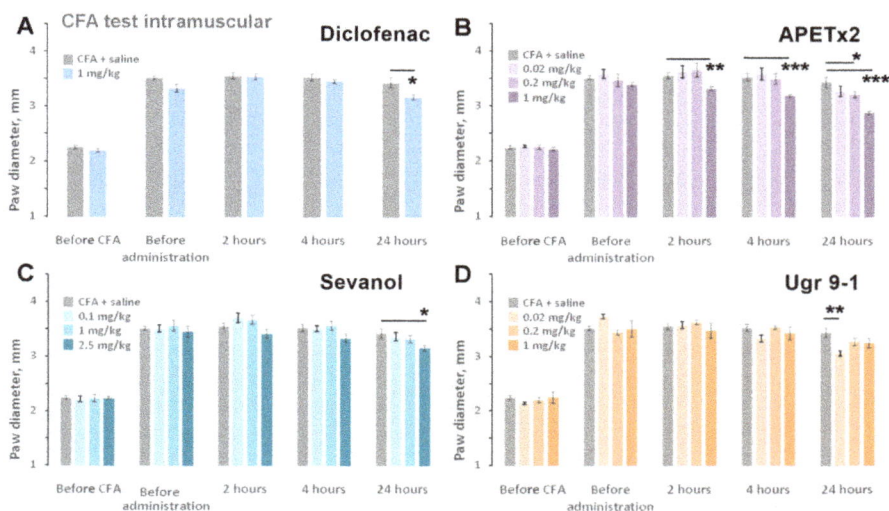

Figure 5. Anti-inflammatory effect of ligands. Paw oedema induced by CFA injection was estimated before the CFA and testing compounds administration and 2, 4, and 24 h after the intramuscular injection of diclofenac (**A**), APETx2 (**B**), sevanol (**C**), and Ugr9-1 (**D**). Results are presented as mean ± SEM (*n* = 7–8). * *p* < 0.05, ** *p* < 0.01, *** *p* < 0.001 versus saline group (ANOVA followed by a Tukey's test).

3. Discussion

ASIC3 channels play an important role in the perception and maintenance of pain signals in peripheral neurons. Several ligands with inhibitory properties were found for this receptor, each of which was able to induce analgesia in animal tests. The most well-known inhibitor APETx2 in various studies has been tested on models of acid-induced muscle pain model, CFA-induced inflammatory pain model (at doses of 0.07, 0.22 and 2.2 μM) [25]. Ugr9-1 was studied in models of CFA-induced thermal hyperalgesia and acetic acid writhing test (at doses of 0.5, 0.1, and 0.01 mg/kg) [22]. Sevanol was studied in CFA-induced thermal hyperalgesia and in response to intraperitoneal administration of acetic acid (at doses of 1 and 10 mg/kg) [19]. Diclofenac significantly reduced CFA-induced thermal hyperalgesia (100 mg/kg i.p.) [28] and inhibited acetic acid-induced writhing (20 mg/kg i.p.) [29]. Therefore, it was extremely interesting to compare these ligands together in the same pain models. A comparison between the antagonists acting on both components of the ASIC3 current and APETx2 inhibiting only the transient current was important for the understanding of their contributions to pain perception.

APETx2 is the most well-studied and well-known inhibitor of ASIC3 channels despite proven inhibitory activity on $Na_V 1.2$ ($IC_{50} \sim 113$ nM) and $Na_V 1.8$ channels ($IC_{50} \sim 55$ nM on *X. laevis* oocytes and ~ 2.6 μM on DRG neurones) [30,31] and the inhibition of hERG channels by reducing the maximal current amplitude and shifting the voltage dependence of activation to more positive potentials [32]. Moreover, APETx2 potentiates rat ASIC1b and ASIC2a at concentrations of 3–10 μM (30–100-fold higher than its ASIC3 inhibitory concentration), which may have implications for its use in in vivo experiments [33]. The possible cumulative effect on pain relief via ASICs and $Na_V 1.8$ channel inhibition increases the apparent efficacy, but masks the real significance of the acid-sensing pathway inhibition in behavioural tests. Moreover, potentiating ASIC1b most likely counteracts the antihyperalgesic effects produced by ASIC3 inhibition [33].

The importance of the ASIC3 channel in nociception was proven by using APETx2 in several animal models of pain. This toxin produced pain relief in bone, tooth, muscle, and skin pain as well as in gastric acidosis and gastric mucosal lesions, osteoarthritis inflammation, fibromyalgia-induced mechanical hyperalgesia, fatigue-enhanced hyperalgesia, and postoperative hyperalgesia [34–41].

Here, we found that in vitro APETx2 was significantly better (IC_{50} was 344 ± 80 nM) at inhibiting the transient current of hASIC3 than the other tested antagonists (Figure 1). The activity of recombinant APETx2 on hASIC3 in the oocyte system could be considered equipotent to the published data, where toxin inhibited human ASIC3 and rat ASIC3 expressed in COS cells (CV-1 (simian) in Origin, and carrying the SV40 genetic material) with the IC_{50} of 175 nM and 63 nM, respectively [20]. Peptide Ugr9-1 and sevanol had the same inhibitory effects as reported earlier [19,22]. Therefore, in vitro potency of compounds to inhibit the transient component of hASIC3 current could be ranged as APETx2 > Ugr9-1 > sevanol. The potency of sustained component inhibition was ranged as Ugr9-1 > sevanol > diclofenac.

Dose-response analysis was used to acquire a clear relationship between a dose and the extent of the response to it. However, in various tests diverse compounds showed so-called "bell-shaped" or "(inverse) U-shaped" dose response. The best example of this effect was the dose dependence of the analgesic effect of APETx2 in the acetic acid writhing test (Figure 3B). The analgesic effect evidently increased up to 75% at 0.2 mg/kg dose, whereas the peptide was significantly less effective at a 1 mg/kg. Many researchers have described this phenomenon [42,43]. This type of dose response was described for micronutrients, endocrine-disrupting chemicals, endogenous hormones, and other drugs.

Several possible mechanisms of this phenomenon were suggested: a high-dose induction of cytotoxicity; the activity of ligand on different receptors or receptors' states depending on concentration following the competition between multiple receptor pathways; and ligand-induced receptor down-regulation at high concentrations. Tested compounds were studied in electrophysiological experiments on *X. laevis* oocytes and Chinese hamster ovary (CHO) cells in various concentrations, and no cytolytic or cytotoxic effects were observed. Therefore, a high concentration of ASIC3 ligand is most likely the result of activity on other targets and/or an unfavourable breakdown of the ASIC3 signalling pathway (e.g., ligand-induced receptor down-regulation and compensation by other receptors). APETx2 at high concentrations is also able to potentiate ASIC1b, which is involved in peripheral nociception in rodents. Many examples demonstrate how positive modulation of the receptor could dramatically change the overall effect of the substance. Potentiation or weak activation of TRPA1 (pain receptor responsible for the detection of harmful chemicals) can surprisingly cause strong analgesia instead of pain [44–46]. Another example, potentiation of TRPV1 weak activation, gives sea anemone peptides APHC1 and APHC3 (inhibitors of TRPV1) an ability to decrease core body temperature in mice, whereas most of the other inhibitors of TRPV1 cause hyperthermia [47,48].

When the pain was induced by an acetic acid injection (acetic acid-induced writhing test), all of the ASIC3 antagonists, including diclofenac, showed high efficacy and the same maximal effect of reducing pain (~75%). The most stable effect was produced by Ugr9-1, and it was slightly more significant in lower doses (0.002 mg/kg). The efficacy of sevanol was also high. Despite the 1000-fold difference in efficacy in vitro with APETx2 and the 35-fold difference with Ugr9-1, sevanol produced an almost equipotent effect in vivo (molecular weight ratio APETx2/sevanol is 6.4 and Ugr9-1/sevanol is 4.4). However, sevanol is also able to inhibit ASIC1a [19] and produce additional analgesic effect. Blockade of ASIC1a in CNS by psalmotoxin 1 was reported to result in an activation of the endogenous enkephalin pathway and potent analgesic effects [49]. Therefore, it is better to compare the effectiveness of peptides Ugr9-1 and APETx2 for contributions of sustained and transient current in the perception of acid-induced pain in the peripheral nervous system. Peptides are usually unable to penetrate through the blood-brain barrier, therefore no CNS targets could be suspected in additional effects. Ugr9-1 had an effective dose 10-times less than APETx2 in acetic acid-induced writhing test pain, whereas it was much less effective (30 times) in inhibition of the transient component of ASIC3 current. Therefore, we can conclude that a sustained component can make a significant contribution to the development of acid-induced pain, and compounds that inhibit both components of ASIC3 channels are more effective for the treatment of acidosis-associated pain conditions.

In the acetic acid-induced writhing test, only APETx2 showed "U-shaped" dose response with maximal effect at 0.2 mg/kg dose. The decrease of effect at a high dose is most likely the result of conflict between inhibition of ASIC3 and enhanced activation of ASIC1b.

CFA-induced inflammation is a general model of inflammatory pain. The TRPV1 receptor is considered to play a leading role in thermal hyperalgesia induced by CFA [50], which could be modulated via other receptors including ASIC3 [51]. All ASIC3 antagonists were capable of completely reversing thermal hyperalgesia. The APETx2 peptide dose-dependently reversed thermal hyperalgesia and reached its maximal effect at 0.2 mg/kg, which corresponds well with previously reported results [24,25]. Despite a great number of described side targets, it is noteworthy that APETx2 showed standard dose response.

Sevanol and Ugr9-1 were more potent in reaching maximal effects in the hyperalgesia tests at doses of 0.01 and 0.02 mg/kg versus the 0.2 mg/kg dose for APETx2. In this test, sevanol and Ugr9-1 showed a nonlinear dose response. Sevanol was unexpectedly more active at a lower dose than peptide Ugr9-1, whereas the peptide showed better inhibition of ASIC3 in vitro. Several explanations could be proposed. First, the result of partial ASIC1a inhibition is unpredictable. Second, better bioavailability of sevanol compared with Ugr9-1 can enhance the effect. Peptides from sea anemones have rather short circulating half-lives (~0.5 h) after subcutaneous or intramuscular administration but could circulate in mammals' blood flow for a long time (over 72 h) before complete elimination [52,53]. It was proposed that the significant part of a peptide could be cleared out from blood by kidneys, whereas a small fraction distributes into some compartment from which the active peptide is released slowly into the blood stream [52]. The low molecular weight compound diclofenac has exponential decrease of concentration to zero with circulating half-life of about 2 h and finally eliminates from the blood flow at 10 h [54]. The stability of sevanol in blood was most likely greater than the rate of elimination/deponation of Ugr9-1. Therefore, a dose of 0.01 mg/kg of sevanol could produce the same analgesic effect in a CFA test as 0.02 mg/kg of Ugr9-1. The absence of the effect at doses 0.001 mg/kg and 0.002 mg/kg for sevanol and Ugr9-1 could be the result of the quick elimination of low doses of compounds.

Therefore, the inhibition of the sustained current should be considered as a major benefit providing effectiveness of sevanol and Ugr9-1 at low doses, but their efficacy significantly decreased at higher doses; the reasons for this remain unclear. The nonspecific actions on other cellular targets and the changes of ASIC3 involvement in the inflammatory process induced by the high antagonists' concentration for 2 h are suspected. We conclude that the inhibition of both components of ASIC3 currents could be beneficial but could be reversed by hormesis in high doses and during a long exposure to an ASIC3 antagonist. The efficacy and final effects of ASIC3 antagonists most likely depend on the route of administration and the time interval before testing. For example, when injected intravenously 30 min before testing, Ugr9-1 was clearly dose-dependent in the CFA thermal hyperalgesia test and showed less efficacy in the acetic writhing test (~50%) [22].

To date, various studies have shown the important role of the sustained component of ASIC3 in inflammatory conditions [24,55,56]. Because a significant qualitative difference between sevanol and Ugr-9-1 versus APETx2 is the inhibition of the sustained component, we have suggested that the more effective anti-inflammatory effect of sevanol and Ugr-9-1 may be a result of sustained component inhibition.

All of the tested compounds displayed poor anti-inflammatory activity. This is most likely because ASIC3 activation plays a significant role only in late phases of paw oedema development [57]. This is well correlated with the observed oedema reduction during the 24-h activity lag. The 1 mg/kg dose of APETx2 was effective 2 h after the injection; however, the effect could be associated with the inhibition of $Na_V1.2$ and 1.8 channels and not a direct action on ASIC3.

Finally, we can assume that all tested antagonists for ASIC3 showed high efficacy in animal models of pain, but could have bell-shaped dose response in some tests in vivo. The higher potency of APETx2 in inhibiting transient currents of ASIC3 gave no advantages in analgesic activity compared to sevanol and Ugr9-1 (inhibitors of both transient and sustained currents) as revealed in the two pain models (acetic acid-induced writhing test and thermal hyperalgesia). The reasons for the bell-shaped dose response of sevanol and Ugr9-1 remain unclear, but this effect should be taken into consideration while testing novel ASIC3 antagonists.

4. Materials and Methods

4.1. Ligands

Peptide Ugr9-1 was obtained by the production of a recombinant analogue in *Escherichia coli* (as described in [22]). Peptide APETx2 was also produced by the heterologous expression in *E. coli* [58]. Synthetic sevanol was obtained from the Laboratory of Biopharmaceutics of the Shemyakin-Ovchinnikov Institute of Bioorganic Chemistry of the Russian Academy of Sciences. Diclofenac was purchased from (Sigma-Aldrich, Moscow, Russia).

4.2. Electrophysiology

X. laevis oocytes were removed surgically and defolliculated by collagenase (Sigma-Aldrich, Moscow, Russia). Oocytes were injected with 2.5 to 10 ng of human ASIC3 cRNA (AF057711.1). The cRNA transcripts were synthesised from a NaeI-linearized ASIC3 cDNA template (pcDNA3.1+humanASIC3 subcloned from clone EX-Q0260- B02 (GeneCopoeia, Inc., Rockville, MD, USA) using a HiScribe T7 High Yield RNA Synthesis Kit (New England Biolabs, Ipswich, MA, USA) according to the manufacturer's protocol for capped transcripts. After the injection, oocytes were kept for 3 to 6 days at 19° in a ND-96 medium containing (in mM) 96 NaCl, 2 KCl, 1.8 $CaCl_2$, 1 $MgCl_2$, and 5 HEPES titrated to pH 7.4 with NaOH supplemented with gentamycin (50 μg/mL). Two-electrode voltage clamp recordings were performed using a GeneClamp 500 amplifier (Axon

Instruments, Union City, CA, USA), and the data were filtered at 20 Hz and digitized at 100 Hz by an AD converter L780 (LCard, Moscow, Russia) using in-house software. To induce transient and/or sustained currents, two different protocols with different conditioning pH were used. Microelectrodes were filled with a 3 M KCl solution. The working buffer solution was ND-96 titrated by NaOH to pH 7.8 or 7.3. The solution for the pH shift was constructed based on the ND-96 solution, in which 5 mM HEPES was replaced with 10 mM acetic acid (pH 4.0) or 10 mM MES (pH 5.5) in a supplementary 0.1% BSA solution. The duration of the activation pulses was 3.5 s.

4.3. Animals

Adult male CD-1 mice (Animal Breeding Facility Branch of Shemyakin-Ovchinnikov Institute of Bioorganic Chemistry, Russian Academy of Sciences, Pushchino, Russia) weighing 20–25 g were used. Animals that originally passed clinical examination that confirmed no deviations in health were divided into groups (at least eight male mice per group) using the principle of randomization. The average body weight of animals in each group was not statistically different between groups. Animals were housed at room temperature ($23 \pm 2\,^\circ$C) and subjected to a 12-h light-dark cycle with food and water available ad libitum. All experiments were performed after receiving approval from the Animal Care and Use Committee of the Branch of the Institute of Bioorganic Chemistry, Russian Academy of Sciences (IBCh RAS) (Pushchino, Russia Federation). The samples were administered intramuscularly 2 h before testing (4 h in the open field test). The initial dose of 1 mg/kg was investigated for all samples, which was further reduced 5, 50, and 500 times for peptides. In the case of sevanol as the least active molecule in vitro, this dose was not only reduced 10, 100, and 1000 times, but was increased to 2.5 or 10 mg/kg in some experiments.

4.3.1. CFA-Induced Thermal Hyperalgesia

CFA suspended in an oil/saline (1:1) emulsion was injected into the dorsal surfaces of the left hind paws of mice (20 µL/paw) 24 h before the samples' intramuscular injection. The control mice received 20 µL of saline (intraplantar). The paw withdrawal latencies to thermal stimulation (53 °C) were measured 2 h after the sample injection. The paw diameter was evaluated before the CFA injection, before the samples and saline administration, and 2, 4, and 24 h after the administration using a digital calliper.

4.3.2. Acetic Acid-Induced Writhing (Abdominal Constriction Test of Visceral Pain)

Separate groups of mice were used. Writhes were caused 2 h after the intramuscular injection of the samples (saline for control mice) with the injection of 0.6% acetic acid in saline (10 mL/kg intraperitoneally). Mice were immediately placed inside transparent glass cylinders, and the latency of a first writhe and the number of writhes were recorded for 15 min.

4.3.3. Open Field Test

In the locomotion measurements, exploration and anxiety were evaluated in the motor activity test on a computerized TSE Multi Conditioning System (TSE Systems GmbH, Bad Homburg, Germany). Four hours after the administration of the sample, the measurement was made, which lasted for 3 min. The animal watching TSE AatiMot programme (TSE Systems GmbH, Bad Homburg, Germany) was used to collect and analyse the control parameters.

4.4. Data Analysis

The analysis of the electrophysiological data was performed using the OriginPro 8.6 programme. The four parameter logistic equation was used for concentration–response curves: $F(x) = ((a1 - a2)/(1 + (x/x0)n)) + a2$, where x is the concentration of sample; $F(x)$ is the response value at given sample concentration; a1 is the control response value (fixed at 100%); x0 is the IC_{50} value; n is the Hill coefficient (slope factor); and a2 is the response value at maximal inhibition (percent of control).

The data significance in animal tests was determined by an analysis of variance followed by a Tukey's test. Data are presented as the mean $\pm$ SEM.

Author Contributions: Conceptualization, Y.A.A. and S.A.K.; Methodology, D.I.O., S.G.K., I.A.D. and Y.A.A.; Experimentation, D.I.O., S.G.K., E.E.M., Y.A.L., V.A.P., Y.A.P. and I.A.D.; Data analysis D.I.O., S.G.K., Y.A.A. and S.A.K.; Writing-Original Draft, Y.A.A., D.I.O. and S.A.K.; Writing-Review & Editing, S.A.K., and Y.A.A.; Supervision, S.A.K.

Funding: This research was funded by Russian Science Foundation, grant No. 18-14-00138.

Acknowledgments: This article is dedicated to the memory of Eugene V. Grishin, without whose guidance this work would be impossible.

Conflicts of Interest: The authors declare no conflict of interest.

References

1. García-Añoveros, J.; Derfler, B.; Neville-Golden, J.; Hyman, B.T.; Corey, D.P. BNaC1 and BNaC2 constitute a new family of human neuronal sodium channels related to degenerins and epithelial sodium channels. *Proc. Natl. Acad. Sci. USA* **1997**, *94*, 1459–1464. [CrossRef] [PubMed]

2. Kellenberger, S.; Schild, L. International Union of Basic and Clinical Pharmacology. XCI. Structure, Function, and Pharmacology of Acid-Sensing Ion Channels and the Epithelial Na+ Channel. *Pharmacol. Rev.* **2015**, *67*, 1–35. [CrossRef] [PubMed]

3. Xiong, Z.-G.; Zhu, X.-M.; Chu, X.-P.; Minami, M.; Hey, J.; Wei, W.-L.; MacDonald, J.F.; Wemmie, J.A.; Price, M.P.; Welsh, M.J.; et al. Neuroprotection in ischemia: Blocking calcium-permeable acid-sensing ion channels. *Cell* **2004**, *118*, 687–698. [CrossRef] [PubMed]

4. Duan, B.; Wu, L.-J.; Yu, Y.-Q.; Ding, Y.; Jing, L.; Xu, L.; Chen, J.; Xu, T.-L. Upregulation of acid-sensing ion channel ASIC1a in spinal dorsal horn neurons contributes to inflammatory pain hypersensitivity. *J. Neurosci.* **2007**, *27*, 11139–11148. [CrossRef] [PubMed]

5. Arias, R.L.; Sung, M.-L.A.; Vasylyev, D.; Zhang, M.-Y.; Albinson, K.; Kubek, K.; Kagan, N.; Beyer, C.; Lin, Q.; Dwyer, J.M.; et al. Amiloride is neuroprotective in an MPTP model of Parkinson's disease. *Neurobiol. Dis.* **2008**, *31*, 334–341. [CrossRef] [PubMed]

6. Komnig, D.; Imgrund, S.; Reich, A.; Gründer, S.; Falkenburger, B.H. ASIC1a Deficient Mice Show Unaltered Neurodegeneration in the Subacute MPTP Model of Parkinson Disease. *PLoS ONE* **2016**, *11*, e0165235. [CrossRef] [PubMed]

7. Deval, E.; Lingueglia, E. Acid-Sensing Ion Channels and nociception in the peripheral and central nervous systems. *Neuropharmacology* **2015**, *94*, 49–57. [CrossRef]

8. Osmakov, D.I.; Andreev, Y.A.; Kozlov, S.A. Acid-sensing ion channels and their modulators. *Biochemistry* **2014**, *79*, 1528–1545. [CrossRef]

9. Babinski, K.; Lê, K.T.; Séguéla, P. Molecular cloning and regional distribution of a human proton receptor subunit with biphasic functional properties. *J. Neurochem.* **1999**, *72*, 51–57. [CrossRef]

10. Price, M.P.; McIlwrath, S.L.; Xie, J.; Cheng, C.; Qiao, J.; Tarr, D.E.; Sluka, K.A.; Brennan, T.J.; Lewin, G.R.; Welsh, M.J. The DRASIC cation channel contributes to the detection of cutaneous touch and acid stimuli in mice. *Neuron* **2001**, *32*, 1071–1083. [CrossRef]

11. Sluka, K.A.; Price, M.P.; Breese, N.M.; Stucky, C.L.; Wemmie, J.A.; Welsh, M.J. Chronic hyperalgesia induced by repeated acid injections in muscle is abolished by the loss of ASIC3, but not ASIC1. *Pain* **2003**, *106*, 229–239. [CrossRef]

12. Andreev, Y.A.; Vassilevski, A.A.; Kozlov, S.A. Molecules to selectively target receptors for treatment of pain and neurogenic inflammation. *Recent Pat Inflamm. Allergy Drug Discov.* **2012**, *6*, 35–45. [CrossRef] [PubMed]

13. Waldmann, R.; Bassilana, F.; de Weille, J.; Champigny, G.; Heurteaux, C.; Lazdunski, M. Molecular cloning of a non-inactivating proton-gated Na+ channel specific for sensory neurons. *J. Biol. Chem.* **1997**, *272*, 20975–20978. [CrossRef] [PubMed]

14. Voilley, N.; de Weille, J.; Mamet, J.; Lazdunski, M. Nonsteroid anti-inflammatory drugs inhibit both the activity and the inflammation-induced expression of acid-sensing ion channels in nociceptors. *J. Neurosci.* **2001**, *21*, 8026–8033. [CrossRef] [PubMed]

15. Leng, T.; Lin, J.; Cottrell, J.E.; Xiong, Z.-G. Subunit and Frequency-Dependent Inhibition of Acid Sensing Ion Channels by Local Anesthetic Tetracaine. *Mol. Pain* **2013**, *9*, 27. [CrossRef] [PubMed]

16. Dubé, G.R.; Lehto, S.G.; Breese, N.M.; Baker, S.J.; Wang, X.; Matulenko, M.A.; Honoré, P.; Stewart, A.O.; Moreland, R.B.; Brioni, J.D. Electrophysiological and in vivo characterization of A-317567, a novel blocker of acid sensing ion channels. *Pain* **2005**, *117*, 88–96. [CrossRef]

17. Liu, T.-T.; Qu, Z.-W.; Qiu, C.-Y.; Qiu, F.; Ren, C.; Gan, X.; Peng, F.; Hu, W.-P. Inhibition of acid-sensing ion channels by levo-tetrahydropalmatine in rat dorsal root ganglion neurons. *J. Neurosci. Res.* **2015**, *93*, 333–339. [CrossRef]

18. He, Q.-L.; Chen, Y.; Qin, J.; Mo, S.-L.; Wei, M.; Zhang, J.-J.; Li, M.-N.; Zou, X.-N.; Zhou, S.-F.; Chen, X.-W.; et al. Osthole, a herbal compound, alleviates nucleus pulposus-evoked nociceptive responses through the suppression of overexpression of acid-sensing ion channel 3 (ASIC3) in rat dorsal root ganglion. *Med. Sci. Monit.* **2012**, *18*, BR229–BR236. [CrossRef]

19. Dubinnyi, M.A.; Osmakov, D.I.; Koshelev, S.G.; Kozlov, S.A.; Andreev, Y.A.; Zakaryan, N.A.; Dyachenko, I.A.; Bondarenko, D.A.; Arseniev, A.S.; Grishin, E.V. Lignan from Thyme Possesses Inhibitory Effect on ASIC3 Channel Current. *J. Biol. Chem.* **2012**, *287*, 32993–33000. [CrossRef]

20. Diochot, S.; Baron, A.; Rash, L.D.; Deval, E.; Escoubas, P.; Scarzello, S.; Salinas, M.; Lazdunski, M. A new sea anemone peptide, APETx2, inhibits ASIC3, a major acid-sensitive channel in sensory neurons. *Embo J.* **2004**, *23*, 1516–1525. [CrossRef]

21. Kozlov, S.A.; Osmakov, D.I.; Andreev, Y.A.; Koshelev, S.G.; Gladkikh, I.N.; Monastyrnaya, M.M.; Kozlovskaya, E.P.; Grishin, E.V. A sea anemone polypeptide toxin inhibiting the ASIC3 acid-sensitive channel. *Russ. J. Bioorganic Chem.* **2012**, *38*, 578–583. [CrossRef]

22. Osmakov, D.I.; Kozlov, S.A.; Andreev, Y.A.; Koshelev, S.G.; Sanamyan, N.P.; Sanamyan, K.E.; Dyachenko, I.A.; Bondarenko, D.A.; Murashev, A.N.; Mineev, K.S.; et al. Sea anemone peptide with uncommon β-hairpin structure inhibits acid-sensing ion channel 3 (ASIC3) and reveals analgesic activity. *J. Biol. Chem.* **2013**, *288*, 23116–23127. [CrossRef]

23. Deval, E.; Noël, J.; Gasull, X.; Delaunay, A.; Alloui, A.; Friend, V.; Eschalier, A.; Lazdunski, M.; Lingueglia, E. Acid-sensing ion channels in postoperative pain. *J. Neurosci.* **2011**, *31*, 6059–6066. [CrossRef] [PubMed]

24. Deval, E.; Noel, J.; Lay, N.; Alloui, A.; Diochot, S.; Friend, V.; Jodar, M.; Lazdunski, M.; Lingueglia, E. ASIC3, a sensor of acidic and primary inflammatory pain. *Embo J.* **2008**, *27*, 3047–3055. [CrossRef] [PubMed]

25. Karczewski, J.; Spencer, R.H.; Garsky, V.M.; Liang, A.; Leitl, M.D.; Cato, M.J.; Cook, S.P.; Kane, S.; Urban, M.O. Reversal of acid-induced and inflammatory pain by the selective ASIC3 inhibitor, APETx2. *Br. J. Pharmacol.* **2010**, *161*, 950–960. [CrossRef] [PubMed]

26. Osmakov, D.I.; Koshelev, S.G.; Andreev, Y.A.; Dyachenko, I.A.; Bondarenko, D.A.; Murashev, A.N.; Grishin, E.V.; Kozlov, S.A. Conversed mutagenesis of an inactive peptide to ASIC3 inhibitor for active sites determination. *Toxicon* **2016**, *116*, 11–16. [CrossRef]

27. Osmakov, D.I.; Koshelev, S.G.; Andreev, Y.A.; Kozlov, S.A. Endogenous isoquinoline alkaloids agonists of acid-sensing ion channel type 3. *Front. Mol. Neurosci.* **2017**, *10*, 282. [CrossRef]

28. Nagakura, Y.; Okada, M.; Kohara, A.; Kiso, T.; Toya, T.; Iwai, A.; Wanibuchi, F.; Yamaguchi, T. Allodynia and Hyperalgesia in Adjuvant-Induced Arthritic Rats: Time Course of Progression and Efficacy of Analgesics. *J. Pharmacol. Exp. Ther.* **2003**, *306*, 490–497. [CrossRef]

29. Gupta, A.K.; Parasar, D.; Sagar, A.; Choudhary, V.; Chopra, B.S.; Garg, R.; Ashish Khatri, N. Analgesic and Anti-Inflammatory Properties of Gelsolin in Acetic Acid Induced Writhing, Tail Immersion and Carrageenan Induced Paw Edema in Mice. *PLoS ONE* **2015**, *10*, e0135558. [CrossRef]

30. Blanchard, M.G.; Rash, L.D.; Kellenberger, S. Inhibition of voltage-gated Na(+) currents in sensory neurones by the sea anemone toxin APETx2. *Br. J. Pharmacol.* **2012**, *165*, 2167–2177. [CrossRef]

31. Peigneur, S.; Beress, L.; Moller, C.; Mari, F.; Forssmann, W.-G.; Tytgat, J. A natural point mutation changes both target selectivity and mechanism of action of sea anemone toxins. *FASEB J.* **2012**, *26*, 5141–5151. [CrossRef] [PubMed]

32. Jensen, J.E.; Cristofori-Armstrong, B.; Anangi, R.; Rosengren, K.J.; Lau, C.H.Y.; Mobli, M.; Brust, A.; Alewood, P.F.; King, G.F.; Rash, L.D. Understanding the molecular basis of toxin promiscuity: The analgesic sea anemone peptide APETx2 interacts with acid-sensing ion channel 3 and hERG channels via overlapping pharmacophores. *J. Med. Chem.* **2014**, *57*, 9195–9203. [CrossRef] [PubMed]

33. Lee, J.Y.P.; Saez, N.J.; Cristofori-Armstrong, B.; Anangi, R.; King, G.F.; Smith, M.T.; Rash, L.D. Inhibition of acid-sensing ion channels by diminazene and APETx2 evoke partial and highly variable antihyperalgesia in a rat model of inflammatory pain. *Br. J. Pharmacol.* **2018**, *175*, 2204–2218. [CrossRef] [PubMed]

34. Hiasa, M.; Okui, T.; Allette, Y.M.; Ripsch, M.S.; Sun-Wada, G.-H.; Wakabayashi, H.; Roodman, G.D.; White, F.A.; Yoneda, T. Bone Pain Induced by Multiple Myeloma Is Reduced by Targeting V-ATPase and ASIC3. *Cancer Res.* **2017**, *77*, 1283–1295. [CrossRef] [PubMed]

35. Kobayashi, Y.; Sekiguchi, M.; Konno, S. Effect of an Acid-sensing Ion Channels Inhibitor on Pain-related Behavior by Nucleus Pulposus Applied on the Nerve Root in Rats. *Spine* **2017**, *42*, E633–E641. [CrossRef] [PubMed]

36. Gao, M.; Long, H.; Ma, W.; Liao, L.; Yang, X.; Zhou, Y.; Shan, D.; Huang, R.; Jian, F.; Wang, Y.; et al. The role of periodontal ASIC3 in orofacial pain induced by experimental tooth movement in rats. *Eur. J. Orthod.* **2016**, *38*, 577–583. [CrossRef] [PubMed]

37. Xu, X.X.; Cao, Y.; Ding, T.T.; Fu, K.Y.; Li, Y.; Xie, Q.F. Role of TRPV1 and ASIC3 channels in experimental occlusal interference-induced hyperalgesia in rat masseter muscle. *Eur. J. Pain* **2016**, *20*, 552–563. [CrossRef] [PubMed]

38. Xu, S.; Tu, W.; Wen, J.; Zhou, H.; Chen, X.; Zhao, G.; Jiang, Q. The selective ASIC3 inhibitor APETx2 alleviates gastric mucosal lesion in the rat. *Pharmazie* **2014**, *69*, 542–546.

39. Izumi, M.; Ikeuchi, M.; Ji, Q.; Tani, T. Local ASIC3 modulates pain and disease progression in a rat model of osteoarthritis. *J. Biomed. Sci.* **2012**, *19*, 77. [CrossRef]

40. Yen, L.-T.; Hsieh, C.-L.; Hsu, H.-C.; Lin, Y.-W. Targeting ASIC3 for Relieving Mice Fibromyalgia Pain: Roles of Electroacupuncture, Opioid, and Adenosine. *Sci. Rep.* **2017**, *7*, 46663. [CrossRef]

41. Gregory, N.S.; Brito, R.G.; Fusaro, M.C.G.O.; Sluka, K.A. ASIC3 Is Required for Development of Fatigue-Induced Hyperalgesia. *Mol. Neurobiol.* **2016**, *53*, 1020–1030. [CrossRef] [PubMed]

42. Calabrese, E.J.; Blain, R.B. The hormesis database: The occurrence of hormetic dose responses in the toxicological literature. *Regul. Toxicol. Pharmacol.* **2011**, *61*, 73–81. [CrossRef] [PubMed]

43. Cookman, C.J.; Belcher, S.M. Classical nuclear hormone receptor activity as a mediator of complex concentration response relationships for endocrine active compounds. *Curr. Opin. Pharmacol.* **2014**, *19*, 112–119. [CrossRef] [PubMed]

44. Materazzi, S.; Benemei, S.; Fusi, C.; Gualdani, R.; De Siena, G.; Vastani, N.; Andersson, D.A.; Trevisan, G.; Moncelli, M.R.; Wei, X.; et al. Parthenolide inhibits nociception and neurogenic vasodilatation in the trigeminovascular system by targeting the TRPA1 channel. *Pain* **2013**, *154*, 2750–2758. [CrossRef] [PubMed]

45. Logashina, Y.A.; Mosharova, I.V.; Korolkova, Y.V.; Shelukhina, I.V.; Dyachenko, I.A.; Palikov, V.A.; Palikova, Y.A.; Murashev, A.N.; Kozlov, S.A.; Stensvåg, K.; et al. Peptide from Sea Anemone *Metridium senile* Affects Transient Receptor Potential Ankyrin-repeat 1 (TRPA1) Function and Produces Analgesic Effect. *J. Biol. Chem.* **2017**, *292*, 2992–3004. [CrossRef] [PubMed]

46. Logashina, Y.A.; Solstad, R.G.; Mineev, K.S.; Korolkova, Y.V.; Mosharova, I.V.; Dyachenko, I.A.; Palikov, V.A.; Palikova, Y.A.; Murashev, A.N.; Arseniev, A.S.; et al. New Disulfide-Stabilized Fold Provides Sea Anemone Peptide to Exhibit Both Antimicrobial and TRPA1 Potentiating Properties. *Toxins* **2017**, *9*, 154. [CrossRef] [PubMed]

47. Nikolaev, M.V.; Dorofeeva, N.A.; Komarova, M.S.; Korolkova, Y.V.; Andreev, Y.A.; Mosharova, I.V.; Grishin, E.V.; Tikhonov, D.B.; Kozlov, S.A. TRPV1 activation power can switch an action mode for its polypeptide ligands. *PLoS ONE* **2017**, *12*, e0177077. [CrossRef] [PubMed]

48. Andreev, Y.A.; Kozlov, S.A.; Korolkova, Y.V.; Dyachenko, I.A.; Bondarenko, D.A.; Skobtsov, D.I.; Murashev, A.N.; Kotova, P.D.; Rogachevskaja, O.A.; Kabanova, N.V.; et al. Polypeptide modulators of TRPV1 produce analgesia without hyperthermia. *Mar. Drugs* **2013**, *11*, 5100–5115. [CrossRef] [PubMed]

49. Mazzuca, M.; Heurteaux, C.; Alloui, A.; Diochot, S.; Baron, A.; Voilley, N.; Blondeau, N.; Escoubas, P.; Gélot, A.; Cupo, A.; et al. A tarantula peptide against pain via ASIC1a channels and opioid mechanisms. *Nat. Neurosci.* **2007**, *10*, 943–945. [CrossRef]

50. Caterina, M.J.; Leffler, A.; Malmberg, A.B.; Martin, W.J.; Trafton, J.; Petersen-Zeitz, K.R.; Koltzenburg, M.; Basbaum, A.I.; Julius, D. Impaired nociception and pain sensation in mice lacking the capsaicin receptor. *Science* **2000**, *288*, 306–313. [CrossRef]

51. Sluka, K.A.; Gregory, N.S. The dichotomized role for acid sensing ion channels in musculoskeletal pain and inflammation. *Neuropharmacology* **2015**, *94*, 58–63. [CrossRef] [PubMed]

52. Pennington, M.W.; Beeton, C.; Galea, C.A.; Smith, B.J.; Chi, V.; Monaghan, K.P.; Garcia, A.; Rangaraju, S.; Giuffrida, A.; Plank, D.; et al. Engineering a stable and selective peptide blocker of the Kv1.3 channel in T lymphocytes. *Mol. Pharmacol.* **2009**, *75*, 762–773. [CrossRef] [PubMed]

53. Jin, L.; Zhou, Q.T.; Chan, H.K.; Larson, I.C.; Pennington, M.W.; Morales, R.A.V.; Boyd, B.J.; Norton, R.S.; Nicolazzo, J.A. Pulmonary Delivery of the Kv1.3-Blocking Peptide HsTX1[R14A] for the Treatment of Autoimmune Diseases. *J. Pharm. Sci.* **2016**, *105*, 650–656. [CrossRef] [PubMed]

54. Hamilton, D.A.; Ernst, C.C.; Kramer, W.G.; Madden, D.; Lang, E.; Liao, E.; Lacouture, P.G.; Ramaiya, A.; Carr, D.B. Pharmacokinetics of Diclofenac and Hydroxypropyl-β-Cyclodextrin (HPβCD) Following Administration of Injectable HPβCD-Diclofenac in Subjects with Mild to Moderate Renal Insufficiency or Mild Hepatic Impairment. *Clin. Pharmacol. Drug Dev.* **2018**, *7*, 110–122. [CrossRef] [PubMed]

55. Deval, E.; Baron, A.; Lingueglia, E.; Mazarguil, H.; Zajac, J.-M.; Lazdunski, M. Effects of neuropeptide SF and related peptides on acid sensing ion channel 3 and sensory neuron excitability. *Neuropharmacology* **2003**, *44*, 662–671. [CrossRef]

56. Yagi, J.; Wenk, H.N.; Naves, L.; McCleskey, E.W. Sustained currents through ASIC3 ion channels at the modest pH changes that occur during myocardial ischemia. *Circ. Res.* **2006**, *99*, 501–509. [CrossRef] [PubMed]

57. Yen, Y.-T.; Tu, P.-H.; Chen, C.-J.; Lin, Y.-W.; Hsieh, S.-T.; Chen, C.-C. Role of acid-sensing ion channel 3 in sub-acute-phase inflammation. *Mol. Pain* **2009**, *5*, 1. [CrossRef] [PubMed]

58. Anangi, R.; Rash, L.D.; Mobli, M.; King, G.F. Functional Expression in Escherichia coli of the Disulfide-Rich Sea Anemone Peptide APETx2, a Potent Blocker of Acid-Sensing Ion Channel 3. *Mar. Drugs* **2012**, *10*, 1605–1618. [CrossRef]

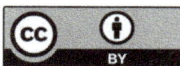

marine drugs

MDPI

Article

Inhibition of Prostate Cancer DU-145 Cells Proliferation by *Anthopleura anjunae* Oligopeptide (YVPGP) via PI3K/AKT/mTOR Signaling Pathway

Xiaojuan Li [1], Yunping Tang [1,*], Fangmiao Yu [1], Yu Sun [2], Fangfang Huang [1], Yan Chen [1], Zuisu Yang [1] and Guofang Ding [1,3,*]

[1] Zhejiang Provincial Engineering Technology Research Center of Marine Biomedical Products, School of Food and Pharmacy, Zhejiang Ocean University, Zhoushan 316022, China; lxj19950329@163.com (X.L.); fmyu@zjou.edu.cn (F.Y.); gracegang@126.com (F.H.); cyancy@zjou.edu.cn (Y.C.); abc1967@126.com (Z.Y.)
[2] Zhejiang Provincial Engineering Technology Research Center of Marine Biomedical Products, Zhejiang Ocean University Donghai Science and Technology College, Zhoushan 316000, China; suny@zjou.edu.cn
[3] Zhejiang Marine Fisheries Research Institution, Zhoushan 316021, China
*   Correspondence: tangyunping1985@zjou.edu.cn (Y.T.); dinggf@zjou.edu.cn (G.D.); Tel.: +86-0580-229-9809 (G.D.); Fax: +86-0580-229-9866 (G.D.)

Received: 13 August 2018; Accepted: 6 September 2018; Published: 11 September 2018

Abstract: We investigated the antitumor mechanism of *Anthopleura anjunae* oligopeptide (AAP-H, YVPGP) in prostate cancer DU-145 cells in vitro and in vivo. Results indicated that AAP-H was nontoxic and exhibited antitumor activities. Cell cycle analysis indicated that AAP-H may arrest DU-145 cells in the S phase. The role of the phosphatidylinositol 3-kinase/protein kinase B/mammalian rapamycin target protein (PI3K/AKT/mTOR) signaling pathway in the antitumor mechanism of APP-H was investigated. Results showed that AAP-H treatment led to dose-dependent reduction in the levels of p-AKT (Ser473), p-PI3K (p85), and p-mTOR (Ser2448), whereas t-AKT and t-PI3K levels remained unaltered compared to the untreated DU-145 cells. Inhibition of PI3K/AKT/mTOR signaling pathway in the DU-145 cells by employing inhibitor LY294002 (10 μM) or rapamycin (20 nM) effectively attenuated AAP-H-induced phosphorylation of AKT and mTOR. At the same time, inhibitor addition further elevated AAP-H-induced cleaved-caspase-3 levels. Furthermore, the effect of AAP-H on tumor growth and the role of the PI3K/AKT/mTOR signaling pathway in nude mouse model were also investigated. Immunohistochemical analysis showed that activated AKT, PI3K, and mTOR levels were reduced in DU-145 xenografts. Western blotting showed that AAP-H treatment resulted in dose-dependent reduction in p-AKT (Ser473), p-PI3K (p85), and p-mTOR (Ser2448) levels, whereas t-AKT and t-PI3K levels remained unaltered. Similarly, Bcl-xL levels decreased, whereas that of Bax increased after AAP-H treatment. AAP-H also increased initiator (caspase 8 and 9) and executor caspase (caspase 3 and 7) levels. Therefore, the antitumor mechanism of APP-H on DU-145 cells may involve regulation of the PI3K/AKT/mTOR signaling pathway, which eventually promotes apoptosis via mitochondrial and death receptor pathways. Thus, the hydrophobic oligopeptide (YVPGP) can be developed as an adjuvant for the prevention or treatment of prostate cancer in the future.

Keywords: prostate cancer; *Anthopleura anjunae* oligopeptide; DU-145 cells; PI3K/AKT/mTOR signaling pathway

1. Introduction

The ocean, with a total area of 360 million square kilometers, accounts for 70% of the earth's surface area. The diversity of the marine environment is crucial for the unique metabolic pathways and genetic background of marine organisms, which produce active substances with special structures and functions [1,2]. Numerous studies have shown that marine organisms possess antithrombotic, antitumor, and antibacterial activities [3]. These unique marine bioactive substances have played significant roles in the development of innovative medicines.

Prostate cancer (PCa) is one of the most common malignancies of the male urinary system and is also the leading cause of cancer-related death in men [4]. In recent years, the incidence and mortality of PCa have increased in both western countries and in Asia [5]. Traditional surgical resection and chemotherapy are often accompanied by side effects, such as low survival rate, poor drug resistance, neurotoxicity, and hematological adverse events [6–8]. Recent studies have shown that bioactive peptides extracted from natural products usually possess low toxicity and anticancer activity [9]. Therefore, development of highly effective anti-prostate cancer peptides of low toxicity from natural products and elucidation of their anticancer mechanisms is urgently required.

Recently, the phosphatidylinositol 3-kinase/protein kinase B/mammalian rapamycin target protein (PI3K/AKT/mTOR) signaling pathway was shown to play a crucial role in malignant transformation and subsequent growth, proliferation, and metastasis of human tumors [10]. Numerous studies have shown that the PI3K signaling pathway is abnormally activated in a variety of cancers [11]. Inhibitors of this pathway are considered as potential drug candidates, and several of them are at different stages of clinical trials [12,13]. Chemical synthesis and extraction of PI3K pathway inhibitors from natural sources are two major methods of generating these inhibitors [14]. The main problems associated with chemical synthesis of inhibitors are their poor water solubility and absorption in the body and toxicity, which are circumvented by further chemically modifying these molecules [15]. Inhibitors from organisms are natural products with negligible toxicity and side effects, structural diversity, and multitarget activity [16,17]. Hence, new inhibitors, such as those targeting the PI3K/AKT/mTOR signaling pathway, are being extensively studied.

Anemones are rich in neurotoxic, cytotoxic, and cytolytic proteins and peptides. Toxic peptides from Sea anemone inhibit growth of various cancer cell lines, but studies on the activity of peptides extracted from sea anemone muscle are limited [18,19]. Previously, we showed that the *Anthopleura anjunae* oligopeptide (APP-H, YVPGP) exhibited anti-prostate cancer effect in vitro, the mechanism of which was also preliminarily investigated [20]. However, the antitumor mechanism of APP-H was not clearly understood. Hence, the antitumor mechanism of *Anthopleura anjunae* oligopeptide (AAP-H) on DU-145 cells, with emphasis on the PI3K/AKT/mTOR signal pathway, was further investigated in vitro and in vivo in this study.

2. Results and Discussion

2.1. Toxicity to Normal Cells

Cell proliferation is the foundation of an organism's growth, development, reproduction, and heredity. Perturbation in the balance between cell proliferation and apoptosis often leads to cancer [21]. Hence, inhibition of cell proliferation is an effective way of controlling cancer. In the previous study, we showed that AAP-H could inhibit the proliferation of prostate cancer DU-145 cells with a half-maximal inhibitory (IC_{50}) concentration of 9.605 mM, 7.910 mM, and 2.298 mM at 24 h, 48 h, and 72 h, respectively [20]. However, the toxicity of AAP-H to normal cells was not studied. In this study, the fibroblast NIH-3T3 cells were used as the normal cells [22], which were added to culture solution containing different concentrations of AAP-H (0, 1, 5, 10, 15, and 20 mM) and incubated for 24 h. As shown in Figure 1, AAP-H showed no inhibitory effect on the fibroblast NIH-3T3 cells.

We observed that the rate of inhibition of DU-145 cells increased in a dose- and time-dependent manner [20], whereas the cell viability of NIH-3T3 cells was not affected under the same concentration. Thus, these observations indicated that AAP-H was nontoxic and exhibited antitumor activities. Huang et al. [23] reported that the inhibitory rate of a tripeptide (QPK) extracted from *Sepia ink* on DU-145 cells is 74.62% at 15 mg/mL. Song et al. [6] reported that the antiproliferative peptide (YALPAH) from *Setipinna taty* inhibited the DU-145 cells with an IC_{50} of 16.9 mM at 48 h. In comparison, the *Anthopleura anjunae* oligopeptides (YVPGP) showed lower IC_{50} values and better anticancer activity.

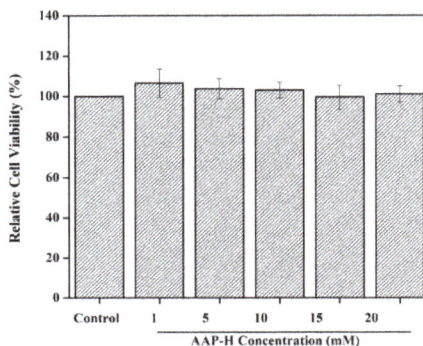

Figure 1. Toxicity of normal liver cells treated with *Anthopleura anjunae* oligopeptide (AAP-H). NIH-3T3 cells were treated with different concentrations of AAP-H (0, 1, 5, 10, 15, and 20 mM) for 24 h and the cell viability was assessed using the 3-(4,5-dimethyl-2 thiazolyl)-2,5-diphenyl-2*H*-tetrazolium bromide (MTT) assay. Each value represents the mean ± SD of three experiments.

2.2. AAP-H Induced Cycle Arrest of DU-145 Cells

The cell cycle is a tightly regulated and ordered event consisting of G1, S, G2, and M phases at the completion of which the newly replicated DNA is equally divided into daughter cells. The morphology and biochemistry of cells undergoing division change accordingly in these four stages [24,25]. The PI3K/AKT signaling pathways activate the cell-cycle-dependent protein kinase 2 (CDK-2) and CDK-4, which induces entry in S phase and DNA synthesis [26]. Evidence shows that AKT can actively and effectively regulate cell cycle progression from G2 to M phase and promote mitosis [27]. To investigate whether AAP-H affects cell cycle progression, DU-145 cells were treated with different concentrations of AAP-H (0, 5, 10, and 15 mM) for 24 h and assessed using flow cytometry. As shown in Figure 2, the number of cells in S phase increased in AAP-H treatment groups ($p < 0.05$) compared to the untreated controls. The percentages of cells in S phase after 24 h of AAP-H treatment (0, 5, 10, and 15 mM) were 7.3 ± 1.5%, 12.2 ± 1.4%, 17 ± 2.1%, and 20.9 ± 1.9%, respectively. To understand the mechanism underlying the AAP-H-induced S phase arrest, western blotting was used to analyze cell cycle regulatory proteins [28]. The levels of cyclin B1, cyclin D1, and CDK2 were dramatically reduced by varying degrees after treatment with high doses of APP-H (10–15 mM) (Figure 2).

Flow cytometric and western blotting analysis showed that AAP-H regulated the cell cycle by altering the distribution of DU-145 cells in different phases of the cycle. Compared to the blank control group, the proportion of G2/M phase cells decreased, whereas that of S phase cells increased. This indicated that AAP-H may block the progression of cancer cells from S to G2/M phase, which eventually leads to apoptosis.

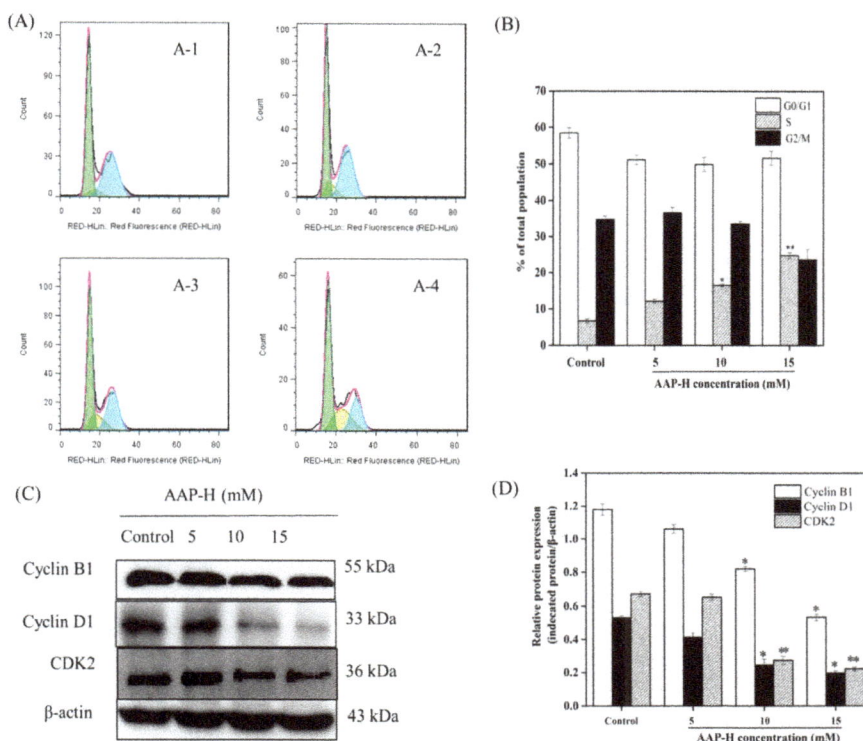

Figure 2. Flow cytometry of cell cycle phases (G0/G1, S and G2/M) distribution. (**A**) Percentage of DU-145 cells in S phase—A-1: control group, 7.3%; A-2: 5 mM AAP-H-treated group, 12.2%; A-3: 10 mM AAP-H-treated group, 17%, and A-4: 15 mM AAP-H-treated group, 20.9%. (**B**) The percentage of each phase in the cell cycle. Each experiment was repeated three times. (**C**) The levels of cyclin B1, cyclin D1, and CDK2 in DU-145 cells detected by western blotting analysis. (**D**) The expression levels of cyclin B1, cyclin D1, and CDK2 in each group analyzed by densitometry normalized to β-actin. * $p < 0.05$ and ** $p < 0.001$ vs. the control group.

2.3. AAP-H Suppressed the PI3K/AKT/mTOR Signaling Pathway in DU-145 Cells

Recent studies have indicated that PCa cells can be inhibited via the PI3K/AKT/mTOR signaling pathway. Meng et al. [29] reported that ursolic acid, a pentacyclic triterpenoid, can inhibit cell growth and induce apoptosis by regulating the PI3K/AKT/mTOR pathway in human PCa cells. Kumar et al. [30] demonstrated that rottlerin (rott), an active molecule isolated from Mallotus philippensis, inhibited autophagy and apoptosis in PCa stem cells. Yasumizu et al. [31] observed that hypoxic microenvironments promoted PI3K/Akt/mTOR signaling pathways and morphological changes in human castration-resistant prostate cancer (CRPC) cells via the PI3K/AKT/mTOR signaling pathway.

Hence, the expression levels of p-PI3K (p85) [32], p-AKT (Ser473) [33], t-PI3K, t-AKT, and p-mTOR (Ser2448) [33] were investigated after 24 h treatment with AAP-H. As shown in Figure 3, AAP-H treatment led to a dose-dependent reduction in the levels of p-AKT (Ser473), p-PI3K (p85), and p-mTOR (Ser2448), whereas t-AKT and t-PI3K levels remained unaltered compared to the nontreated group. Multiple signaling pathways operate and cross-talk inside cells; hence, when one pathway is stimulated, the levels of proteins related to that pathway, as well as other associated pathways, change concomitantly [34].

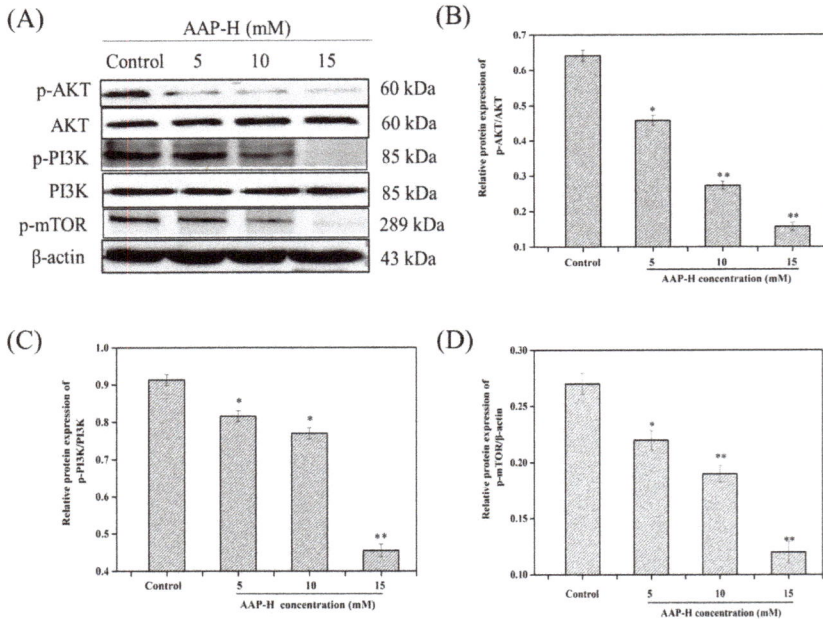

Figure 3. The changes of phosphatidylinositol 3-kinase/protein kinase B/mammalian rapamycin target protein (PI3K/AKT/mTOR) signaling pathway proteins—p-PI3K (p85), p-AKT (Ser473), p-mTOR (Ser2448), PI3K, AKT—in DU-145 cells after treating with AAP-H for 24 h. (**A**) The level of p-PI3K (p85), p-AKT (Ser473), p-mTOR (Ser2448) decreased in a dose-dependent way, and total PI3K and AKT were not changed compared to control groups. β-actin as a house-keeping protein was used for loading control. (**B**) Protein expression level of p-PI3K (p85) and PI3K that presented in AAP-H-treated DU-145 cells. (**C**) Protein expression level of p-AKT (Ser473) and AKT that presented in AAP-H-treated DU-145 cells. (**D**) Protein expression level of p-mTOR (Ser2448) that presented in AAP-H-treated DU-145 cells. * $p < 0.05$ and ** $p < 0.001$ vs. control.

2.4. PI3K/AKT/mTOR Signaling Involved in AAP-H-Induced Apoptosis

To further investigate whether AAP-H-induced apoptosis involves the PI3K/AKT/mTOR signaling pathway, the levels of p-AKT (Ser473), t-AKT, and cleaved-PARP were assessed using western blotting after DU-145 were treated with 10 mM AAP-H for 0, 2, 4, 8, 12, 18, and 24 h [35,36]. Results revealed that AAP-H reduced AKT phosphorylation in a time-dependent manner; however, AKT level remained unchanged. Cleaved-PARP level also increased in a time-dependent manner. Importantly, cleaved-PARP level started increasing concomitantly with decrease in AKT phosphorylation (Figure 4). These results indicated that PI3K/AKT/mTOR inhibition was an early event that was initiated prior to cell death induction.

Furthermore, LY294002 [37] and rapamycin [38], were used to specifically inhibit the PI3K/AKT/mTOR signaling [39]. Figure 5 shows that the levels of phosphorylated AKT and mTOR were significantly reduced after treatment with LY294002 (10 μM) and rapamycin (20 nM), respectively. In addition, pretreatment with LY294002 and rapamycin effectively attenuated AAP-H-induced phosphorylation of AKT and mTOR. At the same time, inhibitor addition further elevated AAP-H-induced cleaved-caspase-3 levels. These results implied that the PI3K/AKT/mTOR signaling pathway is one of the potential mechanisms via which APP-H induces DU-145 cell apoptosis.

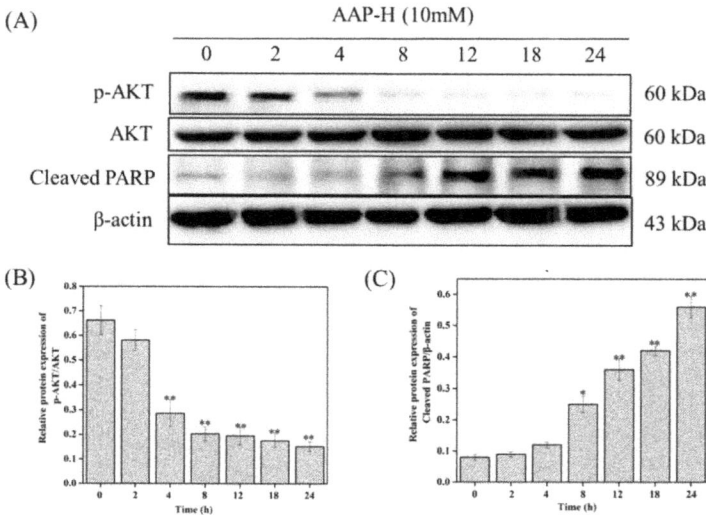

Figure 4. AAP-H affects PI3K/AKT/mTOR signaling pathway in different time points. (**A**) The protein expression level in the DU-145 cells treated with 10 mM AAP-H for 0, 2, 4, 8, 12, 18, and 24 h. (**B**) The expression levels of AKT/p-AKT (Ser473) analyzed using western blotting. (**C**) The expression levels of cleaved-PARP analyzed using western blotting. * $p < 0.05$ and ** $p < 0.001$ vs. control.

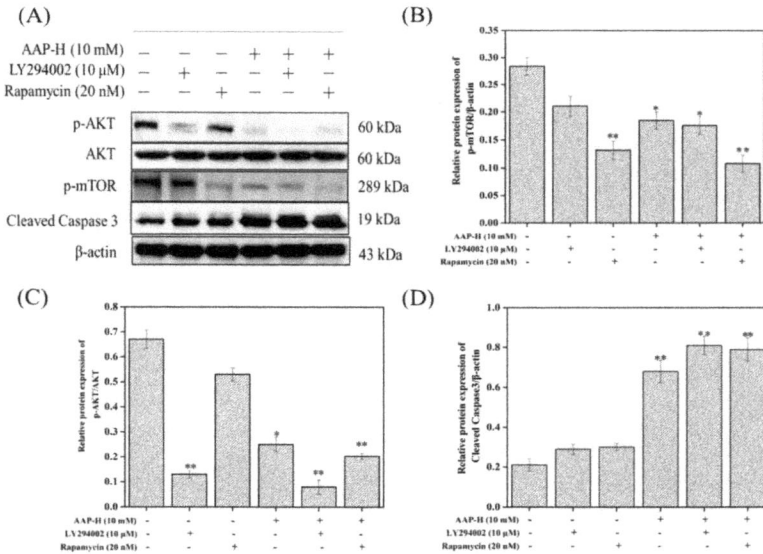

Figure 5. Effects of LY294002 or rapamycin on AAP-H-mediated alterations in PI3K/AKT/mTOR signaling and apoptosis-related protein. The DU-145 cells were preincubated with LY294002 (10 μM) or rapamycin (20 nM) for 2 h and then treated with 10 mM AAP-H for 24 h. (**A**) Western blot analysis of p-AKT, AKT, p-mTOR and Cleaved Caspase-3 levels. β-Actin as a house-keeping protein was used as the loading control. (**B**) The expression levels of p-mTOR analyzed using western blotting. (**C**) The expression levels of p-AKT/AKT analyzed using western blotting. (**D**) The expression levels of Cleaved Caspase-3 analyzed using western blotting. * $p < 0.05$ and ** $p < 0.001$ vs. control.

2.5. Effect of AAP-H on DU-145 Xenografts

To investigate the anticancer effects of AAP-H on DU-145 xenografts, physiological saline, AAP-H, and DDP were injected in nude mice for 14 days. Mice body weight and tumor volume were determined every three days. As shown in the Figure 6A, the growth rate of tumor volume in the AAP-H and DDP treatment groups was slower than that of the control group. The inhibition rate was $36.93 \pm 3.9\%$ in the AAP-H low dose group, $62.22 \pm 6.2\%$ in the AAP-H high dose group, and $66.96 \pm 5.7\%$ in the DDP group. Although DDP had the best inhibitory effect (Figure 6B), it elicited obvious toxic effects in nude mice. AAP-H not only reduced tumor weight but also slightly increased body weight and quality of life of nude mice during medication. Thus, we preliminarily concluded that AAP-H has no harmful effect on nude mice.

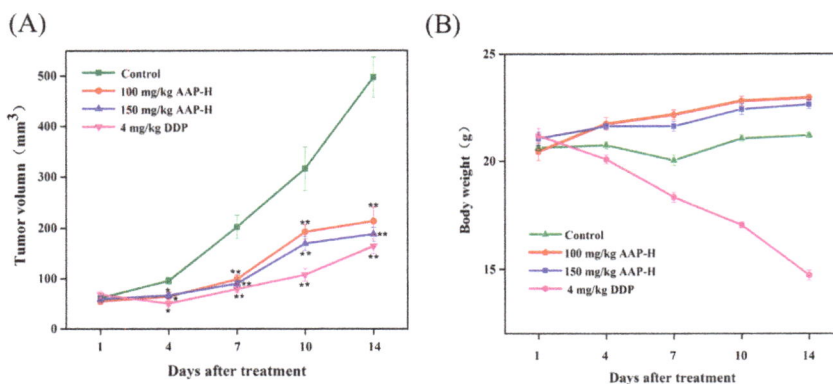

Figure 6. Inhibition of DU-145 prostate tumor growth by the APP-H. Compared to the control group, AAP-H exerted (**A**) antiproliferative effect on DU-145 cells in nude mice and (**B**) slightly increased mice body weight. Nude mice of control group, AAP-H group, and positive control group orally received saline, AAP-H (100 or 150 mg/kg/d), and DDP (4 mg/kg/d) for 14 days, respectively. * $p < 0.05$ and ** $p < 0.001$ vs. control.

2.6. Immunocytochemistry

The expression of members of the PI3K/AKT/mTOR signaling pathway (p-AKT (Ser473), p-PI3K (p85) and p-mTOR (Ser2448)) in tumor tissue from nude mice was examined using immunocytochemistry assay [33]. As shown in Figure 7, p-AKT (Ser473), p-PI3K (p85), and p-mTOR (Ser2448) were detected in the cytoplasm and nucleus of the tumors; however, no expression was observed in the negative control group, whereas strong expression was observed in the positive control group. The positive expression started to decrease in the group treated with low dose of AAP-H (100 mg/kg). p-AKT (Ser473), p-PI3K (p85), and p-mTOR (Ser2448) levels were negligible and cell morphology was poor when the concentration of AAP-H was increased to 150 mg/kg. The results of immunohistochemistry were further confirmed by western blotting analysis.

Recent studies have shown that mutations in PI3KCA of PI3K play crucial roles in the formation of human tumors [40]. Phosphorylated PI3K triggers the production of the second messenger inositol triphosphate, further activating AKT, which can phosphorylate a variety of downstream factors such as enzymes, kinases, and transcription factors to promote tumor production [41]. AKT is an evolutionarily conserved serine/threonine kinase with three subtypes that are expressed to varying degrees in most human tissues. p-AKT is a typical pro-cancer factor, which can promote proliferation of tumor cells via p21, p27, and p53, inhibiting apoptosis, and promoting invasion, metastasis, and angiogenesis of tumor cells. Reports show that p-AKT is expressed in various malignancies, such as oral cancer, breast cancer, and non-small cell lung cancer [42–44]. mTOR is a direct substrate of AKT kinase, and serine 2480 is the site of phosphorylation of the latter on mTOR; the deletion of the residue in the C terminal regulatory region of the protein increases mTOR activity [41]. Hence, immunocytochemistry was used in this study to detect p-AKT in DU-145 cells. Our results showed that the expression of activated AKT, PI3K, and mTOR was increased in DU-145 xenografts, which resulted in continuous activation of the PI3K/AKT/mTOR pathway and rapid cell proliferation, thereby promoting tumor malignancy.

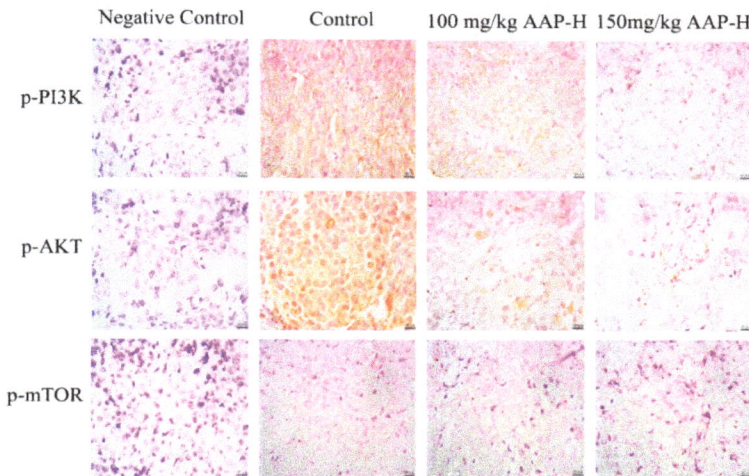

Figure 7. Expression of p-PI3K (p85), p-AKT (Ser473), and p-mTOR (Ser2448) in tumors was detected using immunocytochemistry. The primary antibody was replaced with phosphate buffered saline (PBS) in the negative control. DU-145 xenografts treated with non-AAP-H presented strong positivity, whereas those treated with 100 mg/kg AAP-H and 150 mg/kg AAP-H showed moderate and low positivity, respectively. Bar = 50 μm, 400×.

2.7. AAP-H Suppressed the PI3K/AKT/mTOR Signaling Pathway in DU-145 Xenografts

The PI3K/AKT/mTOR signaling pathway plays a crucial role in growth, proliferation, metastasis, and malignant transformation in human cancer [45]. It can induce tumor formation via the following mechanisms: (1) It inhibits autophagy [46]. For example, mTOR is a key regulator of the initiation stage of autophagy, and its activation inhibits autophagy [47]. (2) Activated AKT inhibits caspases 3 and 9 by phosphorylating their Ser196 and ultimately inhibiting apoptosis [48,49]. Furthermore, it inhibits the Bcl-2 family of proteins. Bad promotes apoptosis with Bcl-2 or Bcl-xL, and activated AKT is a highly effective Bad kinase that can be blocked by phosphorylation of Ser136 to induce apoptosis. (3) Promotion of tumor metastasis, cell movement, and angiogenesis are related to PI3K/AKT signal transduction. The above observations suggest that the PI3K/AKT/mTOR pathway is closely related to the caspase and Bcl-2 signaling pathways. Changes in the levels of key proteins of the PI3K/AKT/mTOR signaling pathway (p-PI3K (p85), p-AKT (Ser473), t-PI3K, t-AKT, and p-mTOR (Ser2448)) in DU-145 xenografts treated with AAP-H for 14 days were analyzed using western blotting. Compared to the control group, AAP-H treatment resulted in dose-dependent reduction in the levels of p-AKT (Ser473), p-PI3K (p85), and p-mTOR (Ser2448), whereas t-AKT and t-PI3K levels remained unaltered (Figure 8). These results were consistent with the in vitro results, indicating that AAP-H may inhibit the activity of DU-145 xenograft by regulating the PI3K/AKT/mTOR signal transduction pathway.

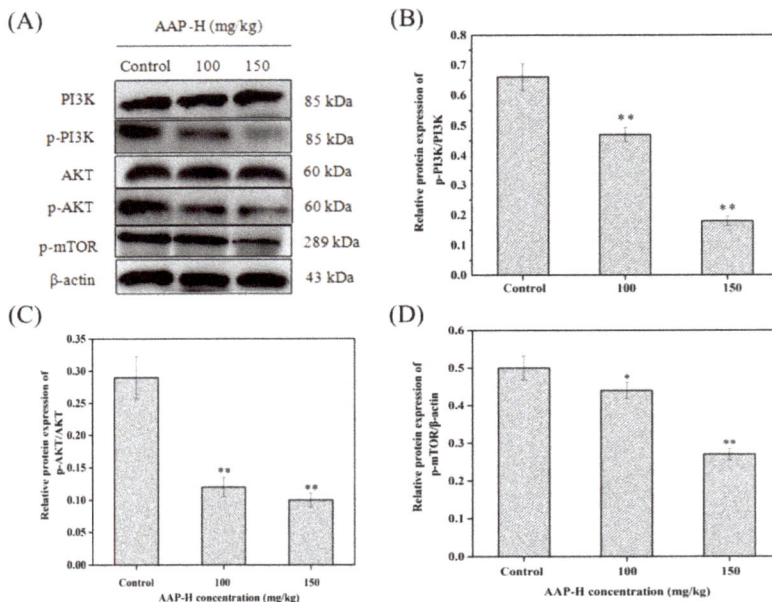

Figure 8. Changes in the levels of PI3K/AKT/mTOR signaling pathway proteins (p-PI3K (p85), p-AKT (Ser473), p-mTOR (Ser2448), PI3K, AKT) in DU-145 xenografts treated with AAP-H for 14 days. (**A**) The level of p-PI3K (p85), p-AKT (Ser473), p-mTOR (Ser2448) were reduced in a dose-dependent manner, whereas total PI3K and AKT were unaltered compared to control groups. β-actin as a house-keeping protein was used as the loading control. (**B**) p-PI3K (p85) and PI3K levels in AAP-H-treated DU-145 cells. (**C**) p-AKT (Ser473) and AKT levels in AAP-H-treated DU-145 cells. (**D**) p-mTOR (Ser2448) level in AAP-H-treated DU-145 cells. * $p < 0.05$ and ** $p < 0.001$ vs. control.

2.8. Western Blotting Analysis of Bcl-2 Family Members

Apoptosis is triggered via the extrinsic (death receptor pathway) and intrinsic (mitochondrial pathway) pathways [50]. The Bcl-2 family of proteins, which regulates the release of cytochrome C from the mitochondria to the cytoplasm, is mainly composed of anti-apoptotic proteins (Bcl-2 and Bcl-xL) and apoptotic proteins (Bax, Bak). Anti-apoptotic and apoptotic proteins play opposite roles during the release of cytochrome C. For example, oligomeric Bax assists cytochrome C and other apoptotic proteins to pass through the mitochondrial membrane. However, Bcl-xL closes the voltage dependent anion channel (VDAC), which inhibits the release of cytochrome C from the Bax/VDAC channel [51]. To investigate whether apoptosis-related proteins participate in AAP-H-induced apoptosis, we analyzed the expression of Bcl-2 family members such as Bcl-xL and Bax. As shown in Figure 9, the level of the anti-apoptotic Bcl-xL was reduced, whereas that of the pro-apoptotic Bax was elevated post-AAP-H treatment. This indicated that AAP-H might affect apoptosis via the mitochondrial pathway.

(A)

AAP-H (mg/kg)

Control   100   150

Bcl-xL   30 kDa

Bax   20 kDa

β-actin   43 kDa

(B)

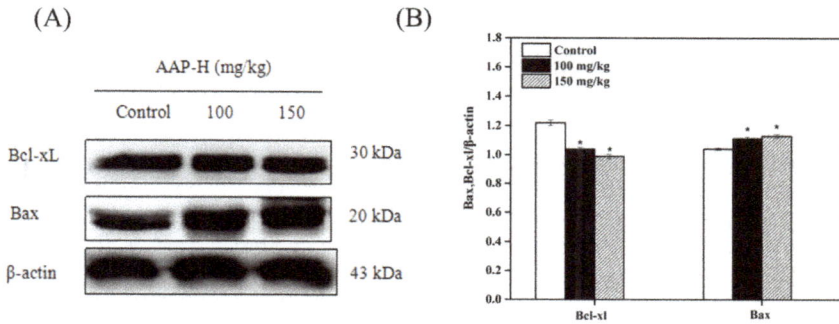

Figure 9. Western blotting showing the expression of Bcl-2 family members (Bcl-xL, Bax) in DU-145 xenografts treated with AAP-H for 14 days. (**A**) Western blotting analysis of Bcl-xL and Bax in DU-145 xenografts treated with AAP-H for 14 days. (**B**) The expression levels of Bcl-xL and Bax analyzed using western blotting. * $p < 0.05$ vs. control.

2.9. Western Blotting of Caspases

The caspase family consists of cysteine-rich proteins, which are divided into initiator caspases (caspases 8 and 9) and executor caspases (caspases 3, 6, and 7). Caspases are activated by two major pathways. One involves the release of cytochrome C from the mitochondria to the cytoplasm, which eventually leads to apoptosis. The other pathway involves the death receptors [50].

Death receptor is a transmembrane protein on the cell membrane, which is responsible for transferring extracellular stimulating signal to the corresponding ligand and inducing apoptosis [52]. Caspase 8, one of the initiators of apoptosis, plays a key role in mediating caspase activation in the death receptor pathway [53] by activating the downstream executors, caspases 3, 6, and 7. However, caspase 8 exists mainly in an inactive state in human cancers. Recently, caspase 8 expression has been analyzed from various perspectives [54,55]. Here, we investigated the levels of initiator and executor caspases in treated and untreated tumors. As shown in Figure 10, initiator caspase 8 and 9 were activated and expressed to similar extents in the presence of 150 mg/kg AAP-H. This was paralleled by increase in the expression of the downstream executor caspase 3 and 7. These results indicated that AAP-H promoted apoptosis of DU-145 cells via both the mitochondrial and death receptor pathways.

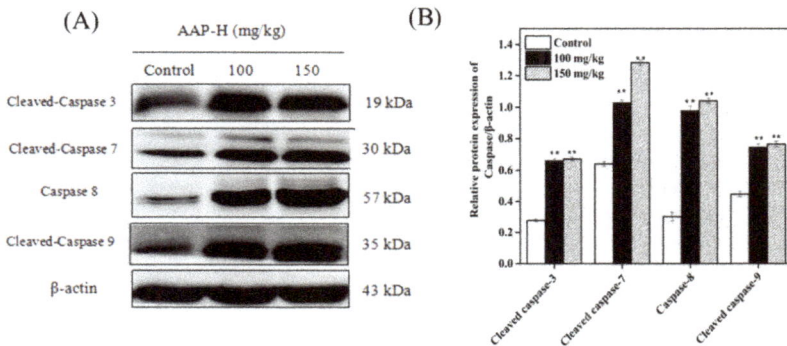

(A)

AAP-H (mg/kg)

Control   100   150

Cleaved-Caspase 3   19 kDa

Cleaved-Caspase 7   30 kDa

Caspase 8   57 kDa

Cleaved-Caspase 9   35 kDa

β-actin   43 kDa

(B)

Figure 10. Western blotting showing the expression of Caspase family members (Caspase 3, 7, 8 and 9) in DU-145 xenografts after being treated with AAP-H for 14 days. (**A**) Western blotting analysis of Caspase 3, 7, 8 and 9 in DU-145 xenografts. (**B**) The expression levels of Caspase 3, 7, 8 and 9 analyzed using western blotting. ** $p < 0.001$ vs. control.

3. Materials and Methods

3.1. Materials and Reagents

The AAP-H (YVPGP) samples were purified from *Anthopleura anjunae* protein hydrolysates as mentioned previously [56] and stored at −20 °C until further use. The DU-145 cell lines and NIH-3T3 cell lines were purchased from the Cell Bank of Chinese Academy of Sciences. Powdered Ham's F12/F-12 nutrient mixture (F12) medium was purchased from Gibco/BRL (Gaithersburg, MD, USA). Fetal bovine serum (FBS) was purchased from Sijiqing Biological Technology Co. (Hangzhou, China). 3-(4,5-dimethyl-2 thiazolyl)-2,5-diphenyl-2*H*-tetrazolium bromide (MTT) kits and cocktail 2 were purchased from Sigma Chemical Co. Ltd. (St. Louis, MO, USA). Antibodies against β-actin (cat. no. 4970S), caspase 3 (cat. no. CST9665T), caspase 7 (cat. no. CST9494S), caspase 8 (cat. no. CST4790T), caspase 9 (cat. no. CST9508T), AKT (cat. no. CST2920ST), p-AKT (Ser473) (cat. no. CST4060T), PI3K (cat. no. CST4257T), p-mTOR (Ser2448) (cat. no. CST5536T), p-PI3K (p85) (cat. no. CST4228T), Bax (cat. no. CST5023T), Bcl-xL (cat. no. CST2764T), PARP (cat. no. CST9532T), CDK2 (cat. no. CST2546T), cyclin D1 (cat. no. CST2978T) and cyclin B1 (cat. no. CST12231T) were purchased from Cell Signaling Technology (Boston, MA, USA). Cell cycle detection kits were purchased from BestBio Biological Technology Co. (Shanghai, China). All other reagents used in the present study were of analytical grade.

3.2. Cell Toxicity Assay

The effect of AAP-H on the toxicity of NIH-3T3 cell viability was detected using the MTT assay according to the method described by Tang et al. [57], with slight modifications. In brief, the NIH-3T3 cells were first seeded in a 96-well (5×105 cell/mL) plate (Costar Corning, Rochester, NY, USA). After incubation for 24 h, 200 μL fresh culture medium containing different final concentrations of AAP-H (0, 1, 5, 10, 15, and 20 mM) was added to each well. After 24 h incubation, the cells were treated with 200 μL MTT reagents and incubated for another 4 h. Finally, the formazan crystals were dissolved in 100 μL dimethyl sulfoxide (DMSO), and the absorbance at 490 nm was recorded using an enzyme-linked immunosorbent assay (ELISA) reader (SpectraMa, Molecular Devices Co., San Jose, CA, USA). Different final concentrations of AAP-H (0, 1, 5, 10, 15, and 20 mM) were used for treatment prior to the MTT assay.

3.3. Determination of Cell Cycle Arrest

To investigate the cytotoxic effect of AAP-H on DU-145 cells, the relative sensitivities of the different phases of the cell cycle were observed using the cell cycle arrest test described by Chen et al. [58], with slight modifications. First, the cells were placed in a 6-well plate and different final concentrations (0, 5, 10, and 15 mM) of APP-H were added when the cells had adhered to the bottom of the plate. After 24 h incubation, the cells were collected by centrifugation, RNase A was added to the cell pellet, and incubated in a water bath at 37 °C for 30 min. Three hundred and fifty microliters of propidium iodide was added to the tubes in dark and incubated at 4 °C for another 40 min. Finally, the cells were sorted using a flow cytometer (Becton Dickinson, NJ, USA).

3.4. Western Blot Analysis

DU-145 cells were treated with culture solution containing different concentrations of AAP-H (0, 5, 10, and 15 mM). Then, the treated cells were incubated in a CO_2 incubator for 24 h. After washing thrice with phosphate buffered saline (PBS) (the tumor tissues were placed in a mortar, liquid nitrogen was added, and the tumor was rapidly ground and collected in a centrifuge tube), 200 μL radioimmunoprecipitation assay (RIPA) lysis solution containing 1% phosphatase inhibitor and phenylmethane sulfonyl fluoride (PMSF) was added to each group. The cracking liquid was transferred into a 1.5 mL centrifuge tube and sonicated for 30 min. Subsequently, the cell lysates were collected by centrifugation at 4 °C (12,000 rpm, 15 min). The total protein content of the supernatant was measured using the bicinchoninic acid (BCA) kit. The samples were then denatured by heating in a boiling water bath for 10 min, and the total protein (50 μg) was separated on preprepared 12% sodium dodecyl sulfate-polyacrylamide gels, followed by transfer to polyvinylidene fluoride membrane (Millipore, Billerica, MA, USA). The membranes were stained with Ponceau S and then blocked with 5% nonfat milk for 1 h. After that, the membranes were incubated with the 1:1000 diluted primary antibodies against caspases 3, 7, 8, and 9, AKT, p-AKT (Ser473), PI3K, p-PI3K (p85), p-mTOR (Ser2448), Bax, Bcl-xL, PARP, CDK2, cyclin B1, and cyclin D1 in 5% w/v nonfat milk at 4 °C with gentle shaking for 16 h. Finally, the 1:1000 diluted secondary antibodies (goat anti-rabbit and goat anti-mouse) were added and incubated at room temperature for 1 h. The target bands were detected using enhanced chemiluminescence and quantified by densitometry as shown in DRAFT-alpha view using the Image J 1.38 software (NIH, Bethesda, MD, USA). β-actin was used as the loading control.

3.5. Effect of AAP-H on DU-145 Xenografts

Male BALB/c nude mice (nu/nu) were obtained from the Zhejiang Laboratory Animal Center (Hangzhou, China) and housed in specific pathogen-free conditions. DU-145 cells were cultured in Ham F12 medium (10% FBS) at 37 °C in a 5% CO_2 incubator. A suspension of DU-145 cells (in the logarithmic growth stage) were then prepared (0.2 mL, with 1×10^6 cells) and injected into the right armpit of nude mice in sterile environment. The tumor nodes appeared after 7 days, which confirmed the successful establishment of the DU-145 tumor-bearing nude mouse model. The body weight was measured after every three days, and the tumor volume was calculated according to the following formula: volume (mm^3) = $1/6 \times \pi \times$ width$^2 \times$ length. When the average tumor volume reached 60 mm^3, the mice were randomly divided into four groups with five mice in each group (negative control, positive control treated with 4 mg/kg cisplatin (DDP), and two treatment groups with 100 mg/kg and 150 mg/kg AAP-H). All mice were injected intraperitoneally for 14 days. The experiments were performed according to the guidelines of the Institutional Animal Care and Use Committee of the Zhejiang Ocean University (SYXK, 2014-0013) and adhered to the code of the World Medical Association (Declaration of Helsinki).

3.6. Immunocytochemistry (IHC)

The animal experiments were divided into four groups, and each group contained five nude mice. All animals were euthanized, and the three transplanted tumors were selected randomly and cut into 1-cm^3 pieces for IHC. IHC was performed as follows: First, the tumors were placed in 4% paraformaldehyde for 24 h and washed with flowing water overnight. Second, the tumors were dehydrated using an ethanol gradient (75%, 95%, and 100%) for 5 min and transparentized with xylene for 40 min. Then, the tumors were put in paraffin to maintain constant temperature (60 °C) for 1 h. Finally, the tumors were put into a square box, fluid wax was poured into these boxes, and the boxes were refrigerated at 4 °C. Subsequently, 4-μm slices were prepared using a Leica slicer (RM2135, Leica Instruments GmbH, Wetzlar, Germany). The adhered slices were peeled off using a spreading machine (III1210, Leica Instruments GmbH, Wetzlar, Germany) and processed using a baking machine (II1220, Leica Instruments GmbH, Wetzlar, Germany). The paraffin section was used for IHC.

IHC for determining the expression of p-PI3K (p85), p-AKT (Ser473), and p-mTOR (Ser2448) was performed according to Luo et al. [59], with minor modifications. Briefly, 4-μm thick sections were dewaxed with xylene for 15 min. Antigen repair of tumor sections was performed using EDTA (pH 8.0) buffer under high temperature and pressure for 3 min. The endogenous biotin in the tumor sections were blocked according to the instructions of the IHC biotin block kit (Maxin Co., Hong Kong, China). Then, the tumor sections were incubated with prediluted primary antibodies against p-PI3K (p85) (1:50), p-AKT (Ser473) (1:50), and p-mTOR (Ser2448) (1:50) in a mixture containing 3% bovine serum albumin (BSA) (w/v), 1× TBS and 0.1% Tween 20 at 4 °C for 16 h. Horse radish peroxidase (HRP)-labeled goat anti-rabbit monoclonal secondary IgG (H + L) against p-PI3K (p85) (1:1000), p-AKT (Ser473) (1:1000), and p-mTOR (Ser2448) (1:1000) were used, and the signal was detected using the

DAB chromogenic kit (Maxin Co., Hong Kong, China). Sections were re-stained with hematoxylin, dehydrated, transparentized with xylene, and sealed with a resin. The primary antibodies were replaced with PBS in the negative control. Antigen expression was analyzed using light microscopy (Olympus, Tokyo, Japan).

4. Conclusions

AAP-H exhibited anticancer activity on DU-145 prostate cancer cells by targeting the PI3K/AKT/mTOR signaling pathway and was not toxic for normal fibroblast cells. In addition, AAP-H showed good antiproliferative effect on DU-145 cells. The antitumor mechanism of APP-H on DU-145 cells may involve regulation of the activity of the PI3K/AKT/mTOR signaling pathway, which eventually promotes apoptosis via both the mitochondrial and death receptor pathways (Figure 11). Therefore, the hydrophobic oligopeptide (YVPGP) will be further studied for use as a functional food or adjuvant for prevention or treatment of prostate cancer.

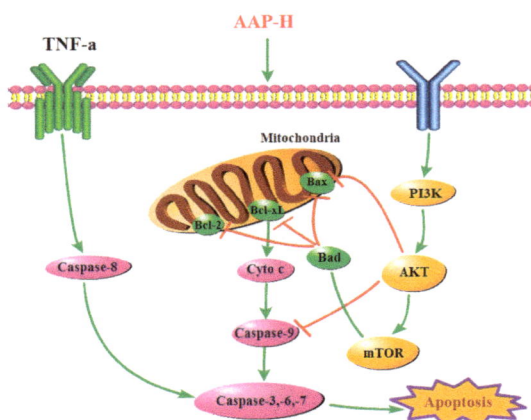

Figure 11. AAP-H inhibits DU-145 cell proliferation via the PI3K/AKT/mTOR signaling pathway.

Author Contributions: G.D. and Y.T. conceived and designed the experiments. X.L. performed the experiments. Y.T., Y.S., F.Y., F.H., Y.C., and Z.Y. carried out statistical analysis of the data. X.L. and Y.T. wrote this paper.

Funding: This work was financially supported by the National Natural Science Foundation of China (grant No. 81773629 and No. 41806153), the Co-innovation of Zhejiang Science and Technology Program (No. 2016F50039) and the Natural Science Foundation of Zhejiang Province (grant No. LQ16H300001 and No. LQ18B060004).

Conflicts of Interest: The authors declare no conflict of interest.

References

1. Kiuru, P.; D'Auria, M.V.; Muller, C.D.; Tammela, P.; Vuorela, H.; Yli-Kauhaluoma, J. Exploring marine resources for bioactive compounds. *Planta Med.* **2014**, *80*, 1234–1246. [CrossRef] [PubMed]
2. Simmons, T.L.; Andrianasolo, E.; Mcphail, K.; Flatt, P.; Gerwick, W.H. Marine natural products as anticancer drugs. *Mol. Cancer Ther.* **2005**, *4*, 333–342. [PubMed]
3. Arumugam, V.; Venkatesan, M.; Ramachandran, S.; Sundaresan, U. Bioactive Peptides from Marine Ascidians and Future Drug Development—A Review. *Int. J. Pept. Res. Ther.* **2017**, *24*, 13–18. [CrossRef]
4. Beltran, H.; Beer, T.M.; Carducci, M.A.; de Bono, J.; Gleave, M.; Hussain, M.; Kelly, W.K.; Saad, F.; Sternberg, C.; Tagawa, S.T. New therapies for castration-resistant prostate cancer: Efficacy and safety. *Eur. Urol.* **2011**, *60*, 279–290. [CrossRef] [PubMed]
5. Ito, K. Prostate cancer in Asian men. *Nat. Rev. Urol.* **2014**, *11*, 197–212. [CrossRef] [PubMed]

6. Song, R.; Wei, R.B.; Luo, H.Y.; Yang, Z.S. Isolation and identification of an antiproliferative peptide derived from heated products of peptic hydrolysates of half-fin anchovy (*Setipinna taty*). *J. Funct. Foods* **2014**, *10*, 104–111. [CrossRef]
7. Karavelioglu, E.; Gonul, Y.; Aksit, H.; Boyaci, M.G.; Karademir, M.; Simsek, N.; Guven, M.; Atalay, T.; Rakip, U. Cabazitaxel causes a dose-dependent central nervous system toxicity in rats. *J. Neurol. Sci.* **2016**, *360*, 66–71. [CrossRef] [PubMed]
8. Frederiks, C.N.; Lam, S.W.; Guchelaar, H.J.; Boven, E. Genetic polymorphisms and paclitaxel- or docetaxel-induced toxicities: A systematic review. *Cancer Treat. Rev.* **2015**, *41*, 935–950. [CrossRef] [PubMed]
9. Li, Z.J.; Cho, C.H. Development of peptides as potential drugs for cancer therapy. *Curr. Pharm. Des.* **2010**, *16*, 1180–1189. [CrossRef] [PubMed]
10. Liu, P.; Cheng, H.; Roberts, T.M.; Zhao, J.J. Targeting the phosphoinositide 3-kinase pathway in cancer. *Nat. Rev. Drug Discov.* **2009**, *8*, 627–644. [CrossRef] [PubMed]
11. Wong, K.K.; Engelman, J.A.; Cantley, L.C. Targeting the PI3K signaling pathway in cancer. *Curr. Opin. Genet. Dev.* **2010**, *20*, 87–90. [CrossRef] [PubMed]
12. Knight, Z.A.; Shokat, K.M. Chemically targeting the PI3K family. *Biochem. Soc. Trans.* **2007**, *35*, 245–249. [CrossRef] [PubMed]
13. Atkins, M.B.; Hidalgo, M.; Stadler, W.M.; Logan, T.F.; Dutcher, J.P.; Hudes, G.R.; Park, Y.; Liou, S.H.; Marshall, B.; Boni, J.P.; et al. Randomized phase II study of multiple dose levels of CCI-779, a novel mammalian target of rapamycin kinase inhibitor, in patients with advanced refractory renal cell carcinoma. *J. Clin. Oncol.* **2004**, *22*, 909–918. [CrossRef] [PubMed]
14. Huang, S. Inhibition of PI3K/Akt/mTOR Signaling by Natural Products. *Anti-Cancer Agent Med. Chem.* **2012**, *13*, 967–970. [CrossRef]
15. Stein, R.C. Prospects for phosphoinositide 3-kinase inhibition as a cancer treatment. *Endocr.-Relat. Cancer* **2001**, *8*, 237–248. [CrossRef] [PubMed]
16. Gharbi, S.I.; Zvelebil, M.J.; Shuttleworth, S.J.; Hancox, T.; Saghir, N.; Timms, J.F.; Waterfield, M.D. Exploring the specificity of the PI3K family inhibitor LY294002. *Biochem. J.* **2007**, *404*, 15–21. [CrossRef] [PubMed]
17. Ben, M.; Rodrigo, D.; Josep, T. Targeting the PI3K/Akt/mTOR Pathway-Beyond Rapalogs. *Oncotarget* **2010**, *1*, 530–543.
18. Maček, P. Polypeptide cytolytic toxins from sea anemones (*Actiniaria*). *Toxicon* **1992**, *40*, 111–124.
19. Ramezanpour, M.; Silva, K.B.D.; Sanderson, B.J. Differential susceptibilities of human lung, breast and skin cancer cell lines to killing by five sea anemone venoms. *J. Venom. Anim. Toxins Incl. Trop. Dis.* **2012**, *18*, 157–163. [CrossRef]
20. Wu, Z.Z.; Ding, G.F.; Huang, F.F.; Yang, Z.S.; Yu, F.M.; Tang, Y.P.; Jia, Y.L.; Zheng, Y.Y.; Chen, R. Anticancer Activity of *Anthopleura anjunae* Oligopeptides in Prostate Cancer DU-145 Cells. *Mar. Drugs* **2018**, *16*, 125. [CrossRef] [PubMed]
21. Vander Heiden, M.G.; Cantley, L.C.; Thompson, C.B. Understanding the Warburg Effect: The Metabolic Requirements of Cell Proliferation. *Science* **2009**, *324*, 1029–1033. [CrossRef] [PubMed]
22. Tang, Y.; Jin, S.; Li, X.; Li, X.; Hu, X.; Chen, Y.; Huang, F.; Yang, Z.; Yu, F.; Ding, G. Physicochemical Properties and Biocompatibility Evaluation of Collagen from the Skin of Giant Croaker (*Nibea japonica*). *Mar. Drugs* **2018**, *16*, 222. [CrossRef] [PubMed]
23. Huang, F.; Yang, Z.; Di, Y.; Wang, J.; Rong, L.; Ding, G. Sepia Ink Oligopeptide Induces Apoptosis in Prostate Cancer Cell Lines via Caspase-3 Activation and Elevation of Bax/Bcl-2 Ratio. *Mar. Drugs* **2012**, *10*, 2153–2165. [CrossRef] [PubMed]
24. Zheng, X.; Wang, Y.; Liu, B.; Liu, C.; Liu, D.; Zhu, J.; Yang, C.; Yan, J.; Liao, X.; Meng, X.; et al. Bmi-1-shRNA Inhibits the Proliferation of Lung Adenocarcinoma Cells by Blocking the G1/S Phase Through Decreasing Cyclin D1 and Increasing p21/p27 Levels. *Nucleic Acid Ther.* **2014**, *24*, 210–216. [CrossRef] [PubMed]
25. Black, A.R.; Black, J.D. Protein kinase C signaling and cell cycle regulation. *Front. Immunol.* **2013**, *3*, 423–440. [CrossRef] [PubMed]
26. Chang, F.; Lee, J.T.; Navolanic, P.M.; Steelman, L.S.; Shelton, J.G.; Blalock, W.L.; Franklin, R.A.; Mccubrey, J.A. Involvement of PI3K/Akt pathway in cell cycle progression, apoptosis, and neoplastic transformation: A target for cancer chemotherapy. *Leukemia* **2003**, *17*, 590–603. [CrossRef] [PubMed]
27. Cammer, M.; Gevrey, J.C.; Lorenz, M.; Dovas, A.; Condeelis, J.; Cox, D. The mechanism of CSF-1 induced wasp activation in vivo: A role for PI 3-kinase and CDC42. *J. Biol. Chem.* **2009**. [CrossRef] [PubMed]

28. Xu, Z.; Zhang, F.; Bai, C.; Yao, C.; Zhong, H.; Zou, C.; Chen, X. Sophoridine induces apoptosis and S phase arrest via ROS-dependent JNK and ERK activation in human pancreatic cancer cells. *J. Exp. Clin. Cancer Res.* **2017**, *36*, 124–134. [CrossRef] [PubMed]

29. Yan, M.; Zhao-Min, L.; Nan, G.; Deng-Lu, Z.; Jie, H.; Feng, K. Ursolic Acid Induces Apoptosis of Prostate Cancer Cells via the PI3K/Akt/mTOR Pathway. *Am. J. Chin. Med.* **2015**, *43*, 1471–1486.

30. Kumar, D.; Shankar, S.; Srivastava, R.K. Rottlerin induces autophagy and apoptosis in prostate cancer stem cells via PI3K/Akt/mTOR signaling pathway. *Cancer Lett.* **2014**, *343*, 179–189. [CrossRef] [PubMed]

31. Yasumizu, Y.; Kosaka, T.; Miyazaki, Y.; Kikuchi, E.; Miyajima, A.; Oya, M. 1318 hypoxic microenvironment promotes PI3K/AKT/mTOR signaling pathways in human castration resistant prostate cancer. *J. Urol.* **2013**, *189*, e539. [CrossRef]

32. Yang, Y.; Liu, L.; Zhang, Y.; Guan, H.; Wu, J.; Zhu, X.; Yuan, J.; Li, M. MiR-503 targets PI3K p85 and IKK-β and suppresses progression of non-small cell lung cancer. *Int. J. Gynecol. Cancer* **2014**, *135*, 1531–1542. [CrossRef] [PubMed]

33. Zhang, H.; Xu, H.L.; Wang, Y.C.; Lu, Z.Y.; Yu, X.F.; Sui, D.Y. 20(S)-Protopanaxadiol-Induced Apoptosis in MCF-7 Breast Cancer Cell Line through the Inhibition of PI3K/AKT/mTOR Signaling Pathway. *Int. J. Mol. Sci.* **2018**, *19*, 1053. [CrossRef] [PubMed]

34. Feng, L.M.; Wang, X.F.; Huang, Q.X. Thymoquinone induces cytotoxicity and reprogramming of EMT in gastric cancer cells by targeting PI3K/Akt/mTOR pathway. *J. Biosci.* **2017**, *42*, 547–554. [CrossRef] [PubMed]

35. Liu, Q.; Hu, S.; Zhang, Y.; Zhang, G.; Liu, S. Lycorine induces apoptosis in human pancreatic cancer cell line PANC-1 via ROS-mediated inactivation of the PI3K/Akt/mTOR signaling pathway. *Int. J. Clin. Lab. Res.* **2016**, *9*, 21048–21056.

36. Song, L.; Chang, J.; Li, Z. A serine protease extracted from Trichosanthes kirilowii induces apoptosis via the PI3K/AKT-mediated mitochondrial pathway in human colorectal adenocarcinoma cells. *Food Funct.* **2015**, *22*, 327–333. [CrossRef] [PubMed]

37. Chen, K.F.; Yeh, P.Y.; Yeh, K.H.; Lu, Y.S.; Huang, S.Y.; Cheng, A.L. Down-regulation of phospho-Akt is a major molecular determinant of bortezomib-induced apoptosis in hepatocellular carcinoma cells. *Cancer Res.* **2008**, *68*, 6698–6707. [CrossRef] [PubMed]

38. Imrali, A.; Mao, X.; Yeste-Velasco, M.; Shamash, J.; Lu, Y. Rapamycin inhibits prostate cancer cell growth through cyclin D1 and enhances the cytotoxic efficacy of cisplatin. *Am. J. Cancer Res.* **2016**, *6*, 1772. [PubMed]

39. Esmaeili, M.A.; Farimani, M.M.; Kiaei, M. Anticancer effect of calycopterin via PI3K/Akt and MAPK signaling pathways, ROS-mediated pathway and mitochondrial dysfunction in hepatoblastoma cancer (HepG2) cells. *Mol. Cell Biochem.* **2014**, *397*, 17–31. [CrossRef] [PubMed]

40. Win, K.T.; Lee, S.W.; Huang, H.Y.; Lin, L.C.; Lin, C.Y.; Hsing, C.H.; Chen, L.T.; Li, C.F. Nicotinamide N-methyltransferase overexpression is associated with Akt phosphorylation and indicates worse prognosis in patients with nasopharyngeal carcinoma. *Tumor Biol.* **2013**, *34*, 3923–3931. [CrossRef] [PubMed]

41. Vivanco, I.; Sawyers, C.L. The phosphatidylinositol 3-Kinase AKT pathway in human cancer. *Nat. Rev. Cancer* **2002**, *2*, 489–501. [CrossRef] [PubMed]

42. Pontes, H.A.R.; Pontes, F.S.C.; de Jesus, A.S.; Soares, M.C.P.; Gonçalves, F.L.N.; de Lucena Botelho, T.; do Carmo Ribeiro, J.; dos Santos Pinto, D., Jr. p-Akt and its relationship with clinicopathological features and survival in oral squamous cell carcinoma: An immunohistochemical study. *J. Oral Pathol. Med.* **2015**, *44*, 532–537. [CrossRef] [PubMed]

43. Wang, K.; Cao, F.; Fang, W.; Hu, Y.; Chen, Y.; Ding, H.; Yu, G. Activation of SNAT1/SLC38A1 in human breast cancer: Correlation with p-Akt overexpression. *BMC Cancer* **2013**, *13*, 343–352. [CrossRef] [PubMed]

44. Lim, W.T.; Zhang, W.H.; Miller, C.R.; Watters, J.W.; Gao, F.; Viswanathan, A.; Govindan, R.; Mcleod, H.L. PTEN and phosphorylated AKT expression and prognosis in early- and late-stage non-small cell lung cancer. *Oncol. Rep.* **2007**, *17*, 853–857. [CrossRef] [PubMed]

45. Morgensztern, D.; Mcleod, H.L. PI3K/Akt/mTOR pathway as a target for cancer therapy. *Anti-Cancer Drug* **2005**, *16*, 797–803. [CrossRef]

46. Hager, M.; Haufe, H.; Kemmerling, R.; Mikuz, G.; Kolbitsch, C.; Moser, P.L. PTEN expression in renal cell carcinoma and oncocytoma and prognosis. *Pathology* **2007**, *39*, 482–485. [CrossRef] [PubMed]

47. Brech, A.; Ahlquist, T.; Lothe, R.A.; Stenmark, H. Autophagy in tumour suppression and promotion. *Mol. Oncol.* **2009**, *3*, 366–375. [CrossRef] [PubMed]

48. Matuzaki, H. Akt phosphorylation site found in human caspase-9 is absent in mouse caspase-9. *Biochem. Biophys. Res. Commun.* **1999**, *264*, 550–555.
49. Goyal, A.; Wang, Y.; Graham, M.M.; Doseff, A.I.; Bhatt, N.Y.; Marsh, C.B. Monocyte survival factors induce Akt activation and suppress caspase-3. *Am. J. Resp. Cell Mol.* **2002**, *26*, 224–230. [CrossRef] [PubMed]
50. Taylor, R.C.; Cullen, S.P.; Martin, S.J. Apoptosis: Controlled demolition at the cellular level. *Nat. Rev. Mol. Cell Biol.* **2008**, *9*, 231–241. [CrossRef] [PubMed]
51. Tomomi, K.; Newmeyer, D.D. Bcl-2-family proteins and the role of mitochondria in apoptosis. *Curr. Opin. Cell Biol.* **2003**, *15*, 691–699.
52. Bosq, D. Targeting IAP proteins for therapeutic intervention in cancer. *Nat. Rev. Drug Discov.* **2012**, *11*, 109.
53. Fulda, S. Caspase-8 in cancer biology and therapy. *Cancer Lett.* **2009**, *281*, 128–133. [CrossRef] [PubMed]
54. Simone, F. Therapeutic opportunities based on caspase modulation. *Cell Dev. Biol.* **2017**. [CrossRef]
55. Fulda, S.; Küfer, M.U.; Meyer, E.; Van, V.F.; Dockhorn-Dworniczak, B.; Debatin, K.M. Sensitization for death receptor- or drug-induced apoptosis by re-expression of caspase-8 through demethylation or gene transfer. *Oncogene* **2001**, *20*, 5865–5877. [CrossRef] [PubMed]
56. Zong-Ze, W.U.; Ding, G.F.; Yang, Z.S.; Fang-Miao, Y.U.; Tang, Y.P.; Jia, Y.L.; Zheng, Y.Y.; Chen, R. Enzymatic preparation of oligopeptide from anthopleura anjunae and its anti-cancer activity of prostate cancer cells. *Oceanol. Limnol. Sin.* **2017**, *48*, 1114–1123.
57. Tang, Y.; Yu, F.; Zhang, G.; Yang, Z.; Huang, F.; Ding, G. A Purified Serine Protease from Nereis virens and Its Impaction of Apoptosis on Human Lung Cancer Cells. *Molecules* **2017**, *22*, 1123. [CrossRef] [PubMed]
58. Chen, J. The Cell-Cycle Arrest and Apoptotic Functions of p53 in Tumor Initiation and Progression. *CSH Perspect. Med.* **2016**, *6*, a026104–a026119. [CrossRef] [PubMed]
59. Luo, W.J.; Xing, X.M.; Wang, C.F.; Hu, L.T.; Zhao, G.Q.; Liu, X.P.; Wu, K.; Li, H. Effect of recombinant human platelet derived growth factor B on cat corneal endothelial cell viability mediated by adeno-associated virus. *Int. J. Ophthalmol.* **2012**, *5*, 419–423. [PubMed]

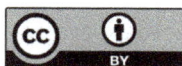

marine drugs

MDPI

Article

Novel Natural Angiotensin Converting Enzyme (ACE)-Inhibitory Peptides Derived from Sea Cucumber-Modified Hydrolysates by Adding Exogenous Proline and a Study of Their Structure–Activity Relationship

Jianpeng Li [1], Zunying Liu [1], Yuanhui Zhao [1,*], Xiaojie Zhu [1], Rilei Yu [2], Shiyuan Dong [1] and Haohao Wu [1]

[1] College of Food Science and Engineering, Ocean University of China, Qingdao 266003, China; changjing@stu.ouc.edu.cn (J.L.); liuzunying@ouc.edu.cn (Z.L.); jie86230@163.com (X.Z.); dongshiyuan@ouc.edu.cn (S.D.); wuhaohao@ouc.edu.cn (H.W.)

[2] School of Medicine and Pharmacy, Ocean University of China, Qingdao 266003, China; ryu@ouc.edu.cn

*   Correspondence: zhaoyuanhui@ouc.edu.cn; Tel./Fax: +86-532-82032400

Received: 13 July 2018; Accepted: 2 August 2018; Published: 4 August 2018

Abstract: Natural angiotensin converting enzyme (ACE)-inhibitory peptides, which are derived from marine products, are useful as antihypertensive drugs. Nevertheless, the activities of these natural peptides are relatively low, which limits their applications. The aim of this study was to prepare efficient ACE-inhibitory peptides from sea cucumber-modified hydrolysates by adding exogenous proline according to a facile plastein reaction. When 40% proline (w/w, proline/free amino groups) was added, the modified hydrolysates exhibited higher ACE-inhibitory activity than the original hydrolysates. Among the modified hydrolysates, two novel efficient ACE-inhibitory peptides, which are namely PNVA and PNLG, were purified and identified by a sequential approach combining a sephadex G-15 gel column, reverse-phase high-performance liquid chromatography (RP-HPLC) and matrix-assisted laser desorption/ionization time-of-flight mass spectrometry (MALDI-TOF/MS), before we conducted confirmatory studies with synthetic peptides. The ACE-inhibitory activity assay showed that PNVA and PNLG exhibited lower IC_{50} values of 8.18 ± 0.24 and 13.16 ± 0.39 μM than their corresponding truncated analogs (NVA and NLG), respectively. Molecular docking showed that PNVA and PNLG formed a larger number of hydrogen bonds with ACE than NVA and NLG, while the proline at the N-terminal of peptides can affect the orientation of the binding site of ACE. The method developed in this study may potentially be applied to prepare efficient ACE-inhibitory peptides, which may play a key role in hypertension management.

Keywords: sea cucumber; ACE-inhibitory peptide; molecular docking; structure-activity relationship; plastein reaction

1. Introduction

Hypertension is one of the leading causes of global disease burden [1]. In 2015, hypertension was estimated to affect 874 million adults worldwide (systolic blood pressure $\geq$ 140 mmHg), causing approximately 4.5 million deaths. Furthermore, the number of patients suffering from hypertension continues to grow [2]. Angiotensin-converting enzyme (ACE) plays a critical role in blood pressure control systems (renin-angiotensin system) as it converts angiotensin I into angiotensin II, leading to the development of hypertension [3,4]. Therefore, it is quite essential to study the inhibition of ACE in order to prevent and manage hypertension.

Currently, chemically synthesized ACE inhibitor drugs, such as captopril, enalapril and lisinopril, are being widely used in clinical applications [5–7]. However, pharmaceutical drugs may lead to some side effects, such as changes in taste, coughs and rashes [8,9]. Consequently, it is important to develop new, efficient and safe natural substitutes to reduce the application of chemical drugs. ACE-inhibitory peptides, which are safer than synthetic ACE inhibitors, have been shown to be useful as antihypertensive drugs [10]. Furthermore, they are found in many food protein sources [4,11,12], including sea cucumber (*Acaudina molpadioidea*). The sea cucumber is a particularly good source of bioactive peptides and is rich in proteins that result in high yields of peptides [13,14]. Recently, it has been reported that efficient ACE-inhibitory peptides can be obtained from *Acaudina molpadioidea* protein hydrolysates by a facile plastein reaction [15–17]. Plastein reaction was first discovered by Danilevski in 1902 when he added chymotrypsin to protein hydrolysates, which is considered to be a reverse enzymatic reaction. Since then, the plastein reaction has been used widely for many purposes [11], including the modification of some protein hydrolysates to improve their antioxidant properties [18] or ACE-inhibitory activity [19].

A number of structure–activity relationship studies have showed that peptides, such as APP [4], KPLL [20] and VYPFPGPIPNSLPQNIPP [21], exhibit high ACE-inhibitory activity, which suggests the importance of proline in controlling the ACE-inhibitory activity. ACE-inhibitory activity could be increased from 27.8% to 76.4% by adding proline to casein hydrolysates [11]. This effect is probably due to the imidazole ring in proline residues exhibiting a strong affinity for the amino acid residues at the active centers of ACE [22], thus resulting in an improvement in the ACE-inhibitory activity. Therefore, it might be reasonable to assume that adding exogenous proline to the plastein reaction system is an effective method to further enhance ACE-inhibitory activity.

Structural bioinformatics show that the activity of ACE-inhibitory peptides is related to both their molecular masses and amino acid sequences [23]. Some studies showed that short-chain polypeptides with low molecular masses exhibited high ACE-inhibitory activity [24,25]. For example, MVGSAPGVL and LGPLGHQ with small molecular masses exhibited high ACE-inhibitory activity [26]. Intriguingly, some studies indicated that the ACE-inhibitory activity of nonapeptide is significantly higher than that of hexapeptide [27], while the inhibitory activity of hexapeptide is also significantly higher than that of tripeptide [11]. Thus, apart from molecular weight, the amino acid sequence also plays an important role in determining the ACE-inhibitory activity of peptides. Many structure–activity relationship studies indicated the importance of the C-terminal of amino acids in determining the ACE-inhibitory activity. The inhibitory activity of polypeptides is higher when the C-terminal amino acids are aromatic amino acids (Trp, Tyr and Phe) or aliphatic amino acids (Ile, Ala, Leu and Met) [28]. However, there are only a few studies examining the influence of N-terminal amino acids on the ACE-inhibitory activity and their ACE-inhibition mechanism has not been clearly elucidated. Molecular docking simulations can provide further insight into peptide−ACE interactions and provide a deeper understanding of the ACE-inhibition mechanism in peptides.

To the best of our knowledge, the addition of exogenous amino acids to *Acaudina molpadioidea* protein hydrolysates to enhance the activity of natural ACE-inhibitory peptides has not been previously discussed. The aim of this study was to prepare efficient ACE-inhibitory peptides from sea cucumber-modified hydrolysates by adding exogenous amino acids according to a facile plastein reaction. Furthermore, we aimed to identify the ACE-inhibitory peptides with high activities by matrix-assisted laser desorption/ionization time-of-flight mass spectrometry (MALDI-TOF/MS). In addition, molecular docking simulations were conducted to investigate the nature of interactions between the peptides and ACE. This study can provide previously unknown information on the effect of exogenous amino acids on the activity of natural ACE-inhibitory peptides and provide an insight into the peptide structure−ACE inhibition relationship.

2. Results and Discussion

2.1. Modification of Acaudina molpadioidea Protein Hydrolysates by Adding Exogenous Amino Acids

As shown in Figure 1A, the ACE-inhibitory activity of modified hydrolysates significantly increased when compared to original hydrolysates in the presence of exogenous Phe, Trp and Pro at 50% weight proportions to free amino groups. After 6 h of reaction, the maximum ACE-inhibitory activity was found in the Pro group ($p < 0.05$). These results demonstrate that the plastein reaction modified by the addition of exogenous Pro was capable of improving ACE-inhibitory activity. The obtained results are consistent with Sun et al. [11], who reported that the ACE-inhibitory activity of casein hydrolysates was enhanced by adding exogenous Pro. In addition, Bougatef et al. [8] reported that the C-terminal domain of ACE exhibited high hydrophobicity. Hydrophobic amino acids play a crucial role in the inhibition of ACE. The exogenous Tyr, Leu, Phe, Trp and Pro used in this study were hydrophobic amino acids. We deduced that the enhancement in ACE-inhibitory activity upon the addition of Pro groups might be due to the assembly of free Pro in ACE-inhibitory peptides. To confirm this hypothesis, the composition of the free amino acids in the reaction system was investigated. As shown in Table 1, the total free amino acid content constantly decreased with an increase in reaction time, which differs from the case of original hydrolysates. This suggests that free amino acids are involved in the synthesis reaction. The single free amino acid content also exhibited a decreasing trend over a period of 4 h. This is especially true in the case of Pro, whose content decreased to (0.23 ± 0.02) g/(100 mL) after 1 h of reaction (Table 1), suggesting that Pro might be incorporated in the peptide chain during the synthesis reaction. In their study, Sun et al. [11] reported that free amino acids could be introduced into the peptide chain through condensation. From these results, it could be assumed that exogenous Pro was integrated into ACE-inhibitory peptides, which could partly contribute to the high ACE-inhibitory activity.

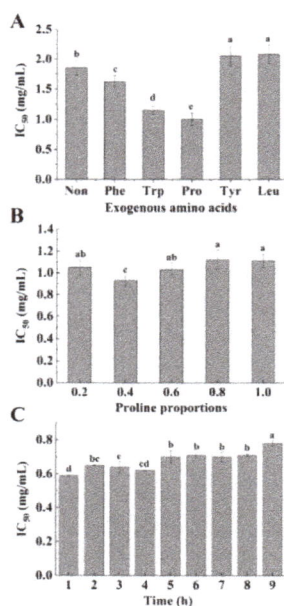

Figure 1. Effect of different amino acids (**A**), proline proportions (**B**) and reaction time (**C**) on the ACE-inhibitory activity. The values of three replicates are shown as mean ± standard deviation. Different lowercase letters indicate significantly different values ($p < 0.05$).

Table 1. The variations of free amino acid groups during plastein reaction.

Amino Acids	Original	1 h g/(100 mL)	4 h g/(100 mL)
Thr	0.05 ± 0.02	0.04 ± 0.01	0.03 ± 0.01
Ser	0.01 ± 0.01	0.01 ± 0.01	0.01 ± 0.01
Glu	0.03 ± 0.01	0.02 ± 0.01	0.02 ± 0.01
Gly	0.05 ± 0.02	0.04 ± 0.02	0.04 ± 0.02
Ala	0.04 ± 0.02	0.03 ± 0.01	0.03 ± 0.01
Cys	0.06 ± 0.02	0.05 ± 0.02	0.05 ± 0.01
Val	0.03 ± 0.01	0.03 ± 0.01	0.02 ± 0.01
Met	0.01 ± 0.01	0.01 ± 0.01	0.01 ± 0.01
Ile	0.02 ± 0.01	0.01 ± 0.02	0.01 ± 0.01
Leu	0.05 ± 0.02	0.04 ± 0.01	0.04 ± 0.02
Tyr	0.03 ± 0.01	0.02 ± 0.01	0.02 ± 0.01
Phe	0.03 ± 0.01	0.02 ± 0.01	0.02 ± 0.01
Lys	0.02 ± 0.01	0.01 ± 0.01	0.02 ± 0.01
His	0.01 ± 0.01	0.01 ± 0.01	0.01 ± 0.01
Arg	0.14 ± 0.03	0.11 ± 0.02	0.11 ± 0.02
Pro	0.29 ± 0.04 [a]	0.23 ± 0.02 [b]	0.2 ± 0.02 [b]
Total	0.90 ± 0.09 [a]	0.69 ± 0.08 [b]	0.66 ± 0.08 [b]

Mean ± SD ($n = 3$). Values with different superscript letters are significantly different ($p < 0.05$).

The plastein reaction is mainly affected by substrate concentration and reaction time [29]. Therefore, the effect of different Pro proportions and reaction time on the ACE-inhibitory activity was determined (Figure 1B,C). When 40% Pro (*w*/*w*, proline/free amino groups) was added, the ACE-inhibitory activity obtained was higher compared to other proportions after 6 h of reaction ($IC_{50} = 0.93 ± 0.05$ mg/mL) ($p < 0.05$) (Figure 1B). Meanwhile, the ACE-inhibitory activity was the highest ($IC_{50} = 0.59 ± 0.03$ mg/mL) after 1 h of reaction (Figure 1C). After this time period, the activity decreased with an increase in reaction time. Our results demonstrate that the ACE-inhibitory activity of hydrolysates can be further improved by optimizing the reaction conditions.

2.2. Isolation and Purification of Modified ACE-Inhibitory Peptides and the ACE-Inhibitory Activity of Each Fraction

Chromatographic fractionation is a method that is often used for peptide elution. A Sephadex G-15 gel column was used to fractionate the ACE-inhibitory peptides, before the fractions were pooled to obtain fractions A−H at 220 nm (Figure 2A). After this, these components were collected for determining the ACE-inhibitory activity. Although ACE-inhibitory activity could be observed in all fractions (Figure 2C), fraction E exhibited higher ACE-inhibitory activity compared to others ($p < 0.05$). The fractions with the same molecular mass peaked at the same time in the Sephadex G-15 gel column [30]. Therefore, it was concluded that fraction E may be a mixture and it required further fractionation by RP-HPLC.

RP-HPLC is a frequently used tool for the isolation and purification of polypeptides. Figure 2B summarizes the RP-HPLC analysis results of fraction E in terms of its absorbance at 220 nm. After 8 min of elution, eight major peaks were detected, among which the peak corresponding to fraction E3 exhibited a relatively high intensity. The different fractions showed different activities (Figure 2D) and fraction E3 exhibited higher activity compared to other fractions ($IC_{50} = 27 ± 2$ µg/mL) ($p < 0.05$). Fraction E3 was purified by 21.85-fold using a two-step purification process (Table 2). This suggests that the ACE-inhibitory activity of *Acaudina molpadioides* peptides can be significantly improved by fractionation and purification.

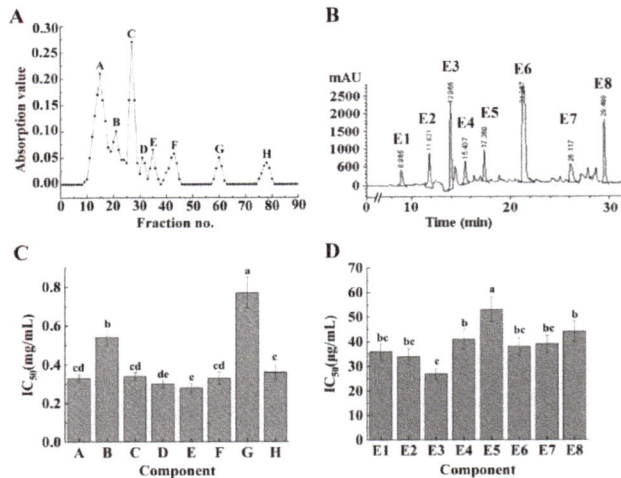

Figure 2. Isolation and purification of modified ACE-inhibitory peptides using a Sephadex G-15 gel column (**A**) and RP-HPLC (**B**). The corresponding ACE-inhibitory activities of each fraction are shown in (**C,D**). Different lowercase letters indicate significantly different values ($p < 0.05$).

Table 2. Purification procedure of ACE-inhibitory peptides.

Component	Purification	IC$_{50}$ (mg/mL)	Purification Fold
Hydrolysates	Ultrafiltration	0.590 ± 0.030 [a]	1.00
E	Sephadex G-15	0.288 ± 0.013 [b]	2.05
E3	RP-HPLC	0.027 ± 0.002 [c]	21.85

Mean $\pm$ SD ($n = 3$). Values with different superscript letters are significantly different ($p < 0.05$).

2.3. Identification of the Purified Peptides and Evaluation of Their ACE-Inhibitory Activity

According to the MALDI-TOF analysis of fraction E3, its mass is 400.0966 Da. Furthermore, different peptides were investigated by MALDI-TOF/MS fragmentation analysis. According to the MS spectral data, the peptide sequences were preliminarily matched with those of NVA and NLG, which had been previously characterized in the database. Subsequently, the N-terminal of the peptides was inferred to be Pro by calculating the molecular mass. From these results, we deduced that the whole peptide sequences were PNVA (Figure 3A) and PNLG (Figure 3B), which did not match with the database. Our results indicate that PNVA and PNLG are novel ACE-inhibitory peptides, which are realized in *Acaudina molpadioidea* protein hydrolysates by adding exogenous Pro. These observations are consistent with the results shown in Figure 1 and Table 1.

Subsequently, four peptides, which were namely PNVA, PNLG, NVA and NLG, were synthesized by a chemical method and their ACE-inhibitory activities were determined. As shown in Table 3, the activity of PNVA (IC$_{50}$ = 8.18 $\pm$ 0.24 μM) was significantly higher than the activity of PNLG (IC$_{50}$ = 13.16 $\pm$ 0.39 μM). Meanwhile, NVA (IC$_{50}$ = 12.69 $\pm$ 1.50 μM) exhibited a significantly higher activity than NLG (IC$_{50}$ = 17.45 $\pm$ 0.89 μM). Our observations are consistent with those of Jang et al. [28], who reported that the presence of aliphatic amino acids at the penultimate C-terminus, which was namely Val, resulted in significantly increased ACE-binding affinity compared to other amino acids. Moreover, Mizuno et al. [31] reported that the presence of hydrophobic amino acids at the C-terminus positively influenced the ACE-inhibitory activity. The hydrophobic parameters of Ala are significantly higher than those of Gly [32], suggesting that the presence of hydrophobic Ala at the C-terminus exerts more influence on the ACE-inhibitory activity than Gly. This report is consistent with our results, which is shown in Table 3. In addition, Table 3 shows that the ACE-inhibitory activity of PNVA is significantly higher than that of NVA. Similarly, the activity of PNLG is significantly higher than that of NLG. The results indicated that Pro at the N-terminus significantly enhanced the ACE-inhibitory activity. Many structure–activity relationship studies highlighted the influence of C-terminal amino acids on the ACE-inhibitory activity [12,28,31,33]. However, there are very few studies examining the effect of N-terminal amino acids on the ACE-inhibitory activity.

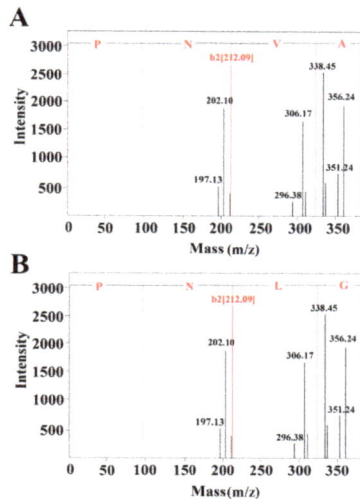

Figure 3. MALDI-TOF/MS spectra of the amino acid sequences of fraction E3. (**A**) peptide PNVA. (**B**) peptide PNLG.

Table 3. IC_{50} values and amino acid sequences of peptides, based on the algorithm for peptide sequencing de novo.

Sequence	Molecular Mass (Da)	ACE IC_{50} (μM) [2]
PNVA [1]	399.45	8.18 ± 0.24 [a]
PNLG [1]	399.45	13.16 ± 0.39 [b]
NVA	302.33	12.69 ± 1.50 [b]
NLG	302.33	17.45 ± 0.89 [c]

[1] peptides from *Acaudina molpadioidea* protein hydrolysates. [2] Mean ± SD ($n = 3$). Values with different superscript letters are significantly different ($p < 0.05$).

2.4. Molecular Docking of ACE-Inhibitory Peptides

To understand the molecular interaction mechanism of the four peptides (PNVA, PNLG, NVA and NLG) against ACE, molecular docking analysis was performed using Molecular Operating Environment (MOE) software. The docking scores of PNVA, PNLG, NVA and NLG were −7.13, −6.77, −5.14 and −5.12 kcal/mol, respectively (Table 4), which suggests that the model can efficiently simulate molecular docking.

The modes of action of ACE-inhibitory peptides include competitive, noncompetitive, uncompetitive and mixed modes. Most ACE-inhibitory peptides act as competitive inhibitors [34]. The binding of ACE to a substrate or competitive inhibitor of amino acid residues is highly specific [11]. Consistent with our experimental studies, the results of molecular docking analysis suggest that the truncation of Pro reduced the binding affinity of PNVA and PNLG as the active peptide PNVA showed the highest binding affinity (Table 4). ACE is a metallo-enzyme with the zinc ion at the active site coordinated by His383, His387 and Glu411 [35]. As shown in Figure 4, PNVA forms eleven hydrogen bonds with the residues Asp354, Thr358, Asp393, His331, His491, Tyr501, Gln259, Tyr498 and Lys489 (Figure 4A,B). Furthermore, PNLG forms ten hydrogen bonds with the residues Asp354, Glu262, Asp255, Ser260, His361, Gln259, Lys489 and His491 (Figure 4C,D). NVA forms seven hydrogen bonds with the residues Glu431, Lys432, Asp391, His331 and Zn1620 (Figure 4E,F), while NLG forms five hydrogen bonds with the residues Asp393, Thr358, His331, His365 and Zn1620 (Figure 4G,H). These results indicate that the ACE active binding sites of different peptides are not identical. This conclusion is consistent with the observations of Liu et al. [35]. Overall, our molecular docking studies indicated that the peptides PNVA and PNLG form more hydrogen bonds with ACE than their corresponding truncated analogs (NVA and NLG), while the four active peptides bind to the catalytic pocket of ACE mainly through a network of hydrogen bonds. The number of hydrogen bonds played an important role in determining the binding affinity of peptides with ACE [17]. For example, lisinopril with higher ACE-inhibitory activity forms nine hydrogen bonds with ACE active residues, which was similar to our results.

Table 4. Docking score and experimental binding affinity of peptides.

Peptide	Docking Score (kcal/mol)	Experimental Binding Affinity (kcal/mol) [1]
PNVA	−7.13	−2.34
PNLG	−6.77	−2.47
NVA	−5.14	−2.46
NLG	−5.12	−2.54

[1] Ligand binding affinities were calculated using the equation: $\Delta G = -RT \ln IC_{50}$, where $R = 8.314 \text{ J} \cdot \text{mol}^{-1} \cdot \text{K}^{-1}$ and $T = 300$ K.

Intriguingly, the Pro of PNVA forms two hydrogen bonds with Asp354 and Thr358, while the Pro of PNLG forms two hydrogen bonds with Asp354 and Glu262. These results indicate that the Pro at the N-terminal of both PNVA and PNLG plays an essential role in determining their binding affinity. Similarly, Min et al. [36] reported that the interactions of the side chains of Leu and Ile with the hydrophobic residues determined the binding positions of N-terminal residues of LKP and IKP. This subsequently influenced the interaction of the residues of LKP and IKP with the active sites of ACE. In addition, the orientations of the last residues of PNVA and PNLG are different from those of NVA and NLG (Figure 4A,C,E,G). The carboxyl groups of the C-terminals, which are namely Ala and Gly, of PNVA and PNLG are oriented towards Lys489 of the ACE, whereas the carboxyl groups of NVA and NLG are oriented towards Zn^{2+}. These results indicate that the Pro at the N-terminal of the peptides could reform the rigid structure of the peptides, further altering the binding sites between peptides and ACE. These are similar to the observations made by Liu et al. [35], who reported that Leu at the N-terminal of LVKF could alter the binding sites of ACE between LVKF and VKF. In summary, our docking studies suggest that Pro at the N-terminal of peptides can affect both the peptide-binding affinity and orientation of the binding site of ACE. The added exogenous Pro was possibly assembled at the N-terminals of their corresponding truncated analogs (NVA and NLG) (Figure 5). Thus, this reforms the rigid structure of the peptides, altering the binding sites and forming a large number of hydrogen bonds with ACE. This subsequently leads to a decrease in the ACE catalytic function.

Numerous studies on hypertensive human volunteers have demonstrated that ACE-inhibitory peptides significantly reduce blood pressure [12]. In addition, some ACE-inhibitory biopeptides have been commercialized [37], which suggests that these biopeptides can be applied for the supplemental treatment of hypertensive patients. In the present study, two novel biopeptides with high ACE-inhibitory activity (PNVA and PNLG) were synthesized by the addition of exogenous Pro. Although the ACE-inhibitory activities of PNVA ($IC_{50} = 8.18 \pm 0.24$ μM) and PNLG ($IC_{50} = 13.16 \pm 0.39$ μM) were much lower than synthetic ACE inhibitor captopril ($IC_{50} = 23$ nM) [5], the peptides from *A. molpadioidea* were characterized as novel peptides, which are derived from a food source that is eaten daily.

Therefore, the ACE-inhibitory peptides (PNVA and PNLG) will be very useful in the preparation of antihypertensive drugs. Meanwhile, their activities were much higher than that of other biopeptides, AGPPGSDGQPGAK (IC_{50} = 420 ± 20 μM) [38], AV (IC_{50} = 956.30 μM) [39] and PPK (IC_{50} > 1000 μM), suggesting the peptides that we prepared have higher ACE-inhibitory activities. The ACE-inhibitory peptides derived from sea cucumber-modified hydrolysates by adding exogenous Pro will play a key role in hypertension management.

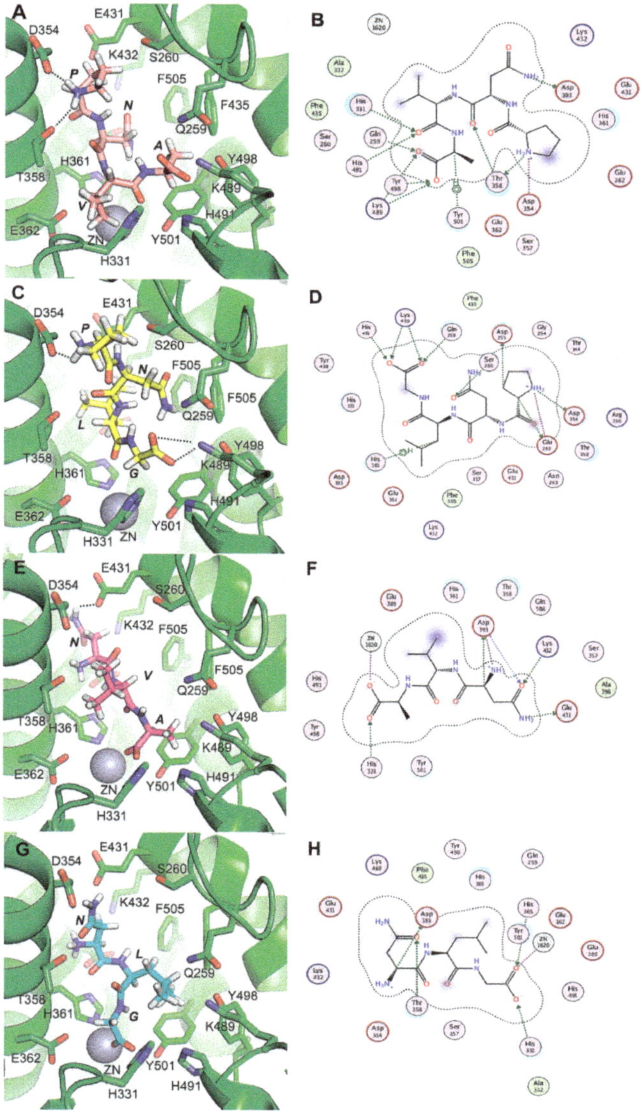

Figure 4. (**A–H**) show the binding modes of PNVA, PNLG, NVA and NLG with the ACE, respectively. (**B,D,F,H**) show 2D schematics of the peptide-binding modes. The dashed lines indicate the hydrogen bonds that were formed between the peptide and residues of the binding sites.

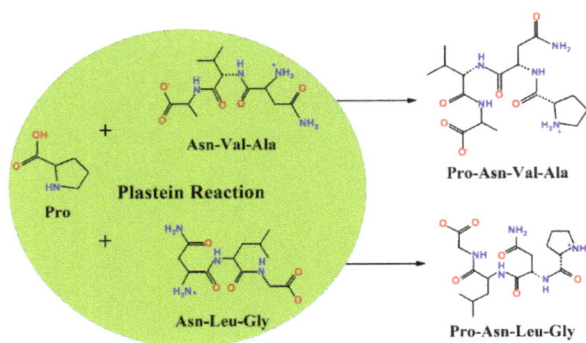

Figure 5. Schematic illustration of the formation of ACE-inhibitory peptides during the plastein reaction.

3. Materials and Methods

3.1. Materials and Chemicals

Sea cucumber (*Acaudina molpadioidea*) was purchased from a local market (Qingdao, China) and its water content was determined to be 12.65% per 20 g on average. Hippuryl histidyl leucine (HHL), rabbit-lung ACE and Sephadex G-15 were purchased from Sigma Chemical Ltd (St. Louis, MO, USA). Papain (from papaya) and trypsin (from bovine sources) were purchased from Nanning Pangbo Biological Engineering Ltd (Nanning, China). O-Pthaldialdehyde (OPA) was purchased from Beijing Soularbio Technology Ltd. (Beijing, China). Proline (PubChem CID 145742), valine (PubChem CID 6287), tyrosine (PubChem CID 6057), tryptophan (PubChem CID 6305), leucine (PubChem CID 6106) and phenylalanine (PubChem CID 6140) were purchased from Sinopharm Chemical Reagent Ltd. (Shanghai, China). All other chemicals were obtained from local commercial sources and were of the highest purity available.

3.2. Acaudina molpadioidea Body Wall Protein Extraction

The protein present in the body wall of *Acaudina molpadioidea* was extracted as described by Jamilah et al. [40]. Briefly, the body wall of *Acaudina molpadioidea* was fully swollen in distilled water over a period of 12 h at 120 °C, before being added to fresh distilled water (10 times in excess) to cut into pieces. During stirring, the protein was extracted at 45 °C over a period of 8 h and centrifuged (10,000× *g*, 20 min) to obtain water-soluble protein solutions. After this, these solutions were freeze-dried using a lyophilizer (Scientz-10nd, Ningbo Scientz Biotechnology Co. Ltd., Ningbo, China).

3.3. Acaudina molpadioidea Protein Hydrolysates Preparation

The freeze-dried *Acaudina molpadioidea* body wall protein was initially dissolved in water and its pH was adjusted to 7.0. After this, trypsin (2.5 kU/g protein) and papain (2.5 kU/g protein) were added to this solution and digested in a 50 °C water bath for 4 h. Subsequently, the enzymes were inactivated at 95 °C for 15 min. The suspension was then centrifuged at 8000× *g* and 4 °C for 20 min, after which the supernatant was removed and ultrafiltration precipitation was carried out with a 5 K membrane (Millipore Isopore, Billerica, MA, USA). The obtained precipitate was freeze-dried (Scientz-10nd, Ningbo Scientz Biotechnology Co. Ltd., Ningbo, China) and stored until further use.

3.4. Modification of Acaudina molpadioidea Protein Hydrolysates by Plastein Reaction

Different concentrations of exogenous Pro, Phe, Trp, Tyr and Leu (at pre-determined weight ratios of exogenous amino acid to free amino groups) were added to the *Acaudina molpadioidea* protein hydrolysates for the plastein reaction. The reaction conditions were as follows: substrate concentration of 40% (*w*/*v*), temperature of 45 °C and papain dosage of 2.5 kU/g protein. Furthermore, the effect of different proportions and reaction time on the ACE-inhibitory activity was determined.

3.5. Changes in the Content of Free Amino Groups during the Plastein Reaction

The OPA method [41], with some modifications, was used to determine the free amino groups in the reaction mixture. The reagent was prepared daily and protected from light. The OPA assay was carried out by adding 3 mL of *Acaudina molpadioidea* hydrolysates to the same volume of OPA reagent (40 mg/mL). After 5 min, the absorbance of the resultant solution was measured at 340 nm using a UV spectrophotometer (UV-2550, Shimadzu, Kyoto, Japan). L-leucine was used as the standard. The equation of the standard curve is $Y = 0.3037X + 0.0078$, where X is the concentration of free amino acids and Y is the absorption value of the sample.

3.6. Determination of the ACE-Inhibitory Activity of Hydrolysates

The ACE-inhibitory activity of the hydrolysates was measured according to a previously reported protocol [14] with slight modifications. Briefly, a sample solution with 40 μL of ACE solution (25 mU/mL) was pre-incubated at 37 °C for 10 min. After this, the mixture was incubated with 50 μL of the substrate (8.3 mM Hip-His-Leu in 50 mM sodium borate buffer containing 0.5 M NaCl at pH of 8.3) for 60 min at the same temperature. The reaction was terminated by the addition of 1.0 M HCl (200 μL). The absorbance of hippuric acid in the incubated solution was determined at 228 nm using a UV-spectrophotometer (UV-2550, Shimadzu, Kyoto, Japan). The IC_{50} value was defined as the concentration of inhibitor that was needed to inhibit 50% of the ACE activity.

3.7. Solvent Fractionation of ACE-Inhibitory Peptides by Chromatography

ACE-inhibitory peptides were purified using a Sephadex G-15 column (2.6 cm × 65 cm) and eluted with double distilled water at a flow rate of 1.2 mL/min. The absorbance of the eluent was monitored at 220 nm.

3.8. Analysis and Purification of ACE-Inhibitory Peptides in Hydrolysates by RP-HPLC

The ACE-inhibitory activity of peptides in the hydrolysates was analyzed by RP-HPLC on a Zorbax SB-C18 column (9.4 mm × 250 mm, Agilent, Santa Clara, CA, USA) equipped with an Agilent 1260 infinity HPLC system (Agilent Technology, Mississauga, ON, Canada) at a flow rate of 1 mL/min. An acetonitrile gradient from 5% to 30% was used for 40 min to separate different groups of peptides. Chromatographic separation was carried out at 35 °C. The components were collected at the absorbance of 220 nm and their ACE-inhibitory activity was measured.

3.9. Mass Spectrometric Analysis and Synthesis of Purified Peptides

The molecular weights of peptides in the filtered hydrolysates were analyzed by MALDI-TOF (TOF 4800, Micromass Company, Manchester, UK). The amino acid sequences were determined in the positive ion mode by de novo sequencing. Subsequently, the peptides were synthesized using the solid phase method and purified by HPLC (ChinaPeptides Co. Ltd., Shanghai, China). The synthesized peptides are listed in Table 3.

3.10. Molecular Docking

The initial peptide structures of PNVA, PNLG, NVA and NLG were produced using the xleap module of AMBER16 (University of California, San Francisco, CA, USA) and were subjected to minimization using the Molecular Operating Environment (MOE) software (version 2016) [42]. Molecular docking was performed by MOE using the AMBER10: EHT force field [42]. The crystal structures of ACE (PDB ID: 2XYD) [17] bound with PNVA, PNLG, NVA and NLG were obtained from the Protein Data Bank (http://www.rcsb.org) for the docking studies. The induced-fit docking approach was applied to analyze the side-chain flexibility of residues at the binding sites.

3.11. Statistical Analysis

All the data (average of three replicates) are reported in the form of mean ± standard deviation and the results were validated by one-way analysis of variance (ANOVA). Significant differences between the means of the parameters were determined by Duncan's multiple range tests ($p < 0.05$).

4. Conclusions

Upon the addition of exogenous amino acids, it was possible to enhance the ACE-inhibitory activity of *Acaudina molpadioidea*-protein hydrolysates. In particular, *Acaudina molpadioidea*-modified hydrolysates with 40% proline (w/w, proline/free amino groups) possessed higher ACE-inhibitory activity than the original hydrolysates. Furthermore, the free proline content in the reaction system decreased significantly ($p < 0.05$). In addition, two novel ACE-inhibitory peptides, PNVA and PNLG with IC_{50} values = 8.18 ± 0.24 and 13.16 ± 0.39 µM, were identified for the first time in *Acaudina molpadioidea* protein hydrolysates. Molecular docking showed that PNVA and PNLG form more hydrogen bonds with ACE than NVA and NLG, while the presence of proline at the N-terminals of the peptides can affect the orientation of the binding sites of ACE, leading to a reduction in ACE activity. The exogenous proline is assembled into ACE-inhibitory peptides, with this phenomenon partially contributing to the increase in the ACE-inhibitory activity of natural peptides. In this study, we demonstrated that the addition of exogenous proline to *Acaudina molpadioidea* protein hydrolysates through the plastein reaction is a promising method to enhance the activity of natural ACE-inhibitory peptides. Further studies are necessary to investigate the detailed assembly of exogenous proline using isotopic tracer methods and to prove the in vivo efficacy of ACE-inhibitory peptides in lowering blood pressure. The results of the present study also highlight the potential applications of plastein reaction in preparing antihypertensive drugs.

Author Contributions: J.L. and Y.Z. designed the experiments. Z.L., X.Z., R.Y., S.D. and H.W. performed data analysis. J.L. wrote the manuscript. All authors commented on the results and modifed the manuscript.

Funding: This project was supported by Qingdao Science and Technology Development Project (No. 17-3-3-46-nsh), Shandong Provincial Key R & D Program (No. 2017GHY15128) and Natural Science Foundation of Shandong Province (No. ZR2015CM011), here the authors are gratefully acknowledged.

Conflicts of Interest: The authors have declared that no conflict of interest exists.

References

1. Kivimäki, M.; Steptoe, A. Effects of stress on the development and progression of cardiovascular disease. *Nat. Rev. Cardiol.* **2018**, *15*, 215–229. [CrossRef] [PubMed]
2. Forouzanfar, M.H.; Liu, P.; Roth, G.A.; Ng, M.; Biryukov, S.; Marczak, L.; Alexander, L.; Estep, K.; Hassen Abate, K.; Akinyemiju, T.F.; et al. Global burden of hypertension and systolic blood pressure of at least 110 to 115 mm Hg, 1990–2015. *JAMA* **2017**, *317*, 165–182. [CrossRef] [PubMed]
3. Bernstein, K.E.; Khan, Z.; Giani, J.F.; Cao, D.Y.; Bernstein, E.A.; Shen, X.Z. Angiotensin-converting enzyme in innate and adaptive immunity. *Nat. Rev. Nephrol.* **2018**, *14*, 325–336. [CrossRef] [PubMed]
4. Sangsawad, P.; Roytrakul, S.; Choowongkomon, K.; Kitts, D.D.; Chen, X.M.; Meng, G.; Lichan, E.; Yongsawatdigul, J. Transepithelial transport across Caco-2 cell monolayers of angiotensin converting enzyme (ACE) inhibitory peptides derived from simulated *in vitro* gastrointestinal digestion of cooked chicken muscles. *Food Chem.* **2018**, *251*, 77–85. [CrossRef] [PubMed]
5. Wood, R. Bronchospasm and cough as adverse reactions to the ACE inhibitors captopril, enalapril and lisinopril. A controlled retrospective cohort study. *Br. J. Clin. Pharmacol.* **1995**, *39*, 265–270. [CrossRef] [PubMed]

6. Yu, Y.; Hu, J.; Miyaguchi, Y.; Bai, X.; Du, Y.; Lin, B. Isolation and characterization of angiotensin I-converting enzyme inhibitory peptides derived from porcine hemoglobin. *Peptides* **2006**, *27*, 2950–2956. [CrossRef] [PubMed]

7. Todd, G.P.; Chadwick, I.G.; Higgins, K.S.; Yeo, W.W.; Jackson, P.R.; Ramsay, L.E. Relation between changes in blood pressure and serum ACE activity after a single dose of enalapril and ACE genotype in healthy subjects. *Br. J. Clin. Pharmacol.* **1995**, *39*, 131–134. [CrossRef] [PubMed]

8. Bougatef, A.; Nedjar-Arroume, N.; Ravallec-Plé, R.; Leroy, Y.; Guillochon, D.; Barkia, A.; Nasri, M. Angiotensin I-converting enzyme (ACE) inhibitory activities of sardinelle (*Sardinella aurita*) by-products protein hydrolysates obtained by treatment with microbial and visceral fish serine proteases. *Food Chem.* **2008**, *111*, 350–356. [CrossRef] [PubMed]

9. Erdmann, K.; Cheung, B.W.; Schröder, H. The possible roles of food-derived bioactive peptides in reducing the risk of cardiovascular disease. *J. Nutr. Biochem.* **2008**, *19*, 643–654. [CrossRef] [PubMed]

10. Raia, J.J., Jr.; Barone, J.A.; Byerly, W.G.; Lacy, C.R. Angiotensin-converting enzyme inhibitors: A comparative review. *Ann. Pharmacother.* **1990**, *24*, 506–525. [CrossRef]

11. Sun, H.; Li, T.J.; Zhao, X.H. ACE inhibition and enzymatic resistance in vitro of a casein hydrolysate subjected to plastein reaction in the presence of extrinsic proline and ethanol- or methanol-eater fractionation. *Int. J. Food Prop.* **2014**, *17*, 386–398. [CrossRef]

12. Corrons, M.A.; Liggieri, C.S.; Trejo, S.A.; Bruno, M.A. ACE-inhibitory peptides from bovine caseins released with peptidases from Maclura pomifera latex. *Food Res. Int.* **2017**, *93*, 8–15. [CrossRef] [PubMed]

13. Ye, L.; Xu, L.; Li, J. Preparation and anticoagulant activity of a fucosylated polysaccharide sulfate from a sea cucumber *Acaudina molpadioidea*. *Carbohyd. Polym.* **2012**, *87*, 2052–2057. [CrossRef]

14. Zhao, Y.; Li, B.; Dong, S.; Liu, Z.; Zhao, X.; Wang, J.; Zeng, M. A novel ACE-inhibitory peptide isolated from *Acaudina molpadioidea* hydrolysate. *Peptides* **2009**, *30*, 1028–1033. [CrossRef] [PubMed]

15. Zhao, Y.H.; Li, B.F.; Ma, J.J.; Dong, S.Y.; Liu, Z.Y.; Zeng, M.Y. Purification and synthesis of ACE-inhibitory peptide from *Acaudina molpadioidea* protein hydrolysate. *Chem. J. Chin. Univ.* **2012**, *33*, 308–312.

16. Zhu, X.J.; Zeng, M.Y.; Ma, G.L.; Zhao, Y.H.; Liu, Z.Y.; Dong, S.Y. Research on plastein reaction-basic modification of *Acaudina molpadioidea* protein hydrolysates and its effects on ACE activity. *Chin. J. Mar. Drugs* **2011**, *30*, 6–12.

17. Shen, Q.; Zeng, M.; Zhao, Y. Modification of *Acaudina molpadioides* hydrolysates by plastein reaction and preparation of ACE-inhibitory peptides. *Chem. J. Chin. Univ.* **2014**, *35*, 965–970.

18. Ono, S.; Kasai, D.; Sugano, T.; Ohba, K.; Takahashi, K. Production of water soluble antioxidative plastein from squid hepatopancreas. *J. Oil Chem. Soc. Jpn.* **2004**, *53*, 267–273. [CrossRef]

19. Xu, W.; Li, T.J.; Zhao, X.H. Coupled neutraseâ catalyzed plastein reaction mediated the ACE-inhibitory activity *in vitro* of casein hydrolysates prepared by alcalase. *Int. J. Food Prop.* **2013**, *16*, 429–443.

20. Sangsawad, P.; Roytrakul, S.; Yongsawatdigul, J. Angiotensin converting enzyme (ACE) inhibitory peptides derived from the simulated *in vitro* gastrointestinal digestion of cooked chicken breast. *J. Funct. Foods* **2017**, *29*, 77–83. [CrossRef]

21. Otte, J.; Shalaby, S.M.; Zakora, M.; Pripp, A.H.; El-Shabrawy, S.A. Angiotensin-converting enzyme inhibitory activity of milk protein hydrolysates: Effect of substrate, enzyme and time of hydrolysis. *Int. Dairy J.* **2007**, *17*, 488–503. [CrossRef]

22. Terashima, M.; Oe, M.; Ogura, K.; Matsumura, S. Inhibition strength of short peptides derived from an ACE-inhibitory peptide. *J. Agric. Food Chem.* **2011**, *59*, 11234–11237. [CrossRef] [PubMed]

23. Wang, X.; Xue, L.; Hu, Z.; Zhang, Q.; Li, Y.; Xia, L. Progress in research on structure–activity relationship of ACE-inhibitory peptides. *Food Sci.* **2017**, *38*, 305–310.

24. Kleekayai, T.; Harnedy, P.A.; O'Keeffe, M.B.; Poyarkov, A.A.; Cunhaneves, A.; Suntornsuk, W.; Fitzgerald, R.J. Extraction of antioxidant and ACE-inhibitory peptides from Thai traditional fermented shrimp pastes. *Food Chem.* **2015**, *176*, 441–447. [CrossRef] [PubMed]

25. Jiang, Z.M.; Bo, T.; Brodkorb, A.; Huo, G.C. Production, analysis and in vivo evaluation of novel angiotensin-I-converting enzyme inhibitory peptides from bovine casein. *Food Chem.* **2010**, *123*, 779–786. [CrossRef]

26. Ngo, D.H.; Ryu, B.; Kim, S.K. Active peptides from skate (*Okamejei kenojei*) skin gelatin diminish angiotensin-I converting enzyme activity and intracellular free radical-mediated oxidation. *Food Chem.* **2014**, *143*, 246–255. [CrossRef] [PubMed]

27. Aluko, R.E.; Girgih, A.T.; He, R.; Malomo, S.; Li, H.; Offengenden, M.; Wu, J. Structural and functional characterization of yellow field pea seed (*Pisum sativum* L.) protein-derived antihypertensive peptides. *Food Res. Int.* **2015**, *77*, 10–16. [CrossRef]

28. Jang, A.; Jo, C.; Kang, K.S.; Lee, M. Antimicrobial and human cancer cell cytotoxic effect of synthetic angiotensin-converting enzyme (ACE) inhibitory peptides. *Food Chem.* **2008**, *107*, 327–336. [CrossRef]

29. Brownsell, V.L.; Williams, R.J.H.; Andrews, A.T. Application of the plastein reaction to mycoprotein. II. plastein properties. *Food Chem.* **2001**, *72*, 337–346. [CrossRef]

30. Zhao, Y.; Ouyang, X.; Chen, J.; Zhao, L.; Qiu, X. Separation of aromatic monomers from oxidatively depolymerized products of lignin by combining sephadex and silica gel column chromatography. *Sep. Purif. Technol.* **2018**, *191*, 250–256. [CrossRef]

31. Aluko, R.E. Antihypertensive peptides from food proteins. *Annu. Rev. Food Sci. Technol.* **2015**, *6*, 235–262. [CrossRef] [PubMed]

32. Charton, M.; Charton, B.I. The structural dependence of amino acid hydrophobicity parameters. *J. Theor. Biol.* **1982**, *99*, 629–644. [CrossRef]

33. Abuohashish, H.M.; Ahmed, M.M.; Sabry, D.; Khattab, M.M.; Al-Rejaie, S.S. ACE-2/Ang1-7/Mas cascade mediates ACE inhibitor, captopril, protective effects in estrogen-deficient osteoporotic rats. *Biomed. Pharmacother.* **2017**, *92*, 58–68. [CrossRef] [PubMed]

34. Rao, S.Q.; Ju, T.; Sun, J.; Su, Y.J.; Xu, R.R.; Yang, Y.J. Purification and characterization of angiotensin I-converting enzyme inhibitory peptides from enzymatic hydrolysate of hen egg white lysozyme. *Food Res. Int.* **2012**, *46*, 127–134. [CrossRef]

35. Liu, R.; Zhu, Y.; Chen, J.; Wu, H.; Shi, L.; Wang, X.; Wang, L. Characterization of ACE-inhibitory peptides from *Mactra veneriformis* hydrolysate by nano-liquid chromatography electrospray ionization mass spectrometry (Nano-LC-ESI-MS) and molecular docking. *Mar. Drugs* **2014**, *12*, 3917–3928. [CrossRef] [PubMed]

36. Zhou, M.; Du, K.; Ji, P.; Feng, W. Molecular mechanism of the interactions between inhibitory tripeptides and angiotensin-converting enzyme. *Biophys. Chem.* **2012**, *168*, 60–66. [CrossRef] [PubMed]

37. Ha, G.E.; Chang, O.K.; Jo, S.M.; Han, G.S.; Park, B.Y.; Ham, J.S.; Jeong, S.G. Identification of antihypertensive peptides derived from low molecular weight casein hydrolysates generated during fermentation by *Bifidobacterium longum* KACC 91563. *Korean J. Food Sci. Anim. Resour.* **2015**, *35*, 738–747. [CrossRef] [PubMed]

38. Chen, J.; Liu, Y.; Wang, G.; Sun, S.; Liu, R.; Hong, B.; Gao, R.; Bai, K. Processing optimization and characterization of angiotensin-I-converting enzyme inhibitory peptides from Lizardfish (*Synodus macrops*) scale gelatin. *Mar. Drugs* **2018**, *16*, 228. [CrossRef] [PubMed]

39. Salampessy, J.; Reddy, N.; Kailasapathy, K.; Phillips, M. Functional and potential therapeutic ACE-inhibitory peptides derived from bromelain hydrolysis of trevally proteins. *J. Funct. Foods* **2015**, *14*, 716–725. [CrossRef]

40. Jamilah, B.; Harvinder, K.G. Properties of gelatins from skins of fish–black tilapia (*Oreochromis mossambicus*) and red tilapia (*Oreochromis nilotica*). *Food Chem.* **2002**, *77*, 81–84. [CrossRef]

41. Spellman, D.; McEvoy, E.; O'Cuinn, G.; Fitzgerald, R.J. Proteinase and exopeptidase hydrolysis of whey protein: Comparison of the TNBS, OPA and pH stat methods for quantification of degree of hydrolysis. *Int. Dairy J.* **2003**, *13*, 447–453. [CrossRef]

42. Vilar, S.; Cozza, G.; Moro, S. Medicinal chemistry and the molecular operating environment (MOE): Application of QSAR and molecular docking to drug discovery. *Curr. Top. Med. Chem.* **2008**, *8*, 1555–1572. [CrossRef] [PubMed]

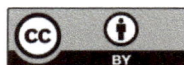

marine drugs

MDPI

Article

A Novel Peptide from Abalone (*Haliotis discus hannai*) to Suppress Metastasis and Vasculogenic Mimicry of Tumor Cells and Enhance Anti-Tumor Effect In Vitro

Fang Gong [1], Mei-Fang Chen [1], Yuan-Yuan Zhang [1], Cheng-Yong Li [2,3], Chun-Xia Zhou [1], Peng-Zhi Hong [1], Sheng-Li Sun [2] and Zhong-Ji Qian [2,3,*]

[1]   College of Food Science and Technology, Guangdong Ocean University, Zhanjiang 524088, China;
      m13025612271@163.com (F.G.); meifangchen93@163.com (M.-F.C.); zyyla92@126.com (Y.-Y.Z.);
      chunxia.zhou@163.com (C.-X.Z.); hongpengzhigdou@163.com (P.-Z.H.)
[2]   School of Chemistry and Environment, Guangdong Ocean University, Zhanjiang 524088, China;
      cyli_ocean@163.com (C.-Y.L.); xinglsun@126.com (S.-L.S.)
[3]   Shenzhen Institute of Guangdong Ocean University, Shenzhen 518114, China
[*]   Correspondence: zjqian78@163.com; Tel.: +86-18607596590

Received: 18 March 2019; Accepted: 19 April 2019; Published: 24 April 2019

Abstract: Vasculogenic mimicry (VM) formed by tumor cells plays a vital role in the progress of tumor, because it provides nutrition for tumor cells and takes away the metabolites. Therefore, the inhibition of VM is crucial to the clinical treatment of tumors. In this study, we investigated the anti-tumor effect of a novel peptide, KVEPQDPSEW (AATP), isolated from abalone (*Haliotis discus hannai*) on HT1080 cells by migration, invasion analysis and the mode of action. The results showed that AATP effectively inhibited MMPs by blocking MAPKs and NF-κB pathways, leading to the downregulation of metastasis of tumor cells. Moreover, AATP significantly inhibited VM and pro-angiogenic factors, including VEGF and MMPs by suppression of AKT/mTOR signaling. In addition, molecular docking was used to study the interaction of AATP and HIF-1α, and the results showed that AATP was combined with an active site of HIF-1α by a hydrogen bond. The effect of AATP on anti-metastatic and anti-vascular in HT1080 cells revealed that AATP may be a potential lead compound for treatment of tumors in the future.

Keywords: abalone; peptide; vasculogenic mimicry; metastasis; MMPs; HIF-1α

1. Introduction

A tumor is a mass or lump formed by cells that have unregulated growth potential [1]. For malignant tumors, tumor cells can distribute diffusely and form the second tumor in distal site [2]. Cancer is a serious threat to human life and health. For cancer patients, metastasis of tumor cells affects the function of other tissues, and results in the death of the patient. In addition, the blood vessels provide the nutrition for the tumor cell's growth in the course of tumorigenesis. Thus, the inhibition of metastasis and angiogenesis of tumor cells is of great significance for clinical treatment of tumors.

The detachment of tumor cells from their primary site, the degradation of basement and extracellular matrix (ECM), and the formation of tumor vessels are significant parts of the process of tumor cells metastasis [3,4]. The secretion of matrix metalloproteinase (MMP) from tumor cells is relevant to the degradation of basement and ECM that resist metastasis of tumor cells. Previous studies have found that MMP-2 and MMP-9 can degrade type IV collagen, which is an important component of ECM [5]. Thus, inhibition of MMPs is extremely crucial in tumor therapy.

Because the unregulated growth of tumor cells needs a large amount of nutrition and oxygen, the formation of new blood vessels is necessary, which not only provides ongoing nutrition and oxygen for tumor growth and takes away metabolites at the same time, but also transports tumor cells to target organs and tissue, which provide a necessary condition for tumor metastasis [6]. Therefore, numerous studies have paid attention as to how to inhibit angiogenesis, which is important for anti-tumor. Besides traditional tumor angiogenesis and vasculogenesis is produced by endothelial cells, vasculogenic mimicry (VM) has attracted attention as a novel blood supply. VM is not found in the healthy body, but is unique to tumor tissue, where it can promote cancer progression by the formation of blood vessel-like structures, independent of vascular endothelial cells [7]. It has been found in various aggressive tumors, such as breast cancer, pancreas cancer, liver cancer and various sarcomas [8]. VM is also implicated in poor patient clinical prognoses, because previous studies have focused on the treatment of blood vessels produced by endothelial cells, rather than VM by tumor cells [9].

The fast growth of tumor cells generally generates a hypoxic microenvironment within the tumor. Under this reduced state of cellular oxygen availability, the hypoxia-inducible factor (HIF)-1α expression is frequently fiercely elevated [10]. HIF-1α is a major transcription factor that mediates oxygen homeostasis, which is disrupted in disorders affecting the circulatory system and in cancer [11]. Increasing evidence is suggesting that HIF-1α could facilitate tumor growth by disrupting metabolic balance, accelerating angiogenesis, increasing cell survival, inhibiting cell apoptosis, as well as increasing drug resistance [12]. Hypoxic induced factor (HIF-1α) overexpression in tumor cells promotes the expression of vascular endothelial growth factor (VEGF), related to VM formation [13,14]. The level of matrix metalloproteinases (MMPs) and the $5\gamma2$ chain of laminin were overexpressed in highly aggressive tumor cells [15]. That excessive expression of MMPs and the presence of laminin receptor on the surface of tumor cells contributes to cells to adhere to more laminin. The activation of MMPs can facilitate the formation of VM by separating laminin [16]. HT1080 is a fibrosarcoma cell line which has been used widely in biomedical research. The cell line was isolated from tissue taken in a biopsy of a fibrosarcoma present in a 35-year-old human male. The sample supplied by the patient had been not subjected to radio or chemotherapy, making it less likely that unwanted mutations were introduced into the cell line. The cell line carries an IDH1 mutation and an activated N-ras oncogene. HT1080 cells are composed of malignant cells, and generally are used to model metastatic cells because MMPs are overexpressed by PMA and other stimulations. In addition, under hypoxic stimulation, HT1080 cells can generate pro-angiogenic factor, including HIF-1α, VEGF and MMPs to promote tumor angiogenesis, and is an ideal model for studying tumor invasion and metastasis.

Marine organisms have attracted intense attention as an effective bioactive source, including sponges, macroalgae, microalgae and bacteria. These creatures are usually made into nutraceuticals and pharmaceuticals. Abalone is a marine gastropod feeding on seaweed, and is commonly considered as very precious food in Asian markets. More and more studies have found that abalone consists of many vital moieties like good protein, fatty acid and polysaccharides, which not only provides the basic nutrition for human health, but possesses the ability for anti-microbial, anti-oxidant, anti-thrombotic, anti-inflammatory and anti-cancer [14–18] uses. Qian [19] found that two peptides from abalone can suppress MMP-2 and MMP-9 expressions to inhibit the migration of HT1080 cells. A novel antimicrobial peptide, Ranatuerin-2PLx, showed inhibitory potential in the proliferation of cancer cells [2]. Peptides have attracted more and more attention as bioactive resources, and are wildly applied in clinical trials because of their high bioactivity and easy synthesis.

The research of abalone in anti-cancer treatment mainly focused on the effect of polysaccharides and the crude extract of abalone, however, and there were few studies about abalone polypeptides. In the present study, HT1080 cells serve as a tumor mold, due to its high metastasis ability, to investigate the anti-tumor effect of a peptide AATP from abalone *haliotis discus hannai*.

2. Results

2.1. Cell Viability and Colony Formation Assay

The peptide AATP (MW = 1214.30 Da) isolated from abalone was obtained according to methods from our previous studies [20]. The amino acid sequence of the purified AATP was determined to be Lys-Val-Asp-Ala-Gln-Asp-Pro-Ser-Glu-Trp (Figure 1a).

Initially, MTT assay was utilized to assess the cytotoxicity of AATP on HT1080 cells and HUVECs. As shown in Figure 1b, there was no significant difference in cell viability between AATP- treated cells and untreated cells. Thus, all tested concentrations (10, 20, 50 and 100 μM) of AATP have no cytotoxicity on HT1080 cells and HUVECs, which revealed that AATP is non-toxic to tumor cells as well as nontumor cells. Therefore, 10–100 μM of AATP could be used for further experiments. The colony formation assay indicated that the number of colonies of HT1080 cells were sharply reduced by AATP treatment compared with the untreated group (Figure 1c), suggesting AATP exerted inhibitory effect on tumor cells.

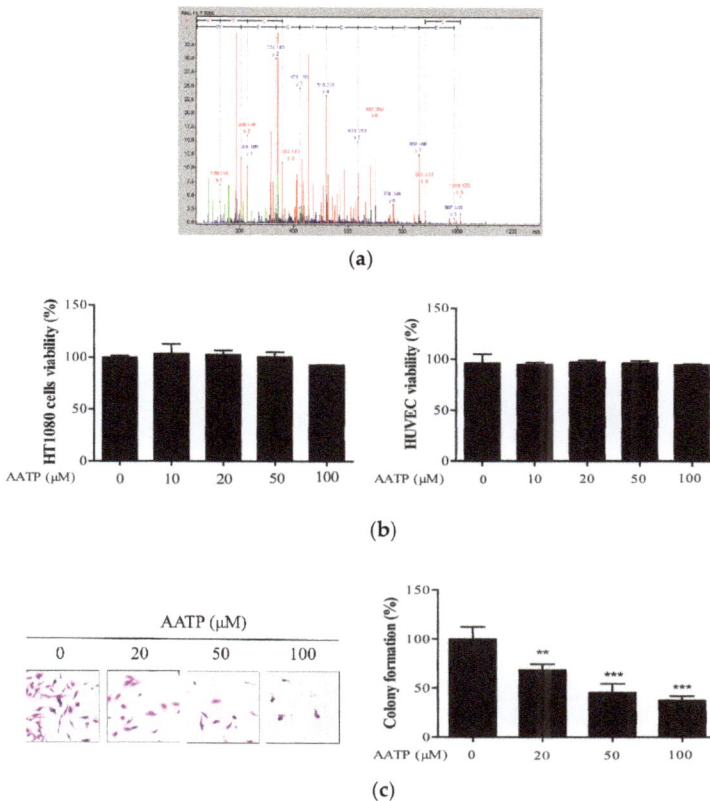

(a)

(b)

(c)

Figure 1. (a) Identification of molecular mass and amino acid sequence of Lys-Val-Glu-Pro-Gln-Asp-Pro-Ser-Glu-Trp (AATP). (b) Effect of AATP on the viability of HT1080 cells and HUVECs. Cells grown were treated with different concentrations of AATP (10, 20, 50 and 100 μM) for 24 h and relative cell viability was assessed by the MTT assay. (c) Anchorage-dependent colony formation in the presence or absence of AATP was visualized by staining with crystal violet solution (*n* = 3 per group). The photographs of tumor cells invasion were taken using inverted microscope at 24 and 48 h and analyzed with ImageJ. ** *p* < 0.01 and *** *p* < 0.001 vs. untreated control.

2.2. AATP Inhibits Tumor Cells Migration and Invasion

The migration assay and cancer cell spheroid assay were carried out to estimate the impact of AATP on cancer cells migration and invasion. As exhibited in Figure 2a, compared with control cells, the migration of cells treated by AATP was obviously down-regulated in a dose- and time-dependent manner. Protease secreted by tumor cells can degrade basement and ECM, which contribute to tumor cells metastasis. In Figure 2b, the invasion area of tumor cells treated with 50 and 100 μM AATP was smaller than the control cells, which suggested that AATP treatment effectively inhibits proteolytic activities implicated in degradation of basement and ECM, and suppresses the cell invasion. The results revealed that AATP may be a potential inhibitor for metastatic therapy.

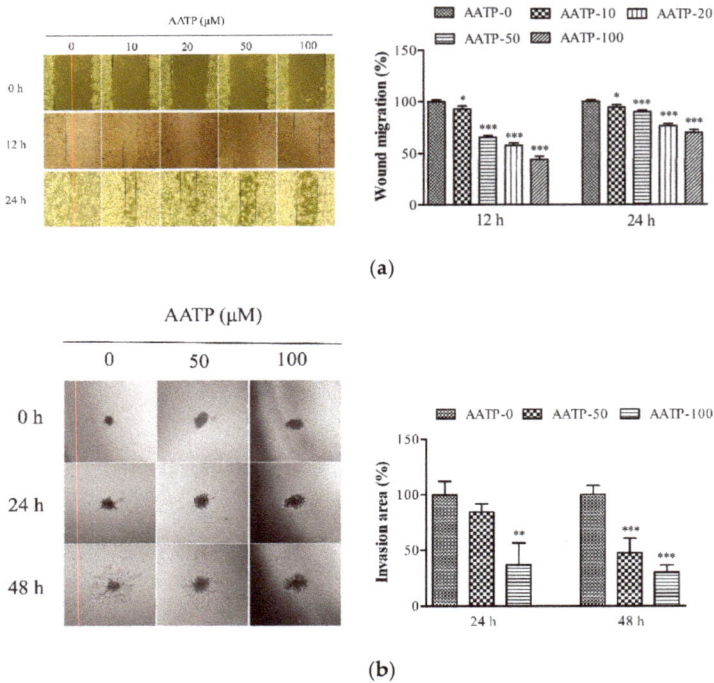

(a)

(b)

Figure 2. (a) Injury lines were made on the confluent cell monolayer, and the effects of AATP on cells migration were monitored for 12 h and 24 h. Cell motility was measured in five selected fields and calculated based on the width of injury at 0 h. (b) AATP inhibits cells invasion in 3D sitting. The mixture of cell spheroid combined with Matrigel and type I collagen was seeded on pre-coated Matrigel 48-well plates for 30min, and incubated with a medium containing 50 and 100 μM AATP. The photographs of tumor cells invasion were taken using inverted microscope at 24 and 48 h and analyzed with ImageJ. * $p < 0.05$, ** $p < 0.01$ and *** $p < 0.001$ vs. untreated control.

2.3. AATP Reduces PMA-induced MMPs Expression and Suppresses Proteolytic Activities in HT1080 Cells

MMPs play an important role in tumor metastasis because MMPs can degrade the surrounding tissue of tumor cells, which creates a place for tumor blood vessels to form. In order to determine the anti-metastatic ability of AATP, we investigated the transcriptional levels of MMPs including MMP-1, -2, -3, -9, -13 as well as activity and protein expression of MMP-2, -9 in HT1080 cells by using Real-Time quantitative reverse transcription-PCR (qPCR), gelatin zymography, and western blotting analysis.

As shown in Figure 3a, PMA stimulation significantly upregulated MMPs RNA expression, whereas AATP treatment efficiently decreased the levels of MMP-1, -2, -3, -9, -13 under PMA stimulation. In zymography analysis and western blotting analysis, we found that AATP treatment significantly suppressed PMA-induced the activities and protein expressions of MMP2 and MMP9 in HT1080 cells in a dose-dependent manner (Figure 3b,c).

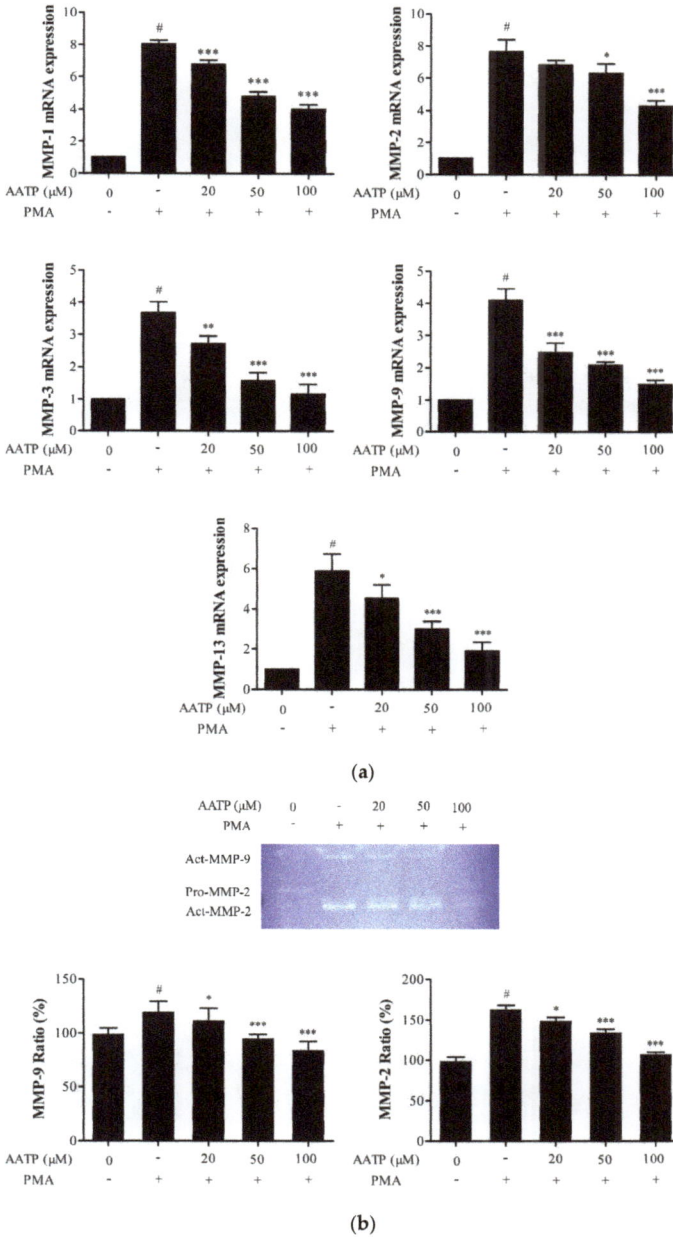

(a)

(b)

Figure 3. *Cont.*

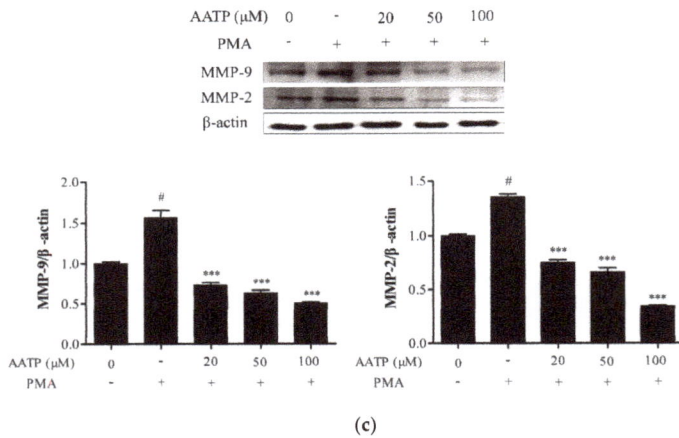

(c)

Figure 3. Effect of AATP treatment on expression of matrix metalloproteinase (MMPs) (**a**) Cells treated with AATP for 1 h were incubated in PMA (10 ng/mL). After 24 h, the expression of MMPs RNA was analyzed by quantitative real time PCR. β-actin was used as a loading control. (**b**) Gelatin zymography for the determination of MMP-2 and MMP-9 activities in AATP-treated HT1080 cells. HT1080 cells were treated with AATP (20, 50, and 100 μM) for 1 h and stimulated by PMA (10 ng/mL) for 72 h. Gelatinolytic activities of MMP-2 and MMP-9 in conditioned media were detected by electrophoresis of soluble protein on a gelatin containing 10% polyacrylamide gel. Untreated control was used as a loading control. (**c**) Expression of MMP-2 and MMP-9 in cell Lysates was detected using western blot analysis. β-actin was used as a loading control. HT1080 cells treated with AATP (20, 50, and 100 μM) for 1 h and stimulated by PMA (10 ng/mL) for 24 h. The relative amounts of MMP-2 and MMP-9 were quantified by densitometry measurement (ImageJ). # $p < 0.001$ vs. untreated control, * $p < 0.05$, ** $p < 0.01$ and *** $p < 0.001$ vs. PMA stimulation.

2.4. AATP Inhibits PMA-induced ERK and JNK Phosphorylation and NF-κB Activation in HT1080 Cells

MAPK and NF-κB signal pathways are related to the expressions of numerous genes that modulate tumor promotion, angiogenesis, metastasis and MMPs expressions. To determine the effect of AATP on MAPK and NF-κB signal pathways in HT1080 cells, the western blotting analysis, p65 translocation and NF-κB activation assay (EMSA) were conducted. As shown in Figure 4a,b, the results of the western blotting assay indicated that AATP treatment markedly suppressed PMA-induced ERK and JNK phosphorylation activation in dose dependent, compared with PMA-induced group. Moreover, the results of p65 translocation and EMSA analysis, the AATP dramatically suppressed p65 nuclear translocation and binding with DNA (Figure 4c,d).

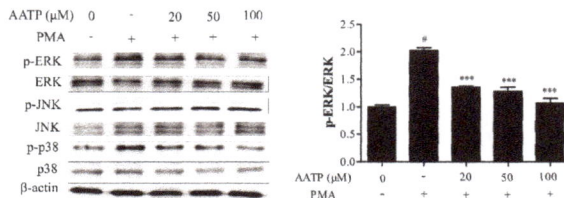

Figure 4. *Cont.*

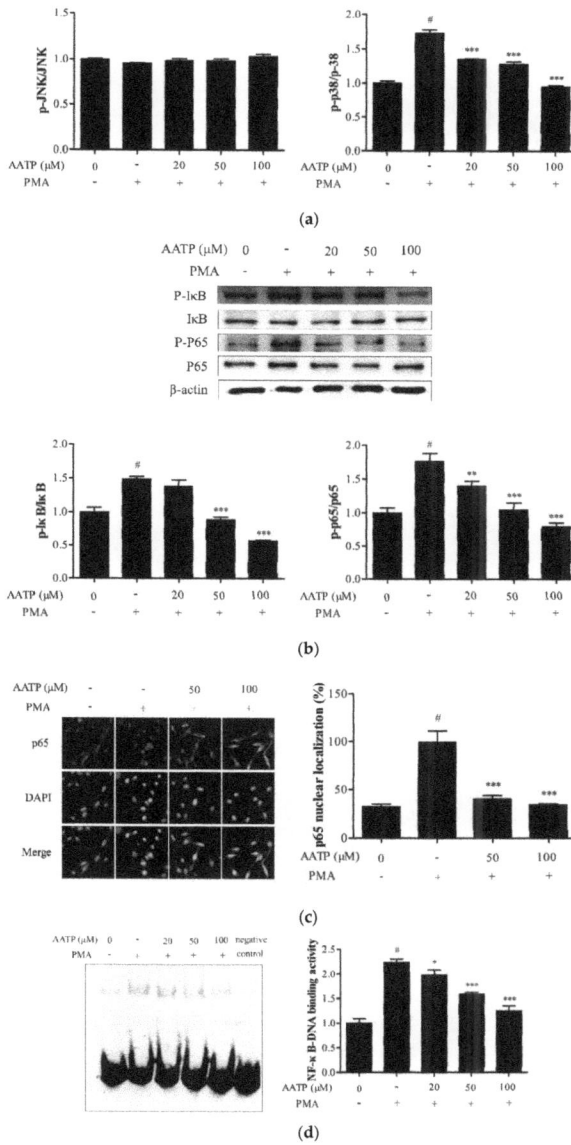

Figure 4. AATP suppressed PMA-induced p-38, ERK, and NF-κB activation in HT1080 cells. After treatment with 20, 50 and 100 μM AATP for 1 h, cells were stimulated with PMA (10 ng/mL) for 24 h. (**a,b**) Total cell lysates were evaluated for MAPKs and NF-κB using western blotting. Band intensities were normalized to β-actin expression, and then the relative ratios of phosphorylated form/total form were calculated. (**c**) NF-κB-DNA binding activity was examined by EMSA. Band intensities were normalized to untreated control. (**d**) Nuclear translocation of NF-κBp65 was monitored by an overlay of blue DAPI staining with green p65 immunofluorescence. p-65 nuclear localization was measured. Untreated control was used as a loading control. # $p < 0.001$ vs. untreated control, * $p < 0.05$, ** $p < 0.01$ and *** $p < 0.001$ vs. PMA stimulation.

2.5. AATP Abolishes VM Formation and Inhibits Secretion of VEGF and Related Protein of Angiogenesis by Suppressing Hypoxia Inducible Factor (HIF)-1α Signal Pathway Under Hypoxic Conditions

The rapid growth and metastasis of tumor cells need adequate nutrition and oxygen. Therefore, VM is necessary for tumor cells' survival, invasion and metastasis. VM formation analysis was employed to investigate the anti-angiogenesis effect of AATP on HT1080 cells. The result showed that VM formation by HT1080 cells on the Matrigel pre-coated wells was abolished through treatment with AATP, as shown in the Figure 5a. VEGF, a pro-angiogenesis protein, is able to promote tumor angiogenesis via stimulating vascular endothelial cells and tumor cells. The level of VEGF secreted by the tumor cell into the medium was determined by ELISA. The ELISA results showed that AATP dose-dependently inhibits the secretion of VEGF from cancer cells (Figure 5b). VEGF is a downstream target of HIF-1α. Therefore, we detected expressions of HIF-1α and AKT/mTOR signal pathway, which is related to angiogenesis. AATP treatment effectively inhibits expression of HIF-1α via blocking AKT/mTOR/p70S6K signaling in a concentration-dependent manner, thus revealing that AATP treatment down-regulated the activation of a pro-angiogenesis factor by suppression of the HIF-1α signal pathway (Figure 5c,d).

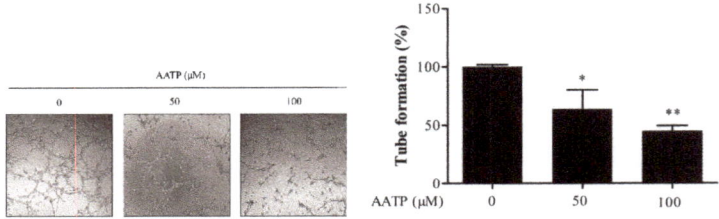

(**a**)

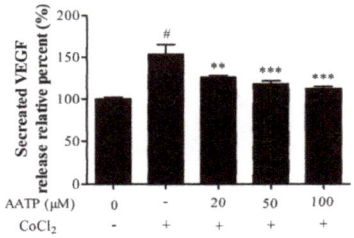

(**b**)

Figure 5. *Cont.*

(c)

(d)

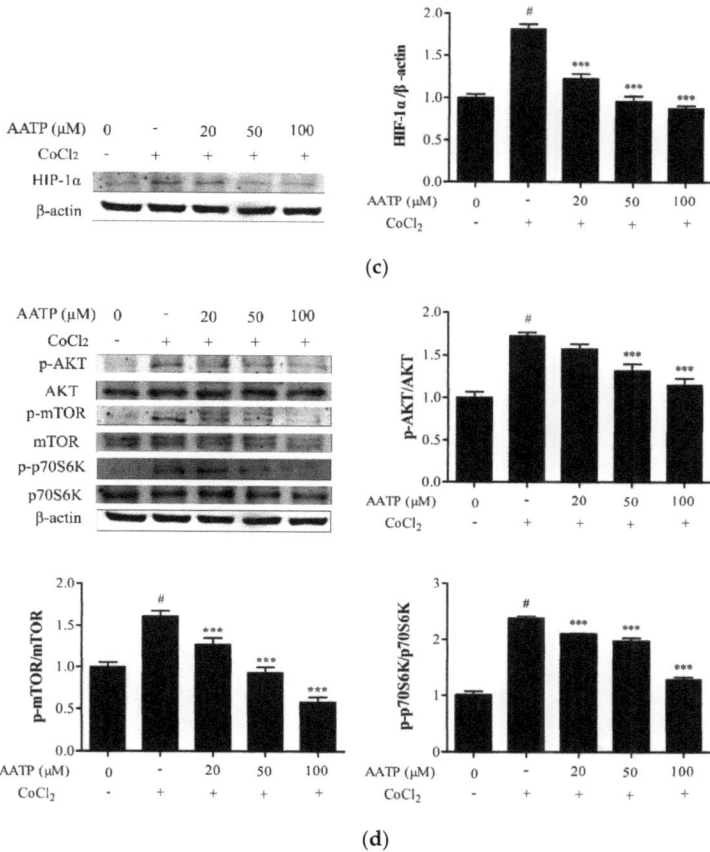

Figure 5. AATP abolishes vasculogenic mimicry (VM) formation and decreases vascular endothelial growth factor (VEGF) secretion in HT1080 cells. (**a**) Cells were seeded on Matrigel pre-coated 96-well plates and incubated in medium containing 50 and 100 μM AATP for 3 h. Then, the photographs of VM formation were taken with an inverted microscope and analyzed by imageJ. (**b**) The cells pre-treated with indicated concentrations AATP for 1 h were stimulated with 100 μM CoCl$_2$ for 24 h. The level of VEGF secretion was detected using ELISA kit. AATP inhibits hypoxia-induced expression of HIF-1α and blocks AKT/mTOR/p70S6K signaling in HT1080 cells. (**c**, **d**) Cells were incubated with 20, 50 and 100 μM AATP for 1 h and stimulated with 100 μM CoCl$_2$ for 24 h. The expression of HIF-1α, p-AKT/AKT, p-mTOR/mTOR and p-p70S6K/p70S6K were determined by western blotting and β-actin was used as loading controls. # $p < 0.001$ vs. untreated control, * $p < 0.05$, ** $p < 0.01$ and *** $p < 0.001$ vs. CoCl$_2$ stimulation.

2.6. Molecular Docking Analysis

HIF-1α plays an important role in the survival, growth and metastasis of tumor cells, suggesting that HIF-1α inhibitors possess effective effect for tumor treatment. Therefore, we investigated the potential of AATP against HIF-1α and binding affinity using molecular docking approach. As depicted in the Figure 6, AATP combined amino acid residues GLY180, GLN181, HIS199, APS201, GLU202 and GLN203 of HIF-1α, and the strong interaction was supported by the formation of a hydrogen bond, and its docking score was -100.21 kcal/mol. The high binding energies between AATP and HIF-1α contribute to suppression of activity of HIF-1α, resulting in downregulation of downstream reactions that relate to tumor metastasis and VM formation.

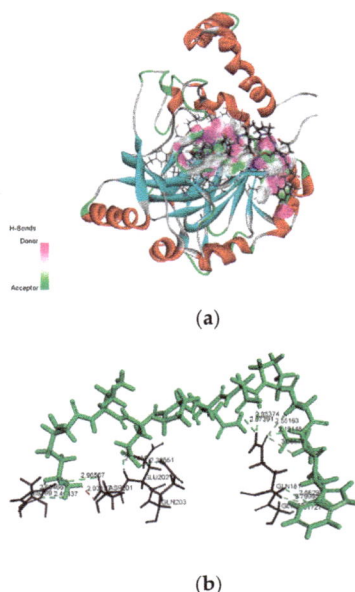

(a)

(b)

Figure 6. Interaction of the AATP with HIF-1α active site. (**a**) Three dimensional representation of Ligand-1H2L hydrogen bonding. (**b**) Two dimensional representation of Ligand-1H2L hydrogen bonding.

3. Discussion

In the present study, we investigated the effect of a polypeptide AATP isolated from abalone on tumor metastasis and VM formation in HT1080 cells. AATP can significantly suppress tumor cells metastasis (Figure 2a,b) and VM formation (Figure 5a), which are essential steps in tumor progression. Previous studies have been found that abalone visceral extracts showed remarkable inhibitory effect on tumor progression by regulating the expressions of tumorigenic factors, such as Cox-2, EGF, VEGF and FGF [21]. It is suggested that the extract obtained from the glycoprotein of *H.discus hannai* possess effective effect on anti-cancer by the host's responses [22], and investigations revealed that water extract from abalone was a source of bioactive molecule against many types of tumors [23]. Currently, the activity of peptides has been paid more and more attention to by researchers. Peptides have advantages in shape to agonist or antagonist bind sites of the receptor, because peptides can bind to a protein receptor and have few off-target effects [24]. Moreover, peptides are applicable as lead compounds for pharmacophores or the design of drug-like molecules with incorporated secondary structural elements [25,26]. Up to now, many marine-derived peptides, such as ziconotide, brentuximab vedotin, kahalalide F, and glembatumumab vedotin, have been used successfully in clinical trials and in the market [24].

The generation of blood vessels is pivotal for tumor cells survival, growth and metastasis. Besides traditional tumor angiogenesis and vasculogenesis, VM, a functional vascular channel developed by tumor cells, is also responsible for the tumor growing and tumor initiation [27]. It can provide nutrition to tumor cells and allow tumor cells to grow through them when the blood vessels by endothelial cells are insufficient to the growth of tumor tissue [28]. Hypoxia within the tumor microenvironment serves as an important causative factor for VM formation because it can increase the generation of pro-angiogenic factors, such as VEGF and MMPs, which facilitate the formation blood vessel and the splitting of pre-existing vessels, respectively [29–31]. Therefore, VM plays a critical role in blood supply in malignant tumors [32], and targeting VM may provide a promising strategy to regulate the spread of tumors.

In this study, under hypoxic conditions, AATP treatment dramatically suppressed expression of HIF-1α induced by hypoxia, and blocked the AKT/mTOR/p70S6K signal pathway related to angiogenesis (Figure 5c,d), which lead to deregulation of VEGF (Figure 5b). Kim [33] found ELH can attenuate HIF-1α accumulation by blocking phosphorylation of AKT/mTOR/p70S6K to inhibit tumor angiogenesis. It has been reported that VEGF can induce cell proliferation, metastasis and tube formation [34], and decreased expression of VEGF lead to suppress angiogenesis in MDA-MB-435 cells [35]. Moreover, AATP markedly downregulated tumor cells metastasis, including migration, invasion and activity of MMPs by MAPKs (p38 and ERK) and NF-κB (p65 and IκB) signaling (Figure 4). It was reported that MAPKs and NF-κB have relationships with the expressions of target genes associated with tumor promotion, angiogenesis, metastasis and MMPs [33–38]. Lu [39] found that emodin could effectively inhibit the anti-inflammatory through blocking NF-κB activation and MAPKs pathway on PMA plus A23187-stimulated BMMCs. Cao [40] exhibited that ginkgetin suppresses growth of breast carcinoma by regulating the MAPKs pathway. And fucoxanthin extract inhibits MMPs by regulating NF-κB and MAPKs pathways in human fibrosarcoma cells [41]. This suggests that regulation of NF-κB and MAPKs pathways are closely related to activity and expression of MMP-2 and MMP-9.

Molecular docking is based on spatial matching and energy matching, simulating the binding ability between ligands and human receptors, and the docking result showed that AATP can combine with GLY180, GLN181, HIS199, APS201, GLU202 and GLN203 of the active site of HIF-1α, leading to the suppression of HIF-1α activity (Figure 6). This suggested that peptide AATP and receptors HIF-1α have a similar key and lock recognition relationship in the configuration, resulting that AATP binds to the active site of the receptor and occupies the spatial position of HIF-1α. Therefore, HIF-1α failed to bind the hypoxia response element of the initiator, leading to downregulation of target genes relevant to tumor metastasis and VM formation. Additionally, the amino acid composition of peptides is responsible for its bioactivity. In the Lys-Val-Asp-Ala-Gln-Asp-Pro-Ser-Glu-Trp (AATP), the amino acids Glu, Asp, Pro and Lys could effectively inhibit activity of MMP-2 and MMPs [42]. In particular, the amino acids Trp, Tyr, Met, Gly, Cys, His, Val and Pro in a peptide can markedly elevate the bioactivity of the peptide and hydrophobic acid residues Val and Pro contribute to the formation of oil-water interfaces, leading to the scavenging of free radicals from the lipid phase [43,44]. Huang found that a novel tripeptide (Gln-Pro-Lys) derived from the sepia ink possesses anti-tumor properties in DU-145 cells [45].

In summary, we demonstrated that AATP isolated from abalone (*Haliotis discus hannai*) suppresses the metastasis and VM formation on HT1080 cells via downregulating MMPs and VEGF. In addition, the result of molecular docking showed that AATP combines with HIF-1α via a hydrogen bond, resulting in suppression of HIF-1α activity, which was accordant with the result of western blotting. Therefore, all results in vitro revealed that AATP can effectively inhibit tumor cells metastasis and VM formation, which provides the basis for the further application of AATP to animal experiments. Furthermore, with regard to the AATP therapeutical setting, there are limitations like most peptides, including delivery, short half-life and orally available as well as clear from kidneys after intravenous administration, which needs to be overcome by using different design strategies in the future.

4. Materials and Methods

4.1. Chemicals and Reagents

Human fibrosarcoma cells (HT1080 cell) and human umbilical vein endothelial cells (HUVEC) were provided by Guangzhou Cellcook Biotech Co., Ltd. (Guangzhou, China). Dulbecco's modified Eagle's minimal essential medium (DMEM) and penicillin/streptomycin were purchased from Gibco (Grand Island, NY, USA). Fetal bovine serum (FBS) was from Vigonob (UY). 3-(4, 5-dimethyl-thiazol-2-yl)-2, 5-diphenyltetrazoliumbromide (MTT) were obtained from Shanghai Aladdin Bio-Chem Technology Co., Ltd. (Shanghai, China). Antibody against p65, p-p65, IκB, p-IκB, ERK, p-ERK, p-38, p-p38, JNK, p-JNK, β-actin, MMP2 and MMP9 were provided by Santa Cruz Biotechnology (Santa Cruz, CA, USA). Antibody HIF-1α, AKT, p-AKT, p-mTOR, mTOR, p-p70S6K, p70S6K and horse anti-mouse IgG were purchased from Cell Signaling Technology (Boston, MA, USA). Matrigel was from BD Biosciences (San Jose, CA, USA). Phorbol 12-myristate 13-acetate (PMA) and $CoCl_2$ were provided by Sigma-Aldrich (St. Louis, MO, USA). The isolated peptide AATP (MW = 1214.30 Da) was from our studies previously [20].

4.2. Cell Viability Assay

HT1080 cells and HUVECs were cultured in 96-well plate in growth medium for 24 h. Then fresh media containing different concentrations (10, 20, 50, and 100 μM) of AATP were added. After 24 h, 100 μL MTT (1 mg/mL) was added into each well for 4 h. Then, adding 100 μL DMSO to dissolve formazan crystals, and the absorbance was measured at 540 nm.

4.3. Colony Formation Assay

HT1080 cells were placed in 6-well plate (500 cells/well) in DMEM containing 10% serum. After 24 h, the medium was replaced with fresh medium containing different concentrations (20, 50 and 100 μM) of AATP, and cultured for 7 days. The colonies were stained with 0.2% crystal violet/methanol (*w/v*) solution for 20 min at room temperature, washed with distilled water and then photographed.

4.4. Cells Migration Assay

The cell migration ability was estimated by injury healing assay. Briefly, HT1080 cells were seeded in a 24-well plate. The cells were scratched using a sterile pipette tip, and then washed with PBS to remove cell debris. Cells were treated with various concentrations of AATP (10, 20, 50 and 100 μM). And the cell migration across injury line was observed using a microscope (JiDi, GD30, Guangzhou, China) and recorded photographically at 0, 12 and 24 h, respectively.

4.5. Cancer Cell Spheroid Invasion Assay

To investigate the inhibitory effect of AATP on cell invasion, the cancer cell spheroid invasion assay was performed to simulate the internal environment and assess invasion in a 3-dimensional (3D) setting. Briefly, single-cell suspension (1×10^5 cells/mL) was seeded in the lid of the dish for 72 h. Next, the spheroids are pooled, and 80 μL cell spheroids were added in 400 μL mixture of Matrigel and type I collagen at 4 °C, plated in 48-well plates and incubated at 37 °C to solidify into a 3D culture. After 30 min, warm media with the indicated concentrations (50 and 100 μM) of AATP was added. The result of cell invasion was observed using a microscope, and recorded at 0, 24, and 48 h.

4.6. RNA Extraction and Quantitative Real Time PCR (qPCR)

Total RNA was extracted and purified using a Nucleic acid purification kit (DSBIO, Guangzhou, China). The purified RNA (1 μg) was reverse transcribed to synthesize cDNA for RT-PCR using the HiScript II 1st Strand cDNA Synthesis Kit (+gDNA wiper) (Vazyme, Nanjing, China). Quantitative PCR reaction was carried out using CFX96 Real-Time System (BIO-RAD, Hercules, CA, USA), and forward and reverse primers of the target gene (MMP-1, MMP-2, MMP-3, MMP-9 and MMP-13) were shown in Table 1. For quantification of target gene, transcript values were analyzed using the $2^{-\Delta\Delta Ct}$ method and β-actin was considered as the reference.

Table 1. Details of primers for quantification of RT-PCR detection.

Primer ID	Primer Sequence (5'→3')
MMP-1	F: 5'-AGCCATCACTTACCTTGCACTGAG-3' R: 5'-RCCACATCAGGCACTCCACATCTG-3'
MMP-2	F: 5'-AGCCAAGCGGTCTAAGTCCAGAG-3' R: 5'-GGAATGAAGCACAGCAGGTCTCAG-3'
MMP-3	F: 5'-ACGCACAGCAACAGTAGGATTGG-3' R: 5'-GAGGCAGGCAAGACAGCAAGG-3'
MMP-9	F: 5'-TCCTGGTGCTCCTGGTGCTG-3' R: 5'-CTGCCTGTCGGTGAGATTGGTTC-3'
MMP-13	F: 5'-AGTCATGGAGCTTGCTGCATTCTC-3' R: 5'-TCCTGGCTGCCTTCCTCTTCTTG-3'
β-actin	F: 5'-CCTGGCACCCAGCACAAT-3' R: 5'-GGGCCGGACTCGTCATAC-3'

4.7. Gelatinolytic Activity

Activities of MMP-2 and -9 of HT1080 cells were determined by gelatin zymography. Briefly, cells were seeded in 24-well plates with a density of 2×10^5 cells/well and pretreated with different concentrations of AATP (20, 50 and 100 μM) for 1 h, and then stimulated by PMA (10 ng/mL) for 72 h. Cell medium was collected to conduct gel electrophoresis. Finally, areas of gelatin hydrolyzed by MMPs were visualized as clear zones against blue backgrounds by Coomassie Blue staining, and the intensities of the bands were estimated by ImageJ software (National Institute of Mental Health, Bethesda, MD, USA).

4.8. Western Blotting

Cellular protein was harvested and lysed using RIPA buffer with 1% PMSF. And then equivalent amounts of proteins (30 μg) were separated using SDS-PAGE, and subsequently transferred to NC membranes. The membrane was blocked with 5% skim milk at room temperature. After 3 h, the membrane was incubated with primary antibodies and secondary antibodies for 2 h respectively at room temperature. Finally, the membrane using enhanced chemiluminescence (ECL) was visualized by detection system (Syngene, Cambridge, UK).

4.9. Immunofluorescence Staining

HT1080 cells treated with AATP (0, 50, and 100 μM) for 1 h were incubated with PMA (10 ng/mL) for 24 h and the medium was discarded. After being fixed with 4% paraformaldehyde (PFA), the cells were permeabilized with 0.2% Triton X-100 for 10 min and washed with PBS thrice. The cells were blocked with 5% BSA at room temperature for 1 h. Then, cells were incubated with diluted anti-p65 antibody overnight at 4 °C, and the primary antibodies were removed. Cells were washed using PBS three times, and incubated with secondary antibody for 2 h. The nuclear was stained with DAPI and images were taken by an inverted fluorescence microscope (Olympus Opticals, Tokyo, Japan).

4.10. NF-κB Activation Assay (Electrophoretic Mobility Shift Assays, EMSA)

The nuclear protein was obtained using the nuclear and cytoplasmic protein extraction kit (Beyotime, Shanghai, China). According to instructions, the complexes of protein and DNA and unbound probes were separated by 6% non-denaturing polyacrylamide gel electrophoresis, and subsequently transferred to Nylon membranes. Membrane was crosslinked for 15 min under UV light and blocked with blocking solution containing streptavidin-HRP conjugate. Then the membrane was balanced with a detection balance solution for 15 min and visualized with an enhanced chemiluminescence (ECL) detection system.

4.11. Assaying the Release of VEGF

Cells were plated at the same density in 6-well plates and treated with various concentrations (20, 50, and 100 μM) of AATP for 1 h and were subsequently stimulated with $CoCl_2$ (100 μM). After 24 h, conditional media were collected, and the quantity of VEGF was analyzed using Elisa Kit (Neobioscience, Shanghai, China).

4.12. Molecular Docking Analysis

The three-dimensional structures of HIF-1α (PDB ID: 1H2L) were obtained from the Protein Data Bank archive (PDB). The structure of AATP and HIF-1α were prepared by Discovery Studio 3.5 software. Molecular docking of AATP and HIF-1α protein binding sites was performed by using CDOCKER protocol of DS 3.5. The small molecule conformation was searched by high temperature dynamics method, and they were optimized in the active sites area of the acceptor by simulated annealing.

4.13. Statistical Analysis

The data were presented as mean ± SD ($n = 3$) and all results were analyzed using the GraphPad Prism 5 software (San Diego, CA, USA). Date was analyzed by one-way ANOVA in the figures, and p value < 0.05 was considered statistically significant.

Author Contributions: F.G. designed the experiments and wrote the original draft of the manuscripts; Z.-J.Q.; and S.-L.S. conceived and designed the research and edited the manuscripts; M.-F.C. and Y.-Y.Z. analyzed the data; C.-Y.L., C.-X.Z., and P.-Z.H. contributed materials and analysis tools. All authors reviewed the final publication.

Funding: The research was funded by the Yangfan Scarce Top Talent Project of Guangdong Province (201433009) and the Program for Postgraduate Courses and Education Reform and Scientific Research Start-Up Funds of Guangdong Ocean University (to Zhong-Ji Qian). The supported by Guangdong Tongde Pharmaceutical Co., Ltd and National Engineering Research Center for Modernization of Traditional Chinese Medicine (Lingnan Medicinal Plant Oil Branch) and funded by Development Project about Marine Economy Demonstration of Zhanjiang City (2017C8B1).

Conflicts of Interest: The authors declare no conflict of interest.

References

1. Kohandel, M.; Kardar, M.; Milosevic, M.; Sivaloganathan, S. Dynamics of tumor growth and combination of anti-angiogenic and cytotoxic therapies. *Phys. Med. Biol.* **2007**, *52*, 3665–3677. [CrossRef]
2. Chen, X.; Zhang, L.; Ma, C.; Zhang, Y.; Xi, X.; Wang, L.; Zhou, M.; Burrows, J.F.; Chen, T. A novel antimicrobial peptide, Ranatuerin-2PLx, showing therapeutic potential in inhibiting proliferation of cancer cells. *Biosci. Rep.* **2018**, *38*, BSR20180710. [CrossRef]
3. Maheswaran, S.; Haber, D.A. Circulating tumor cells: A window into cancer biology and metastasis. *Curr. Opin. Genet. Dev.* **2010**, *20*, 96–99. [CrossRef]
4. Sahai, E. Mechanisms of cancer cell invasion. *Curr. Opin. Genet. Dev.* **2005**, *15*, 87–96. [CrossRef] [PubMed]
5. Mook, O.R.F.; Frederiks, W.M.; Van Noorden, C.J.F. The role of gelatinases in colorectal cancer progression and metastasis. *Biochim. Biophys. Acta BBA Rev. Cancer* **2004**, *1705*, 69–89. [CrossRef]
6. Li, S.; Zhang, Q.; Zhou, L.; Guan, Y.; Chen, S.; Zhang, Y.; Han, X. Inhibitory effects of compound DMBT on hypoxia-induced vasculogenic mimicry in human breast cancer. *Biomed. Pharmacother.* **2017**, *96*, 982–992. [CrossRef] [PubMed]
7. Kawahara, R.; Niwa, Y.; Simizu, S. Integrin β1 is an essential factor in vasculogenic mimicry of human cancer cells. *Cancer Sci.* **2018**, *109*, 2490–2496. [CrossRef]
8. Liu, T.J.; Sun, B.C.; Zhao, X.L.; Zhao, X.M.; Sun, T.; Gu, Q.; Yao, Z.; Dong, X.Y.; Zhao, N.; Liu, N. CD133+ cells with cancer stem cell characteristics associates with vasculogenic mimicry in triple-negative breast cancer. *Oncogene* **2013**, *32*, 544–553. [CrossRef]
9. Niland, S.; Komljenovic, D.; Macas, J.; Bracht, T.; Bäuerle, T.; Liebner, S.; Eble, J.A. Rhodocetin-αβ selectively breaks the endothelial barrier of the tumor vasculature in HT1080 fibrosarcoma and A431 epidermoid carcinoma tumor models. *Oncotarget* **2018**, *9*. [CrossRef] [PubMed]

10. Semenza, G.L. HIF-1 mediates metabolic responses to intratumoral hypoxia and oncogenic mutations. *J. Clin. Invest.* **2013**, *123*, 3664–3671. [CrossRef]

11. Keith, B.; Johnson, R.S.; Simon, M.C. HIF1α and HIF2α: Sibling rivalry in hypoxic tumour growth and progression. *Nat. Rev. Cancer* **2012**, *12*, 9–22. [CrossRef]

12. Ghattass, K.; Assah, R.; El-Sabban, M.; Gali-Muhtasib, H. Targeting Hypoxia for Sensitization of Tumors to Radio- and Chemotherapy. *Curr. Cancer Drug Targets* **2013**, *13*, 670–685. [CrossRef]

13. Lv, Y.; Zhao, S.; Han, J.; Zheng, L.; Yang, Z.; Zhao, L. Hypoxia-inducible factor-1α induces multidrug resistance protein in colon cancer. *OncoTargets Ther.* **2015**, *1941*. [CrossRef]

14. Olenyuk, B.Z.; Zhang, G.-J.; Klco, J.M.; Nickols, N.G.; Kaelin, W.G.; Dervan, P.B. Inhibition of Vascular Endothelial Growth Factor with a Sequence-Specific Hypoxia Response Element Antagonist. *Proc. Natl. Acad. Sci. USA* **2004**, *101*, 16768–16773. [CrossRef]

15. Seftor, R.E.B.; Seftor, E.A.; Koshikawa, N.; Meltzer, P.S.; Gardner, L.M.G.; Bilban, M.; Stetler-Stevenson, W.G.; Quaranta, V.; Hendrix, M.J.C. Cooperative Interactions of Laminin 5 γ2 Chain, Matrix Metalloproteinase-2, and Membrane Type-1-Matrix/Metalloproteinase Are Required for Mimicry of Embryonic Vasculogenesis by Aggressive Melanoma. *Cancer Res.* **2001**, *61*, 6322–6327. [CrossRef] [PubMed]

16. Heitzer, E.; Haque, I.S.; Roberts, C.E.S.; Speicher, M.R. Current and future perspectives of liquid biopsies in genomics-driven oncology. *Nat. Rev. Genet.* **2019**, *20*, 71–88. [CrossRef]

17. De Zoysa, M.; Nikapitiya, C.; Whang, I.; Lee, J.-S.; Lee, J. Abhisin: A potential antimicrobial peptide derived from histone H2A of disk abalone (Haliotis discus discus). *Fish Shellfish Immunol.* **2009**, *27*, 639–646. [CrossRef]

18. Li, J.; Tong, T.; Ko, D.-O.; Kang, S.-G. Antithrombotic potential of extracts from abalone, Haliotis Discus Hannai Ino: In vitro and animal studies. *Food Sci. Biotechnol.* **2013**, *22*, 471–476. [CrossRef]

19. Nguyen, V.-T.; Qian, Z.-J.; Jung, W.-K. Abalone Haliotis discus hannai Intestine Digests with Different Molecule Weights Inhibit MMP-2 and MMP-9 Expression in Human Fibrosarcoma Cells. *Fish. Aquat. Sci.* **2012**, *15*, 137–143. [CrossRef]

20. Qian, Z.-J.; Ryu, B.; Park, W.S.; Choi, I.-W.; Jung, W.-K. Inhibitory Effects and Molecular Mechanism of an Anti-inflammatory Peptide Isolated from Intestine of Abalone, Haliotis Discus Hannai on LPS-Induced Cytokine Production via the p-p38/p-JNK Pathways in RAW264.7 Macrophages. *J. Food Nutr. Res.* **2016**, *4*, 690–698. [CrossRef]

21. Lee, C.-G.; Kwon, H.-K.; Ryu, J.H.; Kang, S.J.; Im, C.-R.; II Kim, J.; Im, S.-H. Abalone visceral extract inhibit tumor growth and metastasis by modulating Cox-2 levels and CD8+ T cell activity. *BMC Complement. Altern. Med.* **2010**, *10*. [CrossRef]

22. Uchida, H.; Sasaki, T.; Uchida, N.; Takasuka, N.; Endo, Y.; Kamiya, H. Oncostatic and immunomodulatory effects of a glycoprotein fraction from water extract of abalone, Haliotis discus hannai. *Cancer Immunol. Immunother.* **1987**, *24*. [CrossRef]

23. Zhu, B.-W.; Zhou, D.-Y.; Yang, J.-F.; Li, D.-M.; Yin, H.-L.; Tada, M. A neutral polysaccharide from the abalone pleopod, Haliotis discus hannai Ino. *Eur. Food Res. Technol.* **2009**, *228*, 591–595. [CrossRef]

24. Sable, R.; Parajuli, P.; Jois, S. Peptides, Peptidomimetics, and Polypeptides from Marine Sources: A Wealth of Natural Sources for Pharmaceutical Applications. *Mar. Drugs* **2017**, *15*, 124. [CrossRef]

25. Jayatunga, M.K.P.; Thompson, S.; Hamilton, A.D. α-Helix mimetics: Outwards and upwards. *Bioorg. Med. Chem. Lett.* **2014**, *24*, 717–724. [CrossRef]

26. Hirschmann, R.F.; Nicolaou, K.C.; Angeles, A.R.; Chen, J.S.; Smith, A.B. The β- D -Glucose Scaffold as a β-Turn Mimetic. *Acc. Chem. Res.* **2009**, *42*, 1511–1520. [CrossRef] [PubMed]

27. Maniotis, A.J.; Folberg, R.; Hess, A.; Seftor, E.A.; Gardner, L.M.G.; Pe'er, J.; Trent, J.M.; Meltzer, P.S.; Hendrix, M.J.C. Vascular Channel Formation by Human Melanoma Cells in Vivo and in Vitro: Vasculogenic Mimicry. *Am. J. Pathol.* **1999**, *155*, 739–752. [CrossRef]

28. Zhang, S.; Zhang, D.; Sun, B. Vasculogenic mimicry: Current status and future prospects. *Cancer Lett.* **2007**, *254*, 157–164. [CrossRef]

29. Yan, C.; Boyd, D.D. Regulation of matrix metalloproteinase gene expression. *J. Cell. Physiol.* **2007**, *211*, 19–26. [CrossRef]

30. Michel, G.; Minet, E.; Ernest, I.; Roland, I.; Durant, F.; Remacle, J.; Michiels, C. A Model for the Complex Between the Hypoxia-Inducible Factor-1 (HIF-1) and its Consensus DNA Sequence. *J. Biomol. Struct. Dyn.* **2000**, *18*, 169–179. [CrossRef]

31. Madanecki, P.; Kapoor, N.; Bebok, Z.; Ochocka, R.; Collawn, J.; Bartoszewski, R. Regulation of angiogenesis by hypoxia: The role of microRNA. *Cell. Mol. Biol. Lett.* **2013**, *18*, 19–26. [CrossRef] [PubMed]
32. Folberg, R.; Hendrix, M.J.C.; Maniotis, A.J. Vasculogenic Mimicry and Tumor Angiogenesis. *Am. J. Pathol.* **2000**, *156*, 361–381. [CrossRef]
33. Kim, A.; Im, M.; Gu, M.J.; Ma, J.Y. Ethanol extract of Lophatheri Herba exhibits anti-cancer activity in human cancer cells by suppression of metastatic and angiogenic potential. *Sci. Rep.* **2016**, *6*. [CrossRef]
34. Shukla, K.; Sonowal, H.; Saxena, A.; Ramana, K.V. Didymin by suppressing NF-κB activation prevents VEGF-induced angiogenesis in vitro and in vivo. *Vascul. Pharmacol.* **2019**. [CrossRef] [PubMed]
35. Dai, X.; Yan, J.; Fu, X.; Pan, Q.; Sun, D.; Xu, Y.; Wang, J.; Nie, L.; Tong, L.; Shen, A.; et al. Aspirin Inhibits Cancer Metastasis and Angiogenesis via Targeting Heparanase. *Clin. Cancer Res.* **2017**, *23*, 6267–6278. [CrossRef] [PubMed]
36. Taylor, C.A.; Zheng, Q.; Liu, Z.; Thompson, J.E. Role of p38 and JNK MAPK signaling pathways and tumor suppressor p53 on induction of apoptosis in response to Ad-eIF5A1 in A549 lung cancer cells. *Mol. Cancer.* **2013**, *12*, 35. [CrossRef]
37. Song, F.-N.; Duan, M.; Liu, L.-Z.; Wang, Z.-C.; Shi, J.-Y.; Yang, L.-X.; Zhou, J.; Fan, J.; Gao, Q.; Wang, X.-Y. RANKL Promotes Migration and Invasion of Hepatocellular Carcinoma Cells via NF-κB-Mediated Epithelial-Mesenchymal Transition. *PLoS ONE.* **2014**, *9*, e108507. [CrossRef] [PubMed]
38. Lee, M.S.; Koh, D.; Kim, G.S.; Lee, S.E.; Noh, H.J.; Kim, S.Y.; Lee, Y.H.; Lim, Y.; Shin, S.Y. 2-Hydroxy-3,4-naphthochalcone (2H-NC) inhibits TNFα-induced tumor invasion through the downregulation of NF-κB-mediated MMP-9 gene expression. *Bioorg. Med. Chem. Lett.* **2015**, *25*, 128–132. [CrossRef]
39. Lu, Y.; Jeong, Y.-T.; Li, X.; Kim, M.J.; Park, P.-H.; Hwang, S.-L.; Son, J.K.; Chang, H.W. Emodin Isolated from Polygoni cuspidati Radix Inhibits TNF-α and IL-6 Release by Blockading NF-κB and MAP Kinase Pathways in Mast Cells Stimulated with PMA Plus A23187. *Biomol. Ther.* **2013**, *21*, 435–441. [CrossRef] [PubMed]
40. Cao, J.; Tong, C.; Liu, Y.; Wang, J.; Ni, X.; Xiong, M. Ginkgetin inhibits growth of breast carcinoma via regulating MAPKs pathway. *Biomed. Pharmacother.* **2017**, *96*, 450–458. [CrossRef]
41. Nguyen, V.-T.; Qian, Z.-J.; Lee, B.; Heo, S.-J.; Kim, K.-N.; Jeon, Y.-J.; Park, W.S.; Choi, I.-W.; Jang, C.H.; Ko, S.-C.; et al. Fucoxanthin derivatives from Sargassum siliquastrum inhibit matrix metalloproteinases by suppressing NF-κB and MAPKs in human fibrosarcoma cells. *ALGAE* **2014**, *29*, 355–366. [CrossRef]
42. Zhu, B.-W.; Wang, L.-S.; Zhou, D.-Y.; Li, D.-M.; Sun, L.-M.; Yang, J.-F.; Wu, H.-T.; Zhou, X.-Q.; Tada, M. Antioxidant activity of sulphated polysaccharide conjugates from abalone (*Haliotis discus hannai Ino*). *Eur. Food Res. Technol.* **2008**, *227*, 1663–1668. [CrossRef]
43. Wu, Z.-Z.; Ding, G.-F.; Huang, F.-F.; Yang, Z.-S.; Yu, F.-M.; Tang, Y.-P.; Jia, Y.-L.; Zheng, Y.-Y.; Chen, R. Anticancer Activity of Anthopleura anjunae Oligopeptides in Prostate Cancer DU-145 Cells. *Mar. Drugs* **2018**, *16*, 125. [CrossRef]
44. Samaranayaka, A.G.P.; Li-Chan, E.C.Y. Food-derived peptidic antioxidants: A review of their production, assessment, and potential applications. *J. Funct. Foods.* **2011**, *3*, 229–254. [CrossRef]
45. Huang, F.; Yang, Z.; Yu, D.; Wang, J.; Li, R.; Ding, G. Sepia Ink Oligopeptide Induces Apoptosis in Prostate Cancer Cell Lines via Caspase-3 Activation and Elevation of Bax/Bcl-2 Ratio. *Mar. Drugs* **2012**, *10*, 2153–2165. [CrossRef] [PubMed]

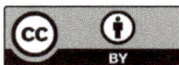

marine drugs

MDPI

Article

Two Novel Multi-Functional Peptides from Meat and Visceral Mass of Marine Snail *Neptunea arthritica cumingii* and Their Activities In Vitro and In Vivo

Shan-Shan Zhang [1,2,†], Li-Wen Han [1,2,†], Yong-Ping Shi [1,2], Xiao-Bin Li [1,2], Xuan-Ming Zhang [1,2], Hai-Rong Hou [1,2], Hou-Wen Lin [3] and Ke-Chun Liu [1,2,*]

[1] Biology Institute, Qilu University of Technology (Shandong Academy of Sciences), Jinan 250103, China; qingshuibaikai@126.com (S.-S.Z.); hanlw@sdas.org (L.-W.H.); syp3317@163.com (Y.-P.S.); bin85666666@163.com (X.-B.L.); lenghanxing_0@163.com (X.-M.Z.); caomu_1314@163.com (H.-R.H.)
[2] Shandong Provncial Engineering Laboratory for Biological Testing Technology, Key Laboratory for Drug Screening Technology of Shandong Academy of Sciences, Jinan 250103, China
[3] Research Center for Marine Drugs, State Key Laboratory of Oncogenes and Related Genes, Department of Pharmacy, School of Medicine, Shanghai Jiao Tong University, Shanghai 200127, China; Franklin67@126.com
*   Correspondence: hliukch@sdas.org; Tel.: +86-531-8260-5352
†   These authors contributed equally to this work.

Received: 31 October 2018; Accepted: 22 November 2018; Published: 27 November 2018

Abstract: *Neptunea arthritica cumingii* (*Nac*) is a marine snail with high nutritional and commercial value; however, little is known about its active peptides. In this study, two multi-functional peptides, YSQLENEFDR (Tyr-Ser-Gln-Leu-Glu-Asn-Glu-Phe-Asp-Arg) and YIAEDAER (Tyr-Ile-Ala-Glu-Asp-Ala-Glu-Arg), were isolated and purified from meat and visceral mass extracts of *Nac* using a multi-bioassay-guided method and were characterized by using liquid chromatography-tandem mass spectrometry. Both peptides showed high antioxidant, angiotensin-converting enzyme (ACE)-inhibitory, and anti-diabetic activities, with half-maximal effective concentrations values less than 1 mM. Antioxidant and ACE-inhibitory activities were significantly higher for YSQLENEFDR than for YIAEDAER. In a zebrafish model, the two peptides exhibited strong scavenging ability for reactive oxygen species and effectively protected skin cells against oxidative damage without toxicity. Molecular docking simulation further predicted the interactions of the two peptides and ACE. Stability analysis study indicated that the two synthetic peptides maintained their activities under thermal stress and simulated gastrointestinal digestion conditions. The low molecular weight, high proportion of hydrophobic and negatively-charged amino acids, and specific C-terminal and N-terminal amino acids may contribute to the observed bio-activities of these two peptides with potential application for the prevention of chronic noncommunicable diseases.

Keywords: *Neptunea arthritica cumingii*; multi-functional peptides; antioxidant activity; ACE-inhibitory activity; anti-diabetic activity

1. Introduction

Marine taxa are rich in bioactive compounds [1] that show antioxidative, antihypertensive, anti-diabetic, antimicrobial, and antitumor bioactivities [2], and are thus potentially valuable for the prevention and treatment of chronic noncommunicable diseases (NCDs) [3,4]. Accordingly, recent research has focused on bioactive peptides isolated from marine organisms [5].

Mollusks are the second largest phylum of the animal kingdom. In addition to their ecological roles, they have great commercial value as food [6]. Mollusks also contain many potential active compounds for the development of dietary supplements, functional foods, nutraceuticals, and medicine [4,7]. However, little is known about these active compounds, and mollusks are a relatively undeveloped resource for high-value products.

Neptunea arthritica cumingii (*Nac*) is a large-sized predatory gastropod belonging to the family Buccinidae, which includes well-known scavengers [8]. It mainly lives in the sea at depths from 10 to 78 m in China, Japan, North Korea, and South Korea. *Nac* has high commercial value owing to its hypertrophic and tendermeat, delicious taste, and high nutritional value, but its low hatching rate limits productivity. Despite studies of its genome, auxanology, reproductive features [9–12], and nutritive composition [13,14], little is known about the active chemical composition of *Nac*. To date, only tetramine, histamine, and choline derivatives with neural activity have been isolated from *Nac* [15,16]. We previously reported peptide extracts from whelks that show ACE-inhibitory activity [17]. Hence, we hypothesized that *Nac* might also contain peptides with activities that have potential for the prevention of NCDs.

To explore this possibility, natural multi-functional peptides were isolated and purified from the meat and visceral mass extracts of *Nac* using a multi-bioassay-guided method. The amino acid sequences of two of the isolated peptides were identified with liquid chromatography–tandem mass spectrometry (LC-MS/MS). The antioxidant, ACE-inhibitory, and anti-diabetic activities were evaluated in vitro, and the bioactivity and toxicity were evaluated in vivo in a zebrafish model (*Danio rerio*). Owing to their rapid organogenesis, transparent embryos, and high genetic similarity with humans [18], zebrafish are used extensively for studies of human diseases and activity screening [19]. Special cells of nitroreductase (NTR)-expressing transgenic zebrafish are efficiently ablated after treatment with metronidazole (MTZ) [20], and reactive oxygen species (ROS) are rapidly generated in specific tissues or cells [21]. Because ROS overproduction can induce apoptosis [22], antioxidants can promote the regeneration of ablated cells by effectively mitigating ROS generation [20,21]. Therefore, an MTZ-treated Tg (*krt4:NTR-hKikGR*)[cy17] zebrafish in which the NTR-hKikGR fusion protein is overexpressed under control of the skin-specific *krt4* promoter [23] was used as an ideal model for studying ROS-related pharmaceutical interventions in vivo. In addition, the molecular mechanisms of interactions between angiotensin-converting enzyme (ACE) and ACE-inhibitory peptides were preliminarily explored using molecular docking. Finally, to examine the therapeutic feasibility, the stabilities of the synthetic peptides for maintaining 2,2-diphenyl-1-(2,4,6-trinitrophenyl) hydrazyl (DPPH) radical scavenging activity and ACE-inhibitory activity under thermal stress and exposure to gastrointestinal digestion were investigated.

2. Results

2.1. Proximate Analysis

The mean ± standard deviation length and width of the shell of *Nac* were 105.33 ± 2.39 mm and 63.17 ± 3.20 mm, respectively. The fresh weight was 103.23 ± 2.30 g, and the weights of the meat and visceral mass were 17.34 ± 3.90 g and 24.41 ± 2.86 g, respectively. The proximate compositions of the meat and visceral mass are summarized in Figure S1 of the Supplementary Materials. The meat contained higher ash and lower fat contents than those of the visceral mass, but there was no significant difference ($p > 0.05$) in protein content between the two samples, suggesting that the meat has better nutritional quality than the visceral mass.

2.2. Bioassay-Guided Isolation of the Active Fraction

The yields of meat and visceral mass extracts were 5.02% and 5.15%, respectively. Fractions with stronger absorbance at 280 nm showed higher biological activities (Figure 1). Significant correlations (Pearson correlation coefficients ranging from 0.766 to 0.942) were observed in the antioxidant, ACE-inhibitory, and α-amylase inhibitory activities among fractions (Table S1 in the Supplementary Materials). The most active fractions 34–36 (M-F) for meat and 37–39 (VM-F) for visceral mass had 2,2-diphenyl-1-(2,4,6-trinitrophenyl) hydrazyl (DPPH) radical scavenging and ACE-inhibitory activities exceeding 80% and α-amylase inhibitory activity exceeding 50%, and they were thus collected for further investigation.

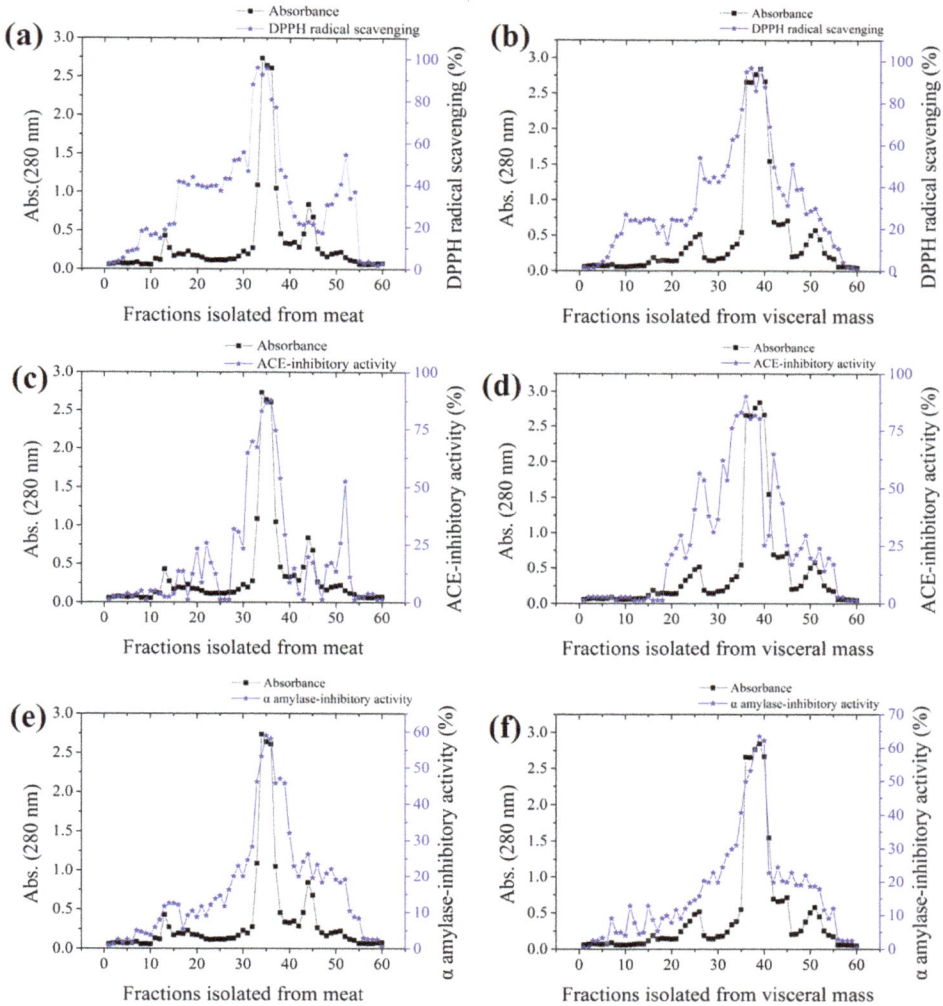

Figure 1. Absorbances and activities of fractions isolated from the meat and visceral mass of *Neptunea arthritica cumingii* (Nac) by using gel filtration column packed with Sephadex G25 gel. (**a**) the 2,2-diphenyl-1-(2,4,6-trinitrophenyl) hydrazyl (DPPH) radical scavenging activity, (**c**) angiotensin-converting enzyme (ACE)-inhibitory activity, and (**e**) α-amylase inhibitory activity of meat fractions; and (**b**) the DPPH radical scavenging activity, (**d**) ACE-inhibitory activity, and (**f**) α-amylase inhibitory activity of visceral mass fractions.

2.3. Molecular Weight Distribution

The molecular weight (MW) profiles of the M-F and VM-F each showed a major peak (more than 90%) in the low-molecular-mass region (Figure S2 in the Supplementary Materials). The average MW of the two major peptides was below 2000 Da (calibration curve molecular weight = 17.50–0.089T, R^2 = 0.9785, where T is the retention time).

2.4. Amino Acid Profile of Active Fractions

Both M-F and VM-F had high contents of hydrophobic and positively/negatively charged amino acids (Table 1). In addition, significant differences between M-F and VM-F were observed with respect to the hydrophobic and aromatic amino acid contents ($p < 0.01$). M-F had higher contents of these amino acids.

Table 1. Amino acid compositions of active fractions ($n = 3$, mean $\pm$ standard deviation (SD)).

Amino Acid	Meat (g/kg)	Visceral Mass (g/kg)
asp	42.24 ± 7.69	73.39 ± 9.67 **
glu	99.87 ± 5.60	65.21 ± 6.73 **
ser	21.82 ± 1.09	24.55 ± 5.99 *
gly	30.65 ± 3.15	36.29 ± 7.46 *
his	31.12 ± 1.03	10.90 ± 3.84 **
arg	388.77 ± 5.93	366.20 ± 8.02
thr	21.78 ± 0.88	18.03 ± 8.46
ala	98.54 ± 5.92	132.58 ± 7.21 **
pro	94.58 ± 5.26	47.18 ± 0.57 **
cys	1.04 ± 0.11	0.72 ± 0.11 *
tyr	5.05 ± 0.67	3.15 ± 5.60 **
val	24.60 ± 2.55	25.50 ± 5.15
met	3.09 ± 0.95	3.24 ± 0.15
lys	14.63 ± 1.25	7.23 ± 1.50 **
ile	18.10 ± 1.16	19.92 ± 4.15
leu	34.87 ± 1.18	32.34 ± 4.81
phe	51.34 ± 1.61	3.98 ± 0.96 **
Sum	982.11 ± 3.20	870.40 ± 2.23 **
EAA	168.42 ± 1.03	110.23 ± 4.43 **
HAA	332. 56 ± 8.61	268.6 ± 3.56 **
AAA	56.40 ± 8.61	7.13 ± 3.83 **
PCAA	434.52 ± 6.95	384.33 ± 5.73
NCAA	140.78 ± 1.81	138.60 ± 6.29

EAA, essential amino acids (ile, leu, lys, met, phe, thr, and val); HAA, hydrophobic amino acids (ala, val, iso, leu, tyr, phe, pro, meth, and cys); AAA, aromatic amino acids (phe and tyr); PCAA, positively charged amino acids (arg, his, and lys); NCAA, negatively charged amino acids (asp and glu). * $p < 0.05$ and ** $p < 0.01$ compared with the active fraction from meat.

2.5. Bioassay-Guided Purification of Active Peptides

The DPPH radical scavenging, ACE-inhibitory and α-amylase inhibitory activities of all purified fractions were determined at the same concentration. As shown in Figure 2a,b, peptides M-P6 and VM-P7 were the main components of the meat and visceral mass. M-P6 and VM-P7 had the strongest activities overall (Table 2), and were thus considered the main active peptides of the meat and visceral mass, respectively, which were subject to further structure characterization and activity determinations.

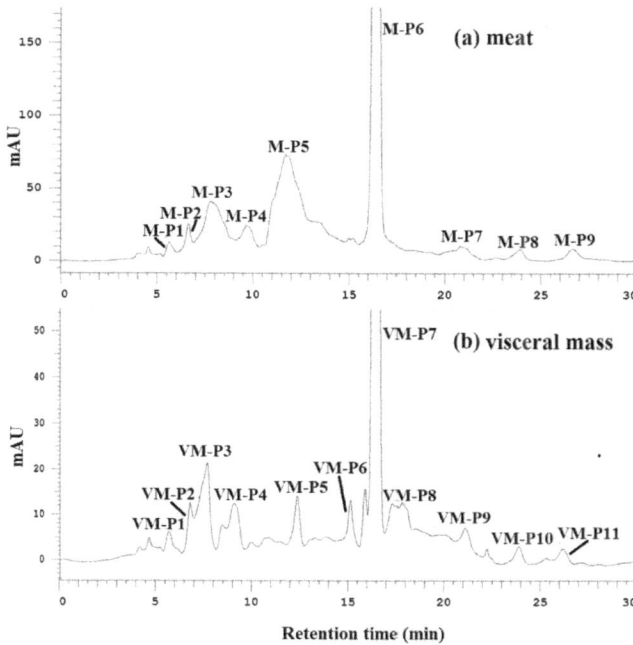

Figure 2. (a) Elution profiles of active fractions from the meat of *Nac* by hydrophilic interaction chromatography (HILIC) at 214 nm; (b) elution profiles of active fractions from the visceral mass of *Nac* by HILIC at 214 nm.

Table 2. The DPPH radical scavenging, ACE-inhibitory, and α-amylase inhibitory activities of fractions purified from M-F and VM-F using HILIC ($n = 3$, mean ± standard deviation).

Origin	Fractions	DPPH Radical Scavenging Activity (%)	ACE-Inhibitory Activity (%)	α-Amylase Inhibitory Activity (%)
M-F	M-P1	14.73 ± 3.36	12.25 ± 1.67	10.25 ± 2.00
	M-P2	25.03 ± 3.11	15.26 ± 3.34	12.55 ± 0.62
	M-P3	20.75 ± 2.39	16.76 ± 3.12	15.26 ± 1.30
	M-P4	27.25 ± 1.82	20.77 ± 0.85	15.76 ± 1.26
	M-P5	33.80 ± 2.93	23.07 ± 2.61	24.55 ± 0.29
	M-P6	91.87 ± 0.62	84.81 ± 0.35	56.15 ± 1.64
	M-P7	34.80 ± 1.22	28.20 ± 3.54	17.85 ± 2.77
	M-P8	32.60 ± 2.17	26.45 ± 1.90	16.45 ± 3.01
	M-P9	35.25 ± 1.40	25.85 ± 1.37	15.85 ± 2.27
VM-F	VM-P1	14.63 ± 3.38	12.50 ± 2.26	11.50 ± 2.46
	VM-P2	17.03 ± 2.07	14.56 ± 2.33	13.55 ± 2.61
	VM-P3	28.70 ± 0.99	20.56 ± 1.10	15.55 ± 1.36
	VM-P4	24.77 ± 3.71	23.85 ± 3.88	16.35 ± 1.34
	VM-P5	33.73 ± 1.47	25.80 ± 3.81	16.30 ± 1.74
	VM-P6	38.40 ± 1.84	28.05 ± 2.80	18.05 ± 4.27
	VM-P7	82.60 ± 0.86	74.95 ± 1.24	53.85 ± 0.92
	VM-P8	35.60 ± 1.99	27.95 ± 0.76	26.95 ± 4.49
	VM-P9	29.93 ± 0.71	24.95 ± 0.85	24.96 ± 0.79
	VM-P10	28.03 ± 3.78	21.55 ± 1.64	11.56 ± 2.87
	VM-P11	32.90 ± 0.86	27.35 ± 3.36	17.91 ± 1.70

2.6. Amino Acid Sequence of Active Peptides

A 10-residue peptide, YSQLENEFDR (Tyr-Ser-Gln-Leu-Glu-Asn-Glu-Phe-Asp-Arg), with a molecular weight of 1299 Da was identified from M-P6 (see the MS/MS spectra in Figure S3A of the Supplementary Materials) according to MS^2 spectra, and an eight-residue peptide, YIAEDAER (Tyr-Ile-Ala-Glu-Asp-Ala-Glu-Arg), with a molecular weight of 965 Da was identified from VM-P7 (see MS/MS spectra in Figure S3B of the Supplementary Materials). The sequences of the two peptides were searched against the BIOPEP database [24], and no reports of the bioactivity of these peptides were found. Hence, the bioactivities of these two active peptides obtained from *Nac* were further investigated through in vitro and in vivo experiments.

2.7. Analyses of Active Peptide Activity

2.7.1. In Vitro Antioxidant Activity

According to the half maximal inhibitory concentration (EC_{50}) values of M-P6 and VM-P7 in three antioxidant assay models (Figure 3a), both two peptides showed high antioxidant activity. Furthermore, although that of M-P6 was significantly higher ($p < 0.01$). The antioxidant activities of M-P6 and VM-P7 showed a concentration-dependent increase from 90 to 4500 µg/mL (Figure 3b–d). At concentrations greater than 1 mg/mL (corresponding to 0.77 mM and 1.04 mM for M-P6 and VM-P7, respectively), the two peptides exhibited similar activity to that of vitamin C.

2.7.2. ACE-Inhibitory Activity

Significantly greater ACE-inhibitory activity was also observed for M-P6 than for VM-P7 ($p < 0.01$, Figure 3a). Furthermore, the ACE-inhibitory activities of the two peptides increased within increasing concentrations but always less than nifepine (Figure 3e).

2.7.3. Anti-Diabetic Activity

The two peptides showed similar anti-diabetic activity (Figure 3a, $p > 0.05$). Compared to the control (acarbose), the α-amylase and α-glucosidase inhibitory activities of the two peptides were relatively poor; however, activities of the two peptides increased as the concentration increased (Figure 3f,g).

2.7.4. In Vivo Antioxidant Activity in Zebrafish Embryos

We next explored the effects of the two active peptides obtained from *Nac* on the mortality and morphology of zebrafish larvae. No death or malformation was observed after exposure to high, medium, and low concentrations of active peptide for 24 h.

For Tg (*krt4:NTR-hKikGR*)[cy17] zebrafish, MTZ treatment can lead to ROS overproduction, apoptosis of skin cells, and reduction of fluorescence spots on skin; thus, this model is used to assess ROS scavenging capacity of sample by measuring the growth rate of fluorescent spots (FS) on the skin of Tg (*krt4:NTR-hKikGR*)[cy17] transgenic zebrafish. Sample with antioxidant activity can remove ROS from transgenic zebrafish and prevent the skin cell apoptosis. Hence, an increased number of FS are observed.

According to visualization of zebrafish skin fluorescence results in Figure 4a, more FS were observed for the sample groups (Figure 4a(D–I)) than the negative control group incubated with MTZ but without peptides (Figure 4a(B)), even at a low concentration. Moreover, the FS number of all samples except VM-P7 at a low concentration showed significant difference ($p < 0.01$) compared with negative control (Figure 4b). There was no significant difference in the number of FS between the VM-P7 at a low concentration and negative control (Figure 4b(G,B)). Furthermore, more FS were detected for M-P6 than VM-P7 at medium and high concentrations ($p < 0.01$).

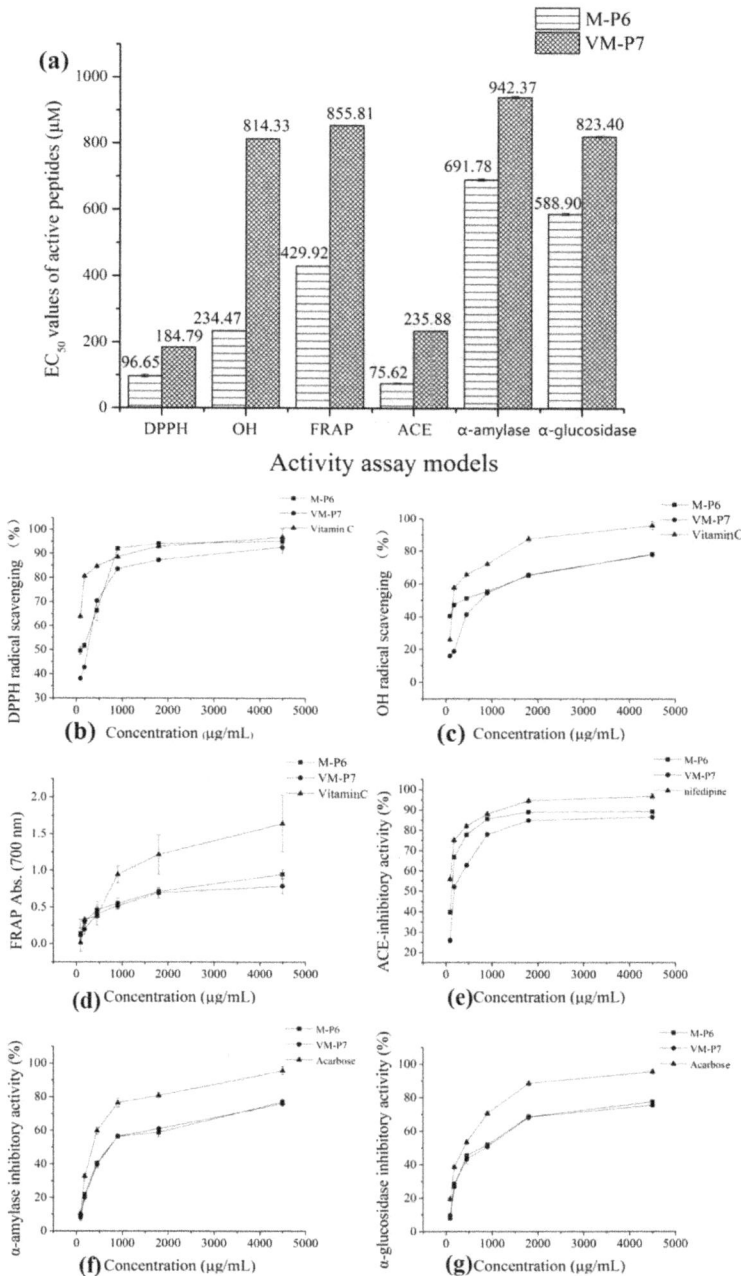

Figure 3. Bioactivities of two peptides. (**a**) half maximal inhibitory concentration (EC$_{50}$) values in different models (** $p < 0.01$ compared with the VM-P7), (**b**) DPPH radical scavenging activity, (**c**) OH radical scavenging activity, (**d**) reducing power, (**e**) ACE-inhibitory activity, (**f**) α-amylase inhibitory activity, and (**g**) α-glucosidase inhibitory activity.

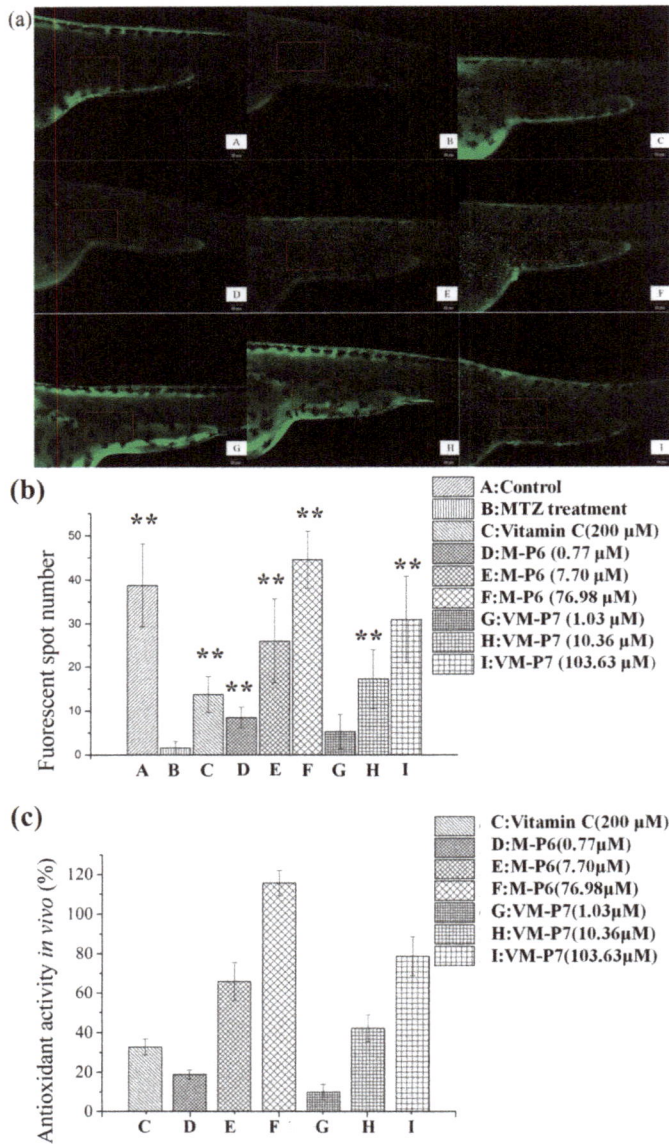

Figure 4. In vivo antioxidant activity of active peptides in zebrafish embryos (*n* = 10, mean ± standard deviation). (**a**) In vivo visualization of zebrafish skin fluorescence treatment with vehicle (A), metronidazole (MTZ; (B)), vitamin C (C), and low (D), medium (E), and high (F) concentrations of M-P6, as well as low (G), medium (H), and high (I) concentrations of VM-P7; (**b**) FS number statistic results of all groups; (**c**) In vivo antioxidant activity of all samples. ** indicates significant differences compared with the MTZ treatment group (*p* < 0.01).

As shown in Figure 4c, the in vivo antioxidant activities of two peptides gradually increased with the increase of concentration. M-P6 showed better antioxidant activity compared with VM-P7. These results were consistent with the findings of in vitro antioxidant activity. In addition, the antioxidant activities of the two peptides at medium and high concentrations were significantly greater than that of the positive control vitamin C at 200 μM ($p < 0.01$). In addition, compared to the control group (no MTZ or peptides), more FS were detected for M-P6 at high concentrations (Figure 4b(F)). The reason for this result may be superior ROS scavenging ability of M-P6 promoting more skin cells regeneration. These results indicated that the two peptides could protect the skin cells of transgenic zebrafish against oxidative damage caused by MTZ.

2.8. Molecular Docking Simulation

CDocker was used to further investigate the intermolecular interactions between the active peptides and ACE. Both peptides showed a stable docking structure with ACE according to the— CDocker energy and—CDocker interaction energy values (Table 3). However, YSQLENEFDR displayed better binding affinity with ACE than YIAEDAER. The docking simulation results of two peptides are shown in Figures 5 and 6. Both peptides successfully entered the channel of ACE after docking (Figure 5a,b). As shown in Figure 6a,b, both active peptides combined with ACE residues through van der Waals interactions, hydrogen bonds, and electrostatic, hydrophobic, and miscellaneous interaction forces. YIAEDAER made contract with the ACE residues His 353, Ala 354, Glu384, and Tyr523 via van der Waals interactions and formed 11 hydrogen bonds with ACE residues Asn66, Asn70, Arg124, Trp220, Lys368, His387, His410, Ser516, Ser517, Pro519, and Arg522, respectively. Electrostatic force were observed between YIAEDAER and the ACE residue Lys368 interacted through an electrostatic force, whereas interactions with Met223, Tyr360, Phe391, and His410 were through the hydrophobic force. YSQLENEFDR made contact with ACE residues Glu384, Lys511, His513, Tyr520, and Tyr523 via the van der Waals force, and formed 13 hydrogen bonds with ACE residues Glu162, Asn277, Gln281, His 353, Ala354, Ala356, Tyr360, San374, Asp377, Glu403, Glu411, Pro519, and Arg522, respectively. YSQLENEFDR and ACE residues Glu162, Asp377, and Glu403 interacted with electrostatic force, whereas a hydrophobic force formed between YSQLENEFDR and ACE residues Val379, His383, and Phe527. Both YIAEDAER and YSQLENEFDR interacted with Zn (II) via miscellaneous force.

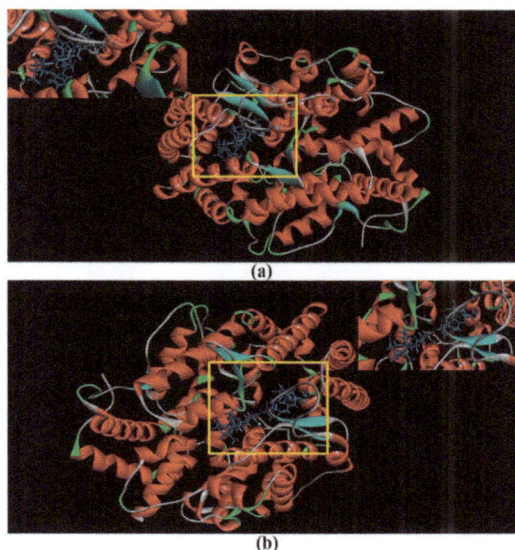

(a)

(b)

Figure 5. The molecular docking of YIAEDAER (a) from visceral mass and YSQLENEFDR (b) from meat to angiotensin-converting enzyme.

Table 3. Docking energies for optimal conformation of two active peptides and ACE. YIAEDAER: Tyr-Ile-Ala-Glu-Asp-Ala-Glu-Arg; YSQLENEFDR: Tyr-Ser-Gln-Leu-Glu-Asn-Glu-Phe-Asp-Arg.

Peptides	- CDocker Energy (kcal/mol)	- CDocker Interaction Energy (kcal/mol)
YIAEDAER	174.672	130.72
YSQLENEFDR	193.884	175.07

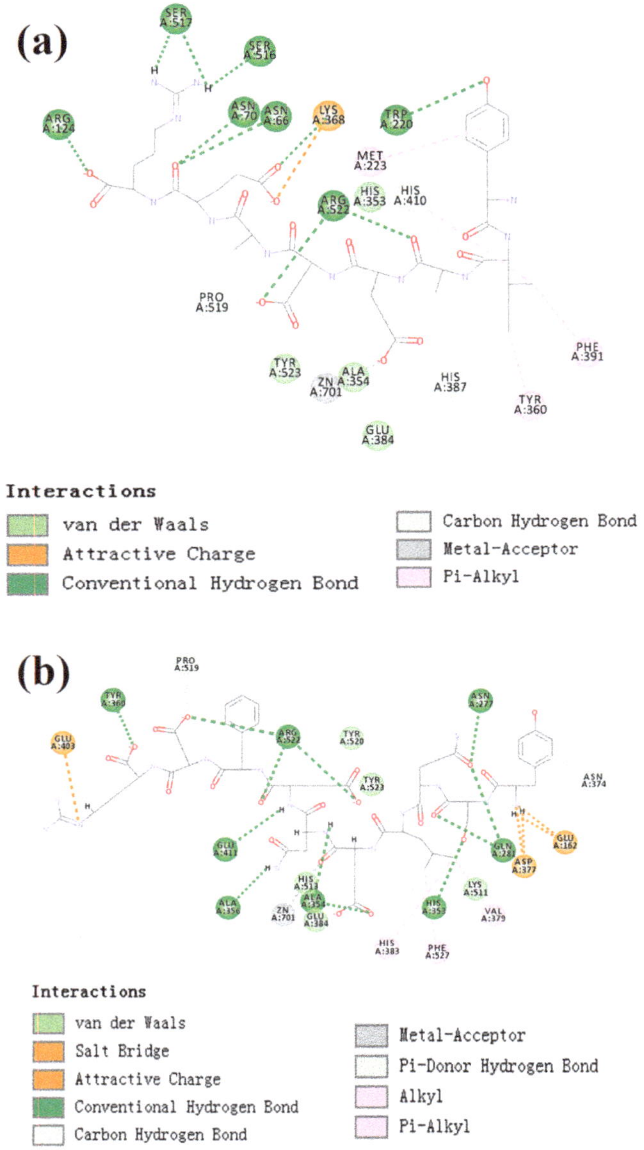

Figure 6. The two-dimensional diagram of molecular docking simulation of YIAEDAER (**a**) from visceral mass and YSQLENEFDR (**b**) from meat to angiotensin-converting enzyme.

2.9. Stablity of Synthetic Peptides against Thermal and Gastrointestinal Digestion Treatments

A series of samples with concentration range from 90 µg/mL (corresponding to 69.28 µM and 93.26 µM for YSQLENEFDR and YIAEDAER, respectively) to 1800µg/mL were used in stability analysis. EC_{50} values (expression in molar concentrations) of active peptide under different treatment conditions were used as evaluation standard.

As shown in Figure 7a,b, the thermal treatments did not significantly affect the DPPH radical scavenging activities or ACE inhibitory activities of both synthetic peptides according to a lack of significant change in EC_{50} values ($p > 0.05$).

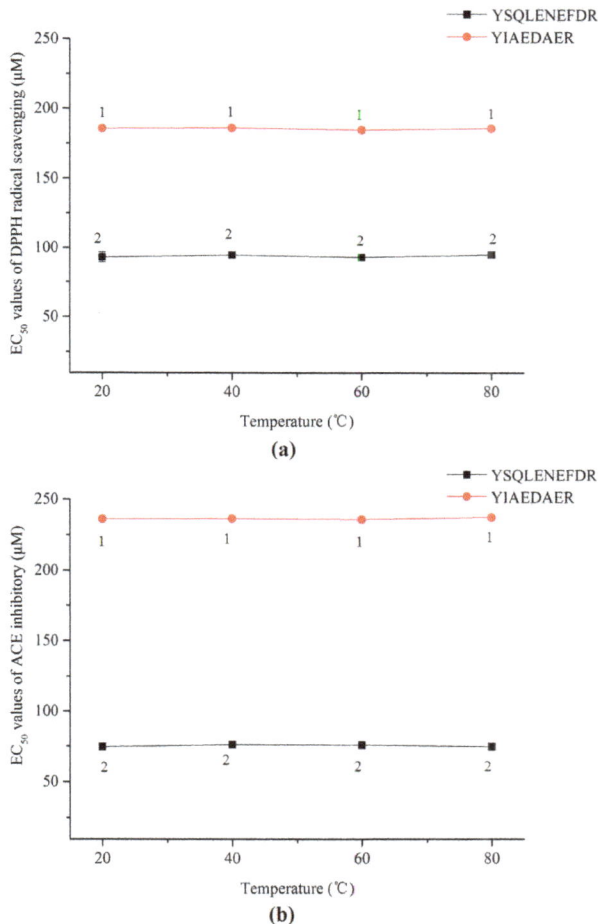

Figure 7. EC_{50} values of DPPH radical scavenging (**a**) and ACE inhibitors (**b**) of two synthetic peptides treated with thermal treatment. The same numbers means no significantly different in a group ($p > 0.05$).

Similar results were observed in the gastrointestinal digestion treatment (Figure 8a,b). The EC_{50} values of DPPH radical scavenging and ACE inhibitory of both peptides slightly increased after digestion but the difference was not significant ($p > 0.05$). These results indicated that the two peptides, YSQLENEFDR and YIAEDAER, have thermal and gastrointestinal stability.

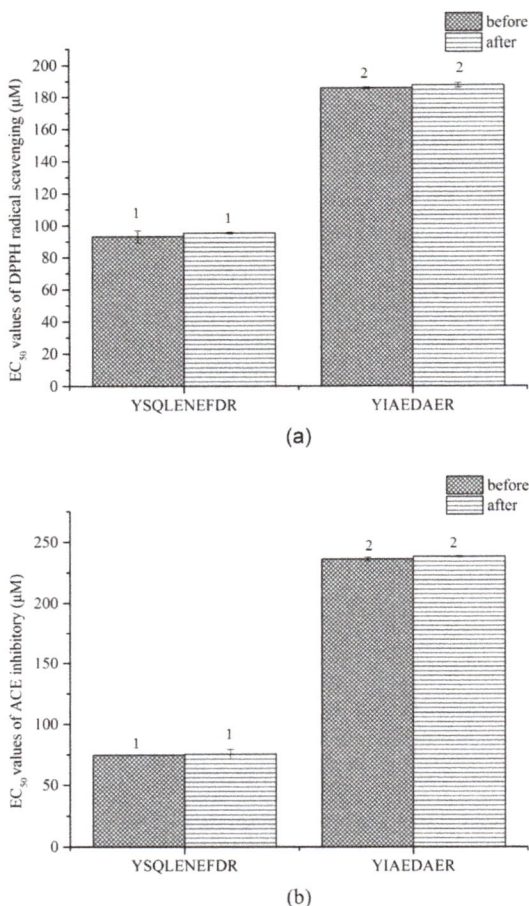

Figure 8. EC$_{50}$ values of DPPH radical scavenging (**a**) and ACE inhibitors (**b**) of two synthetic peptides treated with gastrointestinal digestion treatment. The same numbers indicate no significant difference in a group ($p > 0.05$).

3. Discussion

Two novel multi-functional peptides, YSQLENEFDR and YIAEDAER, were isolated, purified and identified from the meat and visceral mass of *Nac* under multi-bioassay guidance using gel filtration chromatography, reversed phase-high-performance liquid chromatography (RP-HPLC), hydrophilic interaction chromatography (HILIC), and LC-MS/MS. The total proportions of hydrophobic and negatively charged amino acids were relative high in sequences of both peptides. Both peptides showed strong in vitro antioxidant, ACE-inhibitory, and anti-diabetic activities, along with potent scavenging ability for ROS and protected skin cells against oxidative damage in a zebrafish model.

These high antioxidant activities of the two peptides could be attributed to their low molecular weight, which facilitates access to oxidant-antioxidant systems [25]. However, the amino acid composition and peptide sequence are also important determinants of antioxidant activity. Peptides of freshwater mussels with a high molecular weight were reported to show relatively high antioxidant activity due to the abundant hydrophobic amino acids [26]. Indeed, hydrophobic and aromatic amino acids are known to play important roles in the antioxidant activity of peptides [27]. Negatively charged amino acids have strong antioxidant effects because the excess electrons are free to interact with free radicals [28]. The position of Tyr at the N terminus and the dipeptide Glu-Leu and Ala-Glu of the peptide sequence can also contribute to antioxidant activity [29]. Moreover, Glu in the peptide sequence increases antioxidant activity via promoting oxidized glutathione production [30]. Therefore, the higher antioxidant activity of YSQLENEFDR may be due to the presence of aliphatic and aromatic amino acids (Tyr, Ser, Leu and Phe), especially Tyr at the N terminus and Glu-Leu, as well as the acidic amino acid Glu. Similarly, the hydrophobic amino acids (Tyr, Ile, Ala) and the acidic amino acid Glu also contributed to the antioxidant activity of YIAEDAER.

ACE catalyzes the conversion of angiotensin I to angiotensin II, a potent vasoconstrictor, and promotes degradation of the vasodilator bradykinin [31]; thus, inhibition of ACE activity may help with reducing blood pressure. Because high-molecular-weight peptides cannot occupy the active site of ACE [32], ACE-inhibitory peptides are typically 2–30 amino acids in length [33]. Moreover, peptides with high aromatic acid contents have been shown to have higher ACE-inhibitory activity [34]. Peptides containing Arg at the C terminus exhibit inhibitory activity due to the positive charge of the guanidine group [35]. Tyr at the N terminus can enhance the activity. This is supported by data recorded in biopep database. Four peptides, YPR, YLYEIAR, YLYEIARR, and YIPIQYVLSR, which possess similar amino acid residues with active peptides from *Nac*, show EC$_{50}$ values of 16.5, 16.00, 86.00 and 132.50 µM. Furthermore, Asn potentially contributes to ACE-inhibitory activity [36]. Hence, Arg in the C terminus, Tyr in the N terminus and the aromatic amino acid residues in YSQLENEFDR and YIAEDAER might explain their potent ACE-inhibitory activities. In addition, the higher inhibitory activity of YSQLENEFDR than YIAEDAER may be attributed to the presence of the Asn residue.

α-Amylase and α-glucosidase are key enzymes for starch and oligosaccharide digestion [37], and their inhibition is an effective method for controlling glucose homeostasis in diabetic patients [38]. Low-molecular-weight peptides (<3 kDa) have potent inhibitory activities of these digestive enzymes [39]. Aromatic and hydrophobic amino acid residues also play important roles in α-amylase and α-glucosidase inhibitory activities [40,41]. Accordingly, the inhibitory activities of YSQLENEFDR and YIAEDAER could be attributed to their low molecular weights along with the presence of Tyr, Glu, and Arg residues.

Moreover, both purified peptides showed good ROS-scavenging ability in zebrafish in vivo with no toxic effects, and could effectively prevent the skin cell damage caused by peroxidation.

There is no detailed information on the molecular mechanisms of interactions between ACE and ACE-inhibitory peptides from *Nac*. Therefore, to facilitate further research and development of active peptides, molecular docking simulation was conducted between ACE and active peptides from different parts of *Nac* as a preliminary analysis using CDOCKER.

ACE contains three main active site pockets: S1, S2, and S1′. The S1 pocket includes the residues Ala354, Glu384, and Tyr523; the S2 pocket contains Gln281, His353, Lys511, His513, and Tyr520; and S1′ contains Glu162 [42]. The molecular docking results clearly showed interactions of the active peptides with these active site residues of ACE, thus contributing to their inhibition activities. YIAEDAER establishes interactions with the S1 pocket (Ala354, Glu384, and Tyr523) and S2 pocket (His 353) of ACE via van der Waals forces, whereas YSQLENEFDR establishes interactions with all active site residues via van der Waals interactions, hydrogen bonds, and electrostatic forces. Moreover, both peptides established hydrogen bonds with the Arg522 of ACE, which has been reported as an imported residue for activity of the enzyme [43]. Addition, both peptides directly interacted with Zn^{2+} at the ACE active site via a miscellaneous force, which likely promoted the ACE-inhibitory activities of peptides since previous work has shown that interactions between ACE inhibitors and Zn^{2+} play an important role in deactivating ACE [44]. Furthermore, more hydrogen bonds were formed between YSQLENEFDR and ACE, and the number of hydrogen bonds plays a major role in determining interactions between inhibition peptides and ACE [45]. Overall, these results indicate that YSQLENEFDR exhibit better ACE inhibition activity, which is attributed to its more effective interaction with the active sites, supporting the results of the in vitro ACE inhibition assay of the active peptides.

Since functional food or drug processing technology may involve thermal sterilization and drying, it is essential to confirm the stability of active peptides against thermal and gastrointestinal digestion treatments for their applications as functional foods or drugs. Our results suggest that the thermal processing technology may not affect the antioxidant and ACE activities of YSQLENEFDR and YIAEDAER. In vitro simulated gastrointestinal digestion is an effective initial assessment method for the bioavailability of active peptides prior to in vivo applications [46]. Although the antioxidant and ACE activities of YSQLENEFDR and YIAEDAER were slightly reduced after gastrointestinal digestion, both synthetic peptides still showed good activity levels, and the activities of YSQLENEFDR were still better than those of YIAEDAER. Furthermore, the two synthetic peptides showed similar bioactivities with respect to the EC_{50} values of natural peptides in DPPH radical scavenging and ACE-inhibitory activities. It is indicated that modification is an effective method to improve stability, boost bioavailability or enhance activities of natural peptides [47]. Thus, these two natural peptides can be used as precursors of peptides therapeutics.

Overall, the study indicates that two novel natural multi-functional peptides isolated from *Nac* show good antioxidant, ACE-inhibitory, and anti-diabetic activities in vitro, as well as strong ROS scavenging ability in vivo without toxicity. The ACE inhibition of the two peptides may be mainly attributed to the interaction with the active site residues of ACE and Zn^{2+}. Furthermore, the DPPH radical scavenging and ACE-inhibitory activities of the two synthetic peptides were stable after thermal treatment (20–80°C) and gastrointestinal digestion. Thus, these two active peptides, YSQLENEFDR and YIAEDAER, have potential for the treatment and prevention of NCDs. For further study, we will focus on the mechanism of action of these peptides.

4. Materials and Methods

4.1. Materials

Live *Nac* samples (see Figure S4A in the Supplementary Materials) of similar sizes were purchased from a market in Jinan, China. The samples were washed with water and the moisture on the shell was removed by drying at 25 °C. The shell and operculum were removed, and the soft body (Figure S4B in Supplementary Materials) was separated into the meat (Figure S4C in Supplementary Materials) and visceral mass (Figure S4D in Supplementary Materials). The samples were freeze-dried, ground into a power, and stored at −20 °C until analysis.

4.2. Reagents and Animals

DPPH, angiotensin-converting enzyme (0.25 U·mL^{-1}, from the rabbit lung), N-hippuryl-His-Leu hydrate (HHL), hippuric acid, and amino acid standards were purchased from Sigma-Aldrich (Shanghai, China). α-Glucosidase protease (50 U/mg, from yeast), α-amylase protease (50 U/mg, from *Bacillus subtilis*), acarbose, 4-nitrophenyl-β-D-galactopyranoside, 6-aminoquinolyl-N-hydroxysuccinimidyl carbamate (AQC), ribonuclease (13,700 Da, from the bovine pancreas), aprotinin hydrochloride (6511 Da, from the bovine lung), angiotensin II (1046 Da), and L-serine (105 Da) were purchased from Yuanye Biological Technology Co. (Shanghai, China). Trypsin (250 U/mg), pepsin (250 U/mg), Sephadex G25 gel, nifedipine, and vitamin C were purchased from Solarbio (Beijing, China). Transgenic zebrafish Tg (*krt4:NTR-hKikGR*)^{cy17} are maintained in our lab. All chemicals and reagents used for HPLC were of chromatographic grade and other chemicals and reagents were of analytical grade.

4.3. Zebrafish Maintenance and Embryo Handling

Adult zebrafish were maintained at 28 °C under a 14/10 h light/dark cycle and supplied with freshwater, aeration, and food. Embryos were obtained from natural spawning; they were collected within 30 min and cultured in an aquarium. The embryos were used within 24 h. The experiments were performed in accordance with standard ethical guidelines. The procedures were approved by the Ethics Committee of the Biology Institute of Shandong Academy of Science.

4.4. Proximate Composition

The proximate compositions of the two parts of *Nac*, including moisture, ash, crude protein, and fat contents, were determined according to the methods of the Association of Official Analytical Chemists [48].

4.5. Peptide Extraction

The ground meat and visceral mass of *Nac* were suspended in 50% (*v*/*v*) ethanol in ultrapure water (sample: solution = 1:10, *w*/*v*), and the pH was adjusted to 5.0 using acetic acid. The mixture was stirred continuously using a magnetic stirrer at 30 °C for 6 h. The suspension was centrifuged at $6000\times g$ for 20 min. The supernatant was concentrated by rotary evaporation to remove ethanol at 40 °C, and then, an equal volume of hexane was added in a separating funnel three times to minimize low polarity interference. The lower layer was freeze-dried and stored at −20 °C until further separation.

4.6. Bioassay-Guided Isolation of Active Fractions

Lyophilized samples were dissolved in 10 mL of 0.01 mol/L HCl at 50 mg/mL. After filtering through a 0.45-μm syringe filter, 5 mL of the sample was loaded onto a gel filtration column packed with Sephadex G25 gel (1.8 cm × 60 cm) pre-equilibrated with 0.01 mol/L HCl. The column was eluted with 0.01 mol/L HCl at a flow rate of 15 mL/h. Fractions were collected every 5 mL and absorbance was measured at 280 nm to measure the in vitro antioxidant, ACE-inhibitory, and α-amylase inhibitory activities of all fractions. Most of the active fractions separated on Sephadex G25 column were freeze-dried for further analysis and purification.

4.7. Molecular Weight Distribution of Active Fractions

The molecular weight distribution of the active fractions obtained from the meat and visceral mass were determined by gel permeation chromatography using a TSK-gel G2000 SWXL column (7.8 mm × 250 mm) (TOSOH, Yamaguchi, Japan) according to previously reported methods [36], except the flow rate was set to 0.2 mL·min^{-1}. The column was calibrated with ribonuclease, aprotinin hydrochloride, angiotensin II, HHL, and L-serine.

4.8. Amino Acid Compositions of Active Fractions

Active fractions were hydrolyzed according to previously reported methods [49]. After acid hydrolysis, samples and amino acid standards were derivatized with AQC and determined by RP-HPLC [50]. The amino acid compositions of the two fractions were identified and quantified from standard curves of amino acid mixtures. All samples were determined in triplicate.

4.9. Bioassay-Guided Purification of Active Peptides

Freeze-dried active fractions were dissolved in 10 mM ammonium acetate buffer (pH 6.0) at 1 mg·mL^{-1}. Samples were filtered through a 0.45-μm microporous membrane and further separated on a Welch HILIC amide column (4.6 mm × 250 mm, 5 μm). The binary mobile phase composed of acetonitrile and 10 mM ammonium acetate buffer (pH 6.0) (80:20 *v*/*v*) was pumped at a flow-rate of 1 mL/min. The injection volume was 20 μL. The absorption peak was monitored at 214 nm and all absorption peaks were collected. The activities of all fractions were then determined. The most active fractions from the two sources were freeze-dried and stored at −20 °C for further identification.

4.10. Identification of Active Peptide Sequences by Nano-LC-LTQ-Orbitrap-MS/MS

The amino acid sequences of active peptides were identified using an EASY-Nlc1000 chromatography system (Thermo Finnigan, Bremen, Germany) coupled to an LTQ Orbitrap Velos Pro mass spectrometer (Thermo Finnigan) according to previously published methods [51], with some modifications. The purified peptides were resolved in ultrapure water with 0.1% trifluoroacetic acid at a concentration of 0.1 mg/mL. Then, 2 μL of the sample was injected into the trap column (100 μm × 20 mm, RP-C_{18}; Thermo Inc.) for preconcentration. The preconcentrated sample was automatically entered into an analysis column (75 μm × 150 mm, RP-C_{18}; Thermo Inc.). The sample was eluted with 0.1% *v/v* formic acid in ultrapure water for 60 min with a flow rate of 300 nL/min at 30 °C. Mascot 2.3 (Matrix Science, Boston, MA, USA) was used for data analysis. The NCBInr database was used for peptide identification with an expected value threshold of less than 0.05.

4.11. Determination of Activities

4.11.1. DPPH Radical Scavenging Activity

The DPPH radical scavenging activity of the two peptide fractions was determined according to the methods described by Lee et al. [52]. Vitamin C was used as a positive control. The EC_{50} values for DPPH radical scavenging was determined.

4.11.2. Ferric Reducing Capacity

The reducing power of the peptide fractions was assayed as described by Moayedi et al. [53]. Vitamin C was used as a positive control. The reducing power of active peptides was assayed by determining EC_{50} values.

4.11.3. Hydroxyl Radical Scavenging Activity

The hydroxyl radical scavenging activity of peptide fractions was determined according to the methods described by Dong et al. [26]. Vitamin C was used as a positive control. The hydroxyl radical activity of active peptides was evaluated by EC_{50}.

4.11.4. Determination of Antioxidative Activity in Zebrafish Embryos

The fluorescence spots on the Tg (*krt4:NTR-hKikGR*)^{cy17} zebrafish skin are significantly reduced after MTZ-treatment due to excessive ROS production. The number of fluorescence spots on the skin will increase after incubation with antioxidant. Thus, we can evaluate the ROS scavenging ability of samples on the basis of changes in the number of fluorescence spots compared with the MTZ-treatment. The in vivo antioxidant activity of the active peptides was evaluated according to previously described methods [54] with some modification using the transgenic zebrafish line Tg (krt4:NTR-hKikGR)^{cy17}. Twenty-four-hour-old transgenic zebrafish embryos were added to 24-well cell culture plates (10 embryos/well) and incubated with 2 mL of 10 mM MTZ (dissolved in fish water) and active peptides for 24 h at 28 °C. Zebrafish treated with fish water without MTZ and peptides were used as controls. Zebrafish treated with MTZ without peptides were used as negative controls. Vitamin C instead of peptides was used as a positive control. After incubation, zebrafish embryos were anesthetized with tricaine (0.16%, *w/v*), and fluorescence was observed using an FSX100 Bio Imaging Navigator instrument. FS were counted using ImagePro-Plus, and the in vivo antioxidant activity (%) of active peptides was determined by Equation 1.

$$\text{Antioxidant activity (\%)} = \{(\text{FSs} - \text{FSnc})/(\text{FSvc} - \text{FSnc})\} \times 100 \tag{1}$$

where FSs indicates the number of FS in the samples, FSnc indicates the number of FSin the negative control, and FSvc indicates the number of FS in the vehicle control.

4.11.5. Determination of ACE-Inhibitory Activity

ACE-inhibitory activity was measured according to the methods of Chen et al. [55]. Nifedipine was used as a positive control. Results were reported as EC_{50} values.

4.11.6. Determination of Anti-Diabetic Activity

α-Amylase and α-glucosidase inhibitory activities were assayed as described by Uraipong et al. [37]. Acarbose was used as a positive control. The inhibitory activity of active peptides was expressed as the EC_{50} value.

4.12. Peptide Synthesis

After identification by nano-LC-ESI-MS/MS, two active peptides (Tyr-Ser-Gln-Leu-Glu-Asn-Glu-Phe-Asp-Arg and Tyr-Ile-Ala-Glu-Asp-Ala-Glu-Arg) were synthesized by Cellmano Biotech Co. Ltd. (Hefei, China) with a purity of 99.02% and 96.43%, respectively.

4.13. Molecular Docking

In the docking study, human ACE was used as receptor. The crystal structure of ACE (1O8A.pdb) was obtained from the Protein Data Bank (https://www.rcsb.org/structure/1O8A). The 3D structure of active peptide was constructed and energy minimized using MM2 molecular mechanics method with Chem3D Pro 14.0 (CambridgeSoft Co., MA, USA). Before docking, the structure of ACE was removed water molecules and inhibitors, retained the cofactors zinc and chloride atoms and cleaned protein. Then, the ACE and two active peptides were energetically minimized by the CHARMm force field, respectively. The automated molecular docking studies of the active peptides at the ACE binding sites were performed using the CDOCKER module according to the method described by Deng et al. [45]. The binding site sphere was set as x:40.302, y:37.243 and z:48.948 with radius of 20 Å. Evaluation of the molecular docking was performed according to values of -CDocker energy and -CDocker interaction energy. The best conformation of peptide and ACE showed the highest values of -CDocker energy and -CDocker interaction energy.

4.14. Stability against Thermal and Gastrointestinal Digestion Treatments

Thermal stability and gastrointestinal digestion stability of two synthetic peptides were determined according to Chen et al. [56]. The incubated temperature for peptide solutions was set as 20, 40, 60, and 80 °C, respectively. DPPH radical scavenging activities and ACE inhibitory activities of the peptide solutions were measured as the above description.

4.15. Statistical Analysis

All tests were repeated three times and results are presented as means ± standard deviation. SPSS 16.0 (SPSS Inc., Chicago, IL, USA) was used for statistical analyses. All figures were generated using Origin 9.0 (Origin Lab, Northampton, MA, USA). One-way analysis of variance was used to analyze differences among groups; $p < 0.05$ was considered statistically significant. Pearson correlation coefficients were used to evaluate correlations among contents and activities. The molecular docking was evaluated and analyzed by Discovery Studio 2.5 (DS2.5, Accelrys, San Diego, CA, USA) and Discovery Studio 4.5 Visualizer (DS4.5, Accelrys, San Diego, CA, USA).

5. Patents

(1) Zhang, S.S.; Liu, K.C.; Han, L.W.; Zhang, X.M.; Li, X.B.; Zhang, Y. Preparation and Application of Peptides with the Function of Repairing Oxidative Damage. Patent No. 201810915407.5.

(2) Han, L.W.; Zhang, S.S.; Liu, K.C.; Li, X.B.; Zhang, X.M.; Hou, H.R; Sun, C. Preparation and Application of Peptides with the Function of Preventing Cardio-Cerebrovascular Disease. Patent No. 201810916171.7.

Supplementary Materials: The following are available online at http://www.mdpi.com/1660-3397/16/12/473/s1. Figure S1: Proximate compositions of the meat and visceral mass of *Nac*. (A) Fresh weight; (B) dry weight. Different letters indicate a significant difference between samples ($p < 0.01$); Figure S2: Molecular weight distribution of the active fraction from meat (A) and visceral mass (B) of *Nac*; Figure S3: MS/MS spectra of active peptides; (A) M-P6 from the meat and (B) VM-P7 from visceral mass of *Nac*. Figure S4: Visualization of *Neptunea arthritica cumingii*. (A) overall appearance, (B) soft body, (C) meat, and (D) visceral mass; Table S1: Pearson correlation coefficients (R) for various activity assays.

Author Contributions: Conceptualization, S.-S.Z., L.-W.H. and K.-C.L.; Data curation, S.-S.Z., Y.-P.S. and H.-R.H.; Formal analysis, X.-B.L. and X.-M.Z.; Funding acquisition, K.-C.L.; Supervision, H.-W.L. and K.-C.L.; Writing—original draft, S.-S.Z.; Writing—review and editing, L.-W.H. and K.-C.L.

Funding: This work was financially supported by the Key Research and Development Plan of Shandong province (grant number 2016GSF121009 and 2017YYSP032), Natural Science Funds of Shandong province (grant number ZR2016YL009), and the Youth fund of Shandong Academy of Sciences (grant number 2018QN0027).

Acknowledgments: We thank Editage (https://www.editage.com/) for the language editing during the manuscript preparation. We thank OE Biotech. Co., Ltd. for help with the amino acid sequence analysis.

Conflicts of Interest: The authors declare no conflict of interest.

References

1. Costa, M.; Costa-Rodrigues, J.; Fernandes, M.H.; Barros, P.; Vasconcelos, V.; Martins, R. Marine cyanobacteria compounds with anticancer properties: A review on the implication of apoptosis. *Mar. Drugs* **2012**, *10*, 2181–2207. [CrossRef] [PubMed]

2. Negi, B.; Kumar, D.; Rawat, D.S. Marine peptides as anticancer agents: A remedy to mankind by nature. *Curr. Protein Pept. Sci.* **2017**, *18*, 1–20. [CrossRef] [PubMed]

3. Pangestuti, R.; Kim, S.K. Bioactive peptide of marine origin for the prevention and treatment of non-communicable diseases. *Mar. Drugs* **2017**, *15*, 67. [CrossRef] [PubMed]

4. Cheung, R.C.; Ng, T.B.; Wong, J.H. Marine peptides: Bioactivities and applications. *Mar. Drugs* **2015**, *13*, 4006–4043. [CrossRef] [PubMed]

5. Guadalupe, M.; Suarez, J.; Armando, B.H.; Josafat, M.; Ezquerra, B. Bioactive peptides and depsipeptides with anticancer potential: Sources from marine animals. *Mar. Drugs* **2012**, *10*, 963–986. [CrossRef]

6. Luo, F.L.; Xing, R.; Wang, X.Q.; Peng, Q.; Li, P. Proximate composition, amino acid and fatty acid profiles of marine snail Rapana venosa meat, visceral mass and operculum. *J. Sci. Food Agric.* **2017**, *97*, 5361–5368. [CrossRef] [PubMed]

7. Turner, A.H.; Craik, D.J.; Kaas, Q.; Schroeder, C.I. Bioactive compounds isolated from neglected predatory marine gastropods. *Mar. Drugs* **2018**, *16*, 118. [CrossRef] [PubMed]

8. Ponder, W.F. A review of the New Zealand recent and fossil species of *Buccinulum deshayes* (*Mollusca: Neogastropoda: Buccinidae*). *J. R. Soc. N. Z.* **1971**, *1*, 231–283. [CrossRef]

9. Hao, Z.L.; Yang, L.M.; Zhan, Y.Y.; Tian, Y.; Mao, J.X.; Wang, L.; Chang, Y.Q. The complete mitochondrial genome of *Neptunea arthritica cumingii* Crosse, (*Gastropoda: Buccinidae*). *Mitochondrial DNA Part B Resour.* **2016**, *1*, 220–221. [CrossRef]

10. Lombardo, R.C.; Goshima, S. Sexual conflict in *Neptunea arthritica*: The power asymmetry and female resistance. *J. Mar. Biol. Assoc.* **2011**, *91*, 251–256. [CrossRef]

11. An, J.E.; Choi, J.D.; Ryu, D.K. Age and Growth of the *Neptunea* (*Barbitonia*) *Arthritica cumingii* in the west sea of Korea. *Korean J. Malacol.* **2014**, *30*, 25–32. [CrossRef]

12. Miranda, R.M.; Fujinaga, K.; Ilano, A.S.; Nakao, S. Effects of imposex and parasite infection on the reproductive features of the Neptune whelk *Neptunea arthritica*. *Mar. Biol. Res.* **2009**, *5*, 268–277. [CrossRef]

13. He, J.Z. Analysis of trace elements and edibleness of *Neptunea cumingi* tissue. *Food Sci.* **2010**, *31*, 181–184. [CrossRef]

14. Esipov, A.V.; Busarova, N.G.; Isai, S.V. Composition and fatty-acid contents of the commercial mollusk *Neptunea arthritica*. *Chem. Nat. Comp.* **2014**, *50*, 1099–1100. [CrossRef]

15. Asano, M.; Ito, M. Occurrence of tetramine and choline compounds in the salivary gland of a marine gastropod *Neptunea arthritica*, Bernardi. *J. Clin. Gastroenterol.* **1959**, *1*, 91–92. [CrossRef]

16. Lloyd, P.E. Cardioactive neuropeptides in gastropods. *Fed. Proc.* **1982**, *41*, 2948–3000. [PubMed]

17. Liu, K.C.; Biology Institute, Qilu University of Technology, Shandong Academy of Sciences, Jinan, China. Personal communication, 2008.

18. Hill, A.; Mesens, N.; Steemans, M.; Xu, J.J.; Aleo, M.D. Comparisons between in vitro whole cell imaging and in vivo zebrafish-based approaches for identifying potential human hepatotoxicants earlier in pharmaceutical development. *Drug. Metab. Rev.* **2012**, *44*, 127–140. [CrossRef] [PubMed]

19. Ingham, P.W. The power of the Zebrafish for disease analysis. *Hum. Mol. Genet.* **2009**, *18*, R107–R112. [CrossRef] [PubMed]

20. Curado, S.; Stainier, D.Y.R.; Anderson, R.M. Nitroreductase-mediated cell/tissue ablation in zebrafish: A spatially and temporally controlled ablation method with applications in developmental and regeneration studies. *Nat. Protoc.* **2018**, *3*, 948–954. [CrossRef] [PubMed]

21. Kulkarni, A.A.; Conteh, A.M.; Sorrell, C.A.; Mirmira, A.; Tersey, S.A.; Mirnira, R.G.; Linnemann, A.K.; Anderson, R.M. An In Vivo Zebrafish Model for Interrogating ROS-Mediated Pancreatic β-Cell Injury, Response, and Prevention. *Oxid. Med. Cell. Long.* **2018**, *2018*, 1324739. [CrossRef] [PubMed]

22. Simon, H.U.; Haj-Yehia, A.; Levi-Schaffer, F. Role of reactive oxygen species (ROS) in apoptosis induction. *Apoptosis* **2000**, *5*, 415–418. [CrossRef] [PubMed]

23. Chen, C.F.; Chu, C.Y.; Chen, T.H.; Lee, S.J.; Shen, C.N.; Ning, C.; Hisiao, C.D. Establishment of a Transgenic Zebrafish Line for Superficial Skin Ablation and Functional Validation of Apoptosis Modulators In Vivo. *PLoS ONE* **2011**, *6*, e20654. [CrossRef] [PubMed]

24. Minkiewicz, P.; Dziuba, J.; Iwaniak, A.; Dziuba, M.; Darewicz, M. BIOPEP database and other programs for processing bioactive peptide sequences. *J. AOAC Int.* **2008**, *91*, 965–980. [CrossRef] [PubMed]

25. Moosman, B.; Behl, C. Secretory peptide hormones are biochemical antioxidants: Structure-activity relationship. *Mol. Pharmacol.* **2002**, *61*, 260–268. [CrossRef]

26. Dong, Z.Y.; Tian, G.; Xu, Z.G.; Li, M.Y.; Zhou, Y.J.; Ren, H. Antioxidant Activities of Peptide Fractions Derived from Freshwater Mussel Protein Using Ultrasound-Assisted Enzymatic Hydrolysis. *Czech J. Food Sci.* **2017**, *35*, 328–338. [CrossRef]

27. Liu, R.; Zheng, W.W.; Li, J.; Wang, L.C.; Wu, H.; Wang, X.Z.; Shi, L. Rapid identification of bioactive peptides with antioxidant activity from the enzymatic hydrolysate of Mactra veneriformis by UHPLC-Q-TOF mass spectrometry. *Food Chem.* **2015**, *167*, 484–489. [CrossRef] [PubMed]

28. Udenigwe, C.C.; Aluko, R.E. Chemometric analysis of the amino acid requirements of antioxidant food protein hydrolysates. *Int. J. Mol. Sci.* **2011**, *12*, 3148–3161. [CrossRef] [PubMed]

29. Dávalos, A.; Miguel, M.; Bartolomé, B.; Lopez-Fandino, R. Antioxidant activity of peptides derived from egg white proteins by enzymatic hydrolysis. *J. Food Protect.* **2004**, *67*, 1939–1944. [CrossRef]

30. Nimalaratne, C.; Bandara, N.; Wu, J.P. Purification and characterization of antioxidant peptides from enzymatically hydrolyzed chicken egg white. *Food Chem.* **2015**, *188*, 467–472. [CrossRef] [PubMed]

31. Soffer, R.L. Angiotensin-converting enzyme and the regulation of vasoactive peptides. *Annu. Rev. Biochem.* **1976**, *45*, 73–94. [CrossRef] [PubMed]

32. Shi, A.M.; Liu, H.Z.; Liu, L.; Hu, H.; Wang, Q.; Adhikari, B. Isolation, Purification and Molecular Mechanism of a Peanut Protein-Derived ACE-Inhibitory Peptide. *PLoS ONE* **2014**, *9*, e111188. [CrossRef] [PubMed]

33. Wilson, J.; Hayes, M.; Carney, B. Angiotensin-I-converting enzyme and prolyl endopeptidase inhibitory peptides from natural sources with a focus on marine processing by-products. *Food Chem.* **2011**, *129*, 235–244. [CrossRef]

34. Segura-Campos, M.R.; Peralta-González, F.; Castellanos-Ruelas, A.; Chel-Guerrero, L.A.; Betancur-Ancona, D.A. Effect of *Jatropha curcas* peptide fractions on the angiotensin I-converting enzyme inhibitory activity. *Biomed. Res. Int.* **2013**, *2013*, 541974. [CrossRef] [PubMed]

35. Murray, B.A.; FitzGerald, R.J. Angiotensin converting enzyme inhibitory peptides derived from food proteins: Biochemistry, bioactivity and production. *Curr. Pharm. Des.* **2007**, *13*, 773–791. [CrossRef] [PubMed]

36. Zhang, C.; Sun, L.C.; Yan, L.J.; Lin, Y.C.; Liu, G.M.; Cao, M.J. Production, optimisation and characterisation of angiotensin converting enzyme inhibitory peptides from sea cucumber (*Stichopus japonicus*) gonad. *Food Funct.* **2018**, *9*, 594–603. [CrossRef] [PubMed]

37. Uraipong, C.; Zhao, J. Rice bran protein hydrolysates exhibit strong in vitro α-amylase, β-glucosidase and ACE-inhibition activities. *J. Sci. Food Agric.* **2016**, *96*, 1101–1110. [CrossRef] [PubMed]

38. Johnson, M.H.; Lucius, A.; Meyer, T.; de Mejia, E.G. Cultivar evaluation and effect of fermentation on antioxidant capacity and in vitro inhibition of a-amylase and a-glucosidase by highbush blueberry (*Vaccinium corombosum*). *J. Agric. Food Chem.* **2011**, *59*, 8923–8930. [CrossRef] [PubMed]

39. Vilcacundo, R.; Martíne-Villaluenga, C.; Hernández-Ledesma, B. Release of dipeptidyl peptidase IV, a-amylase and a-glucosidase inhibitory peptides from quinoa (*Chenopodium quinoa* Willd.) during in vitro simulated gastrointestinal digestion. *J. Funct. Foods* **2017**, *35*, 531–539. [CrossRef]

40. Siow, H.L.; Gan, C.Y. Extraction, identification, and structure-activity relationships of antioxidative and a-amylase inhibitory peptides from cumin seeds (*Cuminum cyminum*). *J. Funct. Foods* **2016**, *22*, 1–12. [CrossRef]

41. Ren, Y.; Liang, K.; Jin, Y.Q.; Zhang, M.M.; Chen, Y.; Wu, H.; Lai, F. Identification and characterization of two novel a-glucosidase inhibitory oligopeptides from hemp (*Cannabis sativa* L.) seed protein. *J. Funct. Foods* **2016**, *26*, 439–450. [CrossRef]

42. Pina, A.S.; Roque, A.C. Studies on the molecular recognition between bioactive peptides and angiotensin-converting enzyme. *J. Mol. Recognit.* **2009**, *22*, 162–168. [CrossRef] [PubMed]

43. Pan, D.D.; Cao, J.X.; Guo, H.Q.; Zhao, B. Studies on purification and the molecular mechanism of a novel ACE inhibitory peptide from whey protein hydrolysate. *Food Chem.* **2012**, *130*, 121–126. [CrossRef]

44. Zhao, Y.H.; Li, B.F.; Liu, Z.Y.; Dong, S.Y.; Zhao, X.; Zeng, M.Y. Antihypertensive effect and purification of an ACE inhibitory peptide from sea cucumber gelatin hydrolysate. *Process Biochem.* **2007**, *42*, 1586–1591. [CrossRef]

45. Deng, Z.Z.; Liu, Y.J.; Wang, J.; Wu, S.H.; Geng, L.H.; Sui, Z.H.; Zhang, Q.B. Antihypertensive Effects of Two Novel Angiotensin I-Converting Enzyme (ACE) Inhibitory Peptides from *Gracilariopsis lemaneiformis* (Rhodophyta) in Spontaneously Hypertensive Rats (SHRs). *Mar. Drugs* **2018**, *16*, 299. [CrossRef] [PubMed]

46. Wu, J.P.; Ding, X.L. Characterization of inhibition and stability of soy-protein derived angiotensin I-converting enzyme inhibitory peptides. *Food Res. Int.* **2002**, *35*, 367–375. [CrossRef]

47. Erak, M.; Bellmann-Sickert, K.; Els-Heindl, S.; Beck-Sickinger, A.G. Peptide chemistry toolbox—Transforming natural peptides into peptides therapeutics. *Bioorg. Med. Chem.* **2018**, *26*, 2759–2765. [CrossRef] [PubMed]

48. AOAC. *Official Methods of Analysis of the Association of Official Analytical Chemists*, 19th ed.; Association of Official Analytical Chemists: Washington, DC, USA, 2005.

49. Chi, C.F.; Hu, F.Y.; Wang, B.; Li, Z.R.; Luo, H.Y. Influence of Amino Acid Compositions and Peptide Profiles on Antioxidant Capacities of Two Protein Hydrolysates from Skipjack Tuna (*Katsuwonus pelamis*) Dark Muscle. *Mar. Drugs* **2015**, *13*, 2580–2601. [CrossRef] [PubMed]

50. Liu, B.; Han, X.D.; Zhang, M.T.; Xu, W.W.; Zhou, W.; Jiao, H. Application AQC as a pre-column derivatization reagent for HPLC determination of free amino acids in *Borojo sorbilis* cuter. *Acta Sci. Nat. Univ. Sunyatseni* **2013**, *52*, 100–104. [CrossRef]

51. Lassoued, I.; Mora, L.; Barkia, A.; Aristory, M.C.; Nasri, M.; Toldráb, F. Bioactive peptides identified in thornback ray skin's gelatin hydrolysates by proteases from *Bacillus subtilis* and *Bacillus amyloliquefaciens*. *J. Proteomic* **2015**, *128*, 8–17. [CrossRef] [PubMed]

52. Lee, J.H.; Moon, S.H.; Kim, H.S.; Park, E.; Ahn, D.; Paik, H.D. Antioxidant and anticancer effects of functional peptides from *Ovotransferrin* hydrolysates. *J. Sci. Food Agric.* **2017**, *97*, 4857–4864. [CrossRef] [PubMed]

53. Moayedi, A.; Mora, L.; Aristoy, M.-C.; Hashemi, M.; Safari, M.; Toldrá, F. ACE inhibitory and antioxidant activities of peptide fragments obtained from tomato processing by-products fermented using Bacillus subtilis: Effect of amino acid composition and peptides molecular mass distribution. *Appl. Biochem. Biotechnol.* **2017**, *181*, 48–64. [CrossRef] [PubMed]

54. Li, Q.G.; Chu, J.; Chen, X.Q.; Wang, J.G.; Wu, X.M.; Liu, K.C. Study on the antioxidant activity evaluation of Jujube(Ziziphus) leaf flavonoids in vitro and zebrafish (*Danio rerio*) with fluorescent skin. *Sci. Technol. Food Ind.* **2014**, *35*, 58–61. [CrossRef]

55. Chen, J.W.; Wang, Y.M.; Zhong, Q.X.; Wu, Y.N.; Xia, W.S. Purification and characterization of a novel angiotensin-I converting enzyme (ACE) inhibitory peptide derived from enzymatic hydrolysate of grass carp protein. *Peptides* **2012**, *33*, 52–58. [CrossRef] [PubMed]

56. Chen, J.D.; Liu, Y.; Wang, G.Y.; Sun, S.S.; Liu, R.; Hong, B.H.; Gao, R.; Bai, K.K. Processing Optimization and Characterization of Angiotensin-I-Converting Enzyme Inhibitory Peptides from Lizardfish (*Synodus macrops*) Scale Gelatin. *Mar. Drugs* **2018**, *16*, 228. [CrossRef] [PubMed]

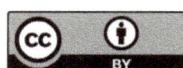

marine drugs

MDPI

Article

Oyster-Derived Zinc-Binding Peptide Modified by Plastein Reaction via Zinc Chelation Promotes the Intestinal Absorption of Zinc

Jianpeng Li [1,†], Chen Gong [1,†], Zaiyang Wang [1], Ruichang Gao [2], Jiaoyan Ren [3], Xiaodong Zhou [4], Haiyan Wang [4], He Xu [5], Feng Xiao [6], Yuhui Cao [1] and Yuanhui Zhao [1,*]

[1] College of Food Science and Engineering, Ocean University of China, Qingdao 266003, China; ljp19881988@126.com (J.L.); 17664076298@163.com (C.G.); wzy13092440827@163.com (Z.W.); caoyuhuijy@126.com (Y.C.)
[2] School of Food and Bioengineering, Jiangsu University, Zhenjiang 212013, China; xiyuan2008@ujs.edu.cn
[3] School of Food Sciences and Engineering, South China University of Technology, Guangzhou 510641, China; renjiaoyanscut@126.com
[4] Hisense (Shandong) Refrigerator Co., Ltd., Qingdao 266100, China; zhouxiaodong@hisense.com (X.Z.); wanghaiyan8@hisense.com (H.W.)
[5] Jiangsu Baoyuan Biotechnology Co., Ltd., Lianyungang 222100, China; xuhe-2001@sohu.com
[6] College of Food and Bioengineering, Henan University of Science and Technology, Luoyang 471023, China; xfeng@haust.edu.cn
*   Correspondence: zhaoyuanhui@ouc.edu.cn; Tel.: +86-532-8203-2400
†   These authors contributed equally to this study.

Received: 13 May 2019; Accepted: 5 June 2019; Published: 8 June 2019

Abstract: Zinc-binding peptides from oyster (*Crassostrea gigas*) have potential effects on zinc supplementation. The aim of this study was to prepare efficient zinc-binding peptides from oyster-modified hydrolysates by adding exogenous glutamate according to the plastein reaction and to further explore the zinc absorption mechanism of the peptide-zinc complex (MZ). The optimum conditions for the plastein reaction were as follows: pH 5.0, 40 °C, substrate concentration of 40%, pepsin dosage of 500 U/g, reaction time of 3 h and L-[1-^{13}C]glutamate concentration of 10 mg/mL. The results of ^{13}C isotope labelling suggested that the addition of L-[1-^{13}C]glutamate contributed to the increase in the zinc-binding capacity of the peptide. The hydrophobic interaction was the main mechanism of action of the plastein reaction. Ultraviolet spectra and scanning electronic microscopy (SEM) revealed that the zinc-binding peptide could bind with zinc and form MZ. Furthermore, MZ could significantly enhance zinc bioavailability in the presence of phytic acid, compared to the commonly used ZnSO$_4$. Additionally, MZ significantly promoted the intestinal absorption of zinc mainly through two pathways, the zinc ion channel and the small peptide transport pathway. Our work attempted to increase the understanding of the zinc absorption mechanism of MZ and to support the potential application of MZ as a supplementary medicine.

Keywords: oyster zinc-binding peptide; peptide-zinc complex; caco-2 cells; intestinal absorption; zinc bioavailability

---

1. Introduction

Zinc, as an essential micronutrient, is essential for human health and participates in numerous enzymatic and metabolic processes in human organisms [1]. The human body mass contains 2–3 g of zinc [2]. In the human body, zinc deficiency usually leads to serious consequences, such as growth defects, hypogonadism, and neurological dysfunctions [3]. As of 2012, zinc deficiency is estimated to affect up to two billion people worldwide [4], which represents a significant global burden. Thus, it is necessary to improve zinc bioavailability and absorption for optimum health. The fortification of food by adding zinc salts or zinc-chelating peptides has promise as an intervention strategy. However, the most commonly used $ZnSO_4$ could irritate the gastrointestinal mucosa and is not safe for long-term intake [5]. In addition, the efficacies of mineral supplements are strongly blocked by mineral absorption inhibitors (such as phytic acid) in daily diets [6]. Thus, searching for both effective and safe components from seafood sources as alternatives to prevent zinc deficiency is a research area with urgent need worldwide.

Oyster (*Crassostrea gigas*), a member of the ostreidae family [7], is a good source of proteins, essential fatty acids, and other nutrients [8]. Many studies have shown that oyster, mainly oyster peptides, has remarkable pharmacological efficacies, including antimicrobial, antihypertensive, anticancer, antioxidant, and antiviral abilities [9–12]. Oysters are usually richer in zinc elements than other seafoods, and zinc is easily combined with proteins or amino acids in oyster soft tissue [13]. The zinc-chelating peptides extracted from oyster have attracted wide attention. Work by Chen et al. demonstrated that the peptide (HLRQEEKEEVTVGSLK) produced from oyster protein hydrolysis has a marked ability to bind zinc [14], and Zhang et al. revealed that the hydrolysate-zinc complex (OPH-Zn) can improve zinc bioaccessibility [15]. However, the zinc absorption mechanism of the oyster-derived peptide-zinc complex has not been fully studied. Thus, exploring the effect of the peptide-zinc complex on zinc supplementation and improving our understanding of the mechanism involved may advance the understanding of oyster peptides as zinc supplementation agents.

Recently, it has been reported that zinc-binding peptides can be obtained from oyster protein hydrolysates by a facile plastein reaction [16]. The plastein reaction was first discovered by Danilevski in 1902 when he added chymotrypsin to protein hydrolysates, and this reaction is considered to be a reverse enzymatic reaction [17]. Under normal conditions, bioactive peptides remain inactive in the sequence of their parent proteins. However, with appropriate enzymatic hydrolysis, the peptides can be released and activated. The plastein reactions provided a possible method to synthesize a multifunctional peptide-based ingredient with desirable bioavailability, safety, and functional properties [18]. However, due to the complexity of the reaction, the mechanism of plastein reactions remains unclear and is still an intellectual curiosity.

In the present study, the efficient zinc-binding peptides were prepared from oyster-modified hydrolysates according to the plastein reaction and the mechanism of the plastein reaction was explored. Then the peptide-zinc complex (MZ) was prepared and characterized. The zinc bioavailability of MZ in the presence of phytic acid was investigated in Caco-2 cells. Subsequently, a possible zinc absorption mechanism of MZ in Caco-2 cells was further explored. This work could provide new information for the potential application of oyster protein-based zinc supplements.

2. Results and Discussion

2.1. Optimization of the Plastein Reaction Conditions

The synthetic reaction dominated the plastein reaction and it inevitably led to a decrease in the free amino acids in the reaction system [17,19]. To improve the efficiency of the plastein reaction, the effects of hydrolysis pH, temperature, substrate concentration, pepsin dosage, reaction time, and glutamate concentration on the decrease in the free amino acid content of the plastein products were optimized in the present study.

The effect of pH on free amino acid reduction was significant, as shown in Figure 1A. With an increase in pH, the reduction of free amino acid presented an upward trend, reaching a maximum value at pH 5.0, and then presented a downward trend at a higher pH. pH can affect the binding efficiency of enzyme molecules and substrates [20]. The suitable pH of pepsin used in this study ranged from 1.5 to 5.5 [21]. Therefore, the optimal hydrolysis pH was 5.0. The free amino acid reduction gradually increased from 20 to 40 °C, and the maximum value was reached at 40 °C (Figure 1B). The possible reason for this finding is that pepsin was gradually activated as the temperature of the enzymatic hydrolysis increased, and the structure of the enzyme protein was affected when the temperature exceeded the optimum temperature. Therefore, the optimal temperature was determined to be 40 °C. Figure 1C shows that when the substrate concentration increased from 25% to 40%, the free amino acid reduction gradually increased, reaching a maximum value at 25 μmol/g. Therefore, the optimal substrate concentration was determined to be 40%. Figure 1D shows that when the pepsin dosage increased from 100 U/g to 500 U/g, the free amino acid reduction gradually increased, which probably meant that the enzyme binding sites were completely occupied by the substrate. With an increase in the reaction time, the free amino acid reduction increased to a maximum value at 3 h (Figure 1E). Therefore, 3 h was selected as the appropriate holding time. The effect of the glutamate concentration on the free amino acid reduction was significant, as shown in Figure 1F, and the optimal glutamate concentration was determined to be 10 mg/mL. The addition of exogenous glutamate during the plastein reaction can effectively increase the efficiency of the plastein reaction.

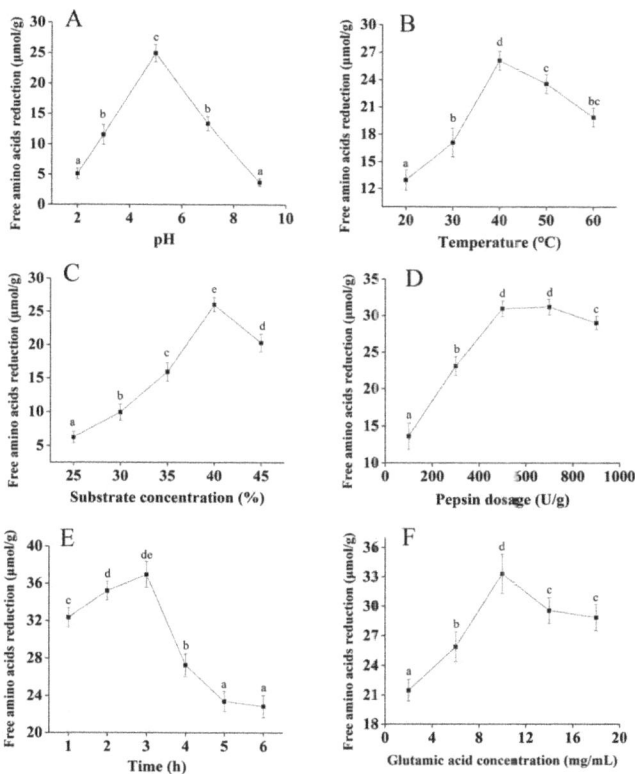

Figure 1. Effects of hydrolysis pH (**A**), temperature (**B**), substrate concentration (**C**), pepsin dosage (**D**), reaction time (**E**), and glutamate concentration (**F**) on free amino acids reduction of the plastein products. Unless otherwise noted, temperate was 40 °C, pH was 5.0, substrate concentration was 40%, pepsin dosage was 500 U/g, reaction time was 3 h, and L-[1-^{13}C]glutamate concentration was 10 mg/mL. Each point is shown as the means ± standard deviation (SD) ($n = 3$). Different letters indicate significant differences ($p < 0.05$).

Overall, the optimum conditions for the free amino acid reduction of the plastein products were obtained at: pH 5.0, 40 °C, substrate concentration of 40%, pepsin dosage of 500 U/g, reaction time of 3 h, and glutamate concentration of 10 mg/mL.

2.2. Change in Zinc-Binding Capacity and Hydrophobicity during the Plastein Reaction

As shown in Figure 2A, the hydrophobicity index of the plastein products steadily increased over 3 h, attaining a maximum of 33.9%. Our results are consistent with those of Jiang et al. [19], who reported that the internal hydrophobic amino acids were exposed during the plastein reaction, indicating that hydrophobic interactions are important forces in the formation of plastein products. Similarly, the zinc-binding capacity of the plastein products continuously increased for 3 h (Figure 2B). This result is consistent with that of Chen et al. [14]. The possible reason for this finding was that the hydrophilic groups (−OH, −NH$_2$, −COOH) were exposed during the reaction, which provided additional binding sites for the zinc ions. In addition, the added exogenous glutamate increased the −COOH content and thus led to an increase in the binding capacity of zinc ions.

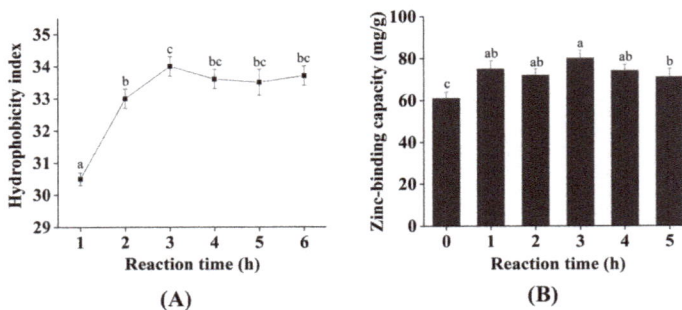

Figure 2. Change in hydrophobicity (**A**) and zinc-binding capacity (**B**) during the plastein reaction. Each point is shown as the means ± SD ($n = 3$). Different letters indicate significant differences ($p < 0.05$).

2.3. The Effects of Protein Denaturants on the Stability of Plastein Products

As shown in Figure 3A, the solubility of the plastein products in the deionized water (DW) and sodium chloride (NaCl) groups was significantly lower than in the hydrolysis products ($p < 0.05$), suggesting that the hydrophobicity of the plastein products was high. Sodium dodecyl sulfate (SDS) and acetic acid (HAc) can destroy the protein structures that are maintained by hydrophobic interactions and then dissolve the plastein products [22]. The solubility of the plastein products in the HAc and SDS groups was significantly higher than the solubility of the hydrolysis products ($p < 0.05$) (Figure 3A), suggesting that the hydrophobic interactions may be primarily responsible for the formation of plastein products, which was consistent with the conclusion of Figure 2A. In addition, high molecular weight proteins have low solubility in trichloroacetic acid (TCA) [23]. The solubility of the plastein products in the TCA group was significantly lower than that of the hydrolysis products ($p < 0.05$) (Figure 3A), suggesting that the plastein products had a higher molecular weight than the hydrolysis products. Urea is a polar molecule that can destroy hydrogen bonds in the protein [24]. As shown in Figure 3B, urea had a significant effect on the turbidity value of the plastein products ($p < 0.05$), which suggested that hydrogen bonds may be partially responsible for the formation of plastein products.

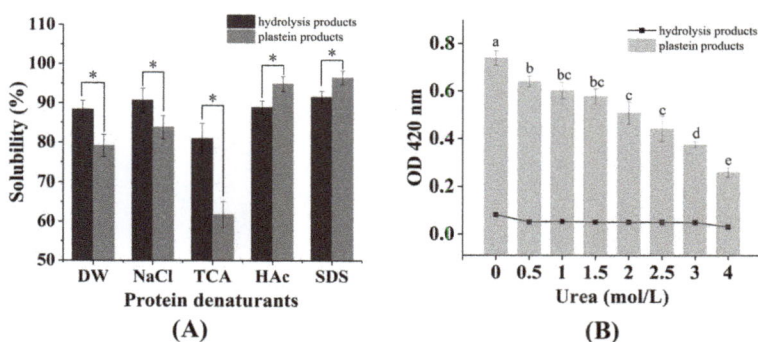

Figure 3. (**A**) Solubility of plastein products in different denaturants; (**B**) effect of urea on the stability of plastein products. Abbreviations: DW, deionized water; NaCl, sodium chloride; TCA, trichloroacetic acid; HAc, acetic acid; SDS, sodium dodecyl sulfate. Each point is shown as the means ± SD ($n = 3$). Asterisk (*) and different letters indicate significant differences ($p < 0.05$).

2.4. Change in Molecular Weight Distribution during the Plastein Reaction

As shown in Figure 4, after the plastein reaction, the content of plastein products with a molecular weight greater than 1000 Da significantly increased, while the content of plastein products with a molecular weight less than 300 Da significantly decreased ($p < 0.05$), indicating that the small molecular weight glutamate and polypeptide were bound to other polypeptide chains by transpeptidation and condensation reactions, thus increasing the percentage of macromolecular polypeptides.

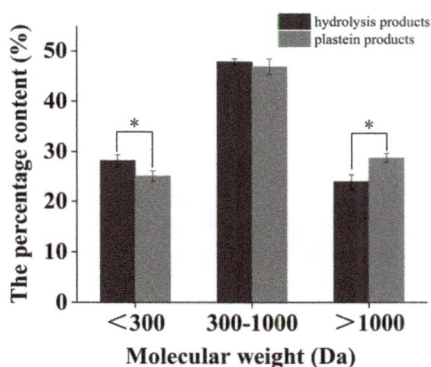

Figure 4. The change of molecular weight distribution during plastein reaction. Each point is shown as the means ± SD ($n = 3$). Asterisk (*) indicate significant differences ($p < 0.05$).

Combined with the above experimental results, it could be demonstrated that the hydrophobic interaction was the main mechanism of action of the plastein reaction and there was also a relatively weak condensation and transpeptidation reaction.

2.5. Zinc-Binding Capacity and L-[1-^{13}C]Glutamate Abundance of Different Components of Plastein Products

The conjugated double bond in the peptides and phenylalanine has an ultraviolet characteristic absorption peak at 220 nm. An aqueous solution of phenylalanine showed an absorption peak between 1.1 and 1.4 h (Figure 5A), indicating that most of the free amino acids eluted with the mobile phase mainly after 1.1 h. The fractions a–d were obtained at 220 nm (Figure 5B). Afterwards, these components were collected to determine the zinc-binding capacity and L-[1-^{13}C]glutamate abundance. The higher the L-[1-^{13}C]glutamate abundance was, the higher the ratio of ^{13}C/^{12}C in the sample. The zinc-binding capacity of a and b components was significantly higher than that of c and d components, meanwhile the L-[1-^{13}C]glutamate abundance of a and b was also significantly higher than that of c and d ($p < 0.05$) (Table 1), suggesting that the addition of exogenous L-[1-^{13}C]glutamate contributed to an increase in the zinc-binding capacity of the peptides.

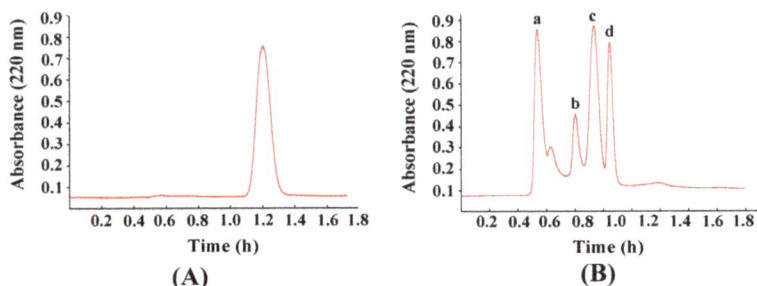

Figure 5. Sephadex G-15 chromatograph of phenylalanine standard (**A**) and different components of plastein products (**B**), a–d mean the fractions that obtained at 220 nm.

Table 1. Zinc-binding capacity and L-[1-^{13}C]glutamate abundance of different components of plastein products. The control group is the plastein products without exogenous L-[1-^{13}C]glutamate added. The different letters indicate significant differences ($p < 0.05$).

Sample Name	Zinc-Binding Capacity (mg/g)	L-[1-^{13}C]glutamate Abundance (‰)
Control	69.12 ± 1.54 [c]	−21.87
a	94.43 ± 2.07 [b]	255.73
b	101.08 ± 3.10 [a]	1108.22
c	72.21 ± 2.68 [c]	7.16
d	26.54 ± 1.43 [d]	−4.54

In addition, the zinc-binding capacity of the d component was significantly lower than that of the b component ($p < 0.05$), which may be related to the molecular weight and spatial structure of the polypeptides. Some macromolecular peptides were aggregated into hydrophobic macromolecular peptides by hydrophobic interactions during the plastein reaction, thereby resulting in the change of structure of the polypeptides and the reduction of binding sites for the zinc ions.

2.6. Scanning electron microscopy (SEM) Photograph and UV-Vis Absorption of the peptide-zinc complex (MZ)

In our previous study, the peptide Glu-Val-Pro-Pro-Glu-Glu-His (M) with high zinc-binding capacity was isolated and purified [16], and we further prepared the MZ in this study. The peptide M showed a sheet appearance with a smooth surface (Figure 6A,C). In contrast, MZ demonstrated a granule-like structure, which was markedly different from the peptide M image (Figure 6B,D). Metal ions can interact with peptides and facilitate peptide aggregation [25]. Zhang et al. [15] reported that zinc ions can promote aggregation by increasing the speed of the dimerization of the peptides. In addition, the carbonyl oxygen and hydroxyl oxygen on the carboxyl group in the peptide chain are involved in the coordination of zinc ions [16], thus promoting the formation of aggregates. The SEM results suggest that the interaction between the peptide and zinc ions could lead to the formation of particles.

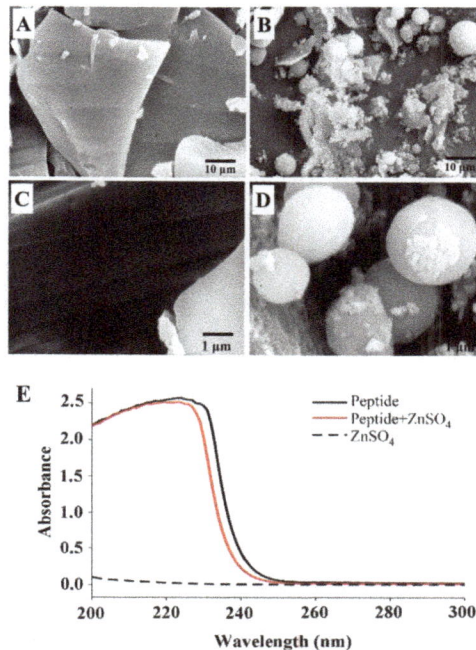

Figure 6. Scanning electron microscopy (SEM) photograph of peptide (**A**,**C**) and peptide-zinc complex (MZ) (**B**,**D**), UV-vis absorption analysis (**E**).

The peptide M had a maximum absorption peak at 223 nm, while the mixture of zinc-binding peptide and $ZnSO_4$ had the maximum absorption peak shifted to 220 nm (Figure 6E). Previous studies have indicated that the addition of zinc ions affected the spatial structure of the peptide [14], thus inducing hypochromicity in the UV absorption spectrum. From these results, it could be concluded that the peptide M could bind with zinc and form the MZ.

2.7. Cytotoxicity of MZ Against Caco-2 Cells

The MZ exhibited no significant cytotoxicity in Caco-2 cells at a concentration of 125 µg/mL or less, however, MZ significantly reduced the viability of Caco-2 cells at concentrations over 125 µg/mL ($p < 0.05$) (Figure 7A). Therefore, subsequent absorption and transport experiments were conducted at a dose of 125 µg/mL.

2.8. Absorption of Zinc from MZ in Caco-2 Cells

Caco-2 cells are similar to intestinal epithelial cells in structure and function, so they are commonly used to simulate the absorption characteristics of intestinal epithelial cells in vitro [26]. Usually, exogenous zinc enters the cellular zinc pool [27]. N,N,N',N'-tetrakis (2-pyridylmethyl)-ethylene-diamine (TPEN), a zinc ion chelator, has frequently been used to consume the initial free zinc in cells [28], and then the Zinquin ethyl ester fluorescent probe is usually used to monitor cellular zinc uptake in real time [29]. As shown in Figure 7B, zinc uptake from $ZnSO_4$ and MZ, at concentrations equivalent to 96 µM zinc, was monitored by the quenching of Zinquin ethyl ester fluorescence. Cellular zinc uptake from $ZnSO_4$ was significantly increased (by 36%), whereas zinc uptake from MZ was only partially increased (by 11%). The reason for this result may be that less free zinc within a certain time was dissociated by MZ than by $ZnSO_4$. In addition, work by Tacnet demonstrated that organic zinc absorption is dependent on a variety of membrane transport mechanisms in pig small intestine [30], including mainly unsaturated diffusion and saturable carrier-mediated mechanisms. Thus, we speculated that the zinc absorption mechanisms of $ZnSO_4$ and MZ were different.

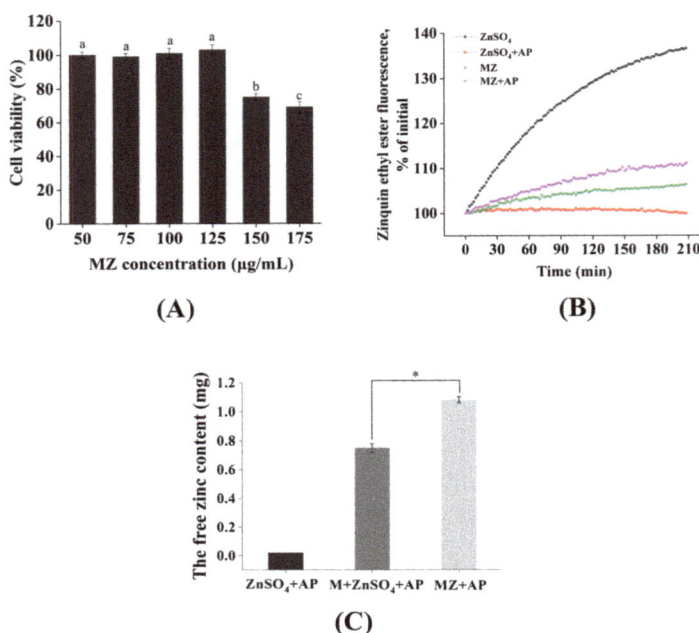

Figure 7. (**A**) Cell viability of Caco-2 cells after being incubated with the MZ at different concentrations. (**B**) Zinc uptake by Caco-2 cell monolayers in the presence of 2:1 molar ratio of zinc/phytic acid. Cellular uptake of exogenous zinc was measured as the quenching of Zinquin ethyl ester fluorescence. (**C**) The free zinc content after phytic acid treatment. M: peptide (EVPPEEH); MZ: peptide-zinc complex; AP: phytic acid. Different lowercase letters and asterisk (*) indicates significant difference between groups ($p < 0.05$).

2.9. The Effect of Phytic Acid on Zinc Bioavailability

Our daily staple foods, such as rice, corn, and cereals, generally contain phytic acid [31], and the phosphate groups of phytic acid can form insoluble complexes with zinc [32], which can significantly affect the absorption and utilization of zinc in the gastrointestinal tract [31]. Therefore, to assess the bioavailability of zinc from MZ, it is necessary to understand the absorption and utilization of zinc in the presence of phytic acid. As shown in Figure 7B, zinc uptake from $ZnSO_4$ and MZ in the presence of a 2:1 molar ratio of zinc/phytic acid was monitored by the quenching of Zinquin ethyl ester fluorescence. The cellular uptake of zinc from $ZnSO_4$ was barely increased, indicating that the absorption of zinc from $ZnSO_4$ was almost completely inhibited by phytic acid. Moreover, the zinc uptake from MZ decreased from 11% (without phytic acid treatment) to 6%, indicating that phytic acid incompletely blocked the zinc uptake from MZ. In other words, MZ showed a certain anti-phytic acid complexation, which reduced the negative effect of phytic acid on zinc absorption.

The free zinc contents of each group after phytic acid treatment are shown in Figure 7C. The free zinc content in the MZ group was significantly higher than that in the $ZnSO_4$ group and in the mixed system of M and $ZnSO_4$ ($p < 0.05$), indicating that the effect of the MZ was more significant against the anti-phytic acid complexation than that of the peptide M. This result is similar to the results of Hansen et al. [33], who reported that a certain amount of casein phosphopeptides (CPP) could overcome the inhibitory effect of phytate on zinc absorption. In addition, Zhu et al. also found that the chelation of zinc with peptides derived from wheat germ protein possessed higher zinc bioavailability than $ZnSO_4$ in Caco-2 cells [34]. Finally, the results revealed that some zinc ions could be "protected" after the combination of peptide M and zinc to avoid the inhibition of zinc absorption by dietary interactions, thereby improving the effective bioavailability of zinc.

2.10. Effect of MZ on hZIP4 and ZnT1 mRNA Levels in Caco-2 Cells

The zinc regulatory protein hZIP4 and the zinc transporter ZnT1 play an important role in maintaining cellular zinc homeostasis [35]. hZIP4 is a member of the ZIP family, mainly located in the apical membrane of small intestinal cells and is mainly used to regulate dietary zinc intake [36]. ZnT1 was the first zinc transporter found in the ZnT family and is mainly located on the basement membrane of intestinal epithelial cells, its main function is to transport zinc out of the cell [35]. As shown in Figure 8A, the hZIP4 level of both the $ZnSO_4$ and MZ groups was significantly reduced compared with that of the control group, while there was no significant difference between the $ZnSO_4$ and MZ groups. The expression of hZIP4 is regulated by intracellular zinc levels, and when the amount of exogenous zinc is sufficient, the cells will reduce the uptake of zinc, which may result in a decrease in hZIP4 expression [36]. Our results indicated that both $ZnSO_4$ and MZ at concentrations equivalent to 96 µM zinc can meet the zinc demand of Caco-2 cells. In addition, the levels of ZnT1 were significantly upregulated in both the $ZnSO_4$ and MZ groups compared with the control group, and the levels of ZnT1 were also significantly increased in the MZ group compared with the control group ($p < 0.05$) (Figure 8B), indicating that MZ is more fully absorbed than ZnSO4 by Caco-2 cells. Overall, it can be seen that cells will not only reduce the intake of zinc but also increase the export of zinc through the zinc ion channel pathway when there is a sufficient supply of exogenous zinc, representing a feedback regulation mechanism for the organism to adapt to changes in external zinc levels.

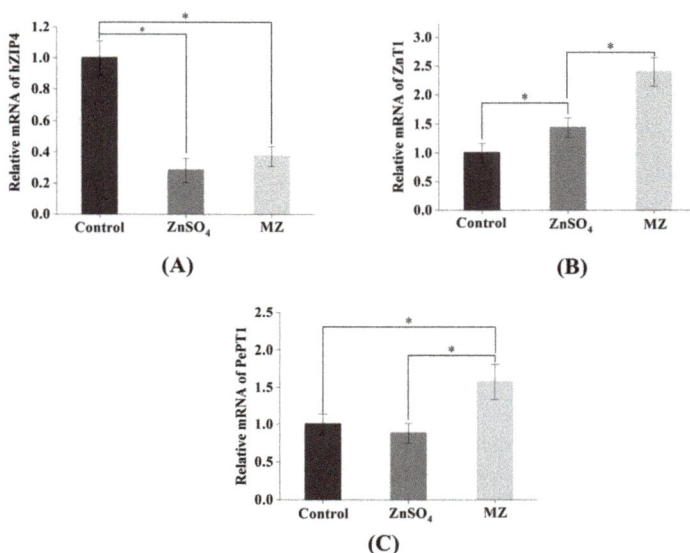

Figure 8. Effects of MZ on the relative level of hZIP4, ZnT1, and PepT1 mRNA in Caco-2 cells. MZ = peptide-zinc complex. Asterisk (*) indicates significant difference between groups ($p < 0.05$).

2.11. Effect of MZ on PePT1 mRNA Levels in Caco-2 Cells

PePT-1 is a member of the oligopeptide transporter family, and its major expression site is on the brush border membrane of intestinal epithelial cells [37]. Maubon et al. found that the expression of PePT1 in Caco-2 cells and small intestinal epithelial cells were quite similar [38]. As shown in Figure 8C, the levels of PePT1 were significantly increased in the MZ group compared with the control and $ZnSO_4$ groups ($p < 0.05$), while there was no significant difference between the $ZnSO_4$ and control groups, suggesting that MZ promoted the expression of PePT1 in Caco-2 cells. Tacnet et al. demonstrated that organic zinc can be absorbed either by the regulation of zinc transporters or by the absorption mechanisms of small peptides or amino acids [30]. Therefore, it is speculated that MZ may be absorbed and utilized by cells through the small peptide transport system.

Based on the above results, we can conclude that the intestinal absorption of MZ may occur mainly through two pathways: the zinc ion channel and the small peptide transport pathway. For the zinc ion channel pathway, MZ promotes the activation of ZnT1 and inhibits the activation of hZIP4, which consequently maintains cellular zinc homeostasis. For the small peptide transport pathway, MZ promotes the activation of PePT1, leading to the promotion of zinc absorption from MZ. The two pathways finally result in the promotion of zinc absorption from MZ (Figure 9).

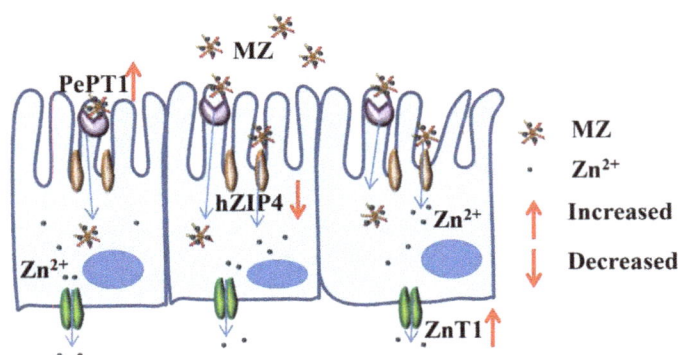

Figure 9. Possible mechanisms of MZ promotes zinc absorption of Caco-2 cells.

3. Materials and Methods

3.1. Materials and Chemicals

Oyster (*Crassostrea gigas*) was obtained from a local market (Qingdao, China). N,N,N',N'-tetrakis (2-pyridylmethyl)-ethylene-diamine (TPEN) and methyl-thiazolyl-diphenyl-tetrazolium bromide (MTT) were obtained from Sigma Chemical Ltd. (St. Louis, MO, USA). Zinquin ethyl ester was purchased from AAT Bioquest Ltd. (Sunnyvale, CA, USA). Dulbecco's modified Eagle's medium (DMEM), N-2-hydroxyethylpiperazine-N-ethane-sulfonicacid (HEPES), Foetal bovine serum (FBS), TrypLE TM Express cell dissociation reagent, Hank's balanced salt solution (HBSS), and Dulbecco's phosphate-buffered saline (DPBS) were procured from Thermo Fisher Ltd. (Waltham, MA, USA). All other reagents used in this study were of analytical grade.

Caco-2 cells preserved in our laboratory [26] were grown in 4.5 g/L of DMEM supplemented with 4 mM glutamine, 25 mM HEPES, 1 mM sodium pyruvate, 10% FBS, and 1% penicillin-streptomycin mixture at 37 °C in a constant temperature incubator containing 5% CO_2.

3.2. Oyster Hydrolysate Preparation

The oyster hydrolysates were prepared in accordance with the method of Chen et al. [14]. Briefly, oyster meat was first homogenized and boiled for 10 min. After cooling, the pH was adjusted to 2.0 with 1 mol/L HCl, pepsin (2500 U/g protein) was added, and the homogenate was digested in a 37 °C water bath for 2.5 h. Afterwards, the pepsin was inactivated at 100 °C for 10 min. Then, the suspension was centrifuged at 6000 r/min for 15 min, after which the supernatant was passed through a 0.45 μm microporous membrane and then desalted by a Chelax-100 exchange resin chromatography column. The obtained hydrolysate products were freeze-dried and stored for further use.

3.3. Modification of Oyster Hydrolysates by Plastein Reaction

The plastein reaction conditions were as follows: exogenous L-[1-^{13}C]glutamate concentration of 2–18 mg/mL; substrate (hydrolysates products) concentration of 25%–45% (w/v); temperature of 20–60 °C; pepsin dosage of 100–900 U/g protein; pH of 2–9; and reaction time of 1–6 h. The free amino acid reduction during the plastein reaction was used as an indicator to optimize the plastein reaction conditions. Afterwards, the plastein products were boiled at 90 °C for 15 min to inactivate the pepsin. Then, the plastein products were further eluted by a Sephadex G-15 gel column (2.6 cm × 65 cm). The absorbance was measured at 220 nm using a UV-2550 spectrophotometer (Shimadzu, Japan), and the components were collected before the peak of 50 mg/mL phenylalanine (as a standard). The obtained components were freeze-dried and stored for further use.

3.4. Free Amino Acids Determination

The free amino acids were detected based on the *O*-phthaldialdehyde (OPA) method [19]. Briefly, 100 μL of oyster plastein products was added to 2 mL of OPA reagent (40 mg/mL). After 2 min of reaction, the absorbance of the resultant solution was measured at 340 nm. Glutamate was used as the standard, and the standard curve was calculated as follows:

$$Y = 0.186X - 0.005 \ (R^2 = 0.997)$$

X indicates the concentration of free amino acids, and Y indicates the absorption value.

3.5. Zinc-Binding Capacity Determination

Ten milligrams of prepared products were dissolved in 5 mL of water, followed by the addition of 5 mL of ammonium chloride buffer, pH 10.0. Then, the chrome black T indicator was added, and ethylenediaminetetraacetate (EDTANa$_2$) was used as a titration solution to determine blue coloration. Afterwards, the consumed EDTANa$_2$ volume was recorded. In addition, the soluble protein content of the plastein products was detected by the Folin-phenol method [39]. The calculation formula was as follows [40]:

$$\text{zinc-binding capacity } (\%) = mV/W$$

where, m (mg/mL) is the zinc mass corresponding to 1 mL of consumed EDTANa$_2$ (0.05 mol/L), V (mL) is the volume of consumed EDTANa$_2$, and W (g) is the soluble protein content of the plastein products.

3.6. Hydrophobic Changes during the Plastein Reaction

The hydrophobic changes were determined by the ANS fluorescence probe method [41]. The plastein products were first dissolved in 0.01 M sodium phosphate buffer to obtain the different concentrations of protein and subsequently, 10 μL ANS was added. The fluorescence intensity was measured at an excitation wavelength of 375 nm and an emission wavelength of 440 nm. The hydrophobicity index was determined by the initial slope of the protein concentration versus fluorescence intensity.

3.7. Effects of Protein Denaturants on Plastein Products

Five hundred milligrams of hydrolysis products and plastein products were dissolved separately in 35 mL ddH$_2$O, 10 mM sodium phosphate buffer, pH 6.0, 10% (v/v) trichloroacetate (TCA), 50% (v/v) acetic acid, and 0.3 M sodium lauryl sulfate (SDS). After a 30 min reaction, the solutions were centrifuged to obtain the supernatant. Afterwards, the protein contents of the supernatant, hydrolysis products and plastein products were determined by the Kjeldahl method according to Hartnett et al. [42].

Protein solubility was expressed as the protein content of the supernatant versus the original products. In addition, the effect of urea on the plastein products was determined as follows: the hydrolysis and plastein products were dissolved in different concentrations of urea (0, 1, 1.5, 2, 2.5, 3, and 4 mol/L), and the corresponding absorbance was measured at 420 nm by a TU-1810 spectrophotometer (Beijing, China).

3.8. Change in the Molecular Weight Distribution Profile

The molecular weight distribution of plastein products was determined by a TSK-Gel 2000 SWXL column (7.8 × 300 mm, Agilent Technologies, Santa Clara, CA, USA) equipped with an ultraviolet detector (LC-20AT, Shimadzu Corp., Tokyo, Japan) system at a flow rate of 0.5 mL/min for 30 min. Acetonitrile, ddH$_2$O and trifluoroacetic acid (*v/v/v*: 45/55/0.1) were used as mobile phases, and the column temperature was 30 °C. Tyrosine (182 Da), glutathione (307 Da), bacitracin (1423 Da), insulin (5733 Da), and cytochrome C (12590 Da) were used as standards. The equation of the standard curve was as follows: Log (Mw) = −0.2249t + 6.6846 (R^2 = 0.9707), where Mw is the molecular weight, and t is the retention time.

3.9. Determination of the Abundance of ʟ-[1-^{13}C]Glutamate

The samples were wrapped in foil and then placed on a burner (1150 °C) of the elemental analyser set to full combustion. Afterwards, the produced gases were placed in a reduction furnace (810 °C) to remove excess oxygen and reduce the nitrogen oxides to N$_2$. Then, a gas chromatographic column was used to purify the gas, and the samples were subsequently placed in the isotope mass spectrometer to determine the ʟ-[1-^{13}C]glutamate abundance of the samples.

3.10. Characterization of the MZ

3.10.1. Preparation of the MZ

The oyster peptide Glu-Val-Pro-Pro-Glu-Glu-His (M) that was isolated and purified in our previous study [16] was dissolved in aqueous ZnSO$_4$ solution, and the mass ratio of the peptide and ZnSO$_4$ was 3:1. Then, the mixture was reacted at 40 °C for 30 min. The solution was filtered by 0.22 μm Millipore filters. Afterwards, anhydrous ethanol was added and centrifuged at 8000 r/min for 10 min to obtain the complex. The MZ was freeze-dried and stored for further use.

3.10.2. UV-Visible

The zinc-binding peptide and MZ were dissolved in ddH$_2$O and filtered through 0.22 μm Millipore filters. The absorption spectra were recorded in the 200–400 nm region with a UV-2550 spectrophotometer (Shimadzu, Japan). ddH$_2$O was used as a reference.

3.10.3. Morphology Analysis

The morphology of the MZ was observed by scanning electronic microscopy (SEM). The lyophilized MZ powder was spread on a glass slide and sputter-coated with gold (JEOL JFC-1200 fine coater, Tokyo, Japan). The SEM was used to observe the film at 15 kV.

3.11. Cytotoxicity of the MZ against Caco-2 Cells

The procedure to construct an in vitro intestinal cell model was performed according to the method described by Zou et al. [43], with some modifications. Briefly, after the fusion degree of Caco-2 cells reached approximately 80%, the growth medium was removed, and the cell monolayers were washed twice with DPBS. Then, the TrypLE TM Express cell dissociation reagent was added to each well. After 7 min of digestion, high-glucose DMEM medium was proportionally gently added with liquid transfer. The suspension was transferred into a 15 mL sterile centrifuge tube for centrifuging, and the supernatant was discarded. The pellet was diluted with high-glucose DMEM medium to prepare a single-cell suspension. Cells were seeded at a density of 1×10^5 cells/well in collagen-coated 24-well plates (BD Biosciences, San Joes, CA, USA). After reaching confluence, the cells were allowed to differentiate in high-glucose DMEM medium for another 10 d, and an in vitro intestinal cell model was obtained.

Cell viability was measured according to the method described by Zou et al. with some modifications [43]. Cells were seeded at a density of 1×10^4 cells/well in collagen-coated 96-well plates incubated for 24 h in a thermostat incubator with a humid atmosphere containing 5% CO_2 at 37 °C. After the medium was removed, 200 µL of the samples at different concentrations were added to each well, and 8–10 parallel wells were prepared for each sample. After 20 h of incubation in a CO_2 incubator at 37 °C, 20 µL of MTT (5 mg/mL) was added to each well. The precipitate was removed by centrifugation after 4 h of incubation. Then, 150 µL of DMSO was added to each well, and the cell culture plate was shaken at low speed for 10 min. The absorbance was measured with a microplate reader at 570 nm. The relative viability of cells (IC) was calculated according to the method of Duan et al. [44]. IC was calculated as follows: IC (%) = (OD sample group − OD blank)/(OD control group − OD blank) × 100%.

3.12. Zinc Absorption Assay in Caco-2 Cells

The zinc absorption experiment was based on the method of Wu et al. and Makhov et al., with some modifications [45,46]. The caco-2 cell medium was first removed, and 10 µM of TPEN was added for a 2 h treatment to consume intracellular zinc reserves after the cells were washed with HBSS 3 times. Then, the supernatant was discarded, the cell sedimentation was washed with HBSS 3 times again, 500 µL of HBSS solution containing 20 µM Zinquin ethyl ester was added, and the samples were incubated for 30 min in a CO_2 thermostat incubator at 37 °C. The supernatant was then discarded, the sample was dissolved in HBSS, and 1 mL of oyster source MZ or $ZnSO_4$ solution was added (the different sample solutions ensured a zinc content of 96 µM). The cell culture plate was immediately placed in a fluorescence microplate reader with Zinquin ethyl ester fluorescence detected every 3 min (360 nm excitation, 480 nm emission).

The effect of phytic acid on zinc absorption was performed according to the method of Sreenivasulu et al., with some modifications [47]. Phytic acid was dissolved in HBSS to prepare a 96 µM stock solution. The phytic acid reserve solution was diluted to 48 µM in MZ and $ZnSO_4$ solutions containing 96 µM Zn^{2+}, such that the molar ratio of Zn^{2+} to phytic acid was 2:1. The mixed samples were placed in a 37 °C incubator and incubated for 1 h. Then, 1 mL of the mixture was added to the differentiated Caco-2 cells. The cell culture plate was immediately placed in a fluorescence microplate reader with Zinquin ethyl ester fluorescence detected every 3 min (360 nm excitation, 480 nm emission). In addition, in vitro experiment, the MZ and $ZnSO_4$ were dissolved in ddH_2O, respectively, then the phytic acid was added to reach a 2:1 molar ratio of Zn^{2+} to phytic acid. The mixed samples were placed in a 37 °C incubator and incubated for 30 min. Then, the precipitate was removed by centrifugation. The zinc content in the supernatant was determined by an atomic absorption spectrophotometer.

3.13. Effect of MZ on hZIP4, PepT-1 and ZnT1 mRNA Levels in Caco-2 Cells

The expression of mRNA was detected according to the methods of Li et al. [48]. Total RNA was extracted as previously described [49]. The primers were designed using Premier 5.0 software (Premier Biosoft International, Palo Alto, CA, USA) (Table 2). RT-qPCR amplifications were performed with 3 biological replicates using a Bio-Rad CFX Connect System (BioRad Laboratories, Inc., San Diego, CA, USA). The housekeeping gene β-actin was chosen to normalize RNA amounts (internal control). The relative expression of the gene = $2^{-\Delta\Delta CT}$; ΔCT = CT of the target gene—CT of β-actin; and ΔΔCT = ΔCT of the observed sample—CT of the control sample.

Table 2. Primers used in this study.

Genes	Oligonucleotide Sequence (5′–3′)
β-actin	Forward GGAGATTACTGCCCTGGCTCCTA Reverse GACTCATCGTACTCCTGCTTGCTG
ZnT1	Forward ATGGGGGCTCTGGTGAACGC Reverse CCTGGTCGGGACCCTGCTCG
PepT1	Forward GCTCTTATCGCCGACTCGTG Reverse GGGTTTGATTCCTCCAGTCC
hZIP4	Forward TGGTCTCTACGTGGCACTC Reverse GGGTCCCGTACTTTCAACATC

3.14. Statistical Analysis

All experiments were carried out in triplicate, and data were expressed as the mean ± standard deviation (SD), unless specifically noted. The least significant difference method (LSD) was used to compare and analyze the difference in mean values with SPSS 20.0 statistical software (SPSS Inc., Chicago, IL, USA) and the significance level was 5%.

4. Conclusions

In this study, the efficient zinc-binding peptides were prepared from oyster-modified hydrolysates by adding exogenous glutamate according to the plastein reaction. The addition of exogenous L-[1-^{13}C]glutamate contributed to an increase in the zinc-binding capacity of the plastein products and that a hydrophobic interaction was the main mechanism of action of the plastein reaction. Structural analyses suggested that zinc-binding peptides could bind with zinc and form the peptide-zinc complex (MZ). Furthermore, the MZ absorption effect and absorption pathway under simulated intestinal epithelial cells were studied. The results showed that the absorption effect of MZ under phytic acid treatment was significantly higher than that of ZnSO$_4$, indicating that the MZ could significantly enhance zinc bioavailability than ZnSO$_4$. Additionally, MZ could regulate the gene expression of hZIP4, ZnT1, and PepT1, indicating that MZ could promote the zinc absorption through the traditional zinc ion channel and small peptide transport pathway. In summary, the plastein reaction could significantly increase the ability of peptides to bind zinc, and the MZ has better absorption and bioavailability than ZnSO$_4$. The MZ exhibits great potential as a functional ingredient in food and nutraceuticals.

Author Contributions: Conceptualization, J.L. and Y.Z.; methodology, C.G.; software, Z.W.; validation, Y.C.; formal analysis, R.G. and J.R.; resources, X.Z and H.W.; data curation, F.X.; writing—original draft preparation, J.L.; writing—review and editing, J.L. and Y.Z.; project administration, Y.Z.; funding acquisition, H.X. and Y.Z.

Funding: This research was funded by National key R & D Program of China, grant number: 2018YFD0901003; Natural Science Foundation of Shandong Province, grant number: ZR201807110008; Shandong Provincial Key R & D Program, grant number: 2017GHY15128; China Agriculture Research System, grant number: CARS-46; Jiangsu Provincial Science and Technology Program, grant number: LYG-SZ201815.

Conflicts of Interest: The authors declare no conflict of interest.

References

1. Prasad, A.S. Zinc: An antioxidant and anti-inflammatory agent: Role of zinc in degenerative disorders of aging. *J. Trace Elem. Med. Biol.* **2014**, *28*, 364–371. [CrossRef] [PubMed]
2. Trame, S.; Wessels, I.; Haase, H.; Rink, L. A short 18 items food frequency questionnaire biochemically validated to estimate zinc status in humans. *J. Trace Elem. Med. Biol.* **2018**, *49*, 285–295. [CrossRef] [PubMed]
3. Spenser, R.; Hadar, N.; Sharon, M.; Glahn, R.P.; Omry, K.; Elad, T. Chronic zinc deficiency alters chick gut microbiota composition and function. *Nutrients* **2015**, *7*, 9768–9784. [CrossRef]
4. Choi, S.; Liu, X.; Pan, Z. Zinc deficiency and cellular oxidative stress: Prognostic implications in cardiovascular diseases. *Acta Pharmacol. Sin.* **2018**, *39*, 1120–1132. [CrossRef] [PubMed]

5. Udechukwu, M.C.; Collins, S.A.; Udenigwe, C.C. Prospects of enhancing dietary zinc bioavailability with food-derived zinc-chelating peptides. *Food Funct.* **2016**, *7*, 4137–4144. [CrossRef] [PubMed]
6. Dostal, A.; Chassard, C.; Hilty, F.M.; Zimmermann, M.B.; Jaeggi, T.; Rossi, S.; Lacroix, C. Iron depletion and repletion with ferrous sulfate or electrolytic iron modifies the composition and metabolic activity of the gut microbiota in rats. *J. Nutr.* **2011**, *142*, 271–277. [CrossRef] [PubMed]
7. Puckett, B.J.; Eggleston, D.B. Oyster demographics in a network of no-take reserves: Recruitment, growth, survival, and density dependence. *Mar. Coast. Fish.* **2012**, *4*, 605–627. [CrossRef]
8. Liu, Z.; Dong, S.; Xu, J.; Zeng, M.; Song, H.; Zhao, Y. Production of cysteine-rich antimicrobial peptide by digestion of oyster (*Crassostrea gigas*) with alcalase and bromelin. *Food Control* **2008**, *19*, 231–235. [CrossRef]
9. Qian, Z.J.; Jung, W.K.; Byun, H.G.; Kim, S.K. Protective effect of an antioxidative peptide purified from gastrointestinal digests of oyster, *Crassostrea gigas* against free radical induced DNA damage. *Bioresour. Technol.* **2008**, *99*, 3365–3371. [CrossRef]
10. Umayaparvathi, S.; Meenakshi, S.; Vimalraj, V.; Arumugam, M.; Sivagami, G.; Balasubramanian, T. Antioxidant activity and anticancer effect of bioactive peptide from enzymatic hydrolysate of oyster (*Saccostrea cucullata*). *Biomed. Prev. Nutr.* **2014**, *4*, 343–353. [CrossRef]
11. Zeng, M.; Cui, W.; Zhao, Y.; Liu, Z.; Dong, S.; Guo, Y. Antiviral active peptide from oyster. *Chin. J. Oceanol. Limn.* **2008**, *26*, 307–312. [CrossRef]
12. Shiozaki, K.; Shiozaki, M.; Masuda, J.; Yamauchi, A.; Ohwada, S.; Nakano, T.; Yamaguchi, T.; Saito, T.; Muramoto, K.; Sato, M. Identification of oyster-derived hypotensive peptide acting as angiotensin-I-converting enzyme inhibitor. *Fish. Sci.* **2010**, *76*, 865–872. [CrossRef]
13. Coombs, T. The distribution of zinc in the oyster *Ostrea edulis* and its relation to enzymic activity and to other metals. *Mar. Biol.* **1972**, *12*, 170–178. [CrossRef]
14. Chen, D.; Liu, Z.; Huang, W.; Zhao, Y.; Dong, S.; Zeng, M. Purification and characterisation of a zinc-binding peptide from oyster protein hydrolysate. *J. Funct. Foods* **2013**, *5*, 689–697. [CrossRef]
15. Zhang, Z.; Zhou, F.; Liu, X.; Zhao, M. Particulate nanocomposite from oyster (*Crassostrea rivularis*) hydrolysates via zinc chelation improves zinc solubility and peptide activity. *Food Chem.* **2018**, *258*, 269–277. [CrossRef] [PubMed]
16. Cao, Y.; Zhang, J.; Wang, Z.; Zhao, Y. Separation and identification of oyster peptide modified by plastein reaction and characterization of peptide-zinc complexes. *Chem. J. Chin. Univ.* **2018**, *39*, 470–475.
17. Li, J.; Liu, Z.; Zhao, Y.; Zhu, X.; Yu, R.; Dong, S.; Wu, H. Novel natural angiotensin converting enzyme (ACE)-inhibitory peptides derived from sea cucumber-modified hydrolysates by adding exogenous proline and a study of their structure–activity relationship. *Mar. Drugs* **2018**, *16*, 271. [CrossRef] [PubMed]
18. Brownsell, V.; Williams, R.; Andrews, A. Application of the plastein reaction to mycoprotein: II. Plastein properties. *Food Chem.* **2001**, *72*, 337–346. [CrossRef]
19. Suisui, J.; Yuanhui, Z.; Qingqing, S.; Xiaojie, Z.; Shiyuan, D.; Zunying, L.; Haohao, W.; Mingyong, Z. Modification of ACE-inhibitory peptides from *Acaudina molpadioidea* using the plastein reaction and examination of its mechanism. *Food Biosci.* **2018**, *26*, 1–7. [CrossRef]
20. Sun, S.; Xu, X.; Sun, X.; Zhang, X.; Chen, X.; Xu, N. Preparation and identification of ACE inhibitory peptides from the marine macroalga ulva intestinalis. *Mar. Drugs* **2019**, *17*, 179. [CrossRef]
21. Piper, D.W.; Fenton, B.H. pH stability and activity curves of pepsin with special reference to their clinical importance. *Gut* **1965**, *6*, 506–508. [CrossRef] [PubMed]
22. Condés, M.C.; Añón, M.C.; Mauri, A.N.; Dufresne, A. Amaranth protein films reinforced with maize starch nanocrystals. *Food Hydrocolloid.* **2015**, *47*, 146–157. [CrossRef]
23. Grallert, A.; Hagan, I.M. Preparation of protein extracts from *Schizosaccharomyces pombe* using trichloroacetic acid precipitation. *Cold Spring Harb. Protoc.* **2017**, 139–143. [CrossRef] [PubMed]
24. Makhatadze, G.I.; Privalov, P.L. Protein interactions with urea and guanidinium chloride: A calorimetric study. *J. Mol. Biol.* **1992**, *226*, 491–505. [CrossRef]
25. Sharma, A.K.; Pavlova, S.T.; Kim, J.; Kim, J.; Mirica, L.M. The effect of Cu^{2+} and Zn^{2+} on the $A\beta_{42}$ peptide aggregation and cellular toxicity. *Metallomics* **2013**, *5*, 1529–1536. [CrossRef] [PubMed]
26. Feng, G.; Feng, Y.; Guo, T.; Yang, Y.; Guo, W.; Huang, M.; Wu, H.; Zeng, M. Biogenic polyphosphate nanoparticles from *Synechococcus sp.* PCC 7002 exhibit intestinal protective potential in human intestinal epithelial cells in vitro and murine small intestine ex vivo. *J. Agric. Food Chem.* **2018**, *66*, 8026–8035. [CrossRef] [PubMed]

27. Ranaldi, G.; Ferruzza, S.; Canali, R.; Leoni, G.; Zalewski, P.D.; Sambuy, Y.; Perozzi, G.; Murgia, C. Intracellular zinc is required for intestinal cell survival signals triggered by the inflammatory cytokine TNFα. *J. Nutr. Biochem.* **2013**, *24*, 967–976. [CrossRef]

28. Fukada, T.; Yamasaki, S.; Nishida, K.; Murakami, M.; Hirano, T. Zinc homeostasis and signaling in health and diseases: Zinc signaling. *J. Biol. Inorg. Chem.* **2011**, *16*, 1123–1134. [CrossRef]

29. Luo, Y.; Wu, C.; Liu, L.; Gong, Y.; Peng, S.; Xie, Y.; Cao, Y. 3-Hydroxyflavone enhances the toxicity of ZnO nanoparticles in vitro. *J. Appl. Toxicol.* **2018**, *38*, 1206–1214. [CrossRef]

30. Tacnet, F.; Lauthier, F.; Ripoche, P. Mechanisms of zinc transport into pig small intestine brush-border membrane vesicles. *J. Physiol.* **1993**, *465*, 57–72. [CrossRef]

31. Cousins, R.J. Gastrointestinal factors influencing zinc absorption and homeostasis. *Int. J. Vitam. Nutr. Res.* **2010**, *80*, 243–248. [CrossRef] [PubMed]

32. Ito, A.; Ojima, K.; Naito, H.; Ichinose, N.; Tateishi, T. Preparation, solubility, and cytocompatibility of zinc-releasing calcium phosphate ceramics. *J. Biomed. Mater. Res. A* **2015**, *50*, 178–183. [CrossRef]

33. Hansen, M.; Sandström, B.; Lönnerdal, B. The effect of casein phosphopetides on zinc and calcium absorption from high phytate infant diets assessed in rat pups and Caco-2 cells. *Pediatr. Res.* **1996**, *40*, 547. [CrossRef] [PubMed]

34. Zhu, K.X.; Wang, X.P.; Guo, X.N. Isolation and characterization of zinc-chelating peptides from wheat germ protein hydrolysates. *J. Funct. Foods* **2015**, *12*, 23–32. [CrossRef]

35. Deng, B.; Zhou, X.; Wu, J.; Long, C.; Yao, Y.; Peng, H.; Wan, D.; Wu, X. Effects of dietary supplementation with tribasic zinc sulfate or zinc sulfate on growth performance, zinc content and expression of zinc transporters in young pigs. *Anim. Sci. J.* **2017**, *88*, 1556–1560. [CrossRef] [PubMed]

36. Beck, F.W.; Prasad, A.S.; Butler, C.E.; Sakr, W.A.; Kucuk, O.; Sarkar, F.H. Differential expression of hZnT-4 in Human prostate tissues. *Prostate* **2004**, *58*, 374–381. [CrossRef] [PubMed]

37. Jappar, D.; Wu, S.P.; Hu, Y.; Smith, D.E. Significance and regional dependency of peptide transporter (PEPT) 1 in the intestinal permeability of glycylsarcosine: In situ single-pass perfusion studies in wild-type and Pept1 knockout mice. *Drug Metab. Dispos.* **2010**, *38*, 1740–1746. [CrossRef] [PubMed]

38. Maubon, N.; Le Vee, M.; Fossati, L.; Audry, M.; Le Ferrec, E.; Bolze, S.; Fardel, O. Analysis of drug transporter expression in human intestinal Caco-2 cells by real-time PCR. *Fund. Clin. Pharmacol.* **2007**, *21*, 659–663. [CrossRef]

39. Ledoux, M.; Lamy, F. Determination of proteins and sulfobetaine with the Folin-phenol reagent. *Anal. Biochem.* **1986**, *157*, 28–31. [CrossRef]

40. Zhang, J.J.; Liu, Z.Y.; Dong, S.Y.; Mao, X.Z.; Zhao, Y.H. Stability of modified peptide using zinc binding and plastein reaction. *Mod. Food Sci. Technol.* **2015**, *31*, 150–154.

41. Moro, A.; Gatti, C.; Delorenzi, N. Hydrophobicity of whey protein concentrates measured by fluorescence quenching and its relation with surface functional properties. *J. Agric. Food Chem.* **2001**, *49*, 4784–4789. [CrossRef] [PubMed]

42. Hartnett, E.K.; Satterlee, L.D. The formation of heat and enzyme induced (plastein) gels from pepsin-hydrolyzed soy protein isolate. *J. Food Biochem.* **2010**, *14*, 1–13. [CrossRef]

43. Zou, Y.; Zhao, L.; Feng, G.; Miao, Y.; Wu, H.; Zeng, M. Characterization of key factors of anchovy (*Engraulis japonicus*) meat in the nanoparticle-mediated enhancement of non-heme iron absorption. *J. Agric. Food Chem.* **2017**, *65*, 11212–11219. [CrossRef] [PubMed]

44. Duan, J.; Xie, Y.; Luo, H.; Li, G.; Wu, T.; Zhang, T. Transport characteristics of isorhamnetin across intestinal Caco-2 cell monolayers and the effects of transporters on it. *Food Chem. Toxicol.* **2014**, *66*, 313–320. [CrossRef] [PubMed]

45. Wu, H.; Zhu, S.; Zeng, M.; Liu, Z.; Dong, S.; Zhao, Y.; Huang, H.; Lo, Y.M. Enhancement of non-heme iron absorption by anchovy (*Engraulis japonicus*) muscle protein hydrolysate involves a nanoparticle-mediated mechanism. *J. Agric. Food Chem.* **2014**, *62*, 8632–8639. [CrossRef]

46. Makhov, P.; Golovine, K.; Uzzo, R.G.; Rothman, J.; Crispen, P.L.; Shaw, T.; Scoll, B.J.; Kolenko, V.M. Zinc chelation induces rapid depletion of the X-linked inhibitor of apoptosis and sensitizes prostate cancer cells to TRAIL-mediated apoptosis. *Cell Death Differ.* **2008**, *15*, 1745–1751. [CrossRef] [PubMed]

47. Sreenivasulu, K.; Raghu, P.; Ravinder, P.; Nair, K.M. Effect of dietary ligands and food matrices on zinc uptake in Caco-2 cells: Implications in assessing zinc bioavailability. *J. Agric. Food Chem.* **2008**, *56*, 10967–10972. [CrossRef]

48. Li, J.; Yang, X.; Shi, G.; Chang, J.; Liu, Z.; Zeng, M. Cooperation of lactic acid bacteria regulated by the AI-2/LuxS system involve in the biopreservation of refrigerated shrimp. *Food Res. Int.* **2019**, *120*, 679–687. [CrossRef]
49. Moslehi-Jenabian, S.; Gori, K.; Jespersen, L. AI-2 signalling is induced by acidic shock in probiotic strains of *Lactobacillus* spp. *Int. J. Food Microbiol.* **2009**, *135*, 295–302. [CrossRef]

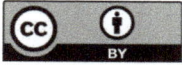

marine drugs

MDPI

Article

Characterization of the First Conotoxin from *Conus ateralbus*, a Vermivorous Cone Snail from the Cabo Verde Archipelago

Jorge L. B. Neves [1,2,3,*], Julita S. Imperial [1], David Morgenstern [4], Beatrix Ueberheide [4], Joanna Gajewiak [1], Agostinho Antunes [2,5], Samuel D. Robinson [1], Samuel Espino [1], Maren Watkins [1], Vitor Vasconcelos [2,5] and Baldomero M. Olivera [1]

[1]   Department of Biology, University of Utah, 257 S 1400 E, Salt Lake City, UT 84112, USA
[2]   CIIMAR/CIMAR—Interdisciplinary Centre of Marine and Environmental Research, Terminal de Cruzeiros, do Porto de Leixões, 4450-208 Porto, Portugal
[3]   FECM—Faculty of Engineering and Marine Science, University of Cabo Verde, Mindelo CP 163, Cabo Verde
[4]   Langone Medical Center, Department of Biochemistry and Molecular Pharmacology, New York University, New York, NY 10016, USA
[5]   Department of Biology, Faculty of Sciences, University of Porto, 4169-007 Porto, Portugal
*   Correspondence: jorgewneves@hotmail.com; Tel.: +351-223401800

Received: 24 April 2019; Accepted: 19 July 2019; Published: 24 July 2019

Abstract: *Conus ateralbus* is a cone snail endemic to the west side of the island of Sal, in the Cabo Verde Archipelago off West Africa. We describe the isolation and characterization of the first bioactive peptide from the venom of this species. This 30AA venom peptide is named conotoxin AtVIA (δ-conotoxin-like). An excitatory activity was manifested by the peptide on a majority of mouse lumbar dorsal root ganglion neurons. An analog of AtVIA with conservative changes on three amino acid residues at the C-terminal region was synthesized and this analog produced an identical effect on the mouse neurons. AtVIA has homology with δ-conotoxins from other worm-hunters, which include conserved sequence elements that are shared with δ-conotoxins from fish-hunting *Conus*. In contrast, there is no comparable sequence similarity with δ-conotoxins from the venoms of molluscivorous *Conus* species. A rationale for the potential presence of δ-conotoxins, that are potent in vertebrate systems in two different lineages of worm-hunting cone snails, is discussed.

Keywords: conotoxin; cone snail; *Conus*; *Conus ateralbus*; Kalloconus

1. Introduction

The cone snails (genus *Conus*) are a biodiverse lineage of venomous predators; most species specialize in envenomating a narrow range of prey. On the basis of their primary prey, species in the genus *Conus* are divided into three broad classes, fish-hunting, snail-hunting and worm-hunting species; the great majority of *Conus* are vermivorous—worm-hunting. Pioneering studies on cone snail venoms by Endean and coworkers [1] demonstrated that the efficacy of the venom observed on particular animals could be correlated to the prey of that species. Fish-hunting cone snail venoms were highly potent on vertebrates, with worm-hunting *Conus* venoms much less so. Snail-hunting *Conus* venoms are extremely potent when tested on gastropods, but much less effective in vertebrate systems. Thus, the venom components that are highly expressed are presumably under strong selection for high potency and efficacy on molecular targets in the prey of each *Conus* species.

The initial characterization of one family of conotoxins, the δ-conotoxins, followed this general pattern. The first venom peptides of this family identified were from snail-hunting *Conus* species, such as *Conus textile* [2] or *Conus gloriamaris* [3]. Although these were highly potent when tested on molluscan systems, they were relatively inactive on vertebrates. In contrast, δ-conotoxins from fish-hunting cones, such as δ-conotoxin PVIA [4], from *Conus purpurascens*, and δ-conotoxin SVIE [5] from *Conus striatus*, were extremely potent when tested on fish or mice.

Thus, it was a surprise to discover a δ-conotoxin from a worm-hunting species, e.g., *Conus tessulatus* and *Conus suturatus*, that was highly potent and efficacious on vertebrate systems [6,7]. Aman et al. (2015) [6] rationalized their discovery by suggesting that the ancestral worm-hunting species that gave rise to fish-hunting lineages of *Conus* had evolved a δ-conotoxin. If a K-channel blocker acting on the same circuitry were subsequently evolved, this would result in a powerful tetanic paralysis of the fish. Major lineages of fish-hunting cone snails have been shown to have both a δ-conotoxin, as well as a κ-conotoxin that blocks K channels, a combination known as the "lightning-strike cabal". Thus, the presence of δ-conotoxins in the ancestral worm-hunting *Conus* was postulated to be critical in the shift from worm hunting to fish hunting. If this ancestor of fish-hunting lineages had indeed evolved a δ-conotoxin effective on fish, then related peptides might still be found in worm-hunting lineages descended from the same ancestral species, such as *Conus tessulatus*.

The present phylogenetic organization [8] of the genus *Conus* is shown in Figure 1. Fish-hunting cone snail lineages are shown underlined, and the position of *Conus tessulatus*, the worm-hunting species in the Tesseliconus lineage that yielded the δ-conotoxin described above, is shown by the red arrow. The phylogeny shown in Figure 1 is consistent with the hypothesis of Aman et al. However, there is a diversity of other worm-hunting lineages that have presumably descended from the same ancestral species, indicated by boxed lineages (mollusc-hunting lineages, marked by checks, are also predicted to have evolved from the same worm-hunting ancestor).

In this report, we demonstrate that one of the other descendant worm-hunting lineages, which is distant from Tesseliconus (the lineage that gave rise to *Conus tessulatus*), and which is presently restricted to an entirely different biogeographic range, does indeed contain a δ-conotoxin-like that is highly potent on vertebrate targets.

This peptide was discovered in a lineage of West African cone snails, the subgenus Kalloconus. A phylogenetic tree showing *Conus ateralbus*, the species analyzed, and other species in the subgenus is shown in Figure 2. This is the first venom characterized from any species in the Kalloconus lineage. The subgenus Kalloconus is restricted to tropical West Africa, from the Islands of Madeira to South Angola (in contrast, Tesseliconus is only found in the Indo-Pacific). Kalloconus species comprise some of the larger *Conus* species found in the Eastern Atlantic, including *Conus pulcher*, the largest species in the entire superfamily Conoidae, growing to a length of 230 mm. Although the shells of Kalloconus species have long been used as cultural objects in northwest Africa, as well as being prized collector's items for many centuries, little was known about their biology and some of the species in this clade have only recently been described [8]. The focus of this article is a single species of Kalloconus, *Conus ateralbus*, and a specific venom component from this species that has broader significance for toxinology.

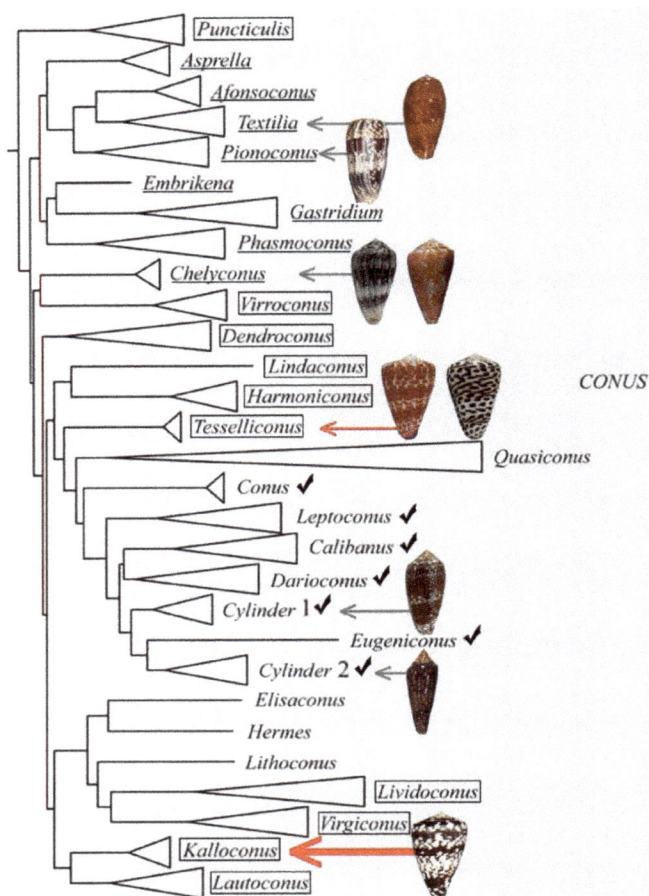

Figure 1. A phylogenetic tree showing the large clade of *Conus* encompassing all lineages that are fish-hunting (underlined) and snail-hunting (checked). Well-established worm-hunting lineages are boxed. δ-conotoxins have been characterized from the nine species figured, including the worm-hunting *Conus tessulatus* (red arrow). In this work, we investigated the venom of *Conus ateralbus* (shown by the thick red arrow), which is in the Kalloconus lineage. This tree was adapted with permission from Puillandre et al. (2014) [8], [*Mol. Phylogenet. Evol.*], [Elsevier Inc.], [2014]. Species discussed in this study whose shells are figured are (from top to bottom): *Conus bullatus* (Textilia); *Conus striatus* (Pionoconus); *Conus ermineus* (l) and *Conus purpurascens* (r) (Chelyconus); *Conus tessulatus* (l) and *Conus eburneus* (r) (Tesseliconus); *Conus textile* and *Conus gloriamaris* (Cylinder); *Conus ateralbus* (Kalloconus).

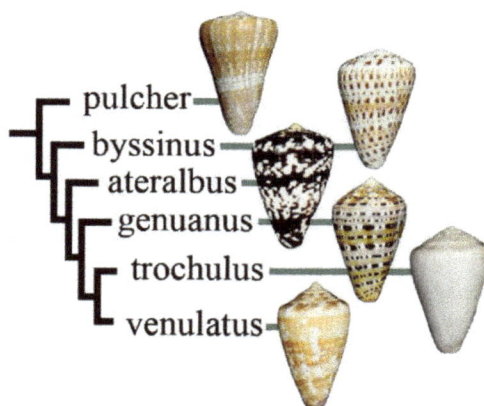

Figure 2. Relationship of species in Kalloconus. Most of the species are approximately the same size (ca. 40 mm), except for *Conus pulcher*, which can be very much larger (up to 230 mm). This tree was adapted with permission from Puillandre et al. (2014) [8], [*Mol. Phylogenet. Evol.*], [Elsevier Inc.], [2014].

This is the first toxinological study on any species in the subgenus Kalloconus. We detail both the collection data and the biological observations made in the field regarding *Conus ateralbus*; some of these may apply more broadly to all Kalloconus species. In contrast to some other species in Kalloconus (e.g., *Conus pulcher* and *Conus genuanus*) that are widely distributed across the West African marine biogeographic province, *Conus ateralbus* is an endemic species in Kalloconus with the narrowest known biogeographical range. It is restricted to the west coast of the Island of Sal, in the Cabo Verde archipelago. It has been suggested that an ancestral Kalloconus from the West African coast colonized the Cabo Verde archipelago relatively recently (4.6 MYA), giving rise to at least five extant species that are endemic to Cabo Verde [9]. The specimens analyzed in this study were collected by the senior author, who also recorded field observations that provide direct evidence for the vermivory of *Conus ateralbus* (and by implication, the entire Kalloconus clade).

2. Results

2.1. Collection of Conus Ateralbus and Venom Fractionation

Specimens of *Conus ateralbus* can be reliably collected on the west coast of the Island of Sal from April to June; the field collection protocol is detailed under Methods. One specimen of *Conus ateralbus* was found consuming a polychaete worm (Figure 3). The specimen did not bury itself as it consumed the worm and it took about one hour—it was thus exposed the entire time it was feeding on its prey. As can be seen in the figure (and in the video supplied as Supplemental Material), the prey was far longer than the cone snail itself.

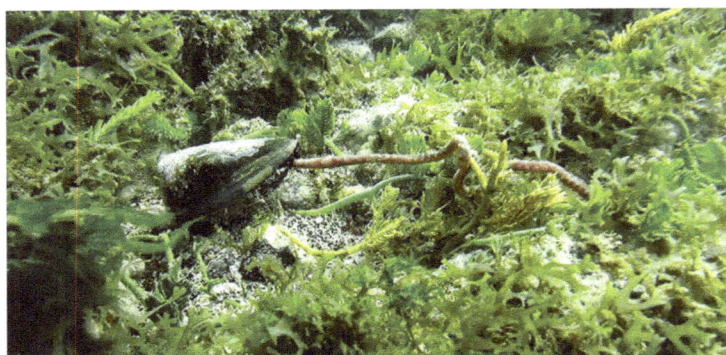

Figure 3. *Conus ateralbus* was observed in the field feeding on a long worm, many times the length of the predatory snail.

Conus ateralbus venom from many specimens was pooled and the venom extract was assayed as described under Methods. The venom extract showed activity on dorsal root ganglion (DRG) neurons and in intracranially-injected mice. The venom extract was fractionated; the HPLC chromatogram is shown in Figure 4A. Several biologically-active fractions were detected; Fraction 38, which showed activity in mice and DRG neurons, was further sub-fractionated and the biologically-active component was purified to homogeneity. The activities on DRG and mice were found in the major peak (Figure 4B); matrix-assisted laser desorption ionization mass spectrometry (MALDI-MS; linear mode) revealed this major peak to be homogeneous with a molecular mass of 3010 Da (Figure 4C). In order to determine the number of cysteine residues, the peptide was reduced with DTT and alkylated with 4-vinylpyridine; the mass increment upon pyridylethylation corresponded to the presence of six cysteine residues.

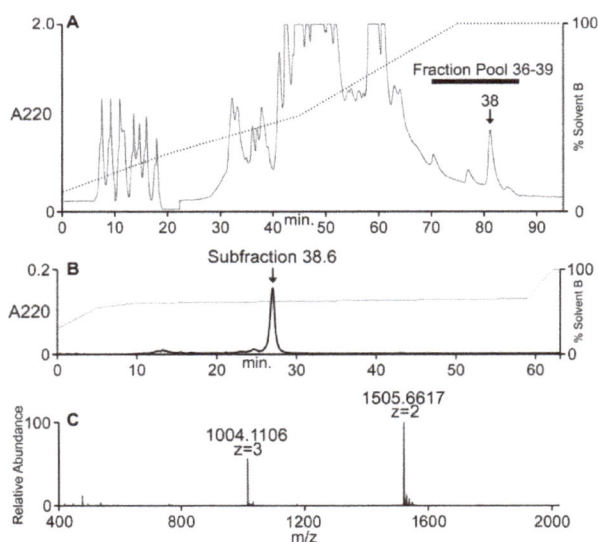

Figure 4. Fractionation of *Conus ateralbus* venom. The peptide characterized in this study was first detected in the pool of fractions shown, 36–39 (**A**). Further purification of the active fraction (fraction 38) yielded the chromatogram shown in (**B**). The major peak (subfraction 38.6) was both biologically active (Figure 5) and gave the results shown in (**C**) upon analysis on an Orbitrap Elite mass spectrometer at 120,000 resolution.

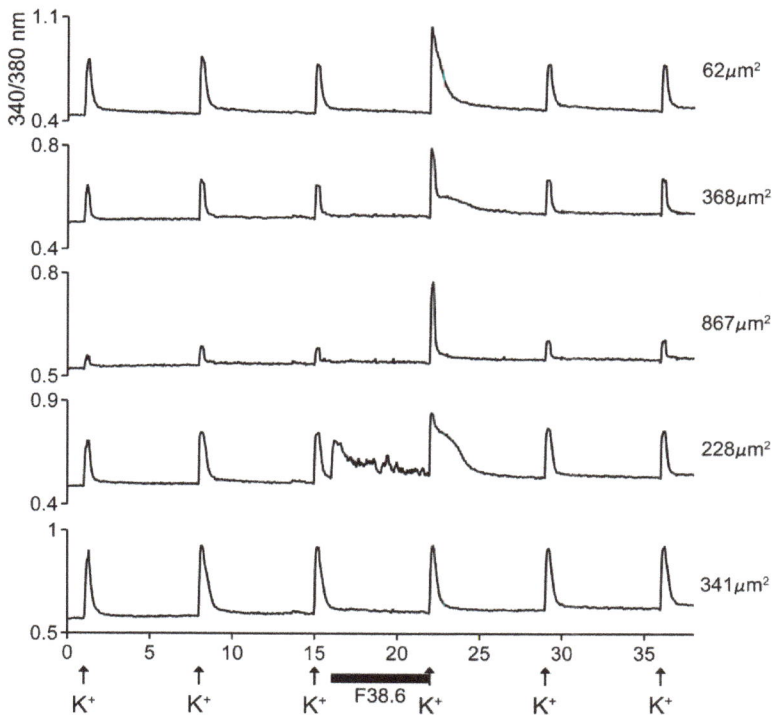

Figure 5. Responses of five different cells to native AtVIA (subfraction 38.6). Shown are the responses of five dorsal root ganglion (DRG) neurons (see Methods); the size of each cell is indicated. A pulse of 25 mM KCl was applied as described under Methods; the horizontal bar indicates when cells were incubated with the purified peptide. The first three cells (from top) show a change in response upon depolarization with KCl. The fourth trace shows a cell that directly increased cytosolic Ca^{++} when the peptide was added, even without KCl depolarization (approximately 26% of neurons responded in this manner) and the bottom trace shows a cell that did not respond (approximately 15% of DRG neurons were non-responsive to the peptide).

2.2. Conus Ateralbus Venom: Biological Activity

The HPLC fractions were assayed using calcium imaging of native DRG neurons [6,10,11] and intracranial injections on mice. The activity that caused excitatory effects on a majority of the DRG cells eluted extremely late (fraction 38), as shown in Figure 4A, suggesting the highly hydrophobic nature of the active component. Compared to control mice, the main behavioral phenotype elicited by the pool fraction, the fraction 38 and the subfraction 38.6 in mice was hypersensitivity to stimuli like touch [12].

The excitatory activity that was purified and characterized affected >80% of DRG neurons. Some of the results with the purified peptide are shown in Figure 5. In the experiment shown, the cells were exposed to 25 mM KCl, which elicited an increase in cytosolic $[Ca^{++}]$. If the cells were preincubated with the purified peptide, a large fraction of the cells responded with an increase in the Ca^{++} influx observed after the KCl pulse (first three traces in Figure 5). A small fraction of the cells responded with an increase in cytosolic $[Ca^{++}]$ even without application of KCl (4th trace, Figure 5), and a minor fraction (~15%) of the cells did not respond to preincubation with the peptide (5th trace, Figure 5). It should be noted that the first three traces show cells of different sizes, and the responses to the peptide differed in detail in these individual cells.

These results are consistent with the activity of a δ-conotoxin that inhibits the inactivation of voltage-gated Na⁺ [6].

2.3. Peptide Sequence Determination

The amino acid sequence of the peptide was determined as described under Methods and is shown in Figure 6. The peptide spectrum is consistent with a 30-amino acid peptide with the following sequence: ZCGADGQFCF(L/I)PG(L/I)G(L/I)NCCSG(L/I)C(L/I)(L/I)VCVPT (where Z is pyroglutamate). It is not possible to differentiate between the isobaric amino acids isoleucine and leucine by mass spectrometry alone and this ambiguity is indicated by (L/I).

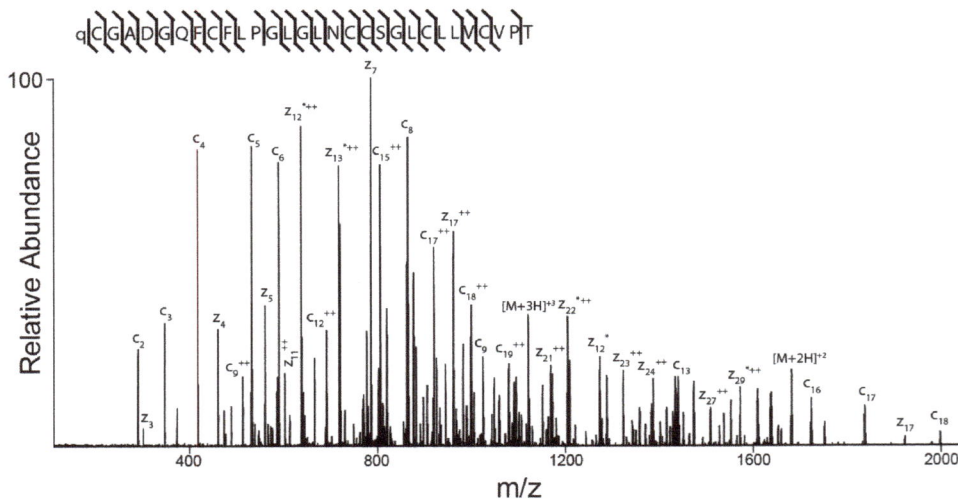

Figure 6. Determination of the sequence of AtVIA by tandem mass spectrometry. MS/MS-electron-transfer dissociation (ETD) spectrum of the (M + 5H) + 5 ion of qCGADGQFCF(L/I)PG(L/I)G(L/I)NCCSG(L/I)C(L/I) (L/I)VCVPT after reduction and alkylation with 2-methylaziridine acquired on the Orbitrap Elite with 15,000 resolution (@ 400 *m/z*). *N*-terminal fragment ions (c-type ions) are indicated by ⌐ and C-terminal fragment ions (z-type ions) are indicated by ⌐. Doubly charged ions are indicated with ++ and z ions resulting from cleavage at cysteine and loss of the cysteine side chain are indicated with *. [M + 5H]+++++•• and [M + 5H]+++++••• indicates quintuply charged precursor ions that captured 2 or 3 electrons, respectively, but have not dissociated into fragment ions. Due to space limitations, not all different charge states of already labeled peptide bond cleavages are indicated in the figure. The mass accuracy for all fragment ions is better than 15 ppm. The mass spectrometer used cannot differentiate between isoleucine or leucine and, for simplicity, leucine is used in the figure to indicate a fragment ion of mass 113.08406.

The arrangement of the six cysteines suggests that this new peptide has an ICK structural motif and belongs to the O-superfamily, with Framework VI (C-C-CC-C-C). As shown in Table 1, the peptide shares significant sequence homology with other δ-conotoxins, e.g., δ-TsVIA, *Conus tessulatus*; δ-ErVIA, *C. eburneus*; δ-SuVIA, *C. suturatus*; δ-EVIA, *C. purpurascens*; and δ-SVIE, *C. striatus*. Together, the activity in DRG neurons and the sequence homology to δ-conotoxin shown in Table 1 are consistent with the peptide being a δ-conotoxin, i.e., inhibiting the inactivation of voltage-gated Na⁺. We, therefore, designate the peptide δ-conotoxin AtVIA.

Table 1. Comparison of δ-AtVIA with δ-conotoxins from various *Conus* species.

Subgenus (Prey)	-Conotoxin	Conus Species	Sequence	Ref.
A.				
Tesseliconus (worm)	-TsVIA	*C. tessulatus*	CAAFGSFCGLPGLVD–CCSGRCFIVCLL	[6]
Tesseliconus (worm)	-ErVIA	*C. eburneus*	CAGIGSFCGLPGLVD–CCSGRCFIVCLP	[6]
Tesseliconus (worm)	SuVIA	*C. suturatus*	CAGIGSFCGLPGLVD–CCSDRCFIVCLP	[7]
Kalloconus (worm)	-AtVIA	*C. ateralbus*	ZCGADGQFCFL-PGLGLNCCSGLCLIVCVPT	This work
B.				
Chelyconus (fish)	PVIA	*C. purpurascens*	EACYAOGTFCGIKOGL—CCSEFCLPGVCFG	[4]
Pionoconus (fish)	SVIE	*C. striatus*	DGCSSGGTFCGIHOGL—CCSEFCF-LWCITFID	[5]
Textilia (fish)	-BuVIA	*C. bullatus*	DECSAOGAFCLIROGL—CCSEFCF-FACF	[13]
Kalloconus (worm)	AtVIA	*C. ateralbus*	ZCGADGQFCFL-PGLGLNCCSGLCL-IVCVPT	This work
Tesseliconus (worm)	TsVIA	*C. tessulatus*	CAAFGSFCGL-PGLVD-CCSGRCF-IVCLL	[6]
Tesseliconus (worm)	ErVIA	*C. eburneus*	CAGIGSFCGL-PGLVD-CCSGRCF-IVCLP	[6]
Tesseliconus (worm)	SuVIA	*C. suturatus*	CAGIGSFCGL-PGLVD-CCSDRCF-IVCLP_	[7]
Cylinder (snail)	TxVIA	*C. textile*	WCKQSGEMCNLLDQN—CCDGYCIVLV-CT	[14]
Cylinder (snail)	GmVIA	*C. gloriamaris*	VKPCRKEGQLCDPIFQN—CCRGWNCVLF-CV	[3]

The identity of the residues identified as (L/I) in δ-AtVIA from mass spectrometric data was resolved by screening for a genomic DNA clone encoding the peptide. The genomic DNA sequence that was obtained, which encoded AtVIA, is: catcgatcatctgtccatccatccatttcattcattcgctgccaaatggaataaatattcgc gtctctctttctgtttgtatctgacagATTGAGCAAGAAGCAGTGCGGGACTGATGGTCAGTTTTGTTTCCTAC CGGGCCTTGGATTGAATTGCTGCAGTGGGCTTTGCTTAATCGTTTGCGTGCCGACATGATGTCT TCTCTTCCCCTC. Translation of the 3′ region (shown above in uppercase letters) gave: LSKKQCGTDGQFCFLPGLGLNCCSGLCLIVCVPT, and the predicted cleavage yields the peptide: QCGTDGQFCFLPGLGLNCCSGLCLIVCVPT. Q (glutamine) is a residue that is prone to spontaneously cyclize to Z (pyroglutamate) when at the *N*-terminus of a peptide [15]. It is apparent that only the (L/I) closest to the C-terminus in the sequence obtained from mass spectrometry is present as I (isoleucine), the rest of the (L/I)'s is present as L (leucine).

2.4. Synthesis and Folding of AtVIA[I25L;V28L;T30S]

The δ-conotoxin family is known to be difficult to synthesize and correctly fold due to their highly hydrophobic character [13,16]. While some of them are relatively easy to handle in linear form (e.g., PVIA), others are not; AtVIA[I25L;V28L;T30S], which was the peptide identified from the early sequencing results, is a good example of such behavior. When suspended in HPLC solvent with high acetonitrile content (>50%) and injected on the C18 column, no peptide peak was observed (Figure 7, Panel A). However, with methane thiosulfonate bromide (MTSET) treatment for 1 h 30 min, a major product appeared (Figure 7, Panel B). Its identity was confirmed by mass spectrometry. Methanethiosulfonate reagents (MTS-R) are known to rapidly and selectively react with cysteine residues forming mixed disulfides [17]. Thus, all 6 cysteines of AtVIA[I25L;V28L;T30S] were modified with thiocholine residues, thereby increasing overall solubility of the peptide, and making it easy to purify by reversed-phase high performance liquid chromatography (RP-HPLC). Such mixed disulfides are reversible and do not interfere with the subsequent oxidative folding reaction, which was shown before [18] for the synthesis and folding of hepcidin via S-sulfonation. Linear AtVIA[I25L;V28L;T30S] with thiocholine-modified cysteine residues folded within 4 h in a buffered solution (pH = 8.7), in the presence of 5% Tween 40 and 1:1 mixture of reduced and oxidized gluthatione with 14% yield (Figure 7, Panel C). The temporary peptide modification with MTS-R reagent can be a useful method for improving the solubility of highly hydrophobic conopeptides, in addition to already existing methods, including recently published approach utilizing an acid-cleavable solubility tag [19].

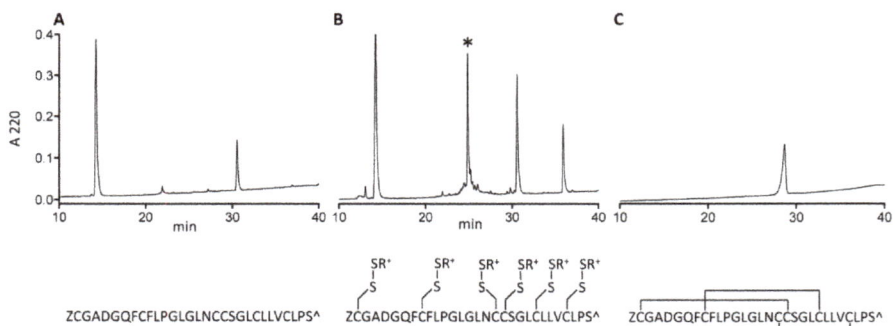

Figure 7. Synthesis of AtVIA[I25L;V28L;T30S]. (**A**) A crude pellet of AtVIA[I25L;V28L;T30S] was suspended in high acetonitrile content HPLC buffer and injected on C18 RP-HPLC. No peak of the desired peptide was observed. (**B**) Methane thiosulfonate bromide (MTS-ET) treatment of the crude peptide led to a S-thiocholine modified peptide (as shown below the HPLC chromatogram); the peak of the temporary S-modified peptide is indicated with an asterisk (*) on the HPLC chromatogram. (**C**) HPLC profile of the folded and purified AtVIA[I25L;V28L;T30S], with an assumed disulfide bond pattern indicated below the HPLC chromatogram.

Biological Activity of AtVIA[I25L;V28L;T30S]

The data obtained by calcium imaging in native DRG neurons in the presence of the AtVIA analog is shown in Figure 8. There is no apparent difference between the indirect effects of the native sample of AtVIA (Figure 5) and that of AtVIA[I25L;V28L;T30S]. However, the direct effects observed on the addition of the native sample of AtVIA were not observed with AtVIA[I25L;V28L;T30S]. These direct effects (Figure 5, 4th trace from the top) could be attributed to the presence of a trace of impurity in the native sample; on the other hand, the absence of these direct effects in the presence of the synthetic sample could also be attributed to any of the substitutions made on the amino acid sequence of native AtVIA.

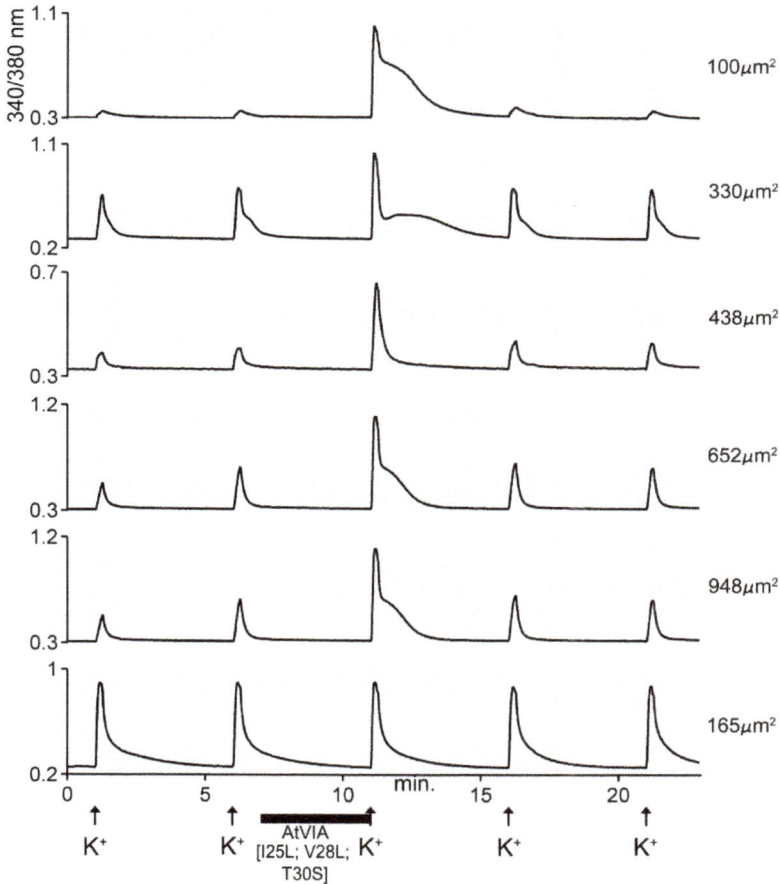

Figure 8. Responses of 6 different cells to AtVIA[I25L;V28L;T30S]. Shown are the responses of 6 DRG neurons, with the size of each indicated. Pulses of 25mM KCl were applied as described under Methods; the horizontal bar indicates where the cells were incubated with the peptide. The first five traces (from top) show a change in response upon depolarization with KCl (~95% of neurons responded in this manner). The bottom trace shows a cell that did not respond (~5% of DRG neurons).

3. Discussion

We report the first peptide isolated and characterized from *Conus ateralbus* venom. *Conus ateralbus* is an endemic cone snail species that belongs to the subgenus Kalloconus from the Cabo Verde Islands, an isolated archipelago in the tropical Atlantic Ocean. This species is only found on Sal Island (Calheta Funda and Mordeira Bays). The phylogenetic tree in Figure 2 shows a close relationship with two other species endemic to the Cabo Verde archipelago, *Conus trochulus* (found only in Boa Vista) and *Conus venulatus* (found on Sal, Boa Vista, Maio and Santiago) [20,21], and with *Conus genuanus* (non endemic). It was previously suggested that *Conus ateralbus* was worm hunting, based on the analysis of the radular teeth [21]; we provide direct field observations that definitively establish *Conus ateralbus* as a worm hunter (Figure 3). Thus, it is likely that all Kalloconus are worm hunting, since specific clades in the genus *Conus* generally sort out on the basis of their primary prey. It is notable that in the phylogenetic tree in Figure 1, there are clusters of worm-hunting lineages that are well separated from each other. *Conus tessulatus*, in the subgenus Tesseliconus clusters with Harmoniconus and Lindaconus. In contrast, Kalloconus clusters with Lautoconus (also West African) and less closely with Virgiconus and Lividoconus (both Indo-Pacific). In the present work, we establish the presence of δ-conotoxins that act on vertebrate Na channels in the two divergent clusters of worm-hunting clades, Kalloconus and Tesseliconus. These δ-conotoxins vary greatly with respect to their sequence similarities (see Table 1A), in a manner concordant with the phylogenetic tree shown in Figure 1.

The *Conus ateralbus* venom peptide, δ-conotoxin-like AtVIA (δ-AtVIA; GenBank accession number is MH025915), was purified to homogeneity and biochemically characterized. A clone was identified in order to sort out the I/L uncertainty that is inherent in sequence data obtained by mass spectrometry. Despite the conservative amino acid substitutions on the C-terminal region based on the early mass spectrometric sequencing data, exhibited indirect effects on mouse DRG responses to depolarization with KCl, which were identical to those of the native δ-AtVIA and δ-TsVIA [6].

Table 1 shows δ-AtVIA and other δ-conotoxin sequences from various subgenera of *Conus*, including fish-hunting, snail-hunting and worm-hunting lineages. As shown in Table 1A, there are conserved sequence features in venom peptides (highlighted in yellow; 52–59% of conserve sequence between δ-AtVIA petide, δ-TsVIA, δ-ErVIA and δ-SuVIA) from the two worm-hunting and three fish-hunting subgenera identified that are not shared by the peptides from snail-hunting species. The conserved sequence features in the fish-hunting and worm-hunting cone snail δ-conotoxins shown in Table 1 are presumably important for targeting these peptides to vertebrate Na channels. In contrast, the sequences of δ-conotoxins from snail-hunting species do not share these consensus sequence features and are not broadly effective on vertebrate Na channels.

It should be noted that although there are conserved sequence features between δ-conotoxins from worm-hunting and fish-hunting species, there are also systematic subgeneric differences between groups of peptides. Thus, the peptide from *Conus ateralbus* is much more divergent (14AA differences) from the three sequences from the three Tesseliconus species (*Conus tessulatus*, *Conus eburneus*, and *Conus suturatus* that differ by 1-4AA from each other). However, δ-conotoxin structures provide amino acids critical for the activity of conotoxins, and it was demonstrated that homologous sequences with large hydrophobic amino acids of δ-conotoxin are very relevant for activity on vertebrate Na channels [13]. Thus, three large hydrophobic amino acids (F, L and I) are conserved in all sequence of the peptides AtVIA, TsVIA, SuVIA and ErVIA, on the first, second and fourth intercysteine loops [6,7]. δ-conotoxin has some other characteristic proprieties, as the HPLC similar profile of the longest retention time and a well-shaped peak in reverse-phase column. In addition, the worm-hunting peptides can be separated from those from fish-hunting cone snail venoms by examining the loop between the second and third Cys residues in these peptides. In all the δ-conotoxins from fish-hunting cones, the third amino acid in this loop is always a positively charged residue (i.e., K in the Chelyconus sequences, H in the Pionoconus peptide and R in the Textilia peptide); this positively charged residue is missing from the peptides from worm-hunting *Conus*. Furthermore, although the proline residue is conserved in this loop, it is post-translationally modified to hydroxyproline in all of the sequences from fish-hunting species but is unmodified in the sequences from worm-hunting species. The differences between the peptides derived from fish-hunting versus worm-hunting *Conus* suggest that the spectrum of voltage gated sodium channels might systematically differ between the two classes of peptides. If this were the case, then δ-conotoxins, such as the peptide we have characterized here from *Conus ateralbus*, may prove to be useful pharmacological reagents for differentiating between the various molecular subtypes of voltage gated sodium channels.

The sequence conservation that is highlighted in Table 1 is consistent with the hypothesis that the last common ancestor of the four fish-hunting species, whose shells are shown in the figure (i.e., *Conus purpurascens*, *Conus ermineus*, *Conus striatus*, and *Conus bullatus*) and the four worm-hunting species (i.e., *Conus eburneus*, *Conus tessulatus*, *Conus suturatus* and *Conus ateralbus*) had already evolved a δ-conotoxin with these consensus sequence features as predicted by the hypothesis detailed by Aman et al., (2015) [6] for the molecular events that accompanied the prey shift from worm hunting to fish hunting. Recently, it was demonstrated that Cone snails specialized in two different evoked venom, the predation region and defense region on the venom gland [22]. Worm-hunting cone snails, as *Conus suturatus*, specialized defensive envenomation strategy in the proximal regions of the venom duct. δ-conotoxins in the defense-evoked of the *Conus* venom gland contribute to the understanding of the evolution from worm-hunting to fish-hunting cone snails [7,22].

As shown in Table 1, two snail-hunting δ-conotoxins from the subgenus Cylinder, δ-TxVIA and δ-GmVIA, do not share these consensus sequence features. Since these snail-hunting species are also descended from the last common ancestor referred to above—this would, therefore, appear to be inconsistent with the hypothesis of Imperial et al., (2007) [23] and Aman et al., (2015) [6].

There are two possible explanations for the observed lack of conservation in δ-conotoxins from the snail-hunting *Conus* species. First, δ-conotoxins play a major role in prey capture; a snail hunter has the biological problem of keeping the envenomated snail outside its shell. A predator striking a snail would elicit the automatic response of the prey withdrawing deeply into the shell; snail-hunting cone snails have no way of breaking the shell of their potential prey. The δ-conotoxins are key to activating motor circuitry so that immediately after envenomation, the body of the prey is extended outside the shell accompanied by spastic, uncoordinated movements, and is unable to withdraw into its shell [24]. This then allows further injection of venom, providing continuous access to the soft parts of the prey without having to break the shell. Thus, the δ-conotoxins from molluscivorous *Conus* that have been purified and characterized seem likely to play a role in prey capture, so it would be expected that these are targeted to molluscan sodium channels and are divergent in sequence from the ancestral δ-conotoxin. Additionally, because the prey of snail-hunting cones has a hard shell, retention of a peptide that deters fish competitors may no longer be required. Thus, these explanations rationalize why δ-conotoxin sequences from *Conus* textile and *Conus* gloriamaris do not have the consensus features of the other δ-conotoxins in Table 1, and why these are not active on vertebrate voltage-gated sodium channels.

4. Materials and Methods

4.1. Field Collection and Venom Extraction

Conus ateralbus specimens were collected in the Calheta Funda Bay, Sal Island, in shallow water (around 2 m deep) in 2013. The specimens were collected in one day, kept alive in seawater and preserved at −20 °C at the end of the day. The venom duct was dissected from each frozen specimen. Venom was obtained from ducts immediately after dissection by placing each duct on an ice-cold metal spatula; the venom was squeezed out using an Eppendorf pipette tip and was lyophilized and stored at −80 °C. Crude venom extracts were prepared using 40% (*v/v*) CH3CN/water acidified with 0.1% (*v/v*) trifluoroacetic acid (TFA). A 36.5 mg portion was resuspended in 15 mL of 40% acetonitrile and 0.1% trifluoroacetic acid (TFA) using a vortex mixer for 2 × 1 min with an interval of 3 min, homogenized in a Wheaton homogenizer and centrifuged in a Beckman Avanti centrifuge (F650 rotor) for 15 min at 13.650 rpm, at 4 °C. The supernatant was centrifuged again to remove all residual particles.

4.2. Venom Fractionation

Crude extract from 36.5 mg of venom was fractionated by reversed-phase high performance liquid chromatography (RP-HPLC) using a C18 Vydac 218TP101522 preparative column. Elution was done at a flow rate of 7 mL/min and a gradient ranging from 10% to 30% of solvent B in 20 min, 30% to 50% in 25 min, 50% to 100% in 30 min, and 100% for 15 min. Solvent B was 90% (*v/v*) CH3CN in 0.1% (*v/v*) aqueous TFA, and solvent A was 0.1% (*v/v*) TFA in water. The subfractionation of the active fraction 38 was done by RP-HPLC using a C18 Vydac monomeric 238EV54 column. The absorbance was monitored at 220 and 280 nm.

4.3. Mass Spectrometry and Sequence Determination

The crude HPLC fractions were analyzed using matrix-assisted laser desorption ionization (MALDI) mass spectrometry. The AtVIA sample (subfraction 38.6, Figure 4B) was dissolved in 100 µL of 0.5% acetic acid; 10 µL of the solution were desalted using POROS R2 beads [25]. An aliquot of the unreduced sample was loaded onto a 0.2 × 25 cm Pepswift EasySpray column. The sample was eluted at a flow rate of 1 µL/min with a gradient of 0–100% of Solvent C (90% (*v/v*) CH3CN in 0.5% acetic acid) in 20 min, a spray voltage of 2.5 kV on an Easy nLC-1000 nanoUHPLC coupled to an Orbitrap Elite mass spectrometer. MS1 scans were acquired at 120,000 resolution (@ 400 *m/z*). For MS2, the most abundant precursor was isolated and fragmented using ETD at 15,000 resolution (@ 400 *m/z*) and 60 msec ion reaction time.

The fraction (subfraction 38.6, Figure 4B) was reconstituted in 100 µL of 0.5% acetic acid. For determination of the accurate mass of the peptide (better than 10 ppm) an aliquot of this fraction (1%) was loaded onto a 200 µm × 25 cm Pepswift EasySpray column using the autosampler of an Easy nLC-1000 nano-HPLC coupled to an Orbitrap Elite mass spectrometer. The sample was eluted using a flow rate of 1ul/min with a gradient of 0–100%B (solvent A = 0.5% acetic acid, solvent B = 90% acetonitrile in 0.5% acetic acid (*v/v*)) in 20 min and a spray voltage of 2.5 kV. MS1 scans were acquired at 120,000 resolution (@ 400 *m/z*). For de novo sequence determination another aliquot of the sample was dried in the speedvac and subsequently reduced and alkylated in vapor using 1% 2-methylaziridine and 2% trimethylphosphine in 50% acetonitrile and 100 mM ammonium bicarbonate (pH 8.4) for 90 min at RT. Alkylation vapor was removed and the sample was reconstituted in 0.5% acetic acid. Aliquots of the now reduced and alkylated samples was loaded onto a 200 m × 25 cm Pepswift EasySpray column using the autosampler of an Easy nLC-1000 nano-HPLC coupled to an Orbitrap Elite mass spectrometer as described above. The gradient was 0–50%B in 50 min. MS1 scans were acquired at 120,000 resolution (@ 400 *m/z*). MS2 was acquired on the top 5 precursors that carry at least 4 charges using the following settings: 4 microscans, 3 *m/z* isolation window, target value of 1e4 ions. Each precursor was subjected to ETD and HCD fragmentation using the following conditions: 15,000 resolution (@ 400 *m/z*), 30 s dynamic exclusion, ETD using 60 ms ion reaction time with supplemental activation, HCD using 27% normalized collision energy. The sequence was obtained by manual de novo sequencing. The measured mass deviates from the theoretical mass by 5.5ppm and is within the mass error of the instrument.

Preparation of Genomic DNA and Characterization of Clones Encoding AtVIA

Genomic DNA was prepared from 20 mg of *Conus ateralbus* venom duct using the Gentra PUREGENE DNA Isolation Kit (Gentra Systems, Minneapolis, MN, USA) according to the manufacturer's standard protocol. *Conus ateralbus* genomic DNA (10 ng) was used as a template for polymerase chain reaction (PCR) with oligonucleotides corresponding to the conserved intron and 3′ UTR sequences of previously isolated δ-conotoxin prepropeptides [26]. The resulting PCR product was purified using the PureLink PCR Purification Kit (Life Technologies, Carlsbad, CA, USA) following the manufacturer's suggested protocol. The eluted DNA fragment was annealed to pNEB206A vector and the products were transformed into competent Esherichia coli DH5α cells, using the USER® Friendly

Cloning Kit (New England Biolabs, Inc., Ipswich, MD, USA) following manufacturer's suggested protocols. The nucleic acid sequence of this δ-conotoxin-encoding clone was determined at the Core Sequencing Facility, University of Utah, USA, following the ABI automated sequencing protocol initiated by the M13 universal reverse primer.

4.4. In Vivo Assay and Calcium Imaging Assay on DRG

Each dried aliquot of HPLC fraction pools or individual fractions was resuspended in 12 µL of normal saline solution (NSS, 0.9% NaCl). Mice (male and female, were 15 days old, 6–8 g of body weight) were intracranially injected using a 0.3 mL insulin syringe (equivalent of 4 µg/µL); the same volume of NSS alone was injected in control mice. After the injection of each sample, the peptide-injected mice were observed side by side with NSS-injected controls, all mice were placed in separate cages for at least 1 h [27].

Lumbar dorsal root ganglia (DRG) were dissected from wild type C57/BL6 mice, dissociated, pooled and cultured overnight for calcium imaging experiments, following previously described protocols [10]. Cells were loaded with Fura-2-AM dye one hour before the experiment. During the experiment, the dye inside the cells was excited alternately with 340 nm and 380 nm light and the ratio of the emissions at 510 nm from both excitations was measured. The ratio of the fluorescence intensity was considered indicative of intracellular calcium concentration. A solution of 25 mM KCl was applied for 15 s every seven minutes to induce neuronal depolarization. After the third KCl pulse, venom extract or HPLC fractions were applied and the effects on intracellular calcium levels, before, during and after depolarization, were monitored. Experimental protocols involving live animals were approved by the Institutional Animal Care and Use Committee of the University of Utah.

4.5. Peptide Synthesis

Based on the early sequencing results, AtVIA[I25L;V28L;T30S], a peptide with the following sequence: ZCGADGQFCFLPGLGLNCCSGLCLLVCLPS-OH (Z = pyroglutamate) was synthesized at 50-µmol scale using an AAPPTec Apex 396 synthesizer (AAPPTec, LLC, Louisville, KY, USA) using standard solid-phase Fmoc (9-fluorenylmethyloxycarbonyl) protocols. Fmoc-protected amino acids were purchased from AAPPTec. The peptide was assembled on pre-loaded Fmoc-L-Ser(tBu)-Wang resin (substitution, 0.53 mmol/g; Peptides International Inc., Louisville, KY, USA). Side-chain protection for each corresponding amino acid was as follows: Asp, O-tert-butyl (OtBu); Ser, tert-butyl (tBu); and Asn, Gln and Cys, trytl (Trt). Coupling of each amino acid was achieved using 1 equivalent of 0.4 M benzotriazol-1-yl-oxytripyrrolidinophosphonium hexafluorophosphate (PyBOP) and 2 equivalents of 2 M *N,N*-diisopropylethyl amine (DIPEA) in *N*-methyl-2-pyrrolidone (NMP). The amino acid amounts used were at ten-fold excess (60 min coupling). Fmoc-protecting groups were removed by a 20-min treatment with 20% (*v/v*) piperidine in dimethylformamide (DMF).

4.5.1. AtVIA[I25L;V28L; T30S] Cleavage, Derivatization and Purification

The peptide was cleaved from 100 mg of resin by treatment with Reagent K (TFA/H_2O/phenol/thioanisole/1,2-ethanedithiol; 82.5/5/5/5/2.5 by volume). After 2.5 h, the crude peptide was separated from the resin by vacuum-filtration. The cleavage product was precipitated in cold methyl-tert-butyl ether (MTBE) and subsequently washed one more time with MTBE. The crude peptide was suspended in 50% (*v/v*) CH3CN in 0.01% aqueous TFA and treated with 55 mg of [2-(Trimethylammonium)ethyl] methane thiosulfonate bromide (MTSET). The pellet was still present in the solution after 30 min, so another portion of MTSET was added (~40 mg) and it was allowed to react for an additional 1h. The modified peptide was then purified by reversed-phase (RP) HPLC in a Vydac C18 semi-preparative column (218TP510, 250 mm × 10 mm, 5 µm particle size) over a linear gradient ranging from 20% to 50% of solvent B in 30 min with a flow rate 4 mL/min. The peptide was quantified by comparing the peak area obtained by analytical RP-HPLC to that of a known amount of a reference peptide, At6A[F8Y;V28L;T30S]. Out of 100 mg cleaved resin, ~500 nmol of thiocholine-modified linear peptide was obtained. The identity of the linear peptide was confirmed using ESI MS: calculated: [M+] = 3717.75, obtained: [M+] = 3717.67.

4.5.2. Oxidative Folding of At6A[I25L;V28L;T30S]

The linear, thiocholine-modified peptide (100 nmol) was re-suspended in 50% (v/v) CH3CN in 0.01% aqueous TFA and added to a solution made up of 4 mL of 0.2 M Tris-HCl—2 mM EDTA pH 8.7, 0.4 mL of (5%) Tween 40, 1.6 mL of a 1:1 mixture of 10 mM GSSG and 10 mM GSH and 1.5 mL of water. Folding reaction was conducted for 4 h at room temperature and quenched by acidification using 8% (v/v) formic acid. Peptide was purified by RP-HPLC on the C18 semipreparative column using two different gradients: 35% to 95% change of solvent B in 15 min (4%/min of gradient change, 4 mL/min of elution rate) and 35% to 95% change of solvent B in 30 min (2%/min; 4 mL/min). The identity of the peptide was confirmed by MALDI-TOF mass analysis; calculated [M + H]$^+$: 3008.29 Da, observed: [M + H]$^+$: 3008.33 Da, but the desired mass was represented by a minor peak. The major peaks observed were: 3030.33 Da and 3046.30 Da which correspond to: [M + Na]$^+$ (calculated: 3030.27 Da) and [M + K]$^+$ (calculated: 3046.25 Da), respectively. There were also masses ranging from 1300 to 1500 Da, indicating traces of Tween (used in the folding reaction) in the sample. The peptide was quantified using amino acid analysis. Out of 1200 nmols of the linear peptide, 174 nmols of the desired folded peptide was obtained.

5. Conclusions

In this work, we report the first venom peptide characterized from any species in the subgenus Kalloconus, δ-conotoxin-like AtVIA from *Conus ateralbus*, an endemic cone snail species from the Cabo Verde Islands. δ-like AtVIA has homology with δ-conotoxins from worm-hunting species in the subgenus Tesseliconus, including conserved sequence elements shared with δ-conotoxins from fish-hunting *Conus*. We provide direct field observations (*Conus ateralbus* filmed eating a worm) that definitely establish *Conus ateralbus* as a vermivorous *Conus* species. The presence of δ-conotoxins that act on vertebrate Na+ channels has thus been established in two divergent worm-hunting clades. The results are consistent with the hypothesis that certain worm-hunting *Conus* evolved δ-conotoxins that act to probably deter competitors in a defensive envenomation strategy, and that this may have been an intermediate evolutionary step in the shift to fish prey within the genus *Conus*.

Supplementary Materials: The following are available online at http://doi.org/10.5281/zenodo.3233739, Video S1: Conus ateralbus eating polychaete worm.

Author Contributions: B.M.O., J.S.I., A.A. and V.V. conceived and designed the experiments; J.L.B.N., J.S.I., D.M., B.U., J.G., S.E. and M.W. performed the experiments; J.L.B.N., J.S.I., D.M., B.U., S.E. and M.W. analyzed the data; B.M.O., J.S.I. and B.U. contributed reagents/materials/analysis tools; B.M.O., S.D.R., J.S.I. and J.L.B.N. wrote the paper with input from all authors.

Funding: This work was supported by grants to BMO from the National Institute of General Medical Science, GM 48677 and GM103362. Partial funding was obtained through a PhD grant to JLBN (SFRH/BD/51477/2011) from the European Regional Development Fund (ERDF) through the COMPETE—Operational Competitiveness Program and from national funds through FCT—Foundation for Science and Technology—under the project FCT Project UID/Multi/04423/ and by the project H2020 RISE project EMERTOX—Emergent Marine Toxins in the North Atlantic and Mediterranean: New Approaches to Assess their Occurrence and Future Scenarios in the Framework of Global Environmental Changes—Grant Agreement No. 778069. The sample collection in Cabo Verde was supported by Fundação Calouste Gulbenkian.

Acknowledgments: We thank Grzegorz Bulaj from the University of Utah for creative discussions on the peptide synthesis, William Low from the Salk Institute for Biological Studies, La Jolla, CA and Krishna Parsawar from the University of Utah HSC Cores for MALDI-MS analyses, Scott Endicott from the University of Utah HSC Cores for amino acid analysis, Manuel B. Aguilar from the Universidad Nacional Autonoma de Mexico for the test peptide sequencing run by Edman degradation, and My Huynh and Terry Merritt for help with the figures and manuscript.

Conflicts of Interest: The authors declare no conflicts of interest.

References

1. Endean, R.; Rudkin, C. Further Studies of the Venoms of Conidae. *Toxicon* **1965**, *2*, 225–249. [CrossRef]
2. Fainzilber, M.; Lodder, J.C.; Kits, K.S.; Kofman, O.; Vinnitsky, I.; Van Rietschoten, J.; Zlotkin, E.; Gordon, D. A new conotoxin affecting sodium current inactivation interacts with the d-conotoxin receptor site. *J. Biol. Chem.* **1995**, *270*, 1123–1129. [CrossRef] [PubMed]
3. Shon, K.J.; Hasson, A.; Spira, M.E.; Cruz, L.J.; Gray, W.R.; Olivera, B.M. Delta-Conotoxin GmVIA, a novel peptide from the venom of *Conus gloriamaris*. *Biochemistry* **1994**, *33*, 11420–11425. [CrossRef] [PubMed]
4. Shon, K.-J.; Grilley, M.M.; Marsh, M.; Yoshikami, D.; Hall, A.R.; Kurz, B.; Gray, W.R.; Imperial, J.S.; Hillyard, D.R.; Olivera, B.M. Purification, Characterization, Synthesis, and Cloning of the Lockjaw Peptide from *Conus purpurascens* Venom. *Biochemistry* **1995**, *34*, 4913–4918. [CrossRef] [PubMed]
5. West, P.J.; Bulaj, G.; Yoshikami, D. Effects of delta-conotoxins PVIA and SVIE on sodium channels in the amphibian sympathetic nervous system. *J. Neurophysiol* **2005**, *94*, 3916–3924. [CrossRef] [PubMed]
6. Aman, J.W.; Imperial, J.; Ueberheide, B.; Zhang, M.-M.; Aguilar, M.; Taylor, D.; Watkins, M.; Yoshikami, D.; Showers-Corneli, P.; Safavi-Hermami, H.; et al. Insights into the origins of fish-hunting in venomous cone snails from studies on *Conus tessulatus*. *Proc. Natl. Acad. Sci. USA* **2015**, *112*, 5087–5092. [CrossRef]
7. Jin, A.-H.; Israel, M.R.; Inserra, M.C.; Smith, J.J.; Lewis, R.J.; Alewood, P.F.; Vetter, I.; Dutertre, S. δ-Conotoxin SuVIA suggests an evolutionary link between ancestral predator defence and the origin of fish-hunting behaviour in carnivorous cone snails. *Proc. R. Soc. B Biol. Sci.* **2015**, *282*, 201508170. [CrossRef] [PubMed]
8. Puillandre, N.; Bouchet, P.; Duda Jr, T.F.; Kauferstein, S.; Kohn, A.J.; Olivera, B.M.; Watkins, M.; Meyer, C. Molecular phylogeny and evolution of the cone snails (*Gastropoda conoidea*). *Mol. Phylogenet. Evol.* **2014**, *78*, 290–303. [CrossRef] [PubMed]
9. Cunha, R.L.; Castilho, R.; Ruber, L.; Zardoya, R. Patterns of cladogenesis in the venomous marine gastropod genus *Conus* from the Cape Verde islands. *Syst. Biol.* **2005**, *54*, 634–650. [CrossRef] [PubMed]
10. Imperial, J.; Cabang, A.; Song, J.; Raghuraman, S.; Gajewiak, J.; Watkins, M.; Showers-Corneli, P.; Fedosov, A.; Concepcion, G.P.; Terlau, H.; et al. A Family of Excitatory Peptide Toxins from Venomous Crassispirine Snails: Using Constellation Pharmacology to Assess Bioactivity. *Toxicon* **2014**, *89*, 45–54. [CrossRef] [PubMed]
11. Teichert, R.W.; Raghuraman, S.; Memon, T.; Cox, J.L.; Foulkes, T.; Rivier, J.E.; Olivera, B.M. Characterization of two neuronal subclasses through constellation pharmacology. *Proc. Natl. Acad. Sci. USA* **2012**, *109*, 12758–12763. [CrossRef]
12. Chen, P.; Garrett, J.E.; Watkins, M.; Olivera, B.M. Purification and characterization of a novel excitatory peptide from *Conus distans* venom that defines a novel gene superfamily of conotoxins. *Toxicon* **2008**, *52*, 139–145. [CrossRef]
13. Bulaj, G.; DeLaCruz, R.; Azimi-Zonooz, A.; West, P.; Watkins, M.; Yoshikami, D.; Olivera, B.M. δ-Conotoxin Structure/Function through a Cladistic Analysis. *Biochemistry* **2001**, *40*, 13201–13208. [CrossRef]
14. Hasson, A.; Fainzilber, M.; Gordon, D.; Zlotkin, E.; Spira, M.E. Alteration of sodium currents by new peptide toxins from the venom of a molluscivorous *Conus* snail. *Eur. J. Neurosci.* **1993**, *5*, 56–64. [CrossRef]
15. Tritsch, G.I.; Moore, G.F. Spontaneous decomposition of glutamine in cell culture media. *Exp. Cell. Res.* **1962**, *28*, 360–364. [CrossRef]
16. DeLa Cruz, R.; Whitby, F.G.; Buczek, O.; Bulaj, G. Detergent-assisted oxidative folding of delta-conotoxins. *J. Pept. Res.* **2003**, *61*, 202–212. [CrossRef]
17. Kenyon, G.L.; Bruice, T.W. Novel sulfhydryl reagents. *Methods Enzymol.* **1977**, *47*, 407–430.
18. Luo, S.; Zhangsun, S.D.; Hu, Y.; Zhu, X.; Wu, Y.; McIntosh, J.M. Alpha-Conotoxin LvIA/LVD21, Its Drugs Combination and Application. Patent CN201210347966.3A, 19 September 2012.
19. Peigneur, S.; Tytgat, J. When cone snails and spiders meet: Design of selective and potent sodium channel inhibitors. *Toxicon* **2014**, *91*, 170. [CrossRef]
20. Duda, T.F., Jr.; Kohn, A.J. Species-level phylogeography and evolutionary history of the hyperdiverse marine gastropod genus *Conus*. *Mol. Phylogenet. Evol.* **2005**, *34*, 257–272. [CrossRef]
21. Cunha, R.L.; Tenorio, M.J.; Afonso, C.; Castilho, R.; Zardoya, R. Replaying the tape: Recurring biogeographical patterns in Cape Verde *Conus* after 12 million years. *Mol. Ecol.* **2008**, *17*, 885–901. [CrossRef]
22. Dutertre, S.; Jin, A.H.; Vetter, I.; Hamilton, B.; Sunagar, K.; Lavergne, V.; Dutertre, V.; Fry, B.G.; Antunes, A.; Venter, D.J.; et al. Evolution of separate predation-and defence-evoked venoms in carnivorous cone snails. *Nat. Commun.* **2014**, *5*, 3521. [CrossRef]

23. Imperial, J.; Silverton, N.; Olivera, B.M.; Bandyopadhyay, P.; Sporning, A.; Ferber, M.; Terlau, H. Using chemistry to reconstruct evolution: On the origins of fish-hunting in venomous cone snails. *Proc. Am. Philos. Soc.* **2007**, *151*, 185–200.

24. Olivera, B.M.; Fedosov, A.; Imperial, J.S.; Kantor, Y. Physiology and Pharmacology of Conoidean Venoms. In *Physiology of Molluscs*; Saleuddin, A.S., Mukai, S.T., Eds.; Apple Academic Press: Palm Bay, FL, USA, 2015.

25. Cotto-Rios, X.M.; Bekes, M.; Chapman, J.; Ueberheide, B.; Huang, T.T. Deubiquitinases as a signaling target of oxidative stress. *Cell Rep.* **2012**, *2*, 1475–1484. [CrossRef]

26. Olivera, B.M.; Walker, C.; Cartier, G.E.; Hooper, D.; Santos, A.D.; Schoenfeld, R.; Shetty, R.; Watkins, M.; Bandyopadhyay, P.; Hillyard, D.R. Speciation of cone snails and interspecific hyperdivergence of their venom peptides. Potential evolutionary significance of introns. *Ann. N. Y. Acad. Sci.* **1999**, *870*, 223–237. [CrossRef]

27. Olivera, B.M.; Cruz, L.J.; Yoskikami, D. Effects of *Conus* peptides on the behavior of mice. *Curr. Opin. Neurobiol.* **1999**, *9*, 772–777. [CrossRef]

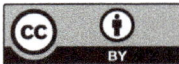

marine drugs

MDPI

Article

High-Throughput Identification and Analysis of Novel Conotoxins from Three Vermivorous Cone Snails by Transcriptome Sequencing

Ge Yao [1,†], Chao Peng [2,†], Yabing Zhu [3], Chongxu Fan [1], Hui Jiang [1], Jisheng Chen [1], Ying Cao [1,*] and Qiong Shi [2,4,*]

[1]   State Key Laboratory of NBC Protection for Civilian, Beijing 102205, China; bzyaoge@163.com (G.Y.); chongxu_fan@hotmail.com (C.F.); jiangtide@sina.cn (H.J.); chenjsh@cae.cn (J.C.)
[2]   Shenzhen Key Lab of Marine Genomics, Guangdong Provincial Key Lab of Molecular Breeding in Marine Economic Animals, BGI Academy of Marine Sciences, BGI Marine, BGI, Shenzhen 518083, China; pengchao@genomics.cn
[3]   BGI Genomics, BGI-Shenzhen, Shenzhen 518083, China; zhuyabing@genomics.cn
[4]   Laboratory of Aquatic Genomics, College of Life Sciences and Oceanography, Shenzhen University, Shenzhen 518060, China
*   Correspondence: caoying01@sina.com (Y.C.); shiqiong@genomics.cn (Q.S.); Tel.: +86-755-3630-7807 (Q.S.)
†   These authors contributed equally to this work.

Received: 21 February 2019; Accepted: 25 March 2019; Published: 26 March 2019

Abstract: The venom of each *Conus* species consists of a diverse array of neurophysiologically active peptides, which are mostly unique to the examined species. In this study, we performed high-throughput transcriptome sequencing to extract and analyze putative conotoxin transcripts from the venom ducts of 3 vermivorous cone snails (*C. caracteristicus*, *C. generalis*, and *C. quercinus*), which are resident in offshore waters of the South China Sea. In total, 118, 61, and 48 putative conotoxins (across 22 superfamilies) were identified from the 3 *Conus* species, respectively; most of them are novel, and some possess new cysteine patterns. Interestingly, a series of 45 unassigned conotoxins presented with a new framework of C-C-C-C-C-C, and their mature regions were sufficiently distinct from any other known conotoxins, most likely representing a new superfamily. O- and M-superfamily conotoxins were the most abundant in transcript number and transcription level, suggesting their critical roles in the venom functions of these vermivorous cone snails. In addition, we identified numerous functional proteins with potential involvement in the biosynthesis, modification, and delivery process of conotoxins, which may shed light on the fundamental mechanisms for the generation of these important conotoxins within the venom duct of cone snails.

Keywords: *Conus*; conotoxin; transcriptome sequencing; phylogeny; venom duct

---

1. Introduction

Cone snail is the common name for predatory marine mollusks in the family Conidae, with over 700 extant species and a categorization of four genera and 71 subgenera [1–3]. Within the *Conus*, the largest genus in the Conidae, 57 subgenera have been recognized [3]. As venomous predators distributed throughout tropical and subtropical coastal waters all over the world, the living cone snails are typically divided into 3 groups based on their feeding habits, including fish hunters, mollusc hunters, and worm hunters [4–6]. Some phylogenetic data have suggested that the ancestral cone snails preyed on marine worms [7,8]. The fish-hunting and mollusc-hunting groups account for ~30% of *Conus* species, and they are assumed to be dangerous to humans; however, the largest worm-hunting group seems to be nonthreatening [5,9,10]. An analysis of 141 human injuries reported from 34 responsible *Conus* species during the period of 1670–2017 [11] supports the fact that the venom of worm-hunting cone snails has only mild effects on humans, compared with those from fish-hunting and mollusc-hunting groups.

Although they are slow-moving creatures, cone snails can defeat fast-moving preys, competitors, and predators because of their specialized envenomation apparatus with potent venom components [12–14]. These venom components are commonly named conotoxins, a unique and remarkably diverse group of bioactive peptides with various pharmacological functions [6,14–17], which target a wide variety of ion channels, receptors, and even their subtypes in preys, predators, and humans with high affinity and specificity [6,18–20]. Consequently, conotoxins have become a research hotspot for the treatment of various neuropathic diseases, such as neuralgia, epilepsy, addiction, and Parkinson's disease [6,21–31].

With popular estimates of 50~200 classical conotoxins in a single *Conus* species, more than 80,000 natural conotoxins may exist in cone snails on a global scale [32–34]. Recent studies have shown that new methods, such as mass spectrometry, next-generation sequencing (NGS), and bioinformatics technologies, have predicted hundreds to thousands of venom peptides or transcripts from a single *Conus* species [34–37]. Therefore, cone snails, a tremendous store of natural conotoxins, are an underexploited resource for the development of potential drug candidates to treat a wide variety of human diseases [38].

Our present work reports a high-throughput transcriptome research on 3 worm hunting *Conus* species, *C. (Puncticulis) caracteristicus* (*C. caracteristicus*), *C. (Lividoconus) quercinus* (*C. quercinus*) and *C. (Strategoconus) generalis* (*C. generalis*), which are resident in offshore waters of the South China Sea. To date, there have been few studies on the screening of conotoxins from cone snails by transcriptome sequencing. One of our earlier studies on *C. quercinus* identified 65, 52, and 55 conotoxins from the venom duct, venom bulb and salivary gland, respectively [39]. Furthermore, only 38 and 4 conotoxins have been previously identified in *C. caracteristicus* and *C. generalis*, with classification into 10 (A, I3, M, O1, O2, O3, Q, S, T and Y) and 2 (D, O1) superfamilies, respectively [40–46]. In order to improve our understanding of the diversity of conotoxins, we performed transcriptome sequencing for the high-throughput identification and analysis of conotoxins from the venom duct of the 3 frequently collected cone snails.

2. Results

2.1. Summary of De Novo Assembled Transcriptome Data

After removal of low-quality reads, ambiguous reads and adapter sequences, we generated 4.57, 3.21, and 4.37 gigabases (Gb) of clean reads (with a mean length of 90 bp) for the venom duct transcriptomes of the 3 *Conus* species. Corresponding quality score 20 (Q20) of these sequencing data were 95.99%, 98.31%, and 96.00% respectively (Table 1). *De novo* assembling of all the high-quality clean reads using SOAPdenovo produced 213 k, 153 k, and 219 k contigs for the 3 species, respectively, which were subsequently assembled into scaffolds and unigenes. In total, the assembly of each transcriptome possessed 72 k, 61 k, and 95 k unigenes. More details of scaffold number, unigene number, mean length, and N50 value are summarized in Table 2.

Table 1. Statistics of venom duct transcriptome sequencing data for the 3 *Conus* species.

Species	Raw Data (Gb)	Clean Data (Gb)	Q20* (%)	Nonsequenced (%)	GC Content (%)
C. caracteristicus	5.51	4.57	95.99	0	47.84
C. quercinus	3.47	3.21	98.31	0.01	47.3
C. generalis	5.32	4.37	96.00	0	47.09

* A quality score for the percentage of incorrect bases at less than 1%.

Table 2. Summary of sequences produced by the assembling for the 3 *Conus* species.

Species	C. caracteristicus	C. generalis	C. quercinus
Clean reads			
Total reads (n)	50,788,576	48,557,734	35,694,024
Base pairs (Mb)	4,570.97	4,370.2	3,212.46
Mean length (bp)	90	90	90
Contigs (≥100 bp)			
Total number	213,155	219,692	153,249
Base pairs (Mb)	47.84	60.75	40.22
Mean length (bp)	224	276	262
N50 (bp)	236	307	313
Scaffolds (≥200bp)			
Total number	79,324	103,682	61,926
Base pairs (Mb)	47.57	65.38	34.96
Mean length (bp)	599	630	564
N50 (bp)	794	891	717
Unigenes (≥200 bp)			
Total number	72,462	95,438	61,002
Base pairs (Mb)	39.61	54.87	33.67
Mean length (bp)	546	574	552
N50 (bp)	670	749	688

2.2. Screening of Conotoxins in the Venom Duct Transcriptomes

To annotate conotoxin coding sequences among the unigenes, we searched all six-frame translations of the unigenes against a local reference database of known conotoxins constructed from the public ConoServer database by running Genewise and Agustus with an E-value cut-off of 1.0×10^{-5} [18], and then manually checked them using the ConoPrec tool [19]. After the removal of the transcripts with duplication, frame-shifting, and truncated mature region sequences, we identified 118, 61, and 48 putative conotoxin sequences from the 3 transcriptome datasets of *C. caracteristicus*, *C. generalis*, and *C. quercinus*, respectively (Tables 3–5). Interestingly, most of these sequences are reported for the first time and some possess new cysteine patterns. We then summarized and named these predicted conotoxins from the 3 *Conus* species as Ca-1 to Ca-118, Ge-1 to Ge-61, and Qu-1 to Qu-48, respectively (see more details in Supplementary Tables S1–S3).

Table 3. Classification and cysteine patterns of the conotoxins identified from *C. caracteristicus*.

Superfamily		Number	Cysteine Pattern (Number of Conotoxins)
A		11	CC-C-C (8), CC-C (3)
B1 (Conantokin)		2	Cysteine free
C (Contulakin)		1	Cysteine free
D		2	C-C-CC-C-C-C-C (1), C-CC-C-CC-C-C-C-C (1)
I	I1	1	C-C-CC-CC-C-C
	I2	6	C-C-CC-CC-C-C (1), C-C-C-C-CC-C-C (4), C-C-CC-C-C (1)
	I3	4	C-C-CC-CC-C-C (3), C-C-CC-C-C (1)
J		7	C-C-C-C
L		4	C-C-C-C
M		6	CC-C-C-CC (5), CC-C-C-C-C-C (1)
O	O1	22	C-C-CC-C-C
	O2	11	C-C-CC-C-C (3), C-C-CC-C-C-C-C (3), C-C (5)
	O3	6	C-C-CC-C-C
S		3	C-C-C-C-C-C-C-C-C
T		9	CC-CC (8), C-C-CC (1)
Y		1	C-C-CC-C-CC-C
Divergent M—L-LTVA		1	C-C-C-C-C-C
Unknown		21	C-C-C-C-C-C (19), C-C-C-C (1), CC-C-C-C-C (1)
Total		**118**	

Table 4. Classification and cysteine patterns of the conotoxins identified from *C. generalis*.

Superfamily			Number	Cysteine Pattern (Number of Conotoxins)
A			2	CC-C-C
B1 (Conantokin)			1	Cysteine free
C (Conotulakin)			1	Cysteine free
D			1	C-CC-C-CC-C-C-C
		I1	1	C-C-CC-CC-C-C
I		I2	4	C-C-CC-CC-C-C (2), C-C-C-C-CC-C-C (2)
		I3	1	C-C-CC-CC-C-C
	L		3	C-C-C-C
	M		4	CC-C-C-CC (3), C-C-CC (1)
		O1	12	C-C-CC-C-C
O		O2	4	C-C-CC-C-C (3), C-C-CC-C-C-C-C (1)
		O3	3	C-C-CC-C-C
	P		2	C-C-C-C-C
	S		1	C-C-C-C-C-C-C-C-C
	T		5	CC-CC
Con-ikot-ikot			1	CC-C-C-C-CC-C-C-C
Conotoxin-like			1	CC-C-C
Divergent MSTLGMTLL-			1	C-C-C-CCC-C-C-C-C
Unknown			13	C-C-C-C-C-C
Total			61	

Table 5. Classification and cysteine patterns of the conotoxins identified from *C. quercinus*.

Superfamily		Number	Cysteine Pattern (Number of Conotoxins)
A		5	CC-C-C
B1 (Conantokin)		3	Cysteine free
I2		3	C-C-CC-CC-C-C (2), C-C-C-C-CC-C-C (1)
M		10	CC-C-C-CC (9), C-C-CC-C-C-C (1)
	O1	8	C-C-CC-C-C
O	O2	3	C-C-CC-C-C
	O3	1	C-C-CC-C-C
T		1	CC-CC
V		3	C-C-CC-C-C-C-C
Y		1	C-C-CC-C-CC-C
Con-ikot-ikot		1	CC-C-C-C-CC-C-C-C-C
Divergent M—L-LTVA		2	C-C-C-C-C
Unknown		7	C-C-C-C-C-C
Total		48	

In this study, each putative conotoxin was assigned to a superfamily based on its percentage of sequence identity to the highly conserved signal region of the known superfamily from the public ConoServer database (Figure 1). Here, among the 118 putative conotoxins in *C. caracteristicus*, 96 sequences were assigned to 16 previously reported superfamilies (A, B1, C, D, I1, I2, I3, J, L, M, O1, O2, O3, S, T, and Y), while only 1 sequence was classified into the "divergent M—L-LTVA" superfamily. In addition, 21 sequences were not assigned to any known superfamily (named "unknown"; see more details in Table 3).

Among the 61 putative conotoxins in *C. generalis*, 46 sequences were classified into 15 known superfamilies (A, B1, C, D, I1, I2, I3, L, M, O1, O2, O3, P, S, and T) and 1 cysteine-rich con-ikot-ikot family. In addition, 1 sequence was assigned to the "divergent MSTLGMTLL-" super-family, 1 was assigned to the conotoxin-like group, and the other 13 sequences were unknown (see more details in Table 4).

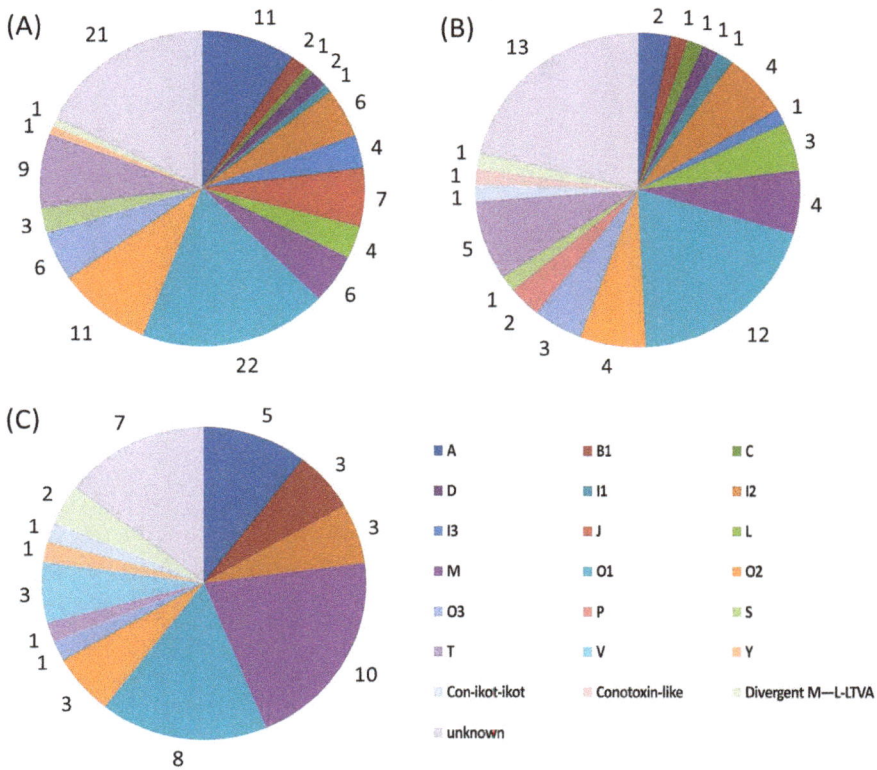

Figure 1. Summary of the conotoxins identified from the 3 *Conus* species. Many superfamilies or groups of conotoxins were classified in (**A**) *C. caracteristicus*, (**B**) *C. generalis*, and (**C**) *C. quercinus*.

Compared with the conotoxin sequences reported in our previous transcriptome study of *C. quercinus* [39], the number of conotoxins from *C. quercinus* in this study was less, with the identification of only 48 putative conotoxins. Among them, 39 sequences were classified into 10 known superfamilies (A, B1, I2, M, O1, O2, O3, T, V, and Y) and the con-ikot-ikot family, 2 sequences were assigned to the "divergent M—L-LTVA" superfamily, and the remaining 7 sequences were unknown (see more details in Table 5).

2.3. Quantification of Conotoxin Abundance

To investigate the transcription levels of conotoxins in each species, we mapped clean reads back to the *de novo* assembled unigenes and calculated the fragments per kilobase of transcript per million mapped fragments (FPKM) values to quantify the abundance of each conotoxin transcript. We screened out those conotoxins with high transcription abundance, and the top 10 (with the highest FPKM values) were selected from each dataset for comparison. The number of mapped reads for the top 10 conotoxins accounted for 60.6%, 84.9%, and 80.4% of the total conotoxin reads from *C. caracteristicus*, *C. generalis*, and *C. quercinus* respectively. Interestingly, O- and M-superfamilies were always the most abundant within each transcriptome dataset (Figure 2, Supplementary Table S4), suggesting their critical roles in predation and defense for the 3 vermivorous *Conus* species.

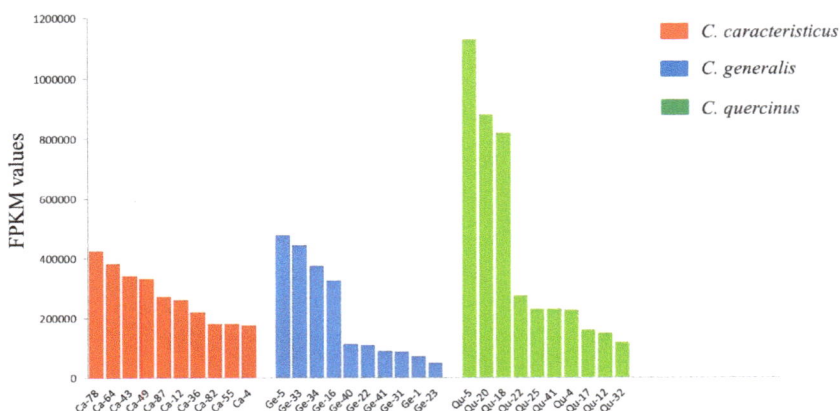

Figure 2. Comparison of the top 10 conotoxins (with the highest FPKM values) from the 3 transcriptome datasets.

The O-superfamily conotoxins specifically target a wide range of ion channels and receptors. In this study, a Bayesian phylogenetic tree was constructed with the Markov Chain Monte Carlo algorithm to analyze the relationships among these predicted O-superfamily conotoxins (Figure 3), in which 14 were presented with known bioactivities (previously reported from different *Conus* species) and 11 demonstrated high transcription levels from this study. Our phylogenetic assessment indicated that the O-superfamily conotoxin clades from the same *Conus* species arise as distinct lineages, suggesting that there was no correlation between the evolution of conotoxin sequences and interspecific genetic relationship (see more details in Figure 3). In turn, Ca-55 and ω-conotoxin PnVIA/PnVIB formed a monophyletic clade [47], and the Posterior probability of Ca-55 and PnVIB was 0.69. Ge-23 and κ-conotoxin PVIIA formed an individual clade [48], and the Posterior probability of both was 0.68. Qc-32 and γ-conotoxin PnVIIA/TxVIIA formed a monophyletic clade [49,50], but the homology between them was not supported by the low Posterior probability; they all exhibited distant evolutionary relationships to the other O-super-family conotoxins. Similarly, Ge-34 and δ-conotoxin TxVIA/TxVIB also formed a separate clade but with low Posterior probability [51].

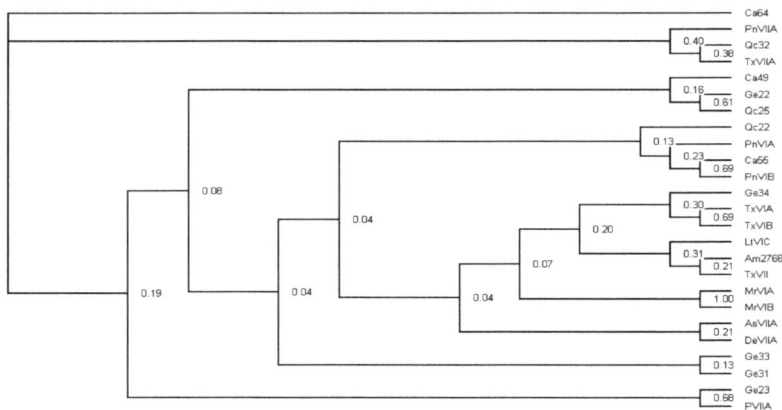

Figure 3. A Bayesian phylogenetic tree of the O-superfamily conotoxins. Posterior probabilities are labeled at each node.

2.4. Diversity of Conotoxin Structures

Among the putative conotoxin sequences in the 3 venom duct transcriptomes, most of them were discovered for the first time, and some possessed new cysteine frameworks or belonged to unknown superfamilies. The O-superfamily, including O1, O2, and O3, was the most abundant group in terms of conotoxin number (Tables 3–5). All of the O1- and O3-superfamily members exhibited the conventional VI/VII (C-C-CC-C-C) cysteine framework, which provides a stable three-disulfide inhibitor cysteine knot (ICK) motif [46]. Four O2-superfamily sequences from *C. caracteristicus* and *C. generalis* exhibited a C-terminal elongated XV (C-C-CC-C-C-C-C) cysteine framework (see Tables 3 and 4), and 5 short single disulfide-containing contryphan peptides with high identity were identified from only *C. caracteristicus* (Table 3). Interestingly, 5 O-superfamily members had the same mature regions as reported sequences from other *Conus* species. For example, Ge-24 from *C. generalis* had exactly the same mature peptide and prepro-region as the reported MgJr94 from piscivorous *C. magus* [52], while Ge-22 and Ge-23 showed mutations in the pro-peptide regions but with identical mature peptides to MiK41 and MiK42 respectively from *C. miles* [53].

The M-superfamily was also the predominant one in terms of transcription abundance and diversity of cysteine frameworks. Besides 17 sequences with the typical III (CC–C–C–CC) cysteine pattern, 3 conotoxins with IV (CC-C-C-C-C), XVI (C-C-CC) and XXVII (C-CC-C-C-C) cysteine frameworks were also observed (Tables 3–5).

For the I-superfamily, a variety of conotoxin (including I1, I2 and I3) transcripts were retrieved from the 3 transcriptomes. A total of 20 members were identified, in which most (13 sequences) belonged to the I2-superfamily and possessed the typical post-peptide and pro-region-free structure. These I-superfamily conotoxins generally had various signal regions and cysteine-rich frameworks, of which 11 exhibited the representative XI (C-C-CC-CC-C-C) pattern and 7 possessed the XII (C-C-C-C-CC-C-C) pattern, whereas only 2 had the framework VI/VII (C-C-CC-C-C) with distinct signal sequences and loop length (Tables 3–5).

Concerning the A-superfamily, 18 conotoxins were determined with 15 sequences of the common I (CC-C-C) pattern, and 3 transcripts with only 3 cysteine residues (the CC-C framework). In contrast to notable abundance and variety of A-superfamily conotoxins in previously reported piscivorous species [54–56], the number and diversity of the A-superfamily identified from these 3 vermivorous species were scarce. Meanwhile, 15 T-superfamily conotoxins were also identified; however, most of them exhibited the simple V (CC-CC) framework with high identity to several known τ-conotoxins, and only one contained the XVI (C-C-CC) framework.

In addition to the abovementioned major superfamilies, many less representative B1 (conontokin)-, C (contulakin)-, D-, J-, L-, P-, S-, V-, Y-superfamilies and the con-ikot-ikot family were also discovered in the 3 transcriptomes. For example, 6 conontokin sequences and 2 contulakin sequences with the cysteine free pattern were identified in this study. Three D-superfamily sequences with the XII (C-CC-C-CC-C-C-C-C) and XV (C-C-CC-C-C-C-C) patterns, 3 V-superfamily sequences with the XV (C-C-CC-C-C-C-C) pattern, and 2 Y-superfamily sequences with the XVII (C-C-CC-C-CC-C) pattern were also observed; interestingly, these 3 superfamilies have been isolated only from vermivorous cone snails to date [57]. Meanwhile, 2 con-ikot-ikot peptides with the novel CC-C-C-C-CC-C-C-C and CC-C-C-C-CC-C-C-C-C frameworks were identified. Con-ikot-ikot toxins were reported to specifically target post-synaptic AMPA receptors [58], but in consideration of the complex cysteine patterns and variable loop length, the functions of both conotoxins with new cysteine frameworks are worth investigating further.

In this study, combined with our published report of *C. betulinus* [32], we also identified 45 putative unassigned conotoxins, which possessed the IX (C-C-C-C-C-C) cysteine framework and loop lengths same as Cal9.1a~d from *Californiconus californicus* [3,59]. In fact, Cal9.1a~d contained unassigned signal peptide sequences, and their loop lengths and mature regions appeared to be sufficiently distinct from other known conotoxins. This group of conotoxins was previously found only in *Californiconus californicus*, an unusual species with special prey-capture behavior and prey preferences, and phylogenetic analysis also indicated that *Californiconus californicus* has large evolutionary distance from the *Conus* species [60]. The experts at WoRMS placed this genus *Californiconus* in the family Conidae, but as indicated it is highly divergent from the Conidae; hence, some researchers have placed this genus in a proposed separate (sub)family [1]. Our present work confirmed that these types of conotoxins are possibly synthesized in various species with different feeding habits; therefore, they may represent a new superfamily with potential specificity in pharmacological activity (Figure 4).

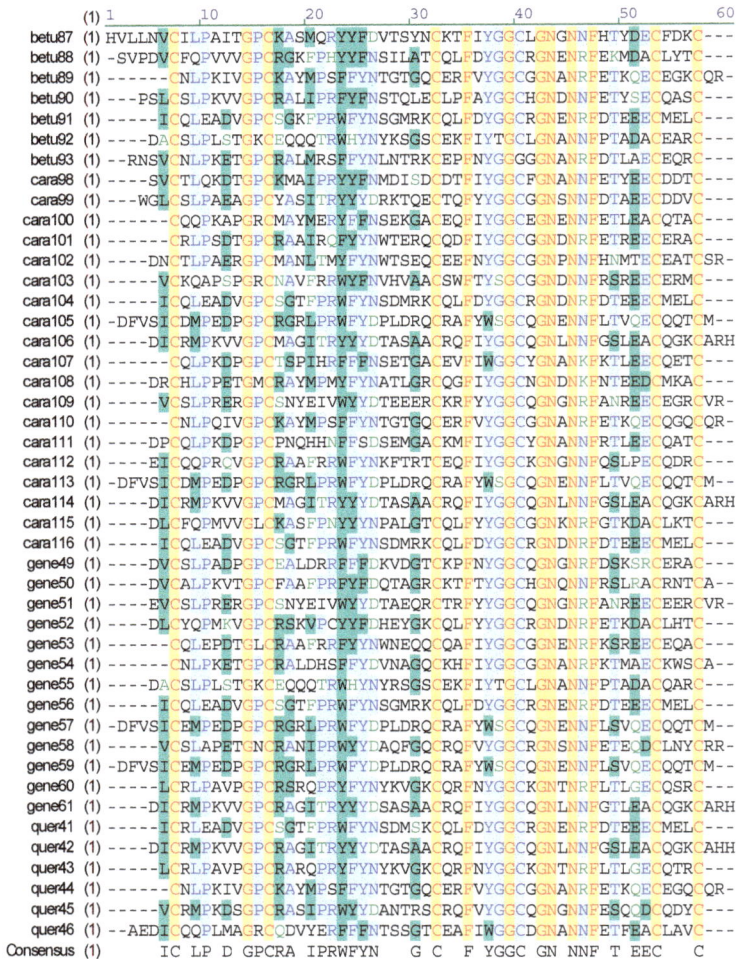

```
              (1) 1        10        20        30        40        50        60
betu87  (1) HVLLNVCILPAITGPCKASMQRYYFDVTSYNCKTFIYGGCLGNGNNFHTYDECFDKC---
betu88  (1) -SVPDVCFQPVVVGPCRGKFPHYYFNSILATCQLFDYGGCRGNENRFEKMDACLYTC---
betu89  (1) ------CNLPKIVGPCKAYMPSFFYNTGTGQCERFVYGGCGGNANRFETKQECEGKCQR-
betu90  (1) ---PSLCSLPKVVGPCRALIPRFYFNSTQLECLPFAYGGCHGNDNNFETYSECQASC---
betu91  (1) -----ICQLEADVGPCSGKFPRWFYNSGMRKCQLFDYGGCRGNENRFDTEEECMELC---
betu92  (1) ----DACSLPLSTGKCEQQQTRWHYNYKSGSCEKFIYTGCLGNANNFPTADACEARC---
betu93  (1) --RNSVCNLPKETGPCRALMRSFFYNLNTRKCEPFNYGGGGNANRFDTLAECEQRC---
cara98  (1) ----SVCTLQKDTGPCKMAIPRYYFNMDISDCDTFIYGGCFGNANNFETYEECDDTC---
cara99  (1) ---WGLCSLPAEAGPCYASITRYYYDRKTQECTQFYYGGCGGNSNNFDTAEECDDVC---
cara100 (1) ------CQQPKAPGRCMAYMERYFFNSEKGACEQFIYGGCENENNFETLEACQTAC---
cara101 (1) ------CRLPSDTGPCRAAIRQFYYNWTERQCQDFIYGGCGNDNRFETREECERAC---
cara102 (1) ----DNCTLPAERGPCMANLTMYFNWTSEQCEEFNYGGCQNPNANRFHNMTECEATCSR-
cara103 (1) -----VCKQAPSPGRCNAVFRRWYFNVHVAACSWFTYSGCGGNDNNFRSREECERMC---
cara104 (1) -----ICQLEADVGPCSGTFPRWFYNSDMRKCQLFDYGGCRGNDNRFDTEEECMELC---
cara105 (1) -DFVSICDMPEDPGPCRGRLPRWFYDPLDRQCRAFYWSGCQGNENNFLTVQECQQTCM--
cara106 (1) ----DICRMPKVVGPCMAGITRYYYDTASAACRQFIYGGCQGNLNNFGSLEACQGKCARH
cara107 (1) ------CQLPKDPGPCTSPIHRFFFNSETGACEVFIWGGCYGNANKFKTLEECQETC---
cara108 (1) ----DRCHLPPETGMCRAYMPMYFYNATLGRCQGFIYGGCNGNDNKFNTEEDCMKAC---
cara109 (1) -----VCSLPRERGPCSNYEIVWYYDTEEERCKRFYYGGCQGNGNRFANREECEGRCVR-
cara110 (1) ------CNLPQIVGPCKAYMPSFFYNTGTGQCERFVYGGCGGNANRFETKQECQGQCQR-
cara111 (1) ----DPCQLPKDPGPCPNQHHNFFSDSEMGACKMFIYGGCYGNANNFRTLEECQATC---
cara112 (1) ----EICQQPRCVGPCRAAFRRWFYNKFTRTCEQFIYGGCKGNGNNFQSLPECQDRC---
cara113 (1) -DFVSICDMPEDPGPCRGRLPRWFYDPLDRQCRAFYWSGCQGNENNFLTVQECQQTCM--
cara114 (1) ----DICRMPKVVGPCMAGITRYYYDTASAACRQFIYGGCQGNLNNFGSLEACQGKCARH
cara115 (1) ----DLCFQPMVVGLCKASFPNYYYNPALGTCQLFYYGGCGSNKNRFGTKDACLKTC---
cara116 (1) -----ICQLEADVGPCSGTFPRWFYNSDMRKCQLFDYGGCRGNDNRFDTEEECMELC---
gene49  (1) ----DVCSLPADPGPCEALDRRFFFDKVDGTCKPFNYGGCQGNENRFDSKSRCERAC---
gene50  (1) ----DVCALPKVTGPCFAAFPRFYFLDQTAGRCKTFTYGGCHGNQNNFRSLRACRNTCA--
gene51  (1) ----EVCSLPRERGPCSNYEIVWYYDTAEQRCTRFYYGGCQGNGNRFANREECEERCVR-
gene52  (1) ----DLCYQPMKVGPCRSKVPCYYFDHEYGKCQLFYYGGCRGNDNRFETKDACLHTC---
gene53  (1) ------CQLEPDTGLCRAAFRRFYYNWNEQQCQAFIYGGCGNENRFKSREECEQAC---
gene54  (1) ------CNLPKETGPCRALDHSFFYLDVNAGQCKHFIYGGCGNANRFKTMAECKWSCA--
gene55  (1) ----DACSLPLSTGKCEQQQTRWHYNYRSGSCEKFIYTGCLGNANNFPTADACQARC---
gene56  (1) -----ICQLEADVGPCSGTFPRWFYNSGMRKCQLFDYGGCRGNENRFDTEEECMELC---
gene57  (1) -DFVSICEMPEDPGPCRGRLPRWFYDPLDRQCRAFYWSGCQGNENNFLSVQECQQTCM--
gene58  (1) -----VCSLAPETGNCRANIPRWYYDAQFGQCRQFVYGGCRGNSNNFETEQDCLNYCRR-
gene59  (1) -DFVSICEMPEDPGPCRGRLPRWFYDPLDRQCRAFYWSGCQGNENNFLSVQECQQTCM--
gene60  (1) ----LCRLPAVPGPCRSRQPRYFYNYKVGKCQRFNYGGCKGNTNRFLTLGECQSRC---
gene61  (1) ----DICRMPKVVGPCRAGITRYYYDSASAACRQFIYGGCQGNLNNFGTLEACQGKCARH
quer41  (1) -----ICRLEADVGPCSGTFPRWFYNSDMSKCQLFDYGGCRGNENRFDTEEECMELC---
quer42  (1) ----DICRMPKVVGPCRAGITRYYYDTASAACRQFIYGGCQGNLNNFGSLEACQGKCAHH
quer43  (1) ----LCRLPAVPGPCRARQPRYFYNYKVGKCQRFNYGGCKGNTNRFLTLGECQTRC---
quer44  (1) ------CNLPKIVGPCKAYMPSFFYNTGTGQCERFVYGGCGGNANRFETKQECEGQCQR-
quer45  (1) -----VCRMPKDSGPCRASIPRWYYDANTRSCRQFVYGGCQNGNGNNFESQQDCQDYC---
quer46  (1) --AEDICQQPLMAGRCQDVYERFFFNTSSGTCEAFIWGGCDGNANNFETFEACLAVC---
Consensus (1)        IC LP D GPCRA IPRWFYN  G C  F YGGC GN NNF T EEC   C
```

Figure 4. Alignment of the achieved new superfamily conotoxins from venom duct transcriptomes of *C. betulinus* [32] (betu), *C. caracteristicus* (cara), *C. generalis* (gene), and *C. quercinus* (quer).

2.5. Identification of Conotoxin Biosynthesis Related Proteins

Transcripts for genes encoding functional proteins that are potentially involved in conotoxin biosynthesis were also annotated in the 3 transcriptome datasets. By homology comparison to known post-translational modification enzymes, we presumed that multiple proteins possess enzymatic activities for involvement in conotoxin maturation and modification in the venom duct lumen. From the transcriptomes, we also identified some isoforms of endoprotease, including sequences with high similarity to Tex31 [61], which has the hydrolytic activity to separate mature conotoxins from the precursor constituents.

Formation of disulfides is the most ubiquitous modification within conotoxins. This process and related proper peptide-folding are mediated by protein disulfide isomerases (PDIs), peptidyl-prolyl cis-trans isomerases, immunoglobulin-binding proteins, and chaperones (e.g., hsp70, hsp60, and calreticulin) [33]. All of these proteins, especially multi-isoforms of PDI were identified (Supplementary Tables S1–S3). Complete sequences of peptidylglycine alpha-amidating monooxygenase with two domains were identified as well, which may mediate the C-terminal amidation process for the full activity of various neuroactive peptides [62]. In addition, other candidate enzymes participating in post- translational modification were also predicted, such as prolyl/lysyl-hydroxylase, vitamin K-dependent γ-carboxylase, and Glutaminyl-peptide cyclotransferase.

Our data also revealed numerous sequences with potential roles in transportation, synergy, and degradation of conotoxins. Translocator-like sequences including the Sec family and diverse transmembrane proteins were discovered. In particular, we predicted several transcripts with high similarity to the Sec61 and Sec14 translocon that were identified in the spider venom duct with the ability to bind specific polypeptide toxins and to induce subsequent localization and transportation [63,64]. Large arrays of conotoxin-related proteins (widely existing in other animal venoms) with high transcription levels were also predicted. These sequences include multiple enzymes, such as the phospholipase A2 (PLA2) family, nucleotidase and hyaluronidase, as most of them may have neurotoxic and cytotoxic activities themselves or participate in anti-hemostatic effects [65], and may enhance the diffusion of conotoxins and cooperate with them for prey capture or synergistic predator defense. Meanwhile, many proteins homologous to the ubiquitin and ubiquitylation system were retrieved from the 3 transcriptome datasets in this study. These proteins may contribute to the degradation of poor-quality conotoxin molecules synthesized in the venom duct, which will ensure the effectiveness of venom to a higher degree in the prey capture process [66] (Supplementary Table S5).

3. Discussion

A total of 118, 61, and 48 putative conotoxin transcripts were identified from the 3 transcriptome datasets of *C. caracteristicus, C. generalis,* and *C. quercinus,* respectively. Given that these *Conus* species have similar feeding habits and distribution (in the offshore waters of the South China Sea), the interspecific divergence in toxin numbers and transcription levels were beyond our expectation. The interspecies variability of venom may contribute to the dietary preferences for different worms. Furthermore, the conotoxin composition in the venom duct of *C. quercinus* from this study was only 23% (11 of 48), identical to our previous report [39]. This remarkable variance of conotoxin types in the same species, especially in the same organ and using the same sequencing method, may be due to differences between *Conus* individuals that were from different geographical populations or at different developmental stages (for a more detailed discussion, please refer to our previous report on *C. betulinus* [32]). The intraspecies variability of venom composition has also been recently observed by other researchers, who recommended sequencing transcriptomes of more than one individual for the solid analysis of the conotoxin inventory in any examined species [67]. In addition, we also identified some identical conotoxin sequences from different *Conus* species; this convergent evolution trend is widespread presented among various *Conus* species with diverse phylogenetic clades. Related biological significance needs more investigation.

Conotoxins have a variety of mechanisms for actions, which however have been limited by the lack of high-throughput functional screening methods; therefore, most of them have not been determined by far. In this study, we attempted to apply the phylogenetic analysis strategy to explore the evolutionary relationships of these highly transcribed O-superfamily members, and then predicted their potential bioactivities. Among the top 10 conotoxins with the highest FPKM values in the 3 *Conus* species, 4 O-superfamily conotoxins formed monophyletic clades with several known pharmacological conotoxins, but the poor Posterior probabilities (0.30~0.69) at the nodes do not support related bioactivity prediction. The detailed functions of these high-abundance conotoxins in predation or defense deserve further investigation (such as by patch-clamp detection). Construction of electrophysiological platforms for the analysis of multiple neural ion channels and receptors is underway in our laboratory, which in turn proposes a potential hope for the development of novel conotoxin-based marine drugs for the treatment of neuroreceptor associated human diseases.

This study also identified many complete and partial sequences of 11 enzymes, which are potentially involved in the post-translational modification of conotoxins, as well as numerous functional proteins that may be related to the conotoxin biosynthesis processes including translation, protein folding, translocation, delivery and degradation. Gene Ontology (GO) functional classification (Supplementary Table S5) showed that conotoxin synthesis may be closely related to binding, catalytic activity, metabolic process and cellular process. The abundance of functional proteins underscores the fact that the venom duct is a metabolically active organ. Although there have been many reports on various novel conotoxins, our present work improves the understanding of conotoxin biosynthesis processes in vivo, which may provide insights into the fundamental mechanisms underlying the generation of complexly modified peptides in general.

4. Materials and Methods

4.1. Sample Collection, RNA Extraction and Sequencing

C. caracteristicus, *C. quercinus*, and *C. generalis* were collected in the offshore areas of Sanya City, Hainan Province, China. Specimen identification (using *COI* gene sequences [39]) was performed after they were collected and dissected on ice. Three intact venom ducts were separated and the total RNAs were extracted using TRIzol® LS Reagent (Invitrogen, Life Technologies, Carlsbad, CA, USA) following the manufacturer's instructions. Total RNAs were further treated with oligo-(dT)- attached magnetic beads (Invitrogen, Life Technologies, Carlsbad, CA, USA) to extract the mRNAs. Three non-normalized Illumina cDNA libraries were constructed separately and sequenced on the Illumina HiSeq2000 platform (Illumina, San Diego, CA, USA) by BGI-Tech (BGI, Shenzhen, China).

4.2. Sequence Analysis and Assembling

Raw sequencing reads from the 3 sets of transcriptome sequencing were cleaned up using SOAPnuke software (BGI, Shenzhen, Guangdong, China) [68] to ensure high quality for downstream analyses. Adapters and reads with over 10% of non-sequenced (N) bases or more than 50% of low-quality bases (base quality ≤ 10) were removed. Then the filtered reads were assembled into unigenes with SOAPdenovo-Trans v1.02 (BGI, Shenzhen, Guangdong, China) for *de novo* transcriptome assembling [69]. The FPKM value, a general parameter for quantification of gene transcription, was calculated for comparison [70].

4.3. Prediction and Identification of Conotoxins

All previously known conotoxins in the ConoServer database [19] were downloaded to construct a local reference dataset for conotoxin prediction from our 3 transcriptome datasets using the traditional homology search method. Subsequently, unigenes from each transcriptome were run against the local conotoxin dataset using Genewise v2.4.1 [71] and Agustus v2.7 [72] with an E-value of 1.0×10^{-5}. Those unigenes with the best hits were translated into peptide sequences. A conotoxin generally consists of a highly conserved N-terminal signal peptide region, a less conserved intervening pro-peptide region, and a hypervariable C-terminal mature peptide region with conserved cysteine patterns [73,74]. A few conotoxins also have a post-peptide region at the C-terminal after the mature peptide region [75]. The predicted conotoxin transcripts were manually inspected using the ConoServer's web-based ConoPrec and NCBI's blastp. Those transcripts with duplication or truncated mature region sequences were removed.

4.4. Classification of Conotoxin Superfamilies

The distinct regions and cysteine frameworks of these predicted conotoxins were analyzed using the ConoServer's web-based ConoPrec. Based on 75% identity in the conserved signal peptide sequences [57], these identified conotoxins could be assigned to most of the 27 known superfamilies in the ConoServer. The particular threshold values for I1, I2, L, M, P, S, con-ikot-ikot and divergent superfamilies were 71.85%, 57.6%, 67.5%, 69.3%, 69.1%, 72.9%, 64.5 $\pm$ 20.2%, and 64.22 $\pm$ 20.53%, respectively [33]. Those conotoxins without signal regions but still showing high similarity either in the proregion or mature region were considered as the "Unknown" group.

4.5. Annotation of Predicted Functional Proteins

Unigenes were firstly translated into amino acids in six frames and aligned with BLASTX to public protein databases (E-value $\leq 1.0 \times 10^{-5}$) including NCBI non-redundant (Nr), Swiss-Prot [76], and Clusters of Orthologous Groups (COG) [77]. The protein with the highest sequence similarity was retrieved and annotated to each unigene. For the Nr annotation, Blast2GO v4.1 (Instituto Valenciano de Investigaciones Agrarias, Moncada, Valencia, Spain) [78] was used to determine GO annotation, which was defined by molecular function, cellular component, and biological process ontologies.

4.6. Phylogenetic Inference of Abundant Conotoxins

Bayesian analyses of the combined data were performed with MrBayes v.2.01 (University of Rochester, Rochester, NY, USA) [79] using the best-fit model indicated by Modeltest 3.06 (Brigham Young University, Provo, UT, USA) [80]. A Metropolis-coupled Markov Chain Monte Carlo algorithm running four Markov chains simultaneously was employed to estimate the posterior probability of phylogenetic trees. Each Markov chain was initiated with a random tree and run for 1,000,000 generations, sampling every 100 generations for a total of 10,000 samples per run. The first 2,500 samples of each run were discarded as burn-in, and the remaining samples were applied to construct a consensus tree using PAUP*4.0 (Florida State University, Tallahassee, FL, USA) [81].

4.7. Availability of Supporting Data

The datasets supporting the results of this article are included within the article and its supplementary files. The transcriptome reads generated in this study have been deposited in China National GeneBank Nucleotide Sequence Archive with accession numbers of CNS0048931 for *C. caracteristicus*, CNS0048933 for *C. generalis*, and CNS0048932 for *C. quercinus* under the project CNP0000360.

5. Conclusions

In this report, we have examined the diverse transcription repertoire in the venom ducts of 3 vermivorous cone snails, which are resident in the offshore waters of the South China Sea. We not only succeeded in characterizing the abundant conotoxin-encoding transcripts across 22 known superfamilies and 1 new superfamily, but also identified a variety of functional proteins that may be responsible for biosynthesis and delivery of these conotoxins. As expected, the majority of the identified conotoxins were novel, based on their transcript sequences, and some possessed new cysteine frameworks and divergent signal regions. Comparison analysis indicated surprising interspecific and intraspecific divergences in the conotoxin numbers and transcription levels, thus we made a primary conclusion that the abundant O-superfamily conotoxins in all 3 venom duct transcriptomes probably play major roles in the prey capture strategy of these vermivorous species. Our study with various cone snail species provides new insights into the complex biosynthesis mechanisms that lead to the remarkable variability of the venom composition. Our present work adds more conotoxins, which will definitely improve our genetic resource to develop new drugs.

Supplementary Materials: The following materials are available online at http://www.mdpi.com/1660-3397/17/3/193/s1. Table S1: Protein sequences of the putative conotoxin transcripts identified from *C. caracteristicus*. Table S2: Protein sequences of the putative conotoxin transcripts identified from *C. generalis*. Table S3: Protein sequences of the putative conotoxin transcripts identified from *C. quercinus*. Table S4: The top 10 conotoxins with the highest FPKM values in the 3 transcriptome datasets. Table S5: Conotoxin biosynthesis-related proteins identified from the 3 venom duct transcriptomes.

Author Contributions: Q.S., Y.C., and J.C. conceived and designed the project; G.Y., C.P., and Y.Z. analyzed the data; G.Y. and C.P. prepared the manuscript; Q.S., Y.C., C.F., and H.J. revised the manuscript. All authors approved submission of the final manuscript.

Funding: This work was supported by Shenzhen Special Project for High-Level Talents (No. SZYSGZZ-2018001), Shenzhen Dapeng Special Program for Industrial Development (No. PT20170302), and China 863 Project (No. 2014AA093501).

Conflicts of Interest: The authors declare no conflict of interest.

References

1. World Register of Marine Species. Available online: http://www.marinespecies.org (accessed on 21 January 2019).
2. Puillandre, N.; Bouchet, P.; Duda, T.F., Jr.; Kauferstein, S.; Kohn, A.J.; Olivera, B.M.; Watkins, M.; Meyer, C. Molecular phylogeny and evolution of the cone snails (Gastropoda, Conoidea). *Mol. Phylogenet. Evol.* **2014**, *78*, 290–303. [CrossRef]
3. Puillandre, N.; Duda, T.F.; Meyer, C.; Olivera, B.M.; Bouchet, P. One, four or 100 genera? A new classification of the cone snails. *J. Molluscan Stud.* **2015**, *81*, 1–23. [CrossRef]
4. Prashanth, J.R.; Dutertre, S.; Jin, A.H.; Lavergne, V.; Hamilton, B.; Cardoso, F.C.; Griffin, J.; Venter, D.J.; Alewood, P.F.; Lewis, R.J. The role of defensive ecological interactions in the evolution of conotoxins. *Mol. Ecol.* **2016**, *25*, 598–615. [CrossRef] [PubMed]
5. Himaya, S.W.; Jin, A.H.; Dutertre, S.; Giacomotto, J.; Mohialdeen, H.; Vetter, I.; Alewood, P.F.; Lewis, R.J. Comparative venomics reveals the complex prey capture strategy of the piscivorous cone snail *Conus catus*. *J. Proteom. Res.* **2015**, *14*, 4372–4381. [CrossRef] [PubMed]
6. Lewis, R.J.; Dutertre, S.; Vetter, I.; Christie, M.J. *Conus* venom peptide pharmacology. *Pharmacol. Rev.* **2012**, *64*, 259–298. [CrossRef]
7. Gao, B.; Peng, C.; Chen, Q.; Zhang, J.; Shi, Q. Mitochondrial genome sequencing of a vermivorous cone snail *Conus quercinus* supports the correlative analysis between phylogenetic relationships and dietary types of *Conus* species. *PLoS ONE* **2018**, *13*, e0193053. [CrossRef]
8. Aman, J.W.; Imperial, J.S.; Ueberheide, B.; Zhang, M.M.; Aguilar, M.; Taylor, D.; Watkins, M.; Yoshikami, D.; Showers-Corneli, P.; Safavi-Hemami, H.; et al. Insights into the origins of fish hunting in venomous cone snails from studies of *Conus tessulatus*. *Proc. Natl. Acad. Sci. USA* **2015**, *112*, 5087–5092. [CrossRef]
9. Robinson, S.D.; Safavi-Hemami, H.; McIntosh, L.D.; Purcell, A.W.; Norton, R.S.; Papenfuss, A.T. Diversity of conotoxin gene superfamilies in the venomous snail, *Conus victoriae*. *PLoS ONE* **2014**, *9*, e87648. [CrossRef] [PubMed]
10. Kumar, P.S.; Kumar, D.S.; Umamaheswari, S. A perspective on toxicology of *Conus* venom peptides. *Asian Pac. J. Trop. Med.* **2015**, *8*, 337–351. [CrossRef]
11. Kohn, A.J. *Conus* envenomation of humans: In fact and fiction. *Toxins* **2019**, *11*, 10. [CrossRef]
12. Olivera, B.M. *Conus* venom peptides, receptor and ion channel targets and drug design: 50 million years of neuropharmacology. *Mol. Biol. Cell.* **1997**, *8*, 2101–2109. [CrossRef] [PubMed]
13. Dutertre, S.; Jin, A.H.; Vetter, I.; Hamilton, B.; Sunagar, K.; Lavergne, V.; Dutertre, V.; Fry, B.G.; Antunes, A.; Venter, D.J.; et al. Evolution of separate predation- and defence-evoked venoms in carnivorous cone snails. *Nat. Commun.* **2014**, *5*, 3521. [CrossRef] [PubMed]
14. Endean, R.; Duchemin, C. The venom apparatus of *Conus magus*. *Toxicon* **1967**, *4*, 275–284. [CrossRef]
15. Safavi-Hemami, H.; Li, Q.; Jackson, R.L.; Song, A.S.; Boomsma, W.; Bandyopadhyay, P.K.; Gruber, C.W.; Purcell, A.W.; Yandell, M.; Olivera, B.M.; et al. Rapid expansion of the protein disulfide isomerase gene family facilitates the folding of venom peptides. *Proc. Natl. Acad. Sci. USA* **2016**, *113*, 3227–3232. [CrossRef] [PubMed]

16. Neves, J.; Campos, A.; Osório, H.; Antunes, A.; Vasconcelos, V. Conopeptides from Cape Verde *Conus crotchii*. *Mar. Drugs* **2013**, *11*, 2203–2215. [CrossRef] [PubMed]

17. Phuong, M.A.; Mahardika, G.N.; Alfaro, M.E. Dietary breadth is positively correlated with venom complexity in cone snails. *BMC Genomics* **2016**, *17*, 401. [CrossRef] [PubMed]

18. Kaas, Q.; Westermann, J.C.; Halai, R.; Wang, C.K.; Craik, D.J. ConoServer, a database for conopeptide sequences and structures. *Bioinformatics* **2007**, *24*, 445–446. [CrossRef] [PubMed]

19. Kaas, Q.; Yu, R.; Jin, A.H.; Dutertre, S.; Craik, D.J. ConoServer: Updated content, knowledge, and discovery tools in the conopeptide database. *Nucleic Acids Res.* **2012**, *40*, D325–D330. [CrossRef]

20. Terlau, H.; Olivera, B.M. *Conus* venoms: A rich source of novel ion channel-targeted peptides. *Physiol. Rev.* **2004**, *84*, 41–68. [CrossRef]

21. Tosti, E.; Boni, R.; Gallo, A. μ-Conotoxins modulating sodium currents in pain perception and transmission: A therapeutic potential. *Mar. Drugs* **2017**, *15*, 295. [CrossRef]

22. Barton, M.E.; White, H.S.; Wilcox, K.S. The effect of CGX-1007 and CI-1041, novel NMDA receptor antagonists, on NMDA receptor-mediated EPSCs. *Epilepsy Res.* **2004**, *59*, 13–24. [CrossRef]

23. Romero, H.K.; Christensen, S.B.; Di Cesare Mannelli, L.; Gajewiak, J.; Ramachandra, R.; Elmslie, K.S.; Vetter, D.E.; Ghelardini, C.; Iadonato, S.P.; Mercado, J.L.; et al. Inhibition of alpha9alpha10 nicotinic acetylcholine receptors prevents chemotherapy-induced neuropathic pain. *Proc. Natl. Acad. Sci. USA* **2017**, *114*, 1825–1832. [CrossRef]

24. Hannon, H.E.; Atchison, W.D. Omega-conotoxins as experimental tools and therapeutics in pain management. *Mar. Drugs* **2013**, *11*, 680. [CrossRef]

25. Crooks, P.A.; Bardo, M.T.; Dwoskin, L.P. Nicotinic receptor antagonists as treatments for nicotine abuse. *Adv. Pharmacol.* **2014**, *69*, 513–551.

26. Gandini, M.A.; Sandoval, A.; Felix, R. Toxins targeting voltage-activated Ca2+ channels and their potential biomedical applications. *Curr. Top. Med. Chem.* **2015**, *15*, 604–616. [CrossRef] [PubMed]

27. Vetter, I.; Lewis, R.J. Therapeutic potential of cone snail venom peptides (conopeptides). *Curr. Top. Med. Chem.* **2012**, *12*, 1546–1552. [CrossRef] [PubMed]

28. Layer, R.T.; Mcintosh, J.M. Conotoxins: Therapeutic potential and application. *Mar. Drugs* **2006**, *4*, 119–142. [CrossRef]

29. Han, T.S.; Teichert, R.W.; Olivera, B.M.; Bulaj, G. *Conus* venoms-a rich source of peptide-based therapeutics. *Curr. Pharm. Des.* **2008**, *14*, 2462–2479. [CrossRef] [PubMed]

30. Olivera, B.M.; Teichert, R.W. Diversity of the neurotoxic *Conus* peptides: A model for concerted pharmacological discovery. *Mol. Interv.* **2007**, *7*, 251–260. [CrossRef]

31. Fedosov, A.E.; Moshkovskii, S.A.; Kuznetsova, K.G.; Olivera, B.M. Conotoxins: From the biodiversity of gastropods to new drugs. *Biomed. Khim.* **2013**, *59*, 267–294. [CrossRef]

32. Peng, C.; Yao, G.; Gao, B.M.; Fan, C.X.; Bian, C.; Wang, J.; Cao, Y.; Wen, B.; Zhu, Y.; Ruan, Z.; et al. High-throughput identification of novel conotoxins from the Chinese tubular cone snail (*Conus betulinus*) by multi-transcriptome sequencing. *Gigascience* **2016**, *5*, 17. [CrossRef] [PubMed]

33. Barghi, N.; Concepcion, G.P.; Olivera, B.M.; Lluisma, A.O. High conopeptide diversity in *Conus tribblei* revealed through analysis of venom duct transcriptome using two high-throughput sequencing platforms. *Mar. Biotechnol.* **2015**, *17*, 81–98. [CrossRef] [PubMed]

34. Dutertre, S.; Jin, A.H.; Kaas, Q.; Jones, A.; Alewood, P.F.; Lewis, R.J. Deep venomics reveals the mechanism for expanded peptide diversity in cone snail venom. *Mol. Cell. Proteom.* **2013**, *12*, 312–329. [CrossRef]

35. Lavergne, V.; Harliwong, I.; Jones, A.; Miller, D.; Taft, R.J.; Alewood, P.F. Optimized deep-targeted proteotranscriptomic profiling reveals unexplored *Conus* toxin diversity and novel cysteine frameworks. *Proc. Natl. Acad. Sci. USA* **2015**, *112*, 3782–3791. [CrossRef] [PubMed]

36. Biass, D.; Dutertre, S.; Gerbault, A.; Menou, J.L.; Offord, R.; Favreau, P.; Stöcklin, R. Comparative proteomic study of the venom of the piscivorous cone snail *Conus consors*. *J. Proteome* **2009**, *72*, 210–218. [CrossRef]

37. Davis, J.; Jones, A.; Lewis, R.J. Remarkable inter- and intra-species complexity of conotoxins revealed by LC/MS. *Peptides* **2009**, *30*, 1222–1227. [CrossRef]

38. Gao, B.; Peng, C.; Yang, J.; Yi, Y.; Zhang, J.; Shi, Q. Cone snails: A big store of conotoxins for novel drug discovery. *Toxins* **2017**, *9*, 397. [CrossRef] [PubMed]

39. Gao, B.; Peng, C.; Zhu, Y.; Sun, Y.; Zhao, T.; Huang, Y.; Shi, Q. High throughput identification of novel conotoxins from the Vermivorous Oak cone snail (*Conus quercinus*) by transcriptome sequencing. *Int. J. Mol. Sci.* **2018**, *19*, 3901. [CrossRef] [PubMed]

40. Zhangsun, D.; Luo, S.; Wu, Y.; Zhu, X.; Hu, Y.; Xie, L. Novel O-superfamily conotoxins identified by cDNA cloning from three vermivorous *Conus* species. *Chem. Biol. Drug Des.* **2006**, *68*, 256–265. [CrossRef] [PubMed]

41. Liu, L.; Wu, X.; Yuan, D.; Chi, C.; Wang, C. Identification of a novel S-superfamily conotoxin from vermivorous *Conus caracteristicus*. *Toxicon* **2008**, *51*, 1331–1337. [CrossRef]

42. Yuan, D.D.; Liu, L.; Shao, X.X.; Peng, C.; Chi, C.W.; Guo, Z.Y. Isolation and cloning of a conotoxin with a novel cysteine pattern from *Conus caracteristicus*. *Peptides* **2008**, *29*, 1521–1525. [CrossRef]

43. Yuan, D.D.; Liu, L.; Shao, X.X.; Peng, C.; Chi, C.W.; Guo, Z.Y. New conotoxins define the novel I3-superfamily. *Peptides* **2009**, *30*, 861–865. [CrossRef]

44. Luo, S.; Zhangsun, D.; Harvey, P.J.; Kaas, Q.; Wu, Y.; Zhu, X.; Hu, Y.; Li, X.; Tsetlin, V.I.; Christensen, S.; et al. Cloning, synthesis, and characterization of αO-conotoxin GeXIVA, a potent α9α10 nicotinic acetylcholine receptor antagonist. *Proc. Natl. Acad. Sci. USA* **2015**, *112*, 4026–4035. [CrossRef]

45. Xu, S.; Zhang, T.; Kompella, S.N.; Yan, M.; Lu, A.; Wang, Y.; Shao, X.; Chi, C.; Adams, D.J.; Ding, J.; et al. Conotoxin αD-GeXXA utilizes a novel strategy to antagonize nicotinic acetylcholine receptors. *Sci. Rep.* **2015**, *5*, 14261. [CrossRef] [PubMed]

46. Jiang, S.; Tae, H.S.; Xu, S.; Shao, X.; Adams, D.J.; Wang, C. Identification of a novel O-conotoxin reveals an unusual and potent inhibitor of the human α9α10 nicotinic acetylcholine receptor. *Mar. Drugs* **2017**, *15*, 170. [CrossRef] [PubMed]

47. Kits, K.S.; Lodder, J.C.; van der Schors, R.C.; Li, K.W.; Geraerts, W.P.; Fainzilber, M. Novel omega-conotoxins block dihydropyridine-insensitive high voltage-activated calcium channels in molluscan neurons. *J. Neurochem.* **1996**, *67*, 2155–2163. [CrossRef]

48. Terlau, H.; Shon, K.J.; Grilley, M.; Stocker, M.; Stuhmer, W.; Olivera, B.M. Strategy for rapid immobilization of prey by a fish-hunting marine snail. *Nature* **1996**, *381*, 148–151. [CrossRef] [PubMed]

49. Fainzilber, M.; Nakamura, T.; Lodder, J.C.; Zlotkin, E.; Kits, K.S.; Burlingame, A.L. gamma-Conotoxin-PnVIIA, a gamma-carboxyglutamate-containing peptide agonist of neuronal pacemaker cation currents. *Biochemistry* **1998**, *37*, 1470–1477. [CrossRef] [PubMed]

50. Fainzilber, M.; Gordon, D.; Hasson, A.; Spira, M.E.; Zlotkin, E. Mollusc-specific toxins from the venom of *Conus textile* neovicarius. *Eur. J. Biochem.* **1991**, *202*, 589–595. [CrossRef]

51. Pi, C.; Liu, J.; Peng, C.; Liu, Y.; Jiang, X.; Zhao, Y.; Tang, S.; Wang, L.; Dong, M.; Chen, S.; et al. Diversity and evolution of conotoxins based on gene expression profiling of *Conus litteratus*. *Genomics* **2006**, *88*, 809–819. [CrossRef]

52. Luo, S.; Zhangsun, D.; Zhang, B.; et al. Novel O-Superfamily conotoxins, and their coding polynucleotides and use. Patent CN (200410103561.0)-A, 30 December 2004.

53. Luo, S.; Zhangsun, D.; Feng, J.; Wu, Y.; Zhu, X.; Hu, Y. Diversity of the O-superfamily conotoxins from *Conus miles*. *J. Pept. Sci.* **2007**, *13*, 44–53. [CrossRef] [PubMed]

54. Hu, H.; Bandyopadhyay, P.K.; Olivera, B.M.; Yandell, M. Characterization of the *Conus bullatus* genome and its venom-duct transcriptome. *BMC Genomics* **2011**, *12*, 60. [CrossRef] [PubMed]

55. Terrat, Y.; Biass, D.; Dutertre, S.; Favreau, P.; Remm, M.; Stöcklin, R.; Piquemal, D.; Ducancel, F. High-resolution picture of a venom duct transcriptome: case study with the marine snail *Conus consors*. *Toxicon* **2012**, *59*, 34–46. [CrossRef]

56. Hu, H.; Bandyopadhyay, P.K.; Olivera, B.M.; Yandell, M. Elucidation of the molecular envenomation strategy of the cone snail *Conus geographus* through transcriptome sequencing of its venom duct. *BMC Genomics* **2012**, *13*, 284. [CrossRef] [PubMed]

57. Kaas, Q.; Westermann, J.C.; Craik, D.J. Conopeptide characterization and classifications: An analysis using ConoServer. *Toxicon* **2010**, *55*, 1491–1509. [CrossRef] [PubMed]

58. Walker, C.S.; Jensen, S.; Ellison, M.; Matta, J.A.; Lee, W.Y.; Imperial, J.S.; Duclos, N.; Brockie, P.J.; Madsen, D.M.; Isaac, J.T.; et al. A novel *Conus* snail polypeptide causes excitotoxicity by blocking desensitization of AMPA receptors. *Curr. Biol.* **2009**, *19*, 900–908. [CrossRef] [PubMed]

59. Elliger, C.A.; Richmond, T.A.; Lebaric, Z.N. Diversity of conotoxin types from *Conus californicus* reflects a diversity of prey types and a novel evolutionary history. *Toxicon* **2011**, *57*, 311–322. [CrossRef] [PubMed]

60. Biggs, J.S.; Watkins, M.; Puillandre, N.; Ownby, J.P.; Lopez-Vera, E.; Christensen, S.; Moreno, K.J.; Bernaldez, J.; Licea-Navarro, A.; Corneli, P.S.; et al. Evolution of *Conus* peptide toxins: analysis of *Conus californicus* Reeve, 1844. *Mol. Phylogenet. Evol.* **2010**, *56*, 1–12. [CrossRef] [PubMed]

61. Milne, T.J.; Abbenante, G.; Tyndall, J.D.; Halliday, J.; Lewis, R.J. Isolation and characterization of a cone snail protease with homology to CRISP proteins of the pathogenesis-related protein superfamily. *J. Biol. Chem.* **2003**, *278*, 31105–31110. [CrossRef] [PubMed]

62. Kang, T.S.; Vivekanandan, S.; Jois, S.D.; Kini, R.M. Effect of C-terminal amidation on folding and disulfide-pairing of alpha-conotoxin ImI. *Angew. Chem. Int. Ed. Engl.* **2005**, *44*, 6333–6337. [CrossRef]

63. Romisch, K. Surfing the Sec61 channel: Bidirectional protein translocation across the ER membrane. *J. Cell Sci.* **1999**, *112*, 4185–4191.

64. Stock, S.D.; Hama, H.; DeWald, D.B. SEC14-dependent secretion in Saccharomyces cerevisiae Nondependence on sphingolipid synthesis-coupled diacylglycerol production. *J. Biol. Chem.* **1999**, *274*, 12979–12983. [CrossRef]

65. Jiang, Y.; Li, Y.; Lee, W. Venom gland transcriptomes of two elapid snakes (*Bungarus multicinctus* and *Naja atra*) and evolution of toxin genes. *BMC Genomics* **2011**, *12*, 1. [CrossRef]

66. Ciechanover, A.; Iwai, K. The ubiquitin system: From basic mechanisms to the patient bed. *IUBMB Life* **2004**, *56*, 193–201. [CrossRef] [PubMed]

67. Abalde, S.; Tenorio, M.J.; Afonso, C.M.L.; Zardoya, R. Conotoxin diversity in *Chelyconus ermineus* (Born, 1778) and the convergent origin of piscivory in the Atlantic and Indo-Pacific cones. *Genome Biol. Evol.* **2018**, *10*, 2643–2662. [CrossRef]

68. Li, R.; Li, Y.; Kristiansen, K.; Wang, J. SOAP: Short oligonucleotide alignment program. *Bioinformatics* **2008**, *24*, 713–714. [CrossRef] [PubMed]

69. Xie, Y.; Wu, G.; Tang, J.; Luo, R.; Patterson, J.; Liu, S.; Zhou, X.; Lam, T.W.; Li, Y.; Xu, X.; et al. SOAPdenovo-Trans: *de novo* transcriptome assembly with short RNA-Seq reads. *Bioinformatics* **2014**, *30*, 1660–1666. [CrossRef]

70. Mortazavi, A.; Williams, B.A.; McCue, K.; Schaeffer, L.; Wold, B. Mapping and quantifying mammalian transcriptomes by RNA-seq. *Nat. Methods* **2008**, *5*, 621–628. [CrossRef]

71. Birney, E.; Clamp, M.; Durbin, R. GeneWise and Genomewise. *Genome Res.* **2004**, *14*, 988–995. [CrossRef] [PubMed]

72. Keller, O.; Kollmar, M.; Stanke, M.; Waack, S. A novel hybrid gene prediction method employing protein multiple sequence alignments. *Bioinformatics* **2011**, *27*, 757–763. [CrossRef]

73. Woodward, S.R.; Cruz, L.J.; Olivera, B.M.; Hillyard, D.R. Constant and hypervariable regions in conotoxin propeptides. *EMBO J.* **1990**, *9*, 1015–1020. [CrossRef] [PubMed]

74. Olivera, B.M.; Walker, C.; Cartier, G.E.; Hooper, D.; Santos, A.D.; Schoenfeld, R.; Shetty, R.; Watkins, M.; Bandyopadhyay, P.; Hillyard, D.R. Speciation of cone snails and interspecific hyperdivergence of their venom peptides. Potential evolutionary significance of introns. *Ann. N.Y. Acad. Sci.* **1999**, *870*, 223–237. [CrossRef] [PubMed]

75. Zamora-Bustillos, R.; Aguilar, M.B.; Falcón, A. Identification, by molecular cloning, of a novel type of I2-superfamily conotoxin precursor and two novel I2-conotoxins from the worm-hunter snail *Conus spurius* from the Gulf of México. *Peptides* **2010**, *31*, 384–393. [CrossRef]

76. Boeckmann, B.; Bairoch, A.; Apweiler, R.; Blatter, M.C.; Estreicher, A.; Gasteiger, E.; Martin, M.J.; Michoud, K.; O'Donovan, C.; Phan, I.; et al. The SWISS-PROT protein knowledgebase and its supplement TrEMBL in 2003. *Nucleic Acids Res.* **2003**, *31*, 365–370. [CrossRef] [PubMed]

77. Tatusov, R.L.; Galperin, M.Y.; Natale, D.A.; Koonin, E.V. The COG database: A tool for genome-scale analysis of protein functions and evolution. *Nucleic Acids Res.* **2000**, *28*, 33–36. [CrossRef] [PubMed]

78. Conesa, A.; Götz, S.; García-Gómez, J.M.; Terol, J.; Talón, M.; Robles, M. Blast2GO: A universal tool for annotation, visualization and analysis in functional genomics research. *Bioinformatics* **2005**, *21*, 3674–3676. [CrossRef]

79. Huelsenbeck, J.P.; Ronquist, F.R. MrBayes: Bayesian inference of phylogenic trees. *Bioinformatics* **2001**, *17*, 754–755. [CrossRef] [PubMed]

80. Posada, D.; Crandall, K.A. Selecting the best-fit model of nucleotide substitution. *Syst. Biol.* **2001**, *50*, 580–601. [CrossRef]

81. Swofford, D.L. *PAUP: Phylogenetic Analysis Using Parsimony (* And Other Methods)*; Version 4.0; Sinauer: Sunderland, MA, USA, 2001.

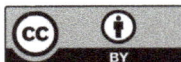

marine drugs

MDPI

Review

Structural and Functional Analyses of Cone Snail Toxins

Harry Morales Duque [1], Simoni Campos Dias [1] and Octávio Luiz Franco [1,2,*]

[1] Centro de Análises Proteômicas e Bioquímicas, Programa de Pós-Graduação em Ciências Genômicas e Biotecnologia, Universidade Católica de Brasília, Brasília-DF 70.790–160, Brazil; hamorales30042033@gmail.com (H.M.D.); si.camposdias@gmail.com (S.C.D.)
[2] S-inova Biotech, Programa de Pós-Graduação em Biotecnologia, Universidade Católica Dom Bosco, Campo Grande-MS 79.117–900, Brazil
* Correspondence: ocfranco@gmail.com

Received: 27 May 2019; Accepted: 17 June 2019; Published: 21 June 2019

Abstract: Cone snails are marine gastropod mollusks with one of the most powerful venoms in nature. The toxins, named conotoxins, must act quickly on the cone snails´ prey due to the fact that snails are extremely slow, reducing their hunting capability. Therefore, the characteristics of conotoxins have become the object of investigation, and as a result medicines have been developed or are in the trialing process. Conotoxins interact with transmembrane proteins, showing specificity and potency. They target ion channels and ionotropic receptors with greater regularity, and when interaction occurs, there is immediate physiological decompensation. In this review we aimed to evaluate the structural features of conotoxins and the relationship with their target types.

Keywords: cone snails; conotoxins; ion channels; function; structure

1. Introduction

Cone snails are marine mollusks from the Conidae family (Fleming, 1822 sensu lato), divided among 152 genera and involving 918 species described until now [1]. They are predatory carnivores that compensate for their slow movement by using hunting strategies with an arsenal of toxic peptides [2]. These molecules are known as conotoxins or conopeptides, with a wide variety of molecular masses ranging from conopressin-S with nine [3], to conkunitzin-S1 with 60, amino acid residues in length [4]. Due to their targets (i.e., Na^+, K^+, and Ca^{++} channels; ligand-gated ion channels; G-coupled proteins; and neurotransmitter transporters), conotoxins produce diverse physiological alterations, principally in excitable tissues [5]. These conotoxins are employed by cone snails to target their prey such as marine worms, snails and fish [6]. Because of the diverse species groups targeted by cone snails, their conotoxins need to act on specific targets of each species (e.g., subtype of ion channels) [7]. As previously studied, cone snails developed their toxins for hunting, but humans are not natural prey for them. However, accidents caused by cone snails' sting have resulted in human injuries, which have been lethal in some cases [8]. Thus it has been demonstrated that *Conus* spp. venom has toxic compounds that also act on specific mammal transmembrane proteins [5]. Transmembrane proteins, such as ion channels or ionotropic receptors, are responsible for basic neurotransmission or signal transduction, which triggers other physiologic functions [9,10]. When these transmembrane proteins are affected, multiple human diseases arise [11–13]. These ion channel disorders are sometimes called channelopathies [14]. The natural capability of conotoxins to target these objectives could be used for disease treatment [15]. Therefore, the pharmacological properties of conotoxins have become a valuable biotechnological tool for potential drug development [16,17].

Conotoxins are structurally variable in reference to their function [18]. Recently, conotoxin classification was addressed by categories (i.e., by gene superfamily or pharmacological family, by cysteine (Cys) framework and connectivity, by loop class, by fold and subfold classes) [19]. The superfamily group was classified based on the nucleic acid sequence from the toxin's signal peptides' identity [20]. Conotoxin cDNAs have been grouped into 41 different superfamilies (Table S1) [21]. The family classification is based on the target type and action mode of conotoxins, independently of their structural features [5]. The present review uses this categorization (Table 1).

Structurally, conotoxins are diverse and categorized by their mature peptide [20,22]. They can be linear peptides without a disulfide bond, like the conantokins [23], or may possess between one and five disulfide bonds [5]. Those with multiple disulfide bonds adopt special three-dimensional conformation due to a different Cys distribution pattern (framework) in the toxin sequence (Table S2) and Cys pair connectivity type [18]. Loop class is a category used to divide the α-conotoxin family into subclasses [24]. This subclassification will be further explained (see α-conotoxin section below) (Table 2). For conotoxins with disulfide bonds, characteristics such as the cysteine framework, their pair connectivity, and number of amino acids provide them with a fold structure that favors their activity [18,19,25]. Conotoxins' structural properties seem to be important for target interaction [25]. Importantly, other features are present in natural conotoxins such as the location of key amino acids on their primary sequence [5] and post-translational modifications, including amidation, sulfation, pyroglutamylation, γ-carboxylation, hydroxylation, O-glycosylation, and bromination [26]. On the whole, these features must be considered when analyzing conotoxin/target interaction.

The structure/function diversity in conotoxins makes research a challenge [27]. Computational analysis has been used improve the cost/benefit ratio in conotoxin studies [28], trying to solve this problem. Due to the variable nature of conotoxins, there is no consensus that allows the mentioned categories to be linked with the family classification (see Table S3) [29]. The distance between the activity and structural variability of conotoxins makes investigation complex [21]. However, it is deduced that for each target there is one conotoxin that has greater potency and affinity than others of its type. In the following section, conotoxin families will be briefly mentioned, emphasizing that these toxins are completely characterized by interaction with their target.

2. Conotoxin Families

With some exceptions, conotoxins are commonly named following a convention [30]. First, a Greek letter makes reference to a family in pharmacology (e.g., α, μ, κ, ω, etc.); the next two letters indicate the initials of the Conus species (e.g., Cg = *Conus geographus*), followed by one Roman number referring to the Cys framework (e.g., I, II, III, IV, etc., as shown in Table S2) and, finally, one uppercase letter indicates the discovery order (e.g., A, B, C, etc.) [18]:

αCgIA

These polypeptides have been divided into families by their pharmacological function [31]. Table 1 shows different family groups indicated by one Greek letter. Among them, the α-conotoxin family is distributed among different Conus species [32]. This toxin group is the most studied [23]. Other toxin groups—the μ-, ω-, and κ-conotoxins—have been the most characterized [33]. In general, some toxins from these family groups show special characteristics than allow specific interaction with their respective target group [5]. Thus, the following sections will describe conotoxins' activity in different ion channels, with special attention to those conotoxins best characterized.

Table 1. Conotoxin family classification.

Family	Target and Mode of Action	Reference
α-conotoxins	Inhibitory competitors of nicotinic acetylcholine receptors (nAChR)	[34]
γ-conotoxins	Acting on neuronal pacemaker currents affecting inward cation currents	[35]
δ-conotoxins	Acting on voltage-gated sodium (Na^+) channel VGSCs, activating and inactivating them	[36]
ε-conotoxins	Acting on G-protein-coupled presynaptic receptors or calcium channels	[37]
ι-conotoxins	Activating VGSCs	[38]
κ-conotoxins	Blocking voltage-gated potassium (K^+) channel VGKCs	[39]
μ-conotoxins	Blocking VGSCs	[40]
ρ-conotoxins	Inhibitors of alpha1-adrenoreceptors (GPCR)	[41]
σ-conotoxins	Acting on serotonin gated ion channels 5-HT3	[42]
τ-conotoxins	Acting on somatostatin receptors	[43]
χ-conotoxins	Inhibitors of neuronal noradrenaline transporters	[41]
ω-conotoxins	Acting on voltage-gated calcium (Ca^{++}) channel VGCCs	[44]

3. Conotoxins Interacting on Nicotinic Acetylcholine Receptors (nAChRs)

Nicotinic acetylcholine receptors (nAChRs) (Figure 1A) are pentameric structures (five subunits surrounding one central filter that allows the flow of Na^+, K^+, and Ca^{++} ions) in which each subunit is composed of four transmembranal segments [45]. There are different subunit types such as α, β, γ, δ, and ε, which can form homomeric (identical subunits) or heteromeric (combination of subunits) nAChRs [46]. These ligand-gated ion channels, expressed in both the nervous system and non-neuronal cells, have a varied number of ligand sites for acetylcholine (ACh) depending on the nAChR subtype [47]. In the nervous system, nAChRs are involved in physiological functions such as analgesia, learning, memory, arousal, and motor control [45], while in the non-neuronal cells, nAChRs promote cell proliferation, secretion, migration, survival, and apoptosis functions [48]. When nAChRs from the nervous system are affected, they generate neuronal disorders such as cognitive disorder, depression, anxiety [11], epilepsy, pain, and diseases, including Parkinson's and Alzheimer's [47]. As seen, nAChRs have been demonstrated to be involved in multiple physiological processes, depending on the nAChR-specific subtype responsible for each activity [49]. Curiously, α-conotoxins have shown target nAChR subtypes [30,34]. They are antagonist competitors from acetylcholine binding sites [50]. As a result, α-conotoxins have become an important research tool to analyze interaction with nAChRs [51].

α-Conotoxins are diverse in structure and have been subclassified by loop class [24]. In this respect, the classification may be based on amino acid number distribution among Cys ($C_1C_2mC_3nC_4$), in which m and n are loops, where n is a defined number (3/m, 4/m, and 5/m) and m is a variable number of amino acids from each α-conotoxin type [18]. However, this classification could be applied for those α-conotoxins from the A superfamily with type I framework (Table 2 and Table S2), which possess Cys (C_1–C_3 and C_2–C_4) globular connectivity [51]. Alternatives for folding (C_1–C_4 and C_2–C_3 and C_1–C_2 and C_3–C_4) of these synthetic toxins are named ribbon and beads, respectively (Figure S1A) [52]. α-conotoxins from other superfamily groups with different frameworks are not included on this list [30]. Below, the structural diversity of α-conotoxins is shown for clarification. These structures allow them to be specific for their target group (Tables 2 and 3). Some α-conotoxins (3/5) are specific for muscle nAChR subtypes, while other (4/3, 4/4, and 4/7) groups are selective for neuronal nAChR subtypes [53]. However, these toxins have shown promiscuous activity in different neuronal nAChR subtypes (Table 3) [51]. The promiscuity of α-conotoxins could be beneficial for these mollusks as a biological function [32], but it is disadvantageous for pharmacological purposes. Thus they need to be re-engineered for development as target-specific tools [54].

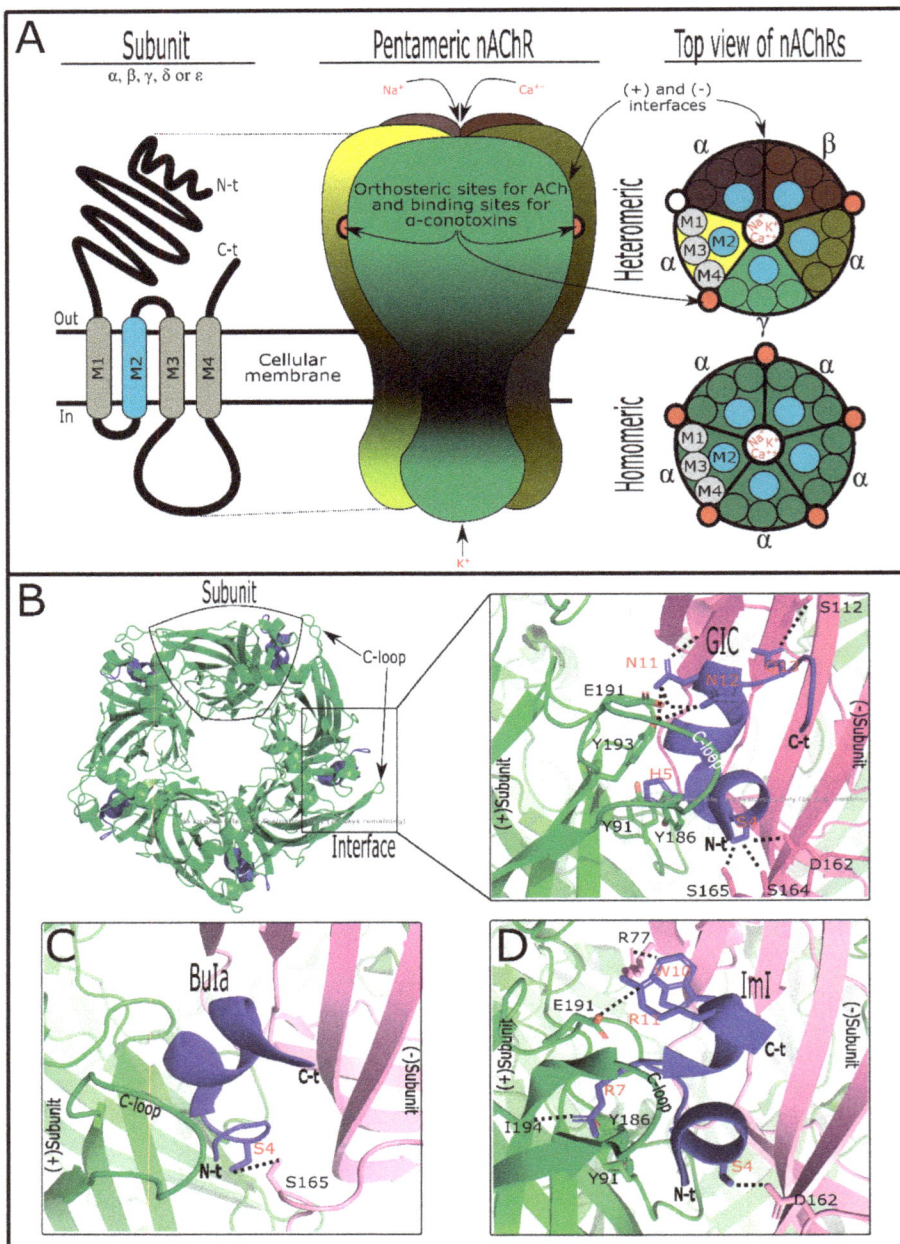

Figure 1. nAChRs and α-conotoxin interactions. (**A**) Basic subunits and pentameric structures of nAChRs. In the "top view" the segments' organization is shown, with segment 2 forming the ion pore. nAChRs could be composed of different subunit types (heteromeric) or identical α-subunits (homomeric). The subunit junctions are the interfaces. (**B**) GIC and Ac-AChBP interaction (PDB: 5CO5) showing top view of this complex. On the left, α-conotoxin GIC (blue) is fitted into the Ac-AChBP interfaces. On the right, specific interaction points between GIC and Ac-AChBP are showed. C-loop

from (+)subunit is highlighted. (**C**) Specific interaction points between BuIa and Ac-AChBP are showed (PDB: 4EZ1). (**D**) Specific interaction points between ImI and Ac-AChBP are showed (PDB: 2C9T). Amino acid residues in α-conotoxins are showed in red. Note that α-conotoxins are similarly oriented when they interact with their targets. nAChR structures were designed as described by the authors in the text.

Table 2. α-Conotoxin subdivisions with representative conotoxins.

α-CTx	Primary Sequence	Loop Class	Reference
Framework	and Cys pair connectivity C₁C₂-*m*-C₃-*n*-C₄	*m/n*	
GI	ECCNPACGRHYSCGK *	3/5	[55]
ImI	GCCSDPRCAWRC *	4/3	[56]
BuIA	GCCSTPPCAVLYC*	4/4	[57]
AuIB	GCCSYPPCFATNPDC *	4/6	[58]
Vc1.1	GCCSDPRCNYDHPEIC *	4/7	[59]
	Other frameworks		
αJ-pl14a	FPRPRICNLACRAGIGHKYPFCHCR *	X	[60]
αS-RVIIIA	KCNFDKCKGTGVYNCG(Gla)SCSC(Gla)GLHS CRCTYNIGSMKSGCACICTYY	X	[61]
αD-VxXXB	DD(Gla)S(Gla)CIINTRDSPWGRCCRTRMCGSM CCPRNGCTCVYHWRRGHGCSCPG (dimer)	X	[62]

Exclusively, α-conotoxins from the A superfamily have Cys framework I (at the top). *m/n* indicates the number of residues among Cys (C₂₋₃ and C₃₋₄, respectively). Only subclass 3/5 targets muscle nAChRs. * C-terminal amidated, (Gla) γ-carboxyglutamate, (dimer) dimerized molecule, X nonidentified.

The capability of α-conotoxins to differentiate between neuronal and muscle nAChRs is due to the subunits' composition in these receptors. Neuronal nAChRs can be homomeric when structured by α-subunits of the same type (α7, -8, or -9) or heteromeric when the α-subunits (α2-10) are combined together or with β-subunits (β2 and β4) [49]. In contrast, muscle nAChRs combine with α1, β1, γ, δ, and ε subunits [46]. They are not shared between tissues, and each subunit possesses its particular feature. So, structurally, α-conotoxins can discriminate among them [63]. Acetylcholine has orthosteric binding to the interface between nAChR subunits [45]. The acetylcholine affinity for these binding sites is due to hydrophilic features from each subunit's nAChR composition [46]. In this way, homomeric subunits (composed of five identical α-subunits) have five binding sites, while heteromeric nAChRs commonly have two binding sites (Figure 1A), in some cases with an accessory binding site for acetylcholine [45,49].

These events have shown differences in activity responses between target nAChR subtypes. It was demonstrated that the acetylcholine concentration in two nAChR isomers, one with double orthosteric interaction points and the other with an additional binding site, stimulated a second phase of macroscopic currents in that nAChR with the third interaction point [64]. Similarly, α-conotoxins interact in nAChRs as antagonist competitors [50]. They bind with diverse affinities on the subunit interfaces, which can vary depending on subunit composition [53]. The variable combination of subunits in nAChRs could explain the promiscuous nature of α-conotoxins (Figure 1A, Table 3). Nevertheless, a certain selectivity of some mutated α-conotoxins in favor of nAChRs containing α3-, α6-, α7-, and α9/α10 interfaces, but not for α2- and α4-interfaces, has been observed [30]. As with acetylcholine, α-conotoxins can interact on various ACh binding sites (i.e., 2, 3, or 6) simultaneously with the same nAChR or homologous AChBP [50,65]. However, it was suggested that only one molecule is enough to inactivate nAChRs [66,67]. Thus, the α-conotoxin/nAChR isoform's stoichiometric interaction could interfere in the real potency of toxin metrics.

Natural α-conotoxins have post-translational modifications (Figure S1B), with C-terminal amidation being the most frequent [63]. Post-translational modifications such as this allow biological activity in these molecules [68]. However, it is not a general rule. It was shown that the presence/absence of sulfated tyrosine in α-AnIB and EpI toxins has no significant biological difference [50,62]. More interestingly, this post-translational modification and the C-terminal amidation together could favor the affinity of α-AnIB for α7 nAChR [62]. These facts show that post-translational modifications in α-conotoxins can interfere in conotoxin/nAChR interactions. Indeed, it was suggested that amidation promotes native folding in this toxin group, leading to their selectivity [26]. Previous experiments showed that the proline from the *m*-loop and C-terminal amidation in α- and χ-conotoxins act as conformational switches [69]. With some exceptions (Figure S1B), the *m*-loop from α-conotoxins possesses one serine followed by one proline [63]. Proline facilitates α-helix formation, while serine provides a hydrophobic patch in these conotoxins' loop [54]. This hydrophobic patch from α-conotoxins could interact with any subunit (-) interface pocket because the nAChR subunits in this site are not very hydrophilic [46]. The (-) here is specified as the subunit receptor interface of anything other than an nAChR α-subunit (Figure 1). In fact, it was suggested that when α-conotoxins interact with their target, they are directionally positioned in a similar manner independently of their amino acid sequence [30]. Similarly, the second loop, the *n*-loop, appears to be involved with the (-) subunit interface due to the presence of key amino acids in α-conotoxins responsible for the interaction [70]. However, the key amino acid in the fifth position of α-conotoxins is important for the (+)α-subunit interface interaction [70]. The (+)α-subunit interface pocket site is more hydrophilic [46] and possesses the C-loop, which plays a significant role in α-conotoxins' interaction [54].

Table 3. α-Conotoxin activity in diverse nAChR subtypes. Some of the α-conotoxins showed different affinities for homomeric or heteromeric nAChRs or both. nAChRs are arranged from greatest to lowest α-conotoxin activity. nAChR subtypes have the first letter indicating the organism's origin, such as h for human, m for mouse, and r for rat origins.

α-Conotoxin	nAChR Type Target (IC$_{50}$)	Reference
ArIB	rα7 (1.81 nM) > rα6/α3β2β3 (6.45 nM) > rα3β2 (60.1 nM)	[71]
BuIA	rα6/α3β2 (0.258 nM) > rα6/α3β4 (1.54 nM) > rα3β2 (5.72 nM) > rα3β4 (27.7 nM)	[57]
GIC	hα3β2 (1.1 nM) > hα4β2 (309 nM) > hα3β4 (755 nM)	[72]
GID	rα3β2 (3.1 nM) > rα7 (4.5 nM) > rα4β2 (152 nM)	[73]
ImI	rα7 (220 nM) > rα7 (1.8 μM) > mα1β1γδ (51 μM)hα3β2 (40.8 nM) > hα7 (595 nM)	[74]
Lt1.3	rα3β2 (44.8 nM)	[75]
MII	rα6/α3β2β3 (0.39 nM) > rα3β2 (2.18 nM)	[76]
PeIA	rα9α10 (6.9 nM) > rα6/α3β2β3 (17.2 nM) > rα3β2 (19.2 nM) > rα3β4 (480 nM)	[77]
PnIA	rα3β2 (9.56 nM) > rα7 (252 nM)	[78]
TxIB	rα6/α3β2β3 (28 nM)	[79]
TxID	rα3β4 (12.5 nM) > rα6/α3β4 (94 nM) > rα3β4 (4.5μM) rα3β4 (3.6 nM) > rα6/α3β4 (34 nM)	[80]
Vc1.1	rα3β4 (4.2 μM) > rα3α5β2 (7.2 μM) > rα3β2 (7.3 μM)	[59]

In some cases, the tertiary structure has been shown to be relevant in α-conotoxins' activity, e.g., the ribbon isomer from native AuIB was seen to be 10-fold more potent in α3β4* nAChRs [50]. Pu1.2, Pn1.2, and Vc1.1 isomers, separately, demonstrated similar activity regarding their targets [52].

The tertiary structure is very important in the function of α-conotoxins because it leads to the spatial amino acid arrangement [18]. Additionally, for an electrostatic surface [18], this offers a special toxin three-dimensional shape that allows it to fit into the nAChR pocket binding site (Figure 1B). C-loops, the local binding site in nAChRs, are considered to be flexible, acting as a hinge that allows the toxin to fit into pocket interface subunits [54,81]. C-loop flexibility is conditioned by amino acid composition, which varies between nAChR subunits [54]. So, α-conotoxin size and shape are important for their interaction. However, α-conotoxins have been shown to be unselective [54]. This probably occurs because the electrostatic surface is able to interact with the nAChR pocket subunits' interface [18]. A basic explanation of this specific phenomenon is that it could occur due to the similarities between the allosteric sites of different receptor subtypes [82]. Interestingly, it was suggested that nAChR orthosteric sites (acetylcholine) are notably conserved among organisms from different taxonomic groups [83].

α-Conotoxins have key residues that recognize their targets' counterparts [54]. These amino acids were detected by scanning mutation [70]. Mutations were developed to enhance the toxin's activity or selectivity [54]. However, this review will only mention the interactions of natural toxins and their targets. As previously mentioned, α-conotoxins show the same spatial position pattern when acting on targets [30]. This is due to the similar point-by-point connection between α-conotoxins and targets [70]. Natural α-conotoxins GIC, BuIA, and ImI, for example, show the characteristics of these interactions (Figure 1B–D). As observed, α-conotoxins recognize the key interaction point of acetylcholine receptor subtypes which are localized in (-) and (+)subunits' interfaces [70]. GIC has the Ser4 common to α-conotoxins [72]. Ser4 and Gln13 interact by hydrogen bond with (Asp162, Ser164, or Ser165) and Ser112 from Ac-AChBP (-)subunits' interface, respectively [84], while residues such as His5 and (Asn11, Asn12) interact with (Tyr91, Tyr186) and (Glu191, Tyr193) from Ac-AChBP (+)subunits' interface, respectively [84]. As happens with Ser4 in α-conotoxins, Asn11 and Asn12 are shared between some of these toxin groups [85] and shown to be significant for toxin interaction on loop C, localized at Ac-AChBPs (+)subunits' interface [70]. By alanine scanning mutation, it was observed that GIC has important residues for interactions with Ac-AChBPs or hα3β2, but not for interactions with hα3β4 subtypes [84,86]. GIC (Gln13Ala) did not appear to be relevant in the interaction with Ac-AChBPs or hα3β2 subtypes [84]. However, Gln13 produced a steric clash on Arg108 from (-)subunits hβ4, preventing affinity with hα3β4 subtypes [84]. These differences are shown in the comparison of acetylcholine receptor subtypes' alignment (Figure S1C)

Similarly, BuIa shares Ser4, which is typical of α-conotoxins [57]. This serine makes a hydrogen bond with Ser165 from Ac-AChBPs (-) subunits' interface, while other residues do not seem to be significant for Ac-AChBPs interaction [70]. However, BuIa shows affinity for neuronal nAChRs containing rα6/α3 and β2 subunits, more than for rα4 or β4 subunit interfaces [57]. Lys185, Thr187, Ile188, Thr198, and Tyr205 from rα6 (+)subunits' interface were seen to be responsible for BuIa interaction [87]. Another α-conotoxin, ImI, was active in homomeric α7 and α9 nAChRs [74,88]. Ser4 from ImI, like GIC and BuIa, is localized spatially, allowing it to interact with Asp162 from the Ac-AChBPs (-)subunit interface [70]. Trp10 of ImI makes contact, by a hydrogen bond, with Arg77 from the same AChBP interface [89]. Arg7 and Arg11 contact (Tyr91, Tyr186, and Ile194) and Glu191 from the Ac-AChBP (+)subunit interface, respectively [70,89].

4. Conotoxins Interacting in Potassium Channels

Potassium channels are the most abundant and varied ion channels in nature [90]. They are responsible for potassium flow across the membrane, allowing cell excitability to be maintained [91]. Other physiological roles of potassium channels involve cell proliferation, apoptosis and hormone secretion [92]. When potassium channel disturbance occurs, autoimmune, chronic inflammatory and metabolic diseases and cancer can develop [12]. Their fundamental organization is a tetrameric structure of α-subunits, which constitutes the K^+ selective filter [93]. Sometimes, α-subunits occur together with accessory subunits (i.e., β) depending on the K^+ channel type [94]. They are grouped in four large families, namely voltage-gated K$^+$-channels (K$_V$) with 12 subfamilies [95], K$^+$-channels activated by calcium (K$_{ca}$) with five subfamilies [96], inwardly rectifying (K$_{ir}$) with seven subfamilies [97], and two-tandem-pore domain K$^+$-Channels (K$_{2P}$) with 16 subfamilies [98]. Conotoxins that interact with potassium channels have demonstrated that they are more active in (K$_V$) channels [99]. Thus, this section will explain the structure of this channel group (Figure 2A,B). K$_V$ channels (VGKCs) are tetramers structured by α-subunits, in which each monomer has six transmembrane segments (S1–S6) [94]. Segments S5 and S6 constitute the ion-selective filter, while segment S4, being positively charged, plays an important role in the channel kinetics [93]. Therefore, voltage sensor S4 segment is responsible for VGKCs' activity [100,101].

Conotoxins that interact with VGKCs are varied in structure, since they are found in various superfamilies (Tables S1–S3). κ-Conotoxins can be disulfide-rich conotoxins shared by A, I, J, M, O superfamilies or conkunitzin-S1, or they can be disulfide-poor conotoxins such as contryphan-Vn [5]. Commonly, the contryphan group possesses a tryptophan or leucine residue in D-configuration and presents variable activity [23]. Among them, contryphan-Vn, a κ-conotoxin with two cysteines, was shown to be active in VGKCs and K$_{ca}$ [102]. Disulfide-rich κ-conotoxins, moreover, show different frameworks (Table S2). This toxin group has some post-translational modifications such as C-terminal amidation, N-terminal pyroglutamylation, γ-carboxylation, hydroxylation, and glycosylation [5]. The last is considered be more frequent in κ-conotoxins than in other conotoxin families [68]. Although its role in κ-conotoxin activity has still not been identified, it is believed that this post-translational modification could increase its half-life in vivo [103]. The role of other post-translational modifications in κ-conotoxins is still unknown.

Disulfide-rich κ-conotoxins have been shown to be preferential blockers [5]. Thus, when interaction occurs, the toxin can decrease K$^+$-currents naturally produced by targeted channels without affecting the action of their molecular mechanism (Figure 2E). An exception for this group is BTX [104]. This toxin, from *C. betulinus* venom, showed K$^+$-currents increasing in a voltage-dependent manner in K$_{ca}$ channels [104]. κ-Conotoxin blockers, however, interact directly with the pore localized in the extracellular vestibule of VGKCs (Figure 2C,D). Conkunitzin-S1, from *C. striatus* venom, inhibited K$^+$-currents from pore-mutated Shaker potassium channels [4]. This toxin was showed to be a specific blocker of mammalian K$_V$1.7 [105]. Similarly, other κ-conotoxins such as RIIIJ and RIIIK from *C. radiatus* [106], SIVA from *C. striatus* [107], pl14a from *C. planorbis* [60], ViTx from *C. virgo* [108], sr11a from *C. spurius* [109], and PVIIA from *C. purpurascens* [110] venoms blocked K$^+$-currents from K$_V$1 and/or related Shaker VGKCs. In this way, it was observed that this toxin group acts in a similar way to other animal toxin blockers [99]. Scorpion K$^+$-blockers (KTx), for example, have at least four interaction modes with their targets [111]. Of these, two interaction models have been demonstrated to be similar to the κ-conotoxins' activity: a dyad and "ring of basic residues" modes. The former was experimentally observed using modeling studies with PVIIA [112–114]. A similar interaction between RIIIJ and K$_V$1.2 channels was also observed [115]. The second model was observed in the interaction of the RIIIK toxin with *TSha1* channels from rainbow trout (*Onchorhynchus mychiis*) [116,117]. Other interaction modes have not yet been clarified for ViTx and sr11a toxins [108,109] because they do not have dyad or "ring of basic residues" characteristics. In all cases, key amino acids localized in the extracellular pore vestibule of K$^+$-channels are necessary for toxin recognition [118].

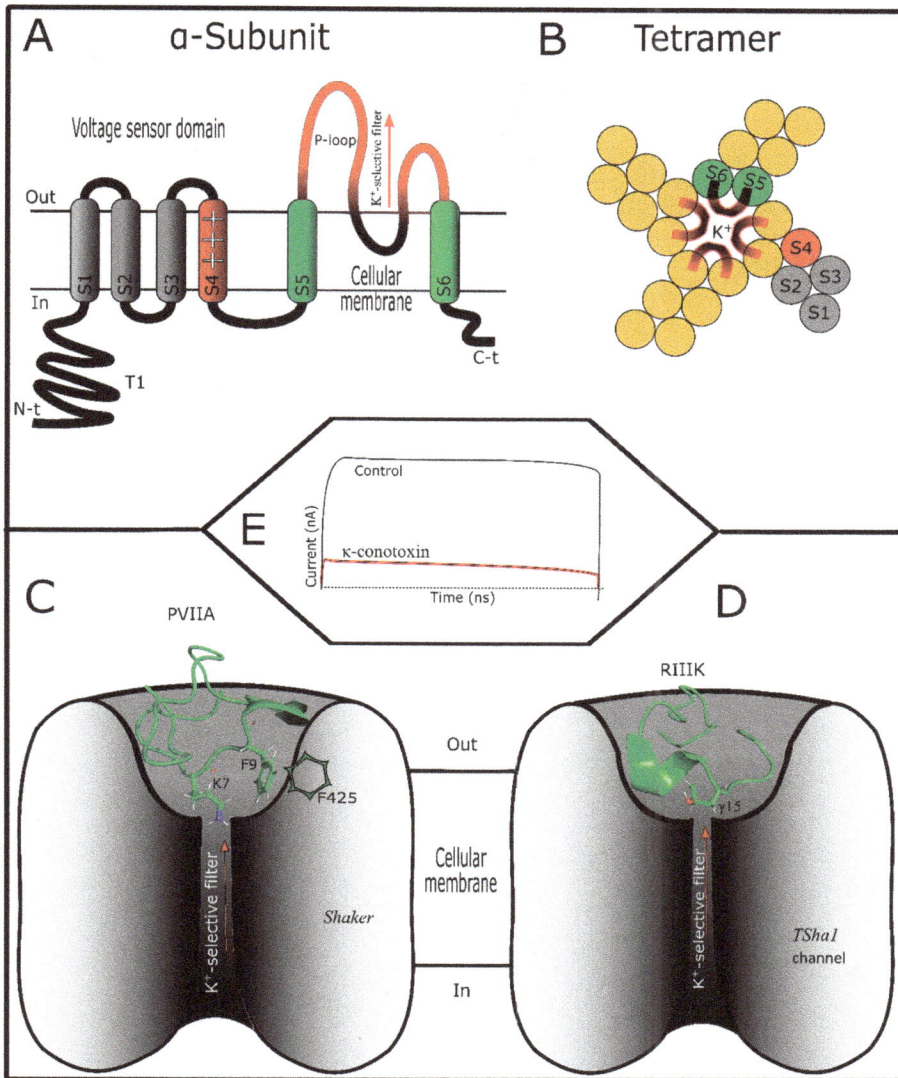

Figure 2. Potassium channels and κ-conotoxin interactions. (**A**) Basic structure of the α-subunit from VGKCs showing segment S4 with positive charges and pore region structured by segments S5 and S6. In this P-loop (highlighted in red) κ-conotoxins interact. Here, accessory subunits are omitted. (**B**) VGKC organization by four α-subunits showing ion pore (P-loops). (**C**) κ-conotoxin PVIIA (PDB: 1AV3) interacting with related Shaker channels. In the dyad model, two amino acids (Lys and Phe) are important for toxin interaction. Lys is inserted in the selective filter of potassium channel. (**D**) RIIIK and related Shaker channel interaction. In this interaction 4-hydroxiproline residue at the 15th position of RIIIK is responsible for the K^+-flow block. (**E**) Typical electrophysiologic record of K^+-currents before (black) and after (red) adding the toxin. It can be observed that K^+-currents decrease after toxin application caused by ion pore obstruction. Here K^+-current types are not considered. VGKC structures were designed as described by the authors in the text.

The dyad model is based on two key amino acid residues (basic and aromatic) strategically distributed in the toxin [119]. κ-Conotoxins, such as PVIIA, show this pattern (Figure 2C). Previously, some notable residues in PVIIA were characterized, including Lys7, Phe9, and Phe23, which are important for channel interaction [112]. K7 is inserted in the ion-selective channel pore, physically preventing ion flow, while the aromatic residues make hydrophobic interactions [113]. Mutagenesis in both the toxin and Shaker channel demonstrated that Phe9 from the toxin is more relevant than Phe23 in the interaction with F425 (loop between S5 and S6 segments) from Shaker VGKCs [112,120]. This interaction affinity occurs due to the structural nature adopted by both toxin and K$^+$-channels, which is related to the distances between residues, inter- and intramolecularly [118]. As an example of this phenomenon, it has been shown that PVIIA is active in Shaker, but not in K$_V$1 channels [120]. This selectivity is based on the structure of each channel subtype. Both VGKC subtypes have one equivalent aromatic residue homologous in interactions with the (Phe9) toxin. Nevertheless, two residues (Thr449 and Asp447) cross-link in *Shaker* channels, favoring Phe23/Phe425 coupling interaction [118]. The natural lack of this cross-linking in K$_V$1 and the mutation in Shaker channels (Thr449Tyr) prevent hydrophobic interactions with Phe23 [118,120]. Other interaction points of PVIIA allow toxin stabilization in the *Shaker* channel vestibule [112,118]. Recently, it was shown that the N-terminal and intramolecular hydrogen bond network of PVIIA are important for toxin stabilization in Shaker channel interaction [114]. In conclusion, PVIIA/Shaker channel interaction is due to two strategically localized residues (Lys7 and Phe9) which allow the toxin activity. Lys7 occludes the pore, preventing K$^+$-flow, while Phe9 fixes the toxin to the K$^+$-channel vestibule (Figure 2C). Other interaction points such as Phe23 or Arg2 are necessary for toxin stabilization [118].

The other model, the "ring of basic residues", is based on the distribution of basic residues (Arg and/or Lys) along the molecule, which are spatially arranged when a disulfide bond occurs, forming the basic ring [111]. In a similar manner, basic residues of RIIIK electrostatically interact with diverse points of the pore region vestibule from *TSha1* channels, and Glu354 in *TSha1* is the most important [117]. Leu1, Arg10, Lys18, and Arg19 showed their importance for RIIIK activity, and it was demonstrated that there is no aromatic residue typical of the dyad model [116]. A mode of interaction between KTx (scorpion toxins) and VGKCs, for example, could explain this phenomenon. It has been suggested than the electrostatic interaction between the basic ring of the KTx and the potassium-channel disrupts K$^+$-flow [111]. However, for this specific case, RIIIK has a post-translational modified residue (4-hydroxiproline at the 15th position, γ15) that interacts with the VGKC, blocking the K$^+$-flow [117]. So, it was suggested that the RIIIK basic ring anchors the toxin to the pore vestibule from *TSha1* channels, while its γ15 residue interacts with carbonyl groups localized on the selectivity filter of VGKCs, altering the normal ionic flow (Figure 2D) [117].

5. Conotoxins Interacting with Voltage-Gated Sodium Channels

Voltage-gated sodium channels (VGSCs) are tetrameric structures that allow the sodium ion to pass through the membrane leading to cell depolarization, which is necessary for physiological activity [121]. VGSCs are responsible for starting action potentials in neurons, muscle and immune system cells, among others [91]. These channels could be classified in nine subtypes (Na$_V$1.1 – Na$_V$1.9) or isoforms, which are distributed among various tissues performing their function [122]. When altered, VGSC subtypes are involved in several diseases such as epilepsy, pain disturbance, autism, and diabetes [14,123]. They are structured by two subunits, the first an α-subunit that composes the ion-selective pore, and the second an accessory β-subunit [121]. The α-subunit is a tetrameric structure made of four domains (DI–DIV), and each domain is structured by six transmembrane segments named (S1–S6) [124,125] (Figure 3A,B). Segments S5 and S6 constitute the Na$^+$-selectivity filter of VGSCs, while S4 segments from each domain are voltage sensors responsible for VGSC activity [121,126]. S4 segments from the DII domain are responsible for VGSC activation while S4 segments from the DIV domain are responsible for fast inactivation [121,127]. VGSCs are the target of diverse toxic compounds and each acts on different points of these channels [128]. Depending on the binding site of VGSCs, the toxins exert different effects on them (Figure 3C–E). For example, scorpion toxins are VGSC modulators because they interact with the loops related to the S4 voltage sensors from DII or DIV; thus, they can modulate activation or fast inactivation of VGSCs, respectively [129]. Depending on the superfamily origin, conotoxins act as modulator or blockers of VGSCs (Table 1, Tables S1 and S3).

Conotoxins acting on VGSCs are divided in four families according to their function, and these are μ-, μO-, δ-, and ι-conotoxins [5]. With the exception of μ-conotoxins, the pharmacophore of these toxins is yet to be identified [130], and interaction experiments with their targets are necessary to enhance understanding in this area. These conotoxin groups will therefore be briefly discussed with special emphasis on μ-conotoxins. Conotoxins that target VGSCs show some post-translational modifications. The most common is C-terminal amidation, but there are others that are less frequent, such as pyroglutamate and hydroxyproline [131]. Despite poor knowledge about post-translational modifications, some investigations have been carried out. For example, some amino acids occur with dextrogyre format in natural ι-conotoxins [132,133]. When a laevogyrate format is substituted by natural D-Phe44 in ι-RXIA, its activity is decreased or lost in VGSCs tested [132,133]. Similarly, two toxins close to ι-RXIA (r11a and r11b) were epimerized [132]. However, only one of them decreased its activity in VGSCs [132]. μ-Conotoxins with natural folding show specific activity in their targets. An experiment made with synthetic cysteine isomers of PIIIA, KIIIA, and KIIIB showed activity in VGSCs, but with diverse affinities [134,135], showing that a defined three-dimensional structure is important for toxin/VGSC interaction [25].

ι-Conotoxins are the least studied group. Only two toxins have been identified [33]. ι-LtIIIA, from *C. litteratus*, has six cysteines, exhibiting a type III framework shown to facilitate sodium currents from root ganglion neurons [136]. ι-RXIA and its analogs from *C. radiatus*, with eight cysteines and framework type XI, elicited action potential in amphibian peripheral axons [137]. Curiously, in spite of structural differences, these two toxins showed equivalent activities [132,136,137]. An interaction analysis made with ι-RXIA showed that this toxin can left-shift the voltage-dependent activation from mammal VGSCs [133]. Although not yet full identified for this toxin group, this phenomenon could occur by interaction with S4 of domain DII from VGSCs [138]. Likewise, ι-conotoxins act like β-toxins from scorpions. β-toxins interact with the S3-S4 loop of DII, trapping the S4 movement in pre-open states from VGSCs [124]. Consequently, it will be necessary to apply less energy to activate VGSCs again, and because of this, the voltage is shifted to hyperpolarizing states (Figure 3A,C).

As with ι-conotoxins, it was suggested that μO-conotoxins interacting with the S3-S4 loop of DII trap the S4 movement from VGSCs, but only inhibit Na$^+$-conductance [138]. Therefore, members of this conotoxin group are modulators but not blockers (Figure 3A,D). μO-conotoxins are hydrophobic polypeptides stabilized by a six-cysteine ICK-motif [139]. These structural and hydrophobic features are challenging due to their synthesis and later folding [5]. Few μO-conotoxins have been described until now, but MrVIA, MrVIB, and MfVIA have been the best studied [5,33,138]. They have showed blocking, preferentially, Na$_v$1.8 subtypes [131]. MrVIA and MrVIB toxins, from *C. marmoreus*, blocked voltage-gated sodium currents from snail neurons [140,141]. MfVIA, from *C. magnificus* and inhibited Na+ currents from human VGSCs [142]. Particularly, it was suggested that loop 2 from the MrVIB structure has some flexibility that allows its interaction with VGSCs [139]. Additionally, by mutagenesis of Na$_v$1.2 and Na$_v$1.4 channels, MrVIA showed interactions with the SS2 pore loop of DIII in Na$_v$1.4 subtypes [143]. Interestingly, MrVIA also interacts with the S4 of DII in VGSCs, therefore also interfering in their activation [144] in a similar way to the activity of β-toxins from scorpion venom. β-toxins could interact with the S3-S4 loop of DII, S2-S3 loop of DII, and SS2 loop of DIII [145,146]. These last interaction points are proposed, anchoring the β-toxin to VGSCs while the interaction with S4 from DII provides its activity [147]. It is possible that, like β-toxins, μO-conotoxins could exert their function by interacting with the S4 loop from DII, while they are anchored to the SS2 pore loop of DIII (Figure 3A). A recent study with MfVIA showed that this conotoxin could interact with voltage sensor points embedded in membrane, generating a voltage shift [148]. On the whole, these findings contribute to the idea that μO-conotoxins could be considered an independent conotoxin family [149]. However, this group is included in the μ-conotoxin group (Table 1), which comprises conotoxin blockers.

Like ι- and μO-conotoxins, δ-conotoxins are VGSC modulators, but they target a different locality from those mentioned regarding other modulators [150,151]. To date, over 22 δ-conotoxins have been described [138]. They have six cysteines with a framework VI/VII pattern stabilized in ICK-motif [5]. Like μO-conotoxins, this toxin group has also been difficult to obtain synthetically and to investigate [5]. This is due to their hydrophobic amino acids distributed along molecules. It was suggested that some of these residues could be important for toxin/VGSCs interaction [138,151]. In fact, three residues (positions 12, 23, and 25) differentiated in δ-CnVIB, δ-CnVIC, and δ-CnVID toxins, respectively, showed selectivity toward mammalian VGSC subtypes [152]. These toxins, from C. *consors*, have residues positioned at (12Ile or 12Phe), (12Phe, 23Phe, and 25Leu), and (25Phe), and they have been seen to be selective to $Na_V1.2$, $Na_V1.3$ and $Na_V1.4$ isoforms, respectively [152]. A previous study made with GmVIA, from C. *gloriamaris*, produced an extended action potential in molluscan neurons [150]. This phenomenon is caused by the modification from fast inactivation in VGSCs, as demonstrated by NgVIA and δ-TxVIA toxins' activity, from C. *nigropunctatus* and C. *textile*, respectively [153]. Indeed, SVIE, from C. *striatus*, interacted with a hydrophobic triad (Tyr-Phe-Val) present at the S4 of DIV from VGSCs [154]. In this interaction (Figure 3A), δ-conotoxins decreased the fast inactivation process by trapping S4, like the interaction mode of α-toxins from scorpions [154]. Recently, an interaction study made with δ-EVIA and $Na_V1.7$ showed that the δ-conotoxin additionally interacted with segment S5 of DI [155]. Identification of one Na^+-current registered when normal kinetic inactivation of VGSCs is affected is shown in Figure 3E.

Differently to previously mentioned modulators, μ-conotoxins inhibit Na+ currents but block VGSCs [40]. More than 20 μ-conotoxins have been described [138], and this group is the most thoroughly characterized among conotoxins that act on VGSCs [5,130,156]. μ-Conotoxins have different cysteine frameworks depending on their superfamily origin [33]. The most common representatives among them are from the M superfamily with six cysteines and type III or IV frameworks [5]. μT-LtVD, from C. *litteratus*, belongs to the T superfamily and has four cysteines with type V framework [157]. See tables (Table 1 and Tables S1–S3) for structure/function. This toxin group is known for targeting VGSCs sensitive to tetrodotoxin (TTX) or saxitoxin (STX) ($Na_V1.1$, $Na_V1.2$, $Na_V1.3$, $Na_V1.4$, $Na_V1.6$, and $Na_V1.7$), but not for ($Na_V1.5$, $Na_V1.8$, or $Na_V1.9$) mammalian subtypes [158]. They interact with overlap sites for TTX or STX in the filter pore from VGSCs [159,160]. μ-conotoxins' activity on insensitive TTX-VGSCs has not yet been described [33]. However, some of them were described as promiscuous and also act on VGKCs. μ-SIIIA and μ-PIIIA blocked $K_V1.1$ and $K_V1.6$ channels [161]. These interactions were identified in in silico studies [162]. Among the VGSCs targeted, μ-conotoxins are more selective toward $Na_V1.4$ and $Na_V1.2$ subtypes, respectively [5]. μ-Conotoxins have basic amino acid distribution, with one of them in the ~13th position key to blocking VGSCs (Figure 3B) [138,163]. Their net positive charge contributes to electrostatic interaction [164]. This facilitates toxin positioning on the local binding site of VGSCs, independently of the basic amino acid distribution [130]. This basic feature of μ-conotoxins could be attracted by the acidic nature of residues localized on outer pore loops of VGSCs [165]. Carboxylates localized in VGSCs' outer filter are responsible for Na+ permeation [166] and they are the target of μ-conotoxins [130], thus blocking ion flow (Figure 3A,B,D).

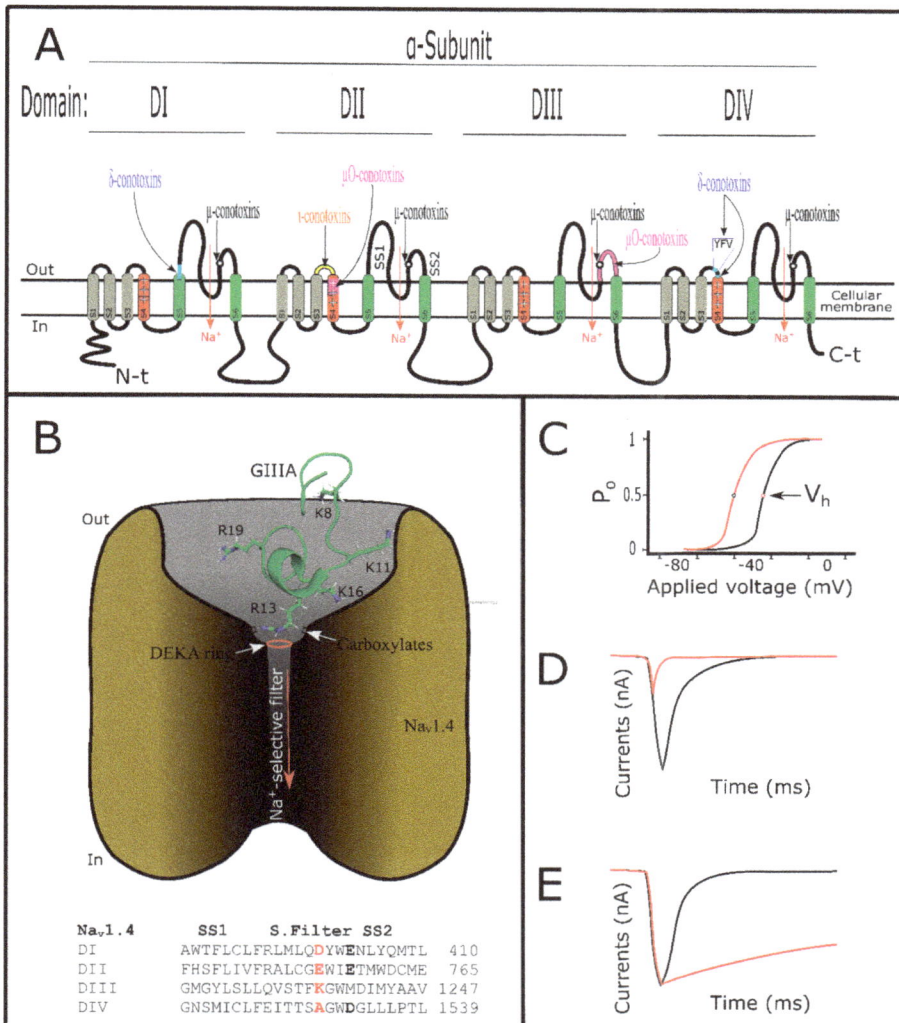

Figure 3. Voltage-gated sodium channels and conotoxins that interact with them. (**A**) Basic structure of the α-subunit of VGSCs. This is constituted by four domains, which compose the Na+ pore. Each domain shows segment S4 with positive charges and pore region structured by segments S5 and S6. Here different interaction localities by conotoxins are showed. Accessory subunits are omitted in this design. (**B**) μ-Conotoxin GIIIA (PDB: 1TCJ) interacting with $Na_V1.4$ channel. Arg13 of GIIIA blocks Na^+-flow by interaction with DEKA ring and outer carboxylates of $Na_V1.4$ (showed in the alignment). Other interaction points are described in the text. (**C**) Representative curve of open kinetic states from VGSCs. Maximal Na^+-current before (black) and after (red) adding the toxin, for each stimulus, with fitted Boltzmann equation. Po is the open probability when a voltage is applied in VGSCs, while V_h is the open probability of 50% of these channels. When voltage sensor S4 of domain II is trapped by the ι-conotoxins a voltage shift for hyperpolarized states is observed. (**D**) Typical electrophysiologic record of Na+ currents before (black) and after (red) adding the toxin. It can be observed that Na+ currents decrease after toxin application. (**E**) Typical electrophysiologic record of Na+ currents before (black) and after (red) adding the toxin. Here VGSCs cannot carry out their fast inactivation. Consequently, these keep their open states for more time. VGSC structures were designed as described by the authors in the text.

GIIIA, KIIIA, BuIIIB, and PIIIA μ-conotoxins have been studied using computational methods which agreed with experimental data [167]. Various models have been tested in the attempt to research μ-conotoxin/VGSC interactions, using elucidated sodium channel structures from bacteria [168,169]. A successful model, using the $Na_v1.4$ subtype created from these basic sodium channel structures, was used [170]. It has led to a better understanding of interactions between μ-conotoxins and VGSCs [167]. To date, GIIIA have been the best characterized (Figure 3B) [130]. Experimentally, this toxin interacted with the four domains of pore vestibule from $Na_v1.4$ channels [163]. Specifically, residues localized in the S5–S6 loop of D2 could be important for μ-conotoxin/VGSC stability [171]. Amino acid interactions for GIIIA/$Na_v1.4$, such as for Lys8/Asp1248, Lys 11/(Asp 1241 and Asp 1532), Lys16/(Glu758 and Asp 1241), and Arg19/(Asp 762), were found [165,169,170]. Arg13 directly interacted with the selective filter (DEKA ring) and outer carboxylates [130,168], Arg13/(Glu 403, Glu 758, and Asp1532), blocking ion flow [165].

6. Conotoxins Interacting with Voltage-Gated Calcium Channels

Like sodium channels, voltage-gated calcium channels (VGCC) are tetramers of four domains (DI–DIV) which constitute the α-subunit (Figure 4A,B) [172,173]. Each domain is structured by six transmembrane segments named (S1–S6), and segments S5–S6 are responsible for the ion flow while S4 is positively charged [172,174]. S4 is a voltage sensor and is responsible for opening and closing the channel's mechanism of action [175]. Furthermore, accessory structures (β, $\alpha_2\delta$, and γ_1) can be present, depending on VGCC subtype [174,176]. VGCCs could be involved in multiple physiological functions such as muscle contraction, hormone and neurotransmitter secretion, enzyme activation, etc. [177]. Their specific function can vary with the VGCC subtype. They are classified as ($Ca_v1.1$–$Ca_v1.4$), ($Ca_v2.1$–$Ca_v2.3$), and ($Ca_v3.1$–$Ca_v3.3$) channels [177]. Ca_v1 and Ca_v2 groups are sensitive to high voltage, while the Ca_v3 group is sensitive to low voltage [13]. ω-conotoxins target $Ca_v2.2$ channels, and thus this toxin group is responsible for affecting N-type currents [33,178]. Other ω-conotoxins are active in P/Q-type Ca^{++} currents [178,179]. These current types are produced by $Ca_v2.1$ channels localized in Purkinge neurons and cerebellar granule cells (P/Q) [176]. $Ca_v2.2$ channel subtypes are known as N-type because they are exclusively neuronal and express a Ca^{++} current component that is different from L-type ($Ca_v1.1$–$Ca_v1.4$) or T-type ($Ca_v3.1$–$Ca_v3.3$) components [176,179]. Thus, these channel subtypes are involved in nociception more than in any other physiologic process [180]. Interestingly, from of MVIIA, a ω-conotoxin purified from *Conus magus* venom, was developed Prialt™ as drug for the treatment of neuropathic pain [181]. Curiously, this is only conotoxin currently guaranteed by the FDA for use [17].

Like κ- or μ-conotoxins, ω-conotoxins are pore-blockers (Figure 4A,B,D), interacting with the outer vestibule of VGCCs [178]. They belong to the O1 superfamily, sharing a three-dimensional structure with other conotoxins (Table S1) [21]. ω-Conotoxins are structured by six cysteines showing β-sheets in their ICK motif [182,183]. They have a type VI/VII Cys framework (Table S2). This configuration confers on ω-conotoxins four variable inter-cysteine loops that allow their affinity [178]. Other characteristics are their net positive charges [184], which are important in interaction with their targets [178]. Conotoxins, with different features, act on VGCCs and have been described. Contryphan-M, a conotoxin from *C. marmoreus*, has only two cysteines and shows activity in L-type currents [185]. Also, RsXXIVA, from *C. regularis*, has eight cysteines without a defined framework and showed activity in the $Ca_v2.2$ channel current [186]. Varied post-translational modifications are not frequent in this conotoxin group (Figure 4C). They show the typical amidated C-terminal found among conotoxins, and some of them have hydroxyproline in their primary sequence [184]. It was detected that substitutions of hydroxyproline by proline did not affect GVIA activity [187]. Studies about the role of post-translational modifications in ω-conotoxins are still needed for more clarification.

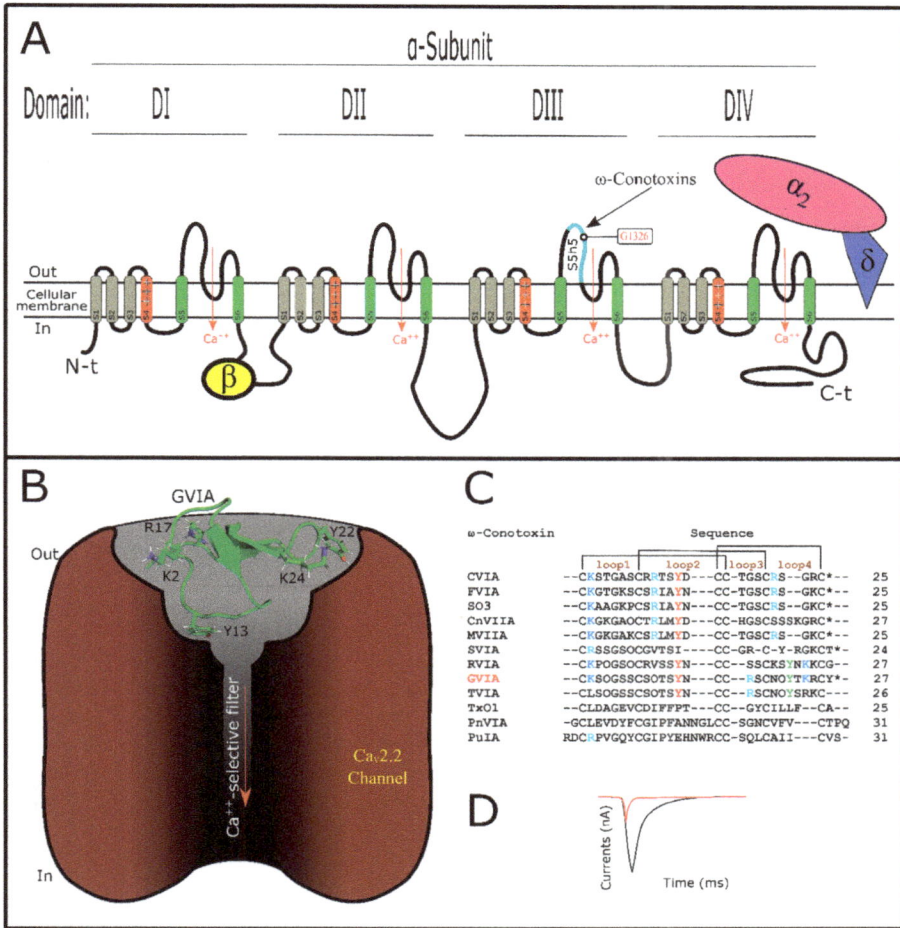

Figure 4. Voltage-gated calcium channels and ω-conotoxin interactions. (**A**) Basic structure of the α-subunit of VGCCs. This is constituted by four domains, which compose the Na+ pore. Each domain shows segment S4 with positive charges and pore region structured by S5 and S6 segments. Here is showed only one known interaction point by ω-conotoxins. Accessory subunits such as β or α₂δ are showed. (**B**) ω-Conotoxin GVIA (PDB: 2CCO) interacting with Ca$_V$2.2 channel. Specific interaction points among them are unknown. (**C**) ω-Conotoxins alignment showing cysteine connectivity and loops. Key amino acids for interaction with their targets are highlighted. * C-terminal amidated, O hydroxyproline. (**D**) Typical electrophysiologic record of Ca++ currents before (black) and after (red) adding the toxin. It can be observed that Ca++ currents decrease after toxin application. Here Ca++ current types are not considered. VGCC structures were designed as described by the authors in the text.

Structurally, ω-conotoxins have some key amino acids distributed in their loops [178]. As a principal residue, Tyr13 (loop 2) is determinant in ω-conotoxin/VGCC interactions, while other residues that are not conserved have affected their affinity [188]. Lys2 (loop1), also conserved among ω-conotoxins (Figure 4C), is important for toxin interaction [187,189,190]. Arg17 (or Arg21 depending on the toxin), Tyr22, and Lys24 in loop 4 are related to binding affinity, while Lys or Arg10 (loop

2) could be related to selectivity toward Ca$_v$2.1 or Ca$_v$2.2, respectively [5]. In contrast, residues localized between the pore region and S5 loop of domain DIII from Ca$_v$2.2 have been shown to be important for ω-conotoxins [191]. One residue from this locality, Gly1326, was key for GVIA and MVIIA recognition [192]. GVIA is the most studied ω-conotoxin; however, to date, the interaction point-by-point of ω-conotoxin/VGCC still needs to be elucidated [31]. In comparison with ω-conotoxins, little has been established about VGCC mutations to evaluate toxin/channel interaction. Consequently, molecular dynamics simulations are restricted [5,193], leaving gaps in the knowledge of this approach.

7. Conclusions

It was observed that conotoxins and their targets have strategic amino acid residues that determine their interaction. Key residues from conotoxins have been demonstrated to be important because they confer activity and specificity. These findings are of extreme importance. Nevertheless, there are other features involved in the toxin/target interaction. For example, the electrostatic surface could define toxin potency. The electrostatic surface is attributed by characteristics such as cysteine framework and pair-linking, post-translational modifications and amino acid composition. However, as regards conotoxins, studies focusing on these characteristics are still under way. Also, each conotoxin has a special three-dimensional structure (shape) that allows them to fit into their target. There are two possible interaction modes between conotoxins and targets. α-Conotoxins show a full superficial interaction with the target because they are inserted into the binding site. In contrast, conotoxins acting on ion channels have one defined interaction patch. In this case, key amino acids that are important for their interaction are spatially site-directed.

In spite of conotoxins' abundance and the structure/function variety, it is curious that only Prialt®, a conotoxin that acts on calcium channels, has been developed as a drug. The promiscuity of conotoxins poses a challenge to their development as future drugs. These findings suggest that the targets' interaction points are very similar among subtype groups. The conotoxin/specific target interactions are closely related. In general, for any protein/protein interaction process, the three-dimensional electrostatic surface of conotoxins and their specific targets' contact area must be carefully analyzed because these features are provided by the space distribution of amino acids. This characteristic determines a key–lock effect which leads to harmonized interactions. For some conotoxin families, such as κ-, ι-, δ-, or ω-conotoxins, more investigation into this area is still necessary.

Supplementary Materials: The following are available online at http://www.mdpi.com/1660-3397/17/6/370/s1, Figure S1: (A) Cysteine connectivity adopts different isomers in α-conotoxins. Structures as described by the authors in the text. (B) Some α-conotoxin alignments showing key amino acid residues highlighted. * C-terminal amidated, O hydroxyproline and γ gamma carboxylic glutamic acid. (C) ACh receptors (-)subunits alignment. Table S1: Conotoxin superfamily classification and families involved. Table S2: Conotoxin Cys framework category and families involved. Table S3: Generic classification and basic structure features from conotoxins.

Author Contributions: H.M.D. designed and wrote the manuscript; S.C.D. and O.L.F. revised the manuscript.

Funding: This research was funded by *Conselho Nacional de Desenvolvimento Científico e Tecnológico-Brasil* CNPq, grant number 380834/2018-9.

Acknowledgments: We thank to pos-graduate program of *Ciências Genômicas e Biotecnologia* by the theory support.

Conflicts of Interest: The authors declare no conflicts of interest.

References

1. Board, W.E. Word Register of Marine Species. Available online: http://www.marinespecies.org (accessed on 14 May 2019).
2. Olivera, B.M.; Seger, J.; Horvath, M.P.; Fedosov, A.E. Prey-capture strategies of fish-hunting cone snails: Behavior, neurobiology and evolution. *Brain Behav. Evolut.* **2015**, *86*, 58–74. [CrossRef] [PubMed]
3. Cruz, L.; De Santos, V.; Zafaralla, G.; Ramilo, C.; Zeikus, R.; Gray, W.; Olivera, B. Invertebrate vasopressin/oxytocin homologs. Characterization of peptides from conus geographus and conus striatus venoms. *J. Biol. Chem.* **1987**, *262*, 15821–15824. [PubMed]

4. Bayrhuber, M.; Vijayan, V.; Ferber, M.; Graf, R.; Korukottu, J.; Imperial, J.; Garrett, J.E.; Olivera, B.M.; Terlau, H.; Zweckstetter, M. Conkunitzin-s1 is the first member of a new kunitz-type neurotoxin family structural and functional characterization. *J. Biol. Chem.* **2005**, *280*, 23766–23770. [CrossRef] [PubMed]

5. Lewis, R.J.; Dutertre, S.; Vetter, I.; Christie, M.J. Conus venom peptide pharmacology. *Pharmacol. Rev.* **2012**, *64*, 259–298. [CrossRef] [PubMed]

6. Duda, T.F., Jr.; Kohn, A.J.; Palumbi, S.R. Origins of diverse feeding ecologies within conus, a genus of venomous marine gastropods. *Biol. J. Linn. Soc.* **2001**, *73*, 391–409. [CrossRef]

7. Bergeron, Z.L.; Chun, J.B.; Baker, M.R.; Sandall, D.W.; Peigneur, S.; Peter, Y.; Thapa, P.; Milisen, J.W.; Tytgat, J.; Livett, B.G. A 'conovenomic'analysis of the milked venom from the mollusk-hunting cone snail conus textile—The pharmacological importance of post-translational modifications. *Peptides* **2013**, *49*, 145–158. [CrossRef] [PubMed]

8. Kohn, A.J. Human injuries and fatalities due to venomous marine snails of the family conidae. *Int. J. Clin. Pharmacol. Ther.* **2016**, *54*, 524. [CrossRef]

9. Dajas-Bailador, F.; Wonnacott, S. Nicotinic acetylcholine receptors and the regulation of neuronal signalling. *Trends Pharmacol. Sci.* **2004**, *25*, 317–324. [CrossRef]

10. Brown, D.A. Regulation of neural ion channels by muscarinic receptors. *Neuropharmacology* **2018**, *136*, 383–400. [CrossRef]

11. Kutlu, M.G.; Gould, T.J. Nicotine modulation of fear memories and anxiety: Implications for learning and anxiety disorders. *Biochem. Pharmacol.* **2015**, *97*, 498–511. [CrossRef]

12. Pérez-Verdaguer, M.; Capera, J.; Serrano-Novillo, C.; Estadella, I.; Sastre, D.; Felipe, A. The voltage-gated potassium channel kv1. 3 is a promising multitherapeutic target against human pathologies. *Expert Opin. Ther. Targets* **2016**, *20*, 577–591. [CrossRef] [PubMed]

13. Zamponi, G.W. A Crash Course in Calcium Channels. *ACS chem neurosci.* **2017**, *8*, 2583–2585. [CrossRef] [PubMed]

14. De Lera Ruiz, M.; Kraus, R.L. Voltage-gated sodium channels: Structure, function, pharmacology, and clinical indications. *J. Med. Chem.* **2015**, *58*, 7093–7118. [CrossRef] [PubMed]

15. Gao, B.; Peng, C.; Yang, J.; Yi, Y.; Zhang, J.; Shi, Q. Cone snails: A big store of conotoxins for novel drug discovery. *Toxins* **2017**, *9*, 397. [CrossRef] [PubMed]

16. Prashanth, J.R.; Brust, A.; Jin, A.-H.; Alewood, P.F.; Dutertre, S.; Lewis, R.J. Cone snail venomics: From novel biology to novel therapeutics. *Future Med. Chem.* **2014**, *6*, 1659–1675. [CrossRef] [PubMed]

17. Bajaj, S.; Han, J. Venom-derived peptide modulators of cation-selective channels: Friend, foe or frenemy. *Front. Pharmacol.* **2019**, *10*, 58. [CrossRef] [PubMed]

18. Akondi, K.B.; Muttenthaler, M.; Dutertre, S.; Kaas, Q.; Craik, D.J.; Lewis, R.J.; Alewood, P.F. Discovery, synthesis, and structure–activity relationships of conotoxins. *Chem. Rev.* **2014**, *114*, 5815–5847. [CrossRef]

19. Mansbach, R.A.; Travers, T.; McMahon, B.H.; Fair, J.M.; Gnanakaran, S. Snails in silico: A review of computational studies on the conopeptides. *Mar. Drugs* **2019**, *17*, 145. [CrossRef]

20. Kaas, Q.; Westermann, J.-C.; Craik, D.J. Conopeptide characterization and classifications: An analysis using conoserver. *Toxicon* **2010**, *55*, 1491–1509. [CrossRef]

21. Robinson, S.; Norton, R. Conotoxin gene superfamilies. *Mar. Drugs* **2014**, *12*, 6058–6101. [CrossRef]

22. Armishaw, C.J.; Alewood, P.F. Conotoxins as research tools and drug leads. *Curr. Protein Pept. Sci.* **2005**, *6*, 221–240. [CrossRef] [PubMed]

23. Lebbe, E.K.; Tytgat, J. In the picture: Disulfide-poor conopeptides, a class of pharmacologically interesting compounds. *J. Venom. Anim. Toxins Incl. Trop. Dis.* **2016**, *22*, 30. [CrossRef] [PubMed]

24. Tsetlin, V.; Utkin, Y.; Kasheverov, I. Polypeptide and peptide toxins, magnifying lenses for binding sites in nicotinic acetylcholine receptors. *Biochem. Pharmacol.* **2009**, *78*, 720–731. [CrossRef] [PubMed]

25. Heimer, P.; Schmitz, T.; Bäuml, C.A.; Imhof, D. Synthesis and structure determination of μ-conotoxin piiia isomers with different disulfide connectivities. *JoVE (J. Vis. Exp.)* **2018**, e58368. [CrossRef] [PubMed]

26. Espiritu, M.J.; Cabalteja, C.C.; Sugai, C.K.; Bingham, J.-P. Incorporation of post-translational modified amino acids as an approach to increase both chemical and biological diversity of conotoxins and conopeptides. *Amino Acids* **2014**, *46*, 125–151. [CrossRef]

27. Craik, Q.K.D. Conoserver, a database for conopeptide sequences and structures. *Bioinformatics* **2007**, *24*, 445–446.

28. Dao, F.-Y.; Yang, H.; Su, Z.-D.; Yang, W.; Wu, Y.; Hui, D.; Chen, W.; Tang, H.; Lin, H. Recent advances in conotoxin classification by using machine learning methods. *Molecules* **2017**, *22*, 1057. [CrossRef] [PubMed]

29. Himaya, S.; Lewis, R. Venomics-accelerated cone snail venom peptide discovery. *Int. J. Mol. Sci.* **2018**, *19*, 788. [CrossRef]

30. Dutertre, S.; Nicke, A.; Tsetlin, V.I. Nicotinic acetylcholine receptor inhibitors derived from snake and snail venoms. *Neuropharmacology* **2017**, *127*, 196–223. [CrossRef]

31. Ramírez, D.; Gonzalez, W.; Fissore, R.; Carvacho, I. Conotoxins as tools to understand the physiological function of voltage-gated calcium (cav) channels. *Mar. Drugs* **2017**, *15*, 313. [CrossRef]

32. Terlau, H.; Olivera, B.M. Conus venoms: A rich source of novel ion channel-targeted peptides. *Physiol. Rev.* **2004**, *84*, 41–68. [CrossRef] [PubMed]

33. Prashanth, J.R.; Dutertre, S.; Lewis, R.J. Pharmacology of predatory and defensive venom peptides in cone snails. *Mol. Biosyst.* **2017**, *13*, 2453–2465. [CrossRef] [PubMed]

34. Gray, W.; Luque, A.; Olivera, B.; Barrett, J.; Cruz, L. Peptide toxins from conus geographus venom. *J. Biol. Chem.* **1981**, *256*, 4734–4740. [PubMed]

35. Fainzilber, M.; Nakamura, T.; Lodder, J.C.; Zlotkin, E.; Kits, K.S.; Burlingame, A.L. Γ-conotoxin-pnviia, a γ-carboxyglutamate-containing peptide agonist of neuronal pacemaker cation currents. *Biochemistry* **1998**, *37*, 1470–1477. [CrossRef] [PubMed]

36. Fainzilber, M.; Gordon, D.; Hasson, A.; Spira, M.E.; Zlotkin, E. Mollusc-specific toxins from the venom of conus textile neovicarius. *Eur. J. Biochem.* **1991**, *202*, 589–595. [CrossRef] [PubMed]

37. Rigby, A.C.; Lucas-Meunier, E.; Kalume, D.E.; Czerwiec, E.; Hambe, B.; Dahlqvist, I.; Fossier, P.; Baux, G.; Roepstorff, P.; Baleja, J.D. A conotoxin from conus textile with unusual posttranslational modifications reduces presynaptic Ca^{2+} influx. *Proc. Natl. Acad. Sci.* **1999**, *96*, 5758–5763. [CrossRef] [PubMed]

38. Buczek, O.; Wei, D.; Babon, J.J.; Yang, X.; Fiedler, B.; Chen, P.; Yoshikami, D.; Olivera, B.M.; Bulaj, G.; Norton, R.S. Structure and sodium channel activity of an excitatory i1-superfamily conotoxin. *Biochemistry* **2007**, *46*, 9929–9940. [CrossRef] [PubMed]

39. Terlau, H.; Shon, K.-J.; Grilley, M.; Stocker, M.; Stühmer, W.; Olivera, B.M. Strategy for rapid immobilization of prey by a fish-hunting marine snail. *Nature* **1996**, *381*, 148. [CrossRef] [PubMed]

40. Cruz, L.; Gray, W.; Olivera, B.; Zeikus, R.; Kerr, L.; Yoshikami, D.; Moczydlowski, E. Conus geographus toxins that discriminate between neuronal and muscle sodium channels. *J. Biol. Chem.* **1985**, *260*, 9280–9288.

41. Sharpe, I.A.; Gehrmann, J.; Loughnan, M.L.; Thomas, L.; Adams, D.A.; Atkins, A.; Palant, E.; Craik, D.J.; Adams, D.J.; Alewood, P.F. Two new classes of conopeptides inhibit the α1-adrenoceptor and noradrenaline transporter. *Nat. Neurosci.* **2001**, *4*, 902. [CrossRef]

42. England, L.J.; Imperial, J.; Jacobsen, R.; Craig, A.G.; Gulyas, J.; Akhtar, M.; Rivier, J.; Julius, D.; Olivera, B.M. Inactivation of a serotonin-gated ion channel by a polypeptide toxin from marine snails. *Science* **1998**, *281*, 575–578. [CrossRef] [PubMed]

43. Petrel, C.; Hocking, H.; Reynaud, M.; Upert, G.; Favreau, P.; Biass, D.; Paolini-Bertrand, M.; Peigneur, S.; Tytgat, J.; Gilles, N. Identification, structural and pharmacological characterization of τ-cnva, a conopeptide that selectively interacts with somatostatin sst3 receptor. *Biochem. Pharmacol.* **2013**, *85*, 1663–1671. [CrossRef] [PubMed]

44. Kerr, L.M.; Yoshikami, D. A venom peptide with a novel presynaptic blocking action. *Nature* **1984**, *308*, 282. [CrossRef] [PubMed]

45. Zoli, M.; Pucci, S.; Vilella, A.; Gotti, C. Neuronal and extraneuronal nicotinic acetylcholine receptors. *Curr. Neuropharmacol.* **2018**, *16*, 338–349. [CrossRef] [PubMed]

46. Millar, N.S.; Gotti, C. Diversity of vertebrate nicotinic acetylcholine receptors. *Neuropharmacology* **2009**, *56*, 237–246. [CrossRef]

47. Gotti, C.; Clementi, F. Neuronal nicotinic receptors: From structure to pathology. *Prog. Neurobiol.* **2004**, *74*, 363–396. [CrossRef]

48. Wessler, I.; Kirkpatrick, C. Acetylcholine beyond neurons: The non-neuronal cholinergic system in humans. *Br. J. Pharmacol.* **2008**, *154*, 1558–1571. [CrossRef]

49. Gotti, C.; Clementi, F.; Fornari, A.; Gaimarri, A.; Guiducci, S.; Manfredi, I.; Moretti, M.; Pedrazzi, P.; Pucci, L.; Zoli, M. Structural and functional diversity of native brain neuronal nicotinic receptors. *Biochem. Pharmacol.* **2009**, *78*, 703–711. [CrossRef]

50. Nicke, A.; Samochocki, M.; Loughnan, M.L.; Bansal, P.S.; Maelicke, A.; Lewis, R.J. A-conotoxins epi and auib switch subtype selectivity and activity in native versus recombinant nicotinic acetylcholine receptors. *FEBS Lett.* **2003**, *554*, 219–223. [CrossRef]

51. Azam, L.; McIntosh, J.M. Alpha-conotoxins as pharmacological probes of nicotinic acetylcholine receptors. *Acta Pharmacol. Sin.* **2009**, *30*, 771. [CrossRef]

52. Carstens, B.B.; Berecki, G.; Daniel, J.T.; Lee, H.S.; Jackson, K.A.; Tae, H.S.; Sadeghi, M.; Castro, J.; O'Donnell, T.; Deiteren, A. Structure–activity studies of cysteine-rich α-conotoxins that inhibit high-voltage-activated calcium channels via gabab receptor activation reveal a minimal functional motif. *Angew. Chem. Int. Ed.* **2016**, *55*, 4692–4696. [CrossRef] [PubMed]

53. Janes, R.W. A-conotoxins as selective probes for nicotinic acetylcholine receptor subclasses. *Curr. Opin. Pharmacol.* **2005**, *5*, 280–292. [CrossRef] [PubMed]

54. Turner, M.W.; Marquart, L.A.; Phillips, P.D.; McDougal, O.M. Mutagenesis of α-conotoxins for enhancing activity and selectivity for nicotinic acetylcholine receptors. *Toxins* **2019**, *11*, 113. [CrossRef] [PubMed]

55. Cruz, L.J.; Gray, W.R.; Olivera, B.M. Purification and properties of a myotoxin from conus geographus venom. *Arch. Biochem. Biophys.* **1978**, *190*, 539–548. [CrossRef]

56. McIntosh, J.M.; Yoshikami, D.; Mahe, E.; Nielsen, D.B.; Rivier, J.E.; Gray, W.R.; Olivera, B.M. A nicotinic acetylcholine receptor ligand of unique specificity, alpha-conotoxin imi. *J. Biol. Chem.* **1994**, *269*, 16733–16739. [PubMed]

57. Azam, L.; Dowell, C.; Watkins, M.; Stitzel, J.A.; Olivera, B.M.; McIntosh, J.M. A-conotoxin buia, a novel peptide from conus bullatus, distinguishes among neuronal nicotinic acetylcholine receptors. *J. Biol. Chem.* **2005**, *280*, 80–87. [CrossRef] [PubMed]

58. Luo, S.; Kulak, J.M.; Cartier, G.E.; Jacobsen, R.B.; Yoshikami, D.; Olivera, B.M.; McIntosh, J.M. A-conotoxin auib selectively blocks α3β4 nicotinic acetylcholine receptors and nicotine-evoked norepinephrine release. *J. Neurosci.* **1998**, *18*, 8571–8579. [CrossRef] [PubMed]

59. Clark, R.J.; Fischer, H.; Nevin, S.T.; Adams, D.J.; Craik, D.J. The synthesis, structural characterization, and receptor specificity of the α-conotoxin vc1. 1. *J. Biol. Chem.* **2006**, *281*, 23254–23263. [CrossRef]

60. Imperial, J.S.; Bansal, P.S.; Alewood, P.F.; Daly, N.L.; Craik, D.J.; Sporning, A.; Terlau, H.; López-Vera, E.; Bandyopadhyay, P.K.; Olivera, B.M. A novel conotoxin inhibitor of kv1. 6 channel and nachr subtypes defines a new superfamily of conotoxins. *Biochemistry* **2006**, *45*, 8331–8340. [CrossRef]

61. Teichert, R.W.; Jimenez, E.C.; Olivera, B.M. As-conotoxin rviiia: A structurally unique conotoxin that broadly targets nicotinic acetylcholine receptors. *Biochemistry* **2005**, *44*, 7897–7902. [CrossRef]

62. Loughnan, M.L.; Nicke, A.; Jones, A.; Adams, D.J.; Alewood, P.F.; Lewis, R.J. Chemical and functional identification and characterization of novel sulfated α-conotoxins from the cone snail conus a nemone. *J. Med. Chem.* **2004**, *47*, 1234–1241. [CrossRef] [PubMed]

63. Armishaw, C.J. Synthetic α-conotoxin mutants as probes for studying nicotinic acetylcholine receptors and in the development of novel drug leads. *Toxins* **2010**, *2*, 1471–1499. [CrossRef] [PubMed]

64. Weltzin, M.M.; George, A.A.; Lukas, R.J.; Whiteaker, P. Distinctive single-channel properties of α4β2-nicotinic acetylcholine receptor isoforms. *PLoS ONE* **2019**, *14*, e0213143. [CrossRef] [PubMed]

65. Lebbe, E.; Peigneur, S.; Wijesekara, I.; Tytgat, J. Conotoxins targeting nicotinic acetylcholine receptors: An overview. *Mar. Drugs* **2014**, *12*, 2970–3004. [CrossRef] [PubMed]

66. Martinez, J.S.; Olivera, B.M.; Gray, W.R.; Craig, A.G.; Groebe, D.R.; Abramson, S.N.; McIntosh, J.M. Alpha.-conotoxin ei, a new nicotinic acetylcholine receptor antagonist with novel selectivity. *Biochemistry* **1995**, *34*, 14519–14526. [CrossRef] [PubMed]

67. Groebe, D.R.; Dumm, J.M.; Levitan, E.S.; Abramson, S.N. Alpha-conotoxins selectively inhibit one of the two acetylcholine binding sites of nicotinic receptors. *Mol. Pharmacol.* **1995**, *48*, 105–111. [PubMed]

68. Gerwig, G.; Hocking, H.; Stöcklin, R.; Kamerling, J.; Boelens, R. Glycosylation of conotoxins. *Mar. Drugs* **2013**, *11*, 623–642. [CrossRef] [PubMed]

69. Kang, T.S.; Radić, Z.; Talley, T.T.; Jois, S.D.; Taylor, P.; Kini, R.M. Protein folding determinants: Structural features determining alternative disulfide pairing in α-and χ/λ-conotoxins. *Biochemistry* **2007**, *46*, 3338–3355. [CrossRef]

70. Lin, B.; Xiang, S.; Li, M. Residues responsible for the selectivity of α-conotoxins for ac-achbp or nachrs. *Mar. Drugs* **2016**, *14*, 173. [CrossRef]

71. Whiteaker, P.; Christensen, S.; Yoshikami, D.; Dowell, C.; Watkins, M.; Gulyas, J.; Rivier, J.; Olivera, B.M.; McIntosh, J.M. Discovery, synthesis, and structure activity of a highly selective α7 nicotinic acetylcholine receptor antagonist. *Biochemistry* **2007**, *46*, 6628–6638. [CrossRef]

72. McIntosh, J.M.; Dowell, C.; Watkins, M.; Garrett, J.E.; Yoshikami, D.; Olivera, B.M. A-conotoxin gic from conus geographus, a novel peptide antagonist of nicotinic acetylcholine receptors. *J. Biol. Chem.* **2002**, *277*, 33610–33615. [CrossRef] [PubMed]

73. Nicke, A.; Loughnan, M.L.; Millard, E.L.; Alewood, P.F.; Adams, D.J.; Daly, N.L.; Craik, D.J.; Lewis, R.J. Isolation, structure, and activity of gid, a novel α4/7-conotoxin with an extended n-terminal sequence. *J. Biol. Chem.* **2003**, *278*, 3137–3144. [CrossRef] [PubMed]

74. Johnson, D.S.; Martinez, J.; Elgoyhen, A.B.; Heinemann, S.F.; McIntosh, J.M. Alpha-conotoxin imi exhibits subtype-specific nicotinic acetylcholine receptor blockade: Preferential inhibition of homomeric alpha 7 and alpha 9 receptors. *Mol. Pharmacol.* **1995**, *48*, 194–199. [PubMed]

75. Chen, J.; Liang, L.; Ning, H.; Cai, F.; Liu, Z.; Zhang, L.; Zhou, L.; Dai, Q. Cloning, synthesis and functional characterization of a novel α-conotoxin lt1. 3. *Mar. Drugs* **2018**, *16*, 112. [CrossRef] [PubMed]

76. McIntosh, J.M.; Azam, L.; Staheli, S.; Dowell, C.; Lindstrom, J.M.; Kuryatov, A.; Garrett, J.E.; Marks, M.J.; Whiteaker, P. Analogs of α-conotoxin mii are selective for α6-containing nicotinic acetylcholine receptors. *Mol. Pharmacol.* **2004**, *65*, 944–952. [CrossRef] [PubMed]

77. Hone, A.J.; Gajewiak, J.; Christensen, S.; Lindstrom, J.; McIntosh, J.M. A-conotoxin peia [s9h, v10a, e14n] potently and selectively blocks α6β2β3 versus α6β4 nicotinic acetylcholine receptors. *Mol. Pharmacol.* **2012**, *82*, 972–982. [CrossRef] [PubMed]

78. Luo, S.; Nguyen, T.; Cartier, G.; Olivera, B.; Yoshikami, D.; McIntosh, J. Single-residue alteration in α-conotoxin pnia switches its nachr subtype selectivity. *Biochemistry* **1999**, *38*, 14542–14548. [CrossRef]

79. Luo, S.; Zhangsun, D.; Wu, Y.; Zhu, X.; Hu, Y.; McIntyre, M.; Christensen, S.; Akcan, M.; Craik, D.J.; McIntosh, J.M. Characterization of a novel α-conotoxin from conus textile that selectively targets α6/α3β2β3 nicotinic acetylcholine receptors. *J. Biol. Chem.* **2013**, *288*, 894–902. [CrossRef]

80. Luo, S.; Zhangsun, D.; Zhu, X.; Wu, Y.; Hu, Y.; Christensen, S.; Harvey, P.J.; Akcan, M.; Craik, D.J.; McIntosh, J.M. Characterization of a novel α-conotoxin txid from conus textile that potently blocks rat α3β4 nicotinic acetylcholine receptors. *J. Med. Chem.* **2013**, *56*, 9655–9663. [CrossRef]

81. Yu, R.; Tabassum, N.; Jiang, T. Investigation of α-conotoxin unbinding using umbrella sampling. *Bioorganic Med. Chem. Lett.* **2016**, *26*, 1296–1300. [CrossRef]

82. Changeux, J.-P. The nicotinic acetylcholine receptor: A typical 'allosteric machine'. *Philos. Trans. R. Soc. B Biol. Sci.* **2018**, *373*, 20170174. [CrossRef] [PubMed]

83. Delbart, F.; Brams, M.; Gruss, F.; Noppen, S.; Peigneur, S.; Boland, S.; Chaltin, P.; Brandao-Neto, J.; von Delft, F.; Touw, W.G. An allosteric binding site of the α7 nicotinic acetylcholine receptor revealed in a humanized acetylcholine-binding protein. *J. Biol. Chem.* **2018**, *293*, 2534–2545. [CrossRef] [PubMed]

84. Lin, B.; Xu, M.; Zhu, X.; Wu, Y.; Liu, X.; Zhangsun, D.; Hu, Y.; Xiang, S.-H.; Kasheverov, I.E.; Tsetlin, V.I. From crystal structure of α-conotoxin gic in complex with ac-achbp to molecular determinants of its high selectivity for α3β2 nachr. *Sci. Rep.* **2016**, *6*, 22349. [CrossRef] [PubMed]

85. Kasheverov, I.E.; Utkin, Y.N.; Tsetlin, V.I. Naturally occurring and synthetic peptides acting on nicotinic acetylcholine receptors. *Curr. Pharm. Des.* **2009**, *15*, 2430–2452. [CrossRef] [PubMed]

86. Seung-Wook, C.; Do-Hyoung, K.; Olivera, B.M.; Mcintosh, J.M.; Kyou-Hoon, H. Solution conformation of alpha-conotoxin gic, a novel potent antagonist of alpha3beta2 nicotinic acetylcholine receptors. *Biochem. J.* **2004**, *380*, 347–352.

87. Kim, H.-W.; McIntosh, J.M. A6 nachr subunit residues that confer α-conotoxin buia selectivity. *FASEB J.* **2012**, *26*, 4102–4110. [CrossRef]

88. Ellison, M.; Gao, F.; Wang, H.-L.; Sine, S.M.; McIntosh, J.M.; Olivera, B.M. A-conotoxins imi and imii target distinct regions of the human α7 nicotinic acetylcholine receptor and distinguish human nicotinic receptor subtypes. *Biochemistry* **2004**, *43*, 16019–16026. [CrossRef]

89. Ulens, C.; Hogg, R.C.; Celie, P.H.; Bertrand, D.; Tsetlin, V.; Smit, A.B.; Sixma, T.K. Structural determinants of selective α-conotoxin binding to a nicotinic acetylcholine receptor homolog achbp. *Proc. Natl. Acad. Sci.* **2006**, *103*, 3615–3620. [CrossRef]

90. Kuo, M.M.-C.; Haynes, W.J.; Loukin, S.H.; Kung, C.; Saimi, Y. Prokaryotic k$^+$ channels: From crystal structures to diversity. *FEMS Microbiol. Rev.* **2005**, *29*, 961–985. [CrossRef]

91. Grider MH, G.C. *Physiology, Action Potential*; StatPearls Publishing LLC: Treasure Island, FL, USA, 2019.
92. Capera, J.; Serrano-Novillo, C.; Navarro-Pérez, M.; Cassinelli, S.; Felipe, A. The potassium channel odyssey: Mechanisms of traffic and membrane arrangement. *Int. J. Mol. Sci.* **2019**, *20*, 734. [CrossRef]
93. Choe, S. Ion channel structure: Potassium channel structures. *Nat. Rev. Neurosci.* **2002**, *3*, 115. [CrossRef] [PubMed]
94. Kuang, Q.; Purhonen, P.; Hebert, H. Structure of potassium channels. *Cell. Mol. Life Sci.* **2015**, *72*, 3677–3693. [CrossRef] [PubMed]
95. Gutman, G.A.; Chandy, K.G.; Grissmer, S.; Lazdunski, M.; Mckinnon, D.; Pardo, L.A.; Robertson, G.A.; Rudy, B.; Sanguinetti, M.C.; Stühmer, W. International union of pharmacology. Liii. Nomenclature and molecular relationships of voltage-gated potassium channels. *Pharmacol. Rev.* **2005**, *57*, 473–508. [CrossRef] [PubMed]
96. Wei, A.D.; Gutman, G.A.; Aldrich, R.; Chandy, K.G.; Grissmer, S.; Wulff, H. International union of pharmacology. Lii. Nomenclature and molecular relationships of calcium-activated potassium channels. *Pharmacol. Rev.* **2005**, *57*, 463–472. [CrossRef] [PubMed]
97. Kubo, Y.; Adelman, J.P.; Clapham, D.E.; Jan, L.Y.; Karschin, A.; Kurachi, Y.; Lazdunski, M.; Nichols, C.G.; Seino, S.; Vandenberg, C.A. International union of pharmacology. Liv. Nomenclature and molecular relationships of inwardly rectifying potassium channels. *Pharmacol. Rev.* **2005**, *57*, 509–526. [CrossRef] [PubMed]
98. Goldstein, S.A.; Bayliss, D.A.; Kim, D.; Lesage, F.; Plant, L.D.; Rajan, S. International union of pharmacology. Lv. Nomenclature and molecular relationships of two-p potassium channels. *Pharmacol. Rev.* **2005**, *57*, 527–540. [CrossRef] [PubMed]
99. Kuzmenkov, A.; Grishin, E.; Vassilevski, A. Diversity of potassium channel ligands: Focus on scorpion toxins. *Biochemistry* **2015**, *80*, 1764–1799. [CrossRef] [PubMed]
100. Miller, C. An overview of the potassium channel family. *Genome Biol.* **2000**, *1*, reviews0004.0001. [CrossRef]
101. Panyi, G.; Deutsch, C. Cross talk between activation and slow inactivation gates of shaker potassium channels. *J. Gen. Physiol.* **2006**, *128*, 547–559. [CrossRef]
102. Massilia, G.R.; Eliseo, T.; Grolleau, F.; Lapied, B.; Barbier, J.; Bournaud, R.; Molgó, J.; Cicero, D.O.; Paci, M.; Schinina, M.E. Contryphan-vn: A modulator of Ca^{2+}-dependent k^+ channels. *Biochem. Biophys. Res. Commun.* **2003**, *303*, 238–246. [CrossRef]
103. Hocking, H.G.; Gerwig, G.J.; Dutertre, S.; Violette, A.; Favreau, P.; Stöcklin, R.; Kamerling, J.P.; Boelens, R. Structure of the o-glycosylated conopeptide cctx from conus consors venom. *Chem. A Eur. J.* **2013**, *19*, 870–879. [CrossRef] [PubMed]
104. Fan, C.-X.; Chen, X.-K.; Zhang, C.; Wang, L.-X.; Duan, K.-L.; He, L.-L.; Cao, Y.; Liu, S.-Y.; Zhong, M.-N.; Ulens, C. A novel conotoxin from conus betulinus, κ-btx, unique in cysteine pattern and in function as a specific bk channel modulator. *J. Biol. Chem.* **2003**, *278*, 12624–12633. [CrossRef] [PubMed]
105. Finol-Urdaneta, R.K.; Remedi, M.S.; Raasch, W.; Becker, S.; Clark, R.B.; Strüver, N.; Pavlov, E.; Nichols, C.G.; French, R.J.; Terlau, H. Block of kv1. 7 potassium currents increases glucose-stimulated insulin secretion. *EMBO Mol. Med.* **2012**, *4*, 424–434. [CrossRef] [PubMed]
106. Chen, P.; Dendorfer, A.; Finol-Urdaneta, R.K.; Terlau, H.; Olivera, B.M. Biochemical characterization of κm-riiij, a kv1. 2 channel blocker evaluation of cardioprotective effects of κm-conotoxins. *J. Biol. Chem.* **2010**, *285*, 14882–14889. [CrossRef]
107. Craig, A.G.; Zafaralla, G.; Cruz, L.J.; Santos, A.D.; Hillyard, D.R.; Dykert, J.; Rivier, J.E.; Gray, W.R.; Imperial, J.; DelaCruz, R.G. An o-glycosylated neuroexcitatory conus peptide. *Biochemistry* **1998**, *37*, 16019–16025. [CrossRef]
108. Kauferstein, S.; Huys, I.; Lamthanh, H.; Stöcklin, R.; Sotto, F.; Menez, A.; Tytgat, J.; Mebs, D. A novel conotoxin inhibiting vertebrate voltage-sensitive potassium channels. *Toxicon* **2003**, *42*, 43–52. [CrossRef]
109. Aguilar, M.B.; Pérez-Reyes, L.I.; López, Z.; de la Cotera, E.P.H.; Falcón, A.; Ayala, C.; Galván, M.; Salvador, C.; Escobar, L.I. Peptide sr11a from conus spurius is a novel peptide blocker for kv1 potassium channels. *Peptides* **2010**, *31*, 1287–1291. [CrossRef]
110. Naranjo, D. Inhibition of single shaker k channels by κ− conotoxin-pviia. *Biophys. J.* **2002**, *82*, 3003–3011. [CrossRef]
111. De la Vega, R.C.R.; Possani, L.D. Current views on scorpion toxins specific for k^+-channels. *Toxicon* **2004**, *43*, 865–875. [CrossRef]

112. Jacobsen, R.B.; Koch, E.D.; Lange-Malecki, B.; Stocker, M.; Verhey, J.; Van Wagoner, R.M.; Vyazovkina, A.; Olivera, B.M.; Terlau, H. Single amino acid substitutions in κ-conotoxin pviia disrupt interaction with the shaker k$^+$ channel. *J. Biol. Chem.* **2000**, *275*, 24639–24644. [CrossRef]

113. Huang, X.; Dong, F.; Zhou, H.-X. Electrostatic recognition and induced fit in the κ-pviia toxin binding to shaker potassium channel. *J. Am. Chem. Soc.* **2005**, *127*, 6836–6849. [CrossRef] [PubMed]

114. Kwon, S.; Bosmans, F.; Kaas, Q.; Cheneval, O.; Conibear, A.C.; Rosengren, K.J.; Wang, C.K.; Schroeder, C.I.; Craik, D.J. Efficient enzymatic cyclization of an inhibitory cystine knot-containing peptide. *Biotechnol. Bioeng.* **2016**, *113*, 2202–2212. [CrossRef] [PubMed]

115. Cordeiro, S.; Finol-Urdaneta, R.K.; Köpfer, D.; Markushina, A.; Song, J.; French, R.J.; Kopec, W.; de Groot, B.L.; Giacobassi, M.J.; Leavitt, L.S. Conotoxin κm-riiij, a tool targeting asymmetric heteromeric kv1 channels. *Proc. Natl. Acad. Sci.* **2019**, *116*, 1059–1064. [CrossRef] [PubMed]

116. Al-Sabi, A.; Lennartz, D.; Ferber, M.; Gulyas, J.; Rivier, J.E.; Olivera, B.M.; Carlomagno, T.; Terlau, H. Km-conotoxin riiik, structural and functional novelty in a k$^+$ channel antagonist. *Biochemistry* **2004**, *43*, 8625–8635. [CrossRef] [PubMed]

117. Verdier, L.; Al-Sabi, A.; Rivier, J.E.; Olivera, B.M.; Terlau, H.; Carlomagno, T. Identification of a novel pharmacophore for peptide toxins interacting with k$^+$ channels. *J. Biol. Chem.* **2005**, *280*, 21246–21255. [CrossRef] [PubMed]

118. Rashid, M.; Mahdavi, S.; Kuyucak, S. Computational studies of marine toxins targeting ion channels. *Mar. Drugs* **2013**, *11*, 848–869. [CrossRef] [PubMed]

119. Dauplais, M.; Lecoq, A.; Song, J.; Cotton, J.; Jamin, N.; Gilquin, B.; Roumestand, C.; Vita, C.; de Medeiros, C.L.; Rowan, E.G. On the convergent evolution of animal toxins conservation of a diad of functional residues in potassium channel-blocking toxins with unrelated structures. *J. Biol. Chem.* **1997**, *272*, 4302–4309. [CrossRef] [PubMed]

120. Shon, K.-J.; Stocker, M.; Terlau, H.; Stühmer, W.; Jacobsen, R.; Walker, C.; Grilley, M.; Watkins, M.; Hillyard, D.R.; Gray, W.R. K-conotoxin pviia is a peptide inhibiting theshaker k$^+$ channel. *J. Biol. Chem.* **1998**, *273*, 33–38. [CrossRef] [PubMed]

121. Catterall, W.A. Voltage-gated sodium channels at 60: Structure, function and pathophysiology. *J. Physiol.* **2012**, *590*, 2577–2589. [CrossRef] [PubMed]

122. Catterall, W.A.; Goldin, A.L.; Waxman, S.G. International union of pharmacology. Xlvii. Nomenclature and structure-function relationships of voltage-gated sodium channels. *Pharmacol. Rev.* **2005**, *57*, 397–409. [CrossRef] [PubMed]

123. Kwong, K.; Carr, M.J. Voltage-gated sodium channels. *Curr. Opin. Pharmacol.* **2015**, *22*, 131–139. [CrossRef] [PubMed]

124. Cestèle, S.; Catterall, W.A. Molecular mechanisms of neurotoxin action on voltage-gated sodium channels. *Biochimie* **2000**, *82*, 883–892. [CrossRef]

125. Payandeh, J.; El-Din, T.M.G.; Scheuer, T.; Zheng, N.; Catterall, W.A. Crystal structure of a voltage-gated sodium channel in two potentially inactivated states. *Nature* **2012**, *486*, 135. [CrossRef] [PubMed]

126. Catterall, W.A. Structure and function of voltage-gated sodium channels at atomic resolution. *Exp. Physiol.* **2014**, *99*, 35–51. [CrossRef] [PubMed]

127. Catterall, W.A. From ionic currents to molecular mechanisms: The structure and function of voltage-gated sodium channels. *Neuron* **2000**, *26*, 13–25. [CrossRef]

128. Zhorov, B.S. Structural models of ligand-bound sodium channels. In *Voltage-Gated Sodium Channels: Structure, Function and Channelopathies*; Springer: New York, NY, USA, 2017; Volume 246, pp. 251–269.

129. Jover, E.; Martin-Moutot, N.; Couraud, F.; Rochat, H. Binding of scorpion toxins to rat brain synaptosomal fraction. Effects of membrane potential, ions, and other neurotoxins. *Biochemistry* **1980**, *19*, 463–467. [CrossRef] [PubMed]

130. Tikhonov, D.B.; Zhorov, B.S. Predicting structural details of the sodium channel pore basing on animal toxin studies. *Front. Pharmacol.* **2018**, *9*, 880. [CrossRef]

131. Ekberg, J.; Craik, D.J.; Adams, D.J. Conotoxin modulation of voltage-gated sodium channels. *Int. J. Biochem. Cell Biol.* **2008**, *40*, 2363–2368. [CrossRef]

132. Buczek, O.; Yoshikami, D.; Bulaj, G.; Jimenez, E.C.; Olivera, B.M. Post-translational amino acid isomerization a functionally important d-amino acid in an excitatory peptide. *J. Biol. Chem.* **2005**, *280*, 4247–4253. [CrossRef]

133. Fiedler, B.; Zhang, M.-M.; Buczek, O.; Azam, L.; Bulaj, G.; Norton, R.S.; Olivera, B.M.; Yoshikami, D. Specificity, affinity and efficacy of iota-conotoxin rxia, an agonist of voltage-gated sodium channels nav1. 2, 1.6 and 1.7. *Biochem. Pharmacol.* **2008**, *75*, 2334–2344. [CrossRef]

134. Tietze, A.A.; Tietze, D.; Ohlenschläger, O.; Leipold, E.; Ullrich, F.; Kühl, T.; Mischo, A.; Buntkowsky, G.; Görlach, M.; Heinemann, S.H. Structurally diverse μ-conotoxin piiia isomers block sodium channel nav1. 4. *Angew. Chem. Int. Ed.* **2012**, *51*, 4058–4061. [CrossRef] [PubMed]

135. Khoo, K.K.; Gupta, K.; Green, B.R.; Zhang, M.-M.; Watkins, M.; Olivera, B.M.; Balaram, P.; Yoshikami, D.; Bulaj, G.; Norton, R.S. Distinct disulfide isomers of μ-conotoxins kiiia and kiiib block voltage-gated sodium channels. *Biochemistry* **2012**, *51*, 9826–9835. [CrossRef] [PubMed]

136. Wang, L.; Liu, J.; Pi, C.; Zeng, X.; Zhou, M.; Jiang, X.; Chen, S.; Ren, Z.; Xu, A. Identification of a novel m-superfamily conotoxin with the ability to enhance tetrodotoxin sensitive sodium currents. *Arch. Toxicol.* **2009**, *83*, 925–932. [CrossRef] [PubMed]

137. Jimenez, E.C.; Shetty, R.P.; Lirazan, M.; Rivier, J.; Walker, C.; Abogadie, F.C.; Yoshikami, D.; Cruz, L.J.; Olivera, B.M. Novel excitatory conus peptides define a new conotoxin superfamily. *J. Neurochem.* **2003**, *85*, 610–621. [CrossRef] [PubMed]

138. Green, B.; Olivera, B. Venom peptides from cone snails: Pharmacological probes for voltage-gated sodium channels. In *Current Topics in Membranes*; Elsevier: Amsterdam, The Netherlands, 2016; Volume 78, pp. 65–86.

139. Daly, N.L.; Ekberg, J.A.; Thomas, L.; Adams, D.J.; Lewis, R.J.; Craik, D.J. Structures of μo-conotoxins from conus marmoreus inhibitors of tetrodotoxin (ttx)-sensitive and ttx-resistant sodium channels in mammalian sensory neurons. *J. Biol. Chem.* **2004**, *279*, 25774–25782. [CrossRef] [PubMed]

140. Fainzilber, M.; van der Schors, R.; Lodder, J.C.; Li, K.W.; Geraerts, W.P.; Kits, K.S. New sodium channel-blocking conotoxins also affect calcium currents in lymnaea neurons. *Biochemistry* **1995**, *34*, 5364–5371. [CrossRef] [PubMed]

141. McIntosh, J.M.; Hasson, A.; Spira, M.E.; Gray, W.R.; Li, W.; Marsh, M.; Hillyard, D.R.; Olivera, B.M. A new family of conotoxins that blocks voltage-gated sodium channels. *J. Biol. Chem.* **1995**, *270*, 16796–16802. [CrossRef] [PubMed]

142. Vetter, I.; Dekan, Z.; Knapp, O.; Adams, D.J.; Alewood, P.F.; Lewis, R.J. Isolation, characterization and total regioselective synthesis of the novel μo-conotoxin mfvia from conus magnificus that targets voltage-gated sodium channels. *Biochem. Pharmacol.* **2012**, *84*, 540–548. [CrossRef]

143. Zorn, S.; Leipold, E.; Hansel, A.; Bulaj, G.; Olivera, B.M.; Terlau, H.; Heinemann, S.H. The μo-conotoxin mrvia inhibits voltage-gated sodium channels by associating with domain-3. *FEBS Lett.* **2006**, *580*, 1360–1364. [CrossRef]

144. Leipold, E.; DeBie, H.; Zorn, S.; Adolfo, B.; Olivera, B.M.; Terlau, H.; Heinemann, S.H. μo-conotoxins inhibit nav channels by interfering with their voltage sensors in domain-2. *Channels* **2007**, *1*, 253–262. [CrossRef]

145. Leipold, E.; Hansel, A.; Borges, A.; Heinemann, S.H. Subtype specificity of scorpion β-toxin tz1 interaction with voltage-gated sodium channels is determined by the pore loop of domain 3. *Mol. Pharmacol.* **2006**, *70*, 340–347. [CrossRef]

146. Cohen, L.; Ilan, N.; Gur, M.; Stühmer, W.; Gordon, D.; Gurevitz, M. Design of a specific activator for skeletal muscle sodium channels uncovers channel architecture. *J. Biol. Chem.* **2007**, *282*, 29424–29430. [CrossRef] [PubMed]

147. Leipold, E.; Borges, A.; Heinemann, S.H. Scorpion β-toxin interference with nav channel voltage sensor gives rise to excitatory and depressant modes. *J. Gen. Physiol.* **2012**, *139*, 305–319. [CrossRef] [PubMed]

148. Deuis, J.R.; Dekan, Z.; Inserra, M.C.; Lee, T.-H.; Aguilar, M.-I.; Craik, D.J.; Lewis, R.J.; Alewood, P.F.; Mobli, M.; Schroeder, C.I. Development of a μo-conotoxin analogue with improved lipid membrane interactions and potency for the analgesic sodium channel nav1. 8. *J. Biol. Chem.* **2016**, *291*, 11829–11842. [CrossRef] [PubMed]

149. Heinemann, S.; Leipold, E. Conotoxins of the o-superfamily affecting voltage-gated sodium channels. *Cell. Mol. Life Sci.* **2007**, *64*, 1329–1340. [CrossRef] [PubMed]

150. Fainzilber, M.; Kofman, O.; Zlotkin, E.; Gordon, D. A new neurotoxin receptor site on sodium channels is identified by a conotoxin that affects sodium channel inactivation in molluscs and acts as an antagonist in rat brain. *J. Biol. Chem.* **1994**, *269*, 2574–2580. [PubMed]

151. Shon, K.-J.; Hasson, A.; Spira, M.E.; Cruz, L.J.; Gray, W.R.; Olivera, B.M. Delta.-conotoxin gmvia, a novel peptide from the venom of conus gloriamaris. *Biochemistry* **1994**, *33*, 11420–11425. [CrossRef] [PubMed]

152. Peigneur, S.; Paolini-Bertrand, M.; Gaertner, H.; Biass, D.; Violette, A.; Stöcklin, R.; Favreau, P.; Tytgat, J.; Hartley, O. Δ-conotoxins synthesized using an acid-cleavable solubility tag approach reveal key structural determinants for nav subtype selectivity. *J. Biol. Chem.* **2014**, *289*, 35341–35350. [CrossRef] [PubMed]

153. Fainzilber, M.; Lodder, J.C.; Kits, K.S.; Kofman, O.; Vinnitsky, I.; Van Rietschoten, J.; Zlotkin, E.; Gordon, D. A new conotoxin affecting sodium current inactivation interacts with the-conotoxin receptor site. *J. Biol. Chem.* **1995**, *270*, 1123–1129. [CrossRef]

154. Leipold, E.; Hansel, A.; Olivera, B.M.; Terlau, H.; Heinemann, S.H. Molecular interaction of δ-conotoxins with voltage-gated sodium channels. *FEBS Lett.* **2005**, *579*, 3881–3884. [CrossRef]

155. Tietze, D.; Leipold, E.; Heimer, P.; Böhm, M.; Winschel, W.; Imhof, D.; Heinemann, S.H.; Tietze, A.A. Molecular interaction of δ-conopeptide evia with voltage-gated na+ channels. *Biochim. Biophys. Acta (BBA)-Gen. Subj.* **2016**, *1860*, 2053–2063. [CrossRef] [PubMed]

156. Green, B.R.; Bulaj, G.; Norton, R.S. Structure and function of μ-conotoxins, peptide-based sodium channel blockers with analgesic activity. *Future Med. Chem.* **2014**, *6*, 1677–1698. [CrossRef] [PubMed]

157. Liu, J.; Wu, Q.; Pi, C.; Zhao, Y.; Zhou, M.; Wang, L.; Chen, S.; Xu, A. Isolation and characterization of a t-superfamily conotoxin from conus litteratus with targeting tetrodotoxin-sensitive sodium channels. *Peptides* **2007**, *28*, 2313–2319. [CrossRef]

158. Norton, R.S. μ-conotoxins as leads in the development of new analgesics. *Molecules* **2010**, *15*, 2825–2844. [CrossRef]

159. Zhang, M.M.; McArthur, J.R.; Azam, L.; Bulaj, G.; Olivera, B.M.; French, R.J.; Yoshikami, D. Unexpected synergism between tetrodotoxin and μ-conotoxin in blocking voltage-gated sodium channels. *Channels* **2009**, *3*, 32–38. [CrossRef]

160. Stephan, M.; Potts, J.; Agnew, W. The μi skeletal muscle sodium channel: Mutation e403q eliminates sensitivity to tetrodotoxin but not to μ-conotoxins giiia and giiib. *J. Membr. Biol.* **1994**, *137*, 1–8. [CrossRef] [PubMed]

161. Leipold, E.; Ullrich, F.; Thiele, M.; Tietze, A.A.; Terlau, H.; Imhof, D.; Heinemann, S.H. Subtype-specific block of voltage-gated k+ channels by μ-conopeptides. *Biochem. Biophys. Res. Commun.* **2017**, *482*, 1135–1140. [CrossRef]

162. Kaufmann, D.; Tietze, A.A.; Tietze, D. In silico analysis of the subtype selective blockage of kcna ion channels through the μ-conotoxins piiia, siiia, and giiia. *Mar. Drugs* **2019**, *17*, 180. [CrossRef]

163. Xue, T.; Ennis, I.L.; Sato, K.; French, R.J.; Li, R.A. Novel interactions identified between μ-conotoxin and the na+ channel domain i p-loop: Implications for toxin-pore binding geometry. *Biophys. J.* **2003**, *85*, 2299–2310. [CrossRef]

164. French, R.J.; Yoshikami, D.; Sheets, M.F.; Olivera, B.M. The tetrodotoxin receptor of voltage-gated sodium channels—Perspectives from interactions with μ-conotoxins. *Mar. Drugs* **2010**, *8*, 2153–2161. [CrossRef]

165. Choudhary, G.; Aliste, M.P.; Tieleman, D.P.; French, R.J.; Dudley, J.; Samuel, C. Docking of μ-conotoxin giiia in the sodium channel outer vestibule. *Channels* **2007**, *1*, 344–352. [CrossRef] [PubMed]

166. Khan, A.; Romantseva, L.; Lam, A.; Lipkind, G.; Fozzard, H. Role of outer ring carboxylates of the rat skeletal muscle sodium channel pore in proton block. *J. Physiol.* **2002**, *543*, 71–84. [CrossRef] [PubMed]

167. Mahdavi, S.; Kuyucak, S. Systematic study of binding of μ-conotoxins to the sodium channel nav1. 4. *Toxins* **2014**, *6*, 3454–3470. [CrossRef] [PubMed]

168. Korkosh, V.S.; Zhorov, B.S.; Tikhonov, D.B. Folding similarity of the outer pore region in prokaryotic and eukaryotic sodium channels revealed by docking of conotoxins giiia, piiia, and kiiia in a navab-based model of nav1. 4. *J. Gen. Physiol.* **2014**, *144*, 231–244. [CrossRef] [PubMed]

169. Patel, D.; Mahdavi, S.; Kuyucak, S. Computational study of binding of μ-conotoxin giiia to bacterial sodium channels navab and navrh. *Biochemistry* **2016**, *55*, 1929–1938. [CrossRef]

170. Mahdavi, S.; Kuyucak, S. Molecular dynamics study of binding of μ-conotoxin giiia to the voltage-gated sodium channel nav1. 4. *PLoS ONE* **2014**, *9*, e105300. [CrossRef]

171. Cummins, T.R.; Aglieco, F.; Dib-Hajj, S.D. Critical molecular determinants of voltage-gated sodium channel sensitivity to μ-conotoxins giiia/b. *Mol. Pharmacol.* **2002**, *61*, 1192–1201. [CrossRef]

172. Catterall, W.A. Structure and regulation of voltage-gated Ca^{2+} channels. *Annu. Rev. Cell Develop. Biol.* **2000**, *16*, 521–555. [CrossRef]

173. Catterall, W.A.; Swanson, T.M. Structural basis for pharmacology of voltage-gated sodium and calcium channels. *Mol. Pharmacol.* **2015**, *88*, 141–150. [CrossRef]

174. Wu, J.; Yan, Z.; Li, Z.; Qian, X.; Lu, S.; Dong, M.; Zhou, Q.; Yan, N. Structure of the voltage-gated calcium channel ca v 1.1 at 3.6 å resolution. *Nature* **2016**, *537*, 191. [CrossRef]
175. Hering, S.; Zangerl-Plessl, E.-M.; Beyl, S.; Hohaus, A.; Andranovits, S.; Timin, E. Calcium channel gating. *Pflügers Archiv-Eur. J. Physiol.* **2018**, *470*, 1291–1309. [CrossRef] [PubMed]
176. Dolphin, A.C. Voltage-gated calcium channels: Their discovery, function and importance as drug targets. *Brain Neurosci. Adv.* **2018**, *2*, 2398212818794805. [CrossRef] [PubMed]
177. Zamponi, G.W.; Striessnig, J.; Koschak, A.; Dolphin, A.C. The physiology, pathology, and pharmacology of voltage-gated calcium channels and their future therapeutic potential. *Pharmacol. Rev.* **2015**, *67*, 821–870. [CrossRef] [PubMed]
178. Nielsen, K.J.; Schroeder, T.; Lewis, R. Structure–activity relationships of ω-conotoxins at n-type voltage-sensitive calcium channels. *J. Mol. Recognit.* **2000**, *13*, 55–70. [CrossRef]
179. Neumaier, F.; Dibue-Adjei, M.; Hescheler, J.; Schneider, T. Voltage-gated calcium channels: Determinants of channel function and modulation by inorganic cations. *Prog. Neurobiol.* **2015**, *129*, 1–36. [CrossRef]
180. Jurkovicova-Tarabova, B.; Lacinova, L. Structure, function and regulation of cav 2.2 n-type calcium channels. *Gen. Physiol. Biophys.* **2019**, *38*, 101–110. [CrossRef] [PubMed]
181. Miljanich, G. Ziconotide: Neuronal calcium channel blocker for treating severe chronic pain. *Curr. Med. Chem.* **2004**, *11*, 3029–3040. [CrossRef]
182. Pallaghy, P.K.; Norton, R.S.; Nielsen, K.J.; Craik, D.J. A common structural motif incorporating a cystine knot and a triple-stranded β-sheet in toxic and inhibitory polypeptides. *Protein Sci.* **1994**, *3*, 1833–1839. [CrossRef]
183. Kohno, T.; Kim, J.I.; Kobayashi, K.; Kodera, Y.; Maeda, T.; Sato, K. Three-dimensional structure in solution of the calcium channel blocker. Omega.-conotoxin mviia. *Biochemistry* **1995**, *34*, 10256–10265. [CrossRef]
184. Adams, D.J.; Berecki, G. Mechanisms of conotoxin inhibition of n-type (cav2. 2) calcium channels. *Biochim. Biophys. Acta (BBA)-Biomembr.* **2013**, *1828*, 1619–1628. [CrossRef]
185. Hansson, K.; Ma, X.; Eliasson, L.; Czerwiec, E.; Furie, B.; Furie, B.C.; Rorsman, P.; Stenflo, J. The first γ-carboxyglutamic acid-containing contryphan a selective l-type calcium ion channel blocker isolated from the venom of conus marmoreus. *J. Biol. Chem.* **2004**, *279*, 32453–32463. [CrossRef] [PubMed]
186. Bernáldez, J.; Román-González, S.; Martínez, O.; Jiménez, S.; Vivas, O.; Arenas, I.; Corzo, G.; Arreguín, R.; García, D.; Possani, L. A conus regularis conotoxin with a novel eight-cysteine framework inhibits cav2. 2 channels and displays an anti-nociceptive activity. *Mar. Drugs* **2013**, *11*, 1188–1202. [CrossRef] [PubMed]
187. Flinn, J.P.; Pallaghy, P.K.; Lew, M.J.; Murphy, R.; Angus, J.A.; Norton, R.S. Roles of key functional groups in ω-conotoxin gvia: Synthesis, structure and functional assay of selected peptide analogues. *Eur. J. Biochem.* **1999**, *262*, 447–455. [CrossRef] [PubMed]
188. Schroeder, C.; Doering, C.; Zamponi, G.; Lewis, R. N-type calcium channel blockers: Novel therapeutics for the treatment of pain. *Med. Chem.* **2006**, *2*, 535–543. [CrossRef] [PubMed]
189. Sato, K.; Park, N.G.; Kohno, T.; Maeda, T.; Kim, J.I.; Kato, R.; Takahashi, M. Role of basic residues for the binding of ω-conotoxin gvia to n-type calcium channels. *Biochem. Biophys. Res. Commun.* **1993**, *194*, 1292–1296. [CrossRef] [PubMed]
190. Lew, M.J.; Flinn, J.P.; Pallaghy, P.K.; Murphy, R.; Whorlow, S.L.; Wright, C.E.; Norton, R.S.; Angus, J.A. Structure-function relationships of ω-conotoxin gvia synthesis, structure, calcium channel binding, and functional assay of alanine-substituted analogues. *J. Biol. Chem.* **1997**, *272*, 12014–12023. [CrossRef] [PubMed]
191. Ellinor, P.T.; Zhang, J.-F.; Horne, W.A.; Tsien, R.W. Structural determinants of the blockade of n-type calcium channels by a peptide neurotoxin. *Nature* **1994**, *372*, 272. [CrossRef] [PubMed]
192. Feng, Z.-P.; Hamid, J.; Doering, C.; Bosey, G.M.; Snutch, T.P.; Zamponi, G.W. Residue gly1326 of the n-type calcium channel α1b subunit controls reversibility of ω-conotoxin gvia and mviia block. *J. Biol. Chem.* **2001**, *276*, 15728–15735. [CrossRef]
193. Chen, R.; Chung, S.-H. Complex structures between the n-type calcium channel (cav2. 2) and ω-conotoxin gvia predicted via molecular dynamics. *Biochemistry* **2013**, *52*, 3765–3772. [CrossRef]

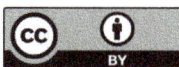

Review

Snails In Silico: A Review of Computational Studies on the Conopeptides

Rachael A. Mansbach [1,†], Timothy Travers [1,2,†,‡], Benjamin H. McMahon [1], Jeanne M. Fair [3] and S. Gnanakaran [1,*]

1   Theoretical Biology and Biophysics Group, Los Alamos National Laboratory, Los Alamos, NM 87545, USA; mansbach@lanl.gov (R.A.M.); tstravers@lanl.gov (T.T.); mcmahon@lanl.gov (B.H.M.)
2   Center for Nonlinear Studies, Los Alamos National Laboratory, Los Alamos, NM 87545, USA
3   Biosecurity and Public Health Group, Los Alamos National Laboratory, Los Alamos, NM 87545, USA; jmfair@lanl.gov
*   Correspondence: gnana@lanl.gov; Tel.: +1-505-665-1923
†   These authors contributed equally to this work.
‡   Current address: New Mexico Consortium and Pebble Labs Inc., Los Alamos, NM 87544, USA.

Received: 18 January 2019; Accepted: 22 February 2019; Published: 1 March 2019

Abstract: Marine cone snails are carnivorous gastropods that use peptide toxins called conopeptides both as a defense mechanism and as a means to immobilize and kill their prey. These peptide toxins exhibit a large chemical diversity that enables exquisite specificity and potency for target receptor proteins. This diversity arises in terms of variations both in amino acid sequence and length, and in posttranslational modifications, particularly the formation of multiple disulfide linkages. Most of the functionally characterized conopeptides target ion channels of animal nervous systems, which has led to research on their therapeutic applications. Many facets of the underlying molecular mechanisms responsible for the specificity and virulence of conopeptides, however, remain poorly understood. In this review, we will explore the chemical diversity of conopeptides from a computational perspective. First, we discuss current approaches used for classifying conopeptides. Next, we review different computational strategies that have been applied to understanding and predicting their structure and function, from machine learning techniques for predictive classification to docking studies and molecular dynamics simulations for molecular-level understanding. We then review recent novel computational approaches for rapid high-throughput screening and chemical design of conopeptides for particular applications. We close with an assessment of the state of the field, emphasizing important questions for future lines of inquiry.

Keywords: conotoxins; conopeptides; computational studies; molecular dynamics; machine learning; docking; review; drug design; ion channels

---

1. Introduction

Marine cone snails from the family *Conidae* capture their prey and defend themselves using venoms containing short proteins called conopeptides [1,2]. The majority of these toxins range in sequence length from 10 to 45 amino acids, with a median size of 26 residues [3]. Every species from the family *Conidae* can produce in excess of a thousand types of conopeptides; it is estimated that that only 5% of the peptides are shared between different species [4]. This large chemical diversity is primarily driven by evolutionary pressure for improving defense and/or prey capture [2], with sudden ecological changes likely driving the selection of new fast-acting conopeptides [5,6]. Although several classes of "disulfide-poor" conopeptides have been recently identified [7,8], the majority of cone snail toxins contain multiple disulfide linkages within a single peptide chain that allow the adoption of highly-ordered structures [9]. In fact, disulfide bond formation is the most prevalent type of posttranslational modification seen in conopeptides [10], although other types of modifications have also been observed, including proline hydroxylation [11], tyrosine sulfation [12], C-terminal amidation [13], O-glycosylation [14], and addition of gamma-carboxyglutamic acid [15].

During the review of the current literature on conopeptides, we noticed that the term "conotoxin" has sometimes been used interchangeably with the term "conopeptide" [15,16]. In this review, following the definition given in [17], we instead draw a distinction and employ the term "conotoxin" to refer to the specific subset of the conopeptides that contain two or more disulfide bonds.

Conopeptides are potent pharmacological agents that bind with high specificity to their target proteins (equilibrium dissociation constants or k_D values in the nM range) [18]. Broadly, the protein families targeted by conopeptides are grouped into the following three categories [19]: (i) ligand-gated channels such as nicotinic acetylcholine receptors (nAChRs) [20]; (ii) voltage-gated channels for sodium [21], potassium [22], and calcium [23]; and (iii) G protein-coupled receptors (GPCRs) [24]. Although these targets belong to various protein families, the same physiological effect is achieved by conopeptide binding: disruption of signaling pathways, which leads to the inhibition of neuromuscular transmission and, ultimately, prey immobilization [25,26].

Due to their highly specific and potent binding modes, conopeptides can exhibit significant toxicity in humans—*Conus geographus* stings have reported fatality rates of 65 percent—which has led to discussions of weaponization potential by biosecurity experts and establishment of USA federal regulations that place restrictions on research into particular conopeptide classes [27–29]. Nevertheless, the conopeptide chemical space is vast and most are not considered to be bioterrorism threats; indeed, conopeptides have become useful research tools for understanding the physiological functions of their target proteins and have emerged as valuable templates for rational drug design of new therapeutic agents in pain management [30–36]. An important milestone was the approval of the conotoxin ω-MVIIA from *Conus magus* as a commercial drug for chronic pain under the name Prialt (generic name ziconotide) [37,38].

Recent years have seen a growing availability and refinement of computational resources and algorithms that can be used for gaining more insights on structure-function relationships in conopeptides. For instance, there is now an increasing emphasis on the use of in silico methods, either alone or in combination with experimental techniques, for molecular-level understanding and protein engineering for drug design [39,40]. The explosion of machine learning (ML) techniques and use-cases has led to a focus on the creation of large databases that can be mined for predictions [41]. Meanwhile, molecular dynamics simulations offer a straightforward and ever-more-efficient method for probing protein conformations in detail [42–44], while docking studies provide a rapid complementary method to predict binding affinities and modes of ligands bound to large complexes [45,46]. Finally, combinations of these methods are being applied to design problems in such disparate areas as the creation of drug-like molecules [47], the identification of antimicrobial peptides [48], and the discovery of novel materials [49].

In this review, we provide an overview of how such computational techniques have been exploited to enrich our understanding of the molecular mechanisms behind conopeptide function and binding, predict their targets and binding affinities, and ultimately design novel conopeptides for specific applications in a rational manner. We begin in Section 2 by discussing the classification and structure of the family of conopeptides in general. In Section 3, we present a detailed review of computational studies that have been performed, ranging from machine learning predictors of conopeptide categories to molecular dynamics and docking studies for structure and folding characterization and binding mode elucidation to large-scale computationally-driven rational design of conopeptides for specific applications. In Section 4, we discuss the current state of the field, and, in Section 5, we briefly conclude.

2. Background

Despite the vast number of different conopeptides and their overall diversity, some similarities do emerge, and it is customary to employ different classification schemes to categorize information about different aspects of these similarities. Since such similarities may arise from different origins—for example, evolutionary similarity versus functional similarity—classification schemes encoding different information do not necessarily provide overlapping categories. In the next sections, we introduce some of the most commonly used schemes and discuss their relationships and some implications for understanding the structures and functions of conopeptides.

2.1. Categories of Conopeptide Classification

Classification schemes exist that describe aspects of conopeptide similarity ranging from those based solely on sequence to those based on a mixture of sequence and structural properties to those based on specific in vivo functionality [3,50], some of which are simple to determine for all conopeptides with known sequence, others of which have only been determined for small subsets of all identified conopeptide sequences (see Table 1 for a summary).

Table 1. Different categories used to classify the conopeptides, along with the basic type of categorization and a brief description.

Category	Type	Description
Gene superfamily	sequence	Clustering of precursor region
Cysteine framework	sequence	Arrangement of cysteines
Loop class	sequence	Number of amino acids between cysteines
Disulfide connectivity	structure	Pattern of disulfide bond formation
Fold	structure	General three-dimensional structure
Subfold	structure	More specific three-dimensional structure
Pharmacological family	action	Target and mode of action (agonist, antagonist, etc.)

2.1.1. Gene Superfamily

Gene superfamily is an evolutionary classification in which conopeptides are assigned a category based on clustering of the slowly evolving region of the precursor protein that is processed by the endoplasmic reticulum [1]. Gene superfamily is strictly a mark of evolutionary similarity within the precursor regions, and is of limited use in finding conservation patterns within the hypervariable regions that are actually transcoded into mature toxins. (See Figure 1 for an example of two conopeptides of gene superfamily A that have highly similar precursor regions but very different mature toxin sequences.)

a)
Ac4.1   MFTVFLLVVLATTLVSIPSDRASDFRNAAVHERQKELVVTATTTCCGYNPMTSCPRCMCDSSCNKKKPGRRND
b)
Ac1.2   MFTVFLLVVLTTTVVSFPSDSASGGRDDEAKDERSDMYELKRNGRCCHPACGGKYVKCGR

Figure 1. Comparison of two conotoxin sequences from Gene Superfamily A. Matching precursor signal sequence regions are in blue, places where the precursor regions do not match are in green, and the mature toxin regions are in red. The remainder of the sequences comprising the N-terminal and C-terminal pro-regions are in black. (**a**) sequence of conotoxin Ac4.1 from *Conus achatinus*; (**b**) sequence of conotoxin Ac1.2 from *Conus achatinus*.

2.1.2. Cysteine Framework and Loop Class

In contrast to the gene superfamily, the cysteine framework of a conopeptide is a category assigned based on the sequence of amino acids of the toxin region itself. It generally refers to the pattern of neighboring and non-neighboring cysteines in the sequence [50] (It should be noted that there has historically been some confusion in the literature over the use of the term "cysteine framework." In addition to the way it is presented here, it has sometimes been used to refer to a more structure-based categorization that includes the pattern of disulfide bonds that form between non-neighboring cysteines. We describe disulfide connectivity separately and adopt the definition of cysteine framework as described by [50]). For example, Figure 2 shows examples of framework I, corresponding to the cysteine pattern CC-C-C, and framework III, corresponding to the cysteine pattern CC-C-C-CC. There is one exception to the general rule for framework definition: peptides with a cysteine pattern of CC-C-C and a hydroxyproline residue between cysteines three and four are assigned to framework X, while all other peptides with a cysteine pattern of CC-C-C are assigned to framework I. Twenty-seven such frameworks are currently recognized (see Table 2), and any new conopeptide may be straightforwardly assigned a framework from knowledge of its amino acid sequence. If, in addition to noting which cysteines are neighboring and which are not, one chooses to classify conopeptides based on intrasequence cysteine distance, one may employ the conopeptide loop class instead of the cysteine framework. A particular loop class is defined by the number of amino acids between the cysteines, where that number is zero for neighboring cysteines (see Figure 2 for two examples).

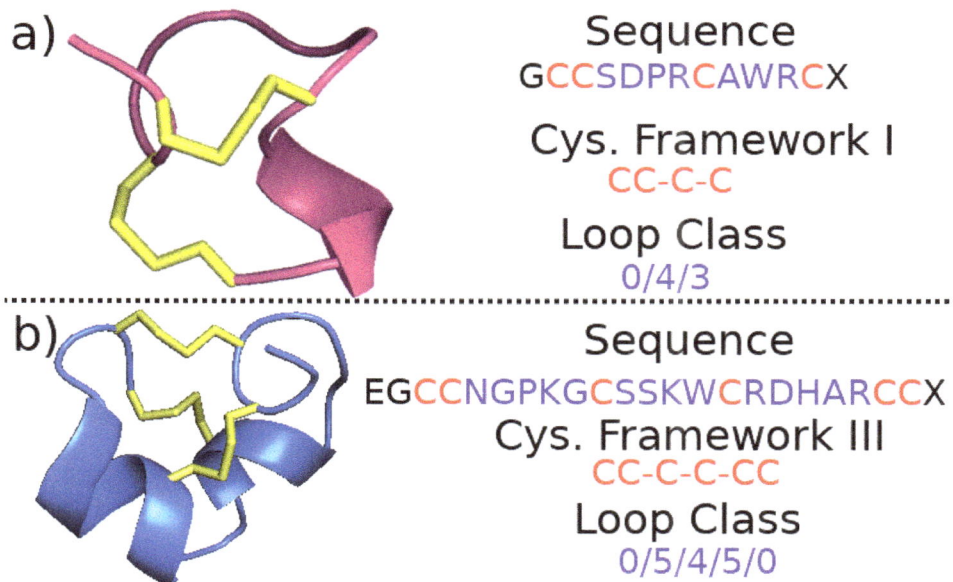

Figure 2. Illustration of sequence, cysteine framework and loop class for (**a**) α-conotoxin ImI (Protein Data Bank or PDB structure 1G2G [51]) and (**b**) µ-conotoxin CnIIIC (PDB structure 2YEN [52]). In the illustrative 3D structures on the left, disulfide bonds are represented as yellow sticks. Images of peptides were generated with Pymol [53].

Table 2. Summary of cysteine frameworks, with defining pattern and number of cysteines. Data compiled from the Conoserver, an automatically-updating online repository of conopeptide data [17,54]. In the entry for framework X, .[PO] represents an interceding hydroxyproline residue.

Framework Name	Pattern	No. Cysteines
I	CC-C-C	4
II	CCC-C-C-C	6
III	CC-C-C-CC	6
IV	CC-C-C-C-C	6
V	CC-CC	4
VI/VII	C-C-CC-C-C	6
VIII	C-C-C-C-C-C-C-C-C-C	10
IX	C-C-C-C-C-C	6
X	CC-C.[PO]C	4
XI	C-C-CC-CC-C-C	8
XII	C-C-C-C-CC-C-C	8
XIII	C-C-C-CC-C-C-C	8
XIV	C-C-C-C	4
XV	C-C-CC-C-C-C-C	8
XVI	C-C-CC	4
XVII	C-C-CC-C-CC-C	8
XVIII	C-C-CC-CC	6
XIX	C-C-C-CCC-C-C-C-C	10
XX	C-CC-C-CC-C-C-C-C	10
XXI	CC-C-C-C-CC-C-C-C	10
XXII	C-C-C-C-C-C-C-C	8
XXIII	C-C-C-CC-C	6
XXIV	C-CC-C	4
XXV	C-C-C-C-CC	6
XXVI	C-C-C-C-CC-CC	8
XXVII	C-CC-C-C-C	6

2.1.3. Fold and Subfold Class

If instead of employing a sequence-based classification, one employs a structure-based scheme, conopeptides may also be divided into different fold and subfold classes due to the high structural similarities that are often enforced by the disulfide connectivities of the cysteines (see also Sections 2.1.4 and 2.2.2). Fold and subfold are structural categorizations for conopeptides that have determined three-dimensional (i.e., secondary and tertiary) structures [3,55], with subfold being a subset of fold class that encompasses finer secondary structural detail. There are 13 folds and 18 subfolds currently defined (see Figure 3), but at the time of this article there are only 161 determined conopeptide structures in the Protein Data Bank (PDB), of which 114 represent unique sequences or post-translationally modified sequences [56], and many fall into only four of the thirteen folds: A, B, C, and D (cf. Figures 3a–d and 6a). For a more detailed discussion of the precise characteristics of each fold and subfold class, the interested reader is referred to Akondi et al. [3].

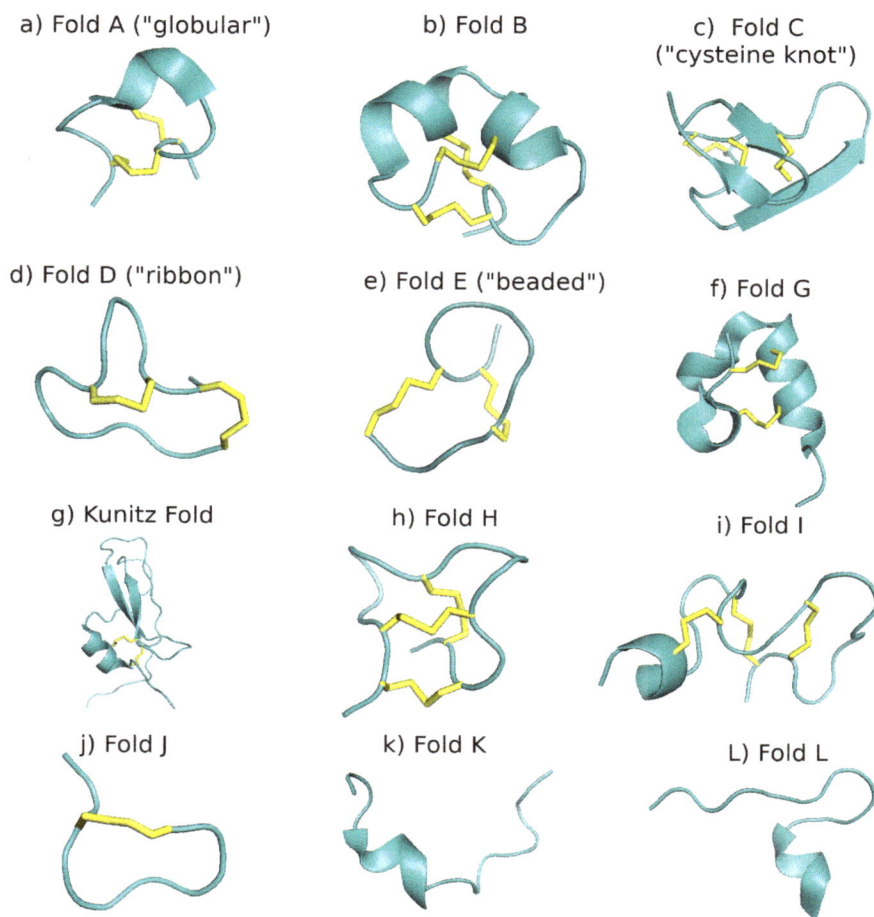

Figure 3. The thirteen major conopeptide folds described in Akondi et al. [3], shown by representative examples from the PDB [56]. Disulfide bonds are represented as yellow sticks. All images rendered in Pymol [53]. (**a**) Fold A, also referred to as the "globular" fold: conotoxin α-RgIA, PDB structure 2JUT [57]; (**b**) Fold B: conotoxin μ-CnIIIC, PDB structure 2YEN [58]; (**c**) Fold C, also referred to as "cysteine knot" fold: conotoxin δ-EVIA, PDB structure 1G1P [59]; (**d**) Fold D, also referred to as "ribbon" fold: ribbon isoform of conotoxin α-GI, PDB structure 1XGB [60]; (**e**) Fold E, also referred to as "beaded" or "beads-on-a-string" fold: conotoxin χ-CMrVIA, PDB structure 2B5Q [61]; (**f**) Fold G: conotoxin κ-PIXIVA, PDB structure 2FQC [62]; (**g**) Kunitz fold: conkunitzin-S2, PDB structure 2J6D [63]; (**h**) Fold H: conotoxin MrIIIe, PDB structure 2EFZ [64]; (**i**) Fold I: Conotoxin α-PIVA, PDB structure 1P1P [65]; (**j**) Fold J: contryphan-Vn, PDB structure 1NXN [66]; (**k**) Fold K: conantokin-G, PDB structure 1AD7 [15]; and (**l**) Fold L: conomarphin, PDB structure 2YYF [67]. There is no representative structure in the PDB for Fold F. The interested reader is referred to the original paper by Zhang et al. [68], which contains the characterization of the only determined structure of this fold.

2.1.4. Disulfide Connectivity

One aspect of conopeptides that has sometimes been employed for their classification is the disulfide connectivity of their cysteines; that is, which cysteines are connected to which via covalent disulfide bonds. Disulfide connectivity is of particular interest for two reasons: (i) patterns of disulfide connectivity in the primary structure of conopeptides play an important role in defining their three-dimensional structure [69] and thus their fold/subfold classes, although the extent to which specific disulfide bonds are important to retaining the native structure can be peptide-dependent [70], and (ii) although it is common to describe conopeptides in terms of their "native" disulfide connectivity, multiple different connectivities for a single peptide have been observed in vitro, which may correspond to stable, metastable, or off-pathway structural isomers, and which often display different properties than the native structure [71] (see Sections 2.2.2 and 4 for further discussion of this point).

In Figure 4, we show the structures resulting from some common disulfide connectivities. For instance, in conopeptides containing four cysteine residues, disulfide formation between cysteines 1–3 and 2–4 leads to the so-called "globular" structure with α-helical content (Figure 4a left and Figure 3a). In contrast, disulfide formation between cysteines 1–4 and 2–3 leads to the so-called "ribbon" structure with β-sheet content (Figure 4a right and Figure 3d). As another example, in conopeptides containing six cysteine residues, disulfide formation between cysteines 1–4, 2–5, and 3–6 leads to a "cysteine knot" structure (Figure 4b left and Figure 3c). However, disulfide formation between cysteines 1–5, 2–4, and 3–6 leads to a different overall tertiary structure (Figure 4b right and Figure 3h).

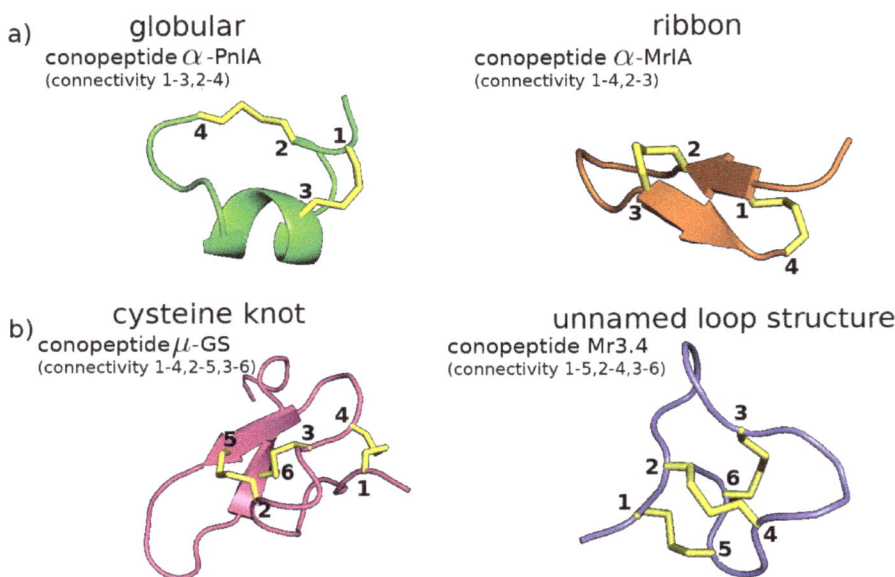

a) **globular**
conopeptide α -PnIA
(connectivity 1-3,2-4)

ribbon
conopeptide α-MrIA
(connectivity 1-4,2-3)

b) **cysteine knot**
conopeptide μ-GS
(connectivity 1-4,2-5,3-6)

unnamed loop structure
conopeptide Mr3.4
(connectivity 1-5,2-4,3-6)

Figure 4. Different disulfide connectivities lead to different conotoxin structures. (**a**) With four cysteines, two different connectivities can lead to either a "globular" structure with α-helical content (left, PDB 1PEN for conotoxin α-PnIA [72]) or a flattened "ribbon" structure which often, but not always, displays β-sheet content (right, PDB 2EW4 for conotoxin α-MrIA [73]). (**b**) With six cysteine residues, two connectivities that differ only in the first two disulfide bonds can lead to either a "cysteine knot" structure with β-sheet content (left, PDB 1AG7 for conotoxin μ-GS [74]) or another structure with no discernable secondary structure content (right, PDB 2EFZ for conotoxin MrIIIe [64]).

2.1.5. Pharmacological Family

Finally, if one chooses to classify conopeptides based on their mode of action, their pharmacological family may be assigned. Pharmacological families group conopeptides based on their target receptor and the type of interaction with this receptor, of which 12 such families are currently recognized [17,54] (see Table 3); however, mode of action is also not a quantity that is straightforward to determine from the sequence, and as of now, only 243 of the more than 6000 sequences downloadable from the Conoserver (an automatically-updating online repository of information about conopeptides [17,54]) have an associated pharmacological family (The Conoserver is the most complete repository of compiled information on the conopeptides the authors of this review were able to find and forms an excellent reference for any researcher in the field; however, it should be noted that there are over 400 sequences that currently appear to be inaccessible via the search function or download. Readers may refer to the Uniprot database as well [75].).

Table 3. Summary of pharmacological families, their targets, and their modes of action. Data compiled from the Conoserver [17,54] and the Uniprot database [75].

Family	Target	Mode of Action
α (alpha)	Nicotinic acetylcholine receptors (nAChRs)	orthosteric, allosteric inhibition
γ (gamma)	Neuronal pacemaker cation currents	increase calcium current
δ (delta)	Voltage-gated sodium channels (VGSCs)	agonist, delayed inactivation
ϵ (epsilon)	Presynaptic calcium channels or G protein-coupled presynaptic receptors (GPCRs)	blocker
ι (iota)	VGSC	agonist, no delayed inactivation
κ (kappa)	Voltage-gated potassium channels (VGPCs)	blocker
μ (mu)	VGSC	antagonist, blocker
ρ (rho)	Alpha-1 adrenergic receptors	allosteric inhibitor
σ (sigma)	Serotonin-gated ion channels	antagonist
τ (tau)	Somatostatin receptor	antagonist
χ (chi)	Neuronal noradrenaline transporter	unknown
ω (omega)	Voltage-gated calcium channels (VGCCs)	blocker

2.2. Relationships between Categories

Knowing how a conopeptide is categorized under one classification scheme is not necessarily indicative of its categorization under another. For example, conopeptides from a particular cysteine framework are not limited to belonging to a single pharmacological family. Conopeptides in framework I can target either nicotinic acetylcholine receptors (nAChRs) or adrenoceptors, while those in framework III can target either nAChRs or sodium/potassium channels. Despite a generally demonstrated selectivity for their targets, certain peptides even display binding affinity for more than one receptor type [76,77]. Nonetheless, there may be similarities between the ways in which different classification schemes group the conopeptides (see Figure 5).

2.2.1. Cysteine Framework, Loop Class, Fold, and Pharmacological Family

To be more specific, in Figure 5a, we demonstrate the similarities and differences between the ways in which conopeptides are grouped when using cysteine framework versus pharmacological family as the classification. We demonstrate groupings for all 243 peptides with defined pharmacological families downloadable from the Conoserver, comprising 137 sequences with four cysteines, 99 sequences with six cysteines, two sequences with eight cysteines, and five sequences with ten cysteines; the image is a visualization of a pairwise matrix of the considered conopeptide dataset. The overall dataset demonstrates that the categories overlap quite strongly, both visually and numerically: 85% of peptide pairs with the same cysteine framework have the same pharmacological target and 88% of peptide pairs with different frameworks have different targets. If we eliminate all frameworks containing four or fewer cysteines (frameworks I and X, comprising about half the dataset, see Figure 5b), however, then only 45% of peptide pairs with the same cysteine framework have the same pharmacological target, although 93% of peptide pairs with different frameworks have different targets. This precipitous drop in categorical overlap for the same frameworks implies that target prediction becomes more difficult as the number of cysteines in the sequence increases, which may be a consequence of the rapidly growing number of possible disulfide bond connectivities for systems with more than four cysteines (see also Section 4 for a brief discussion of this point).

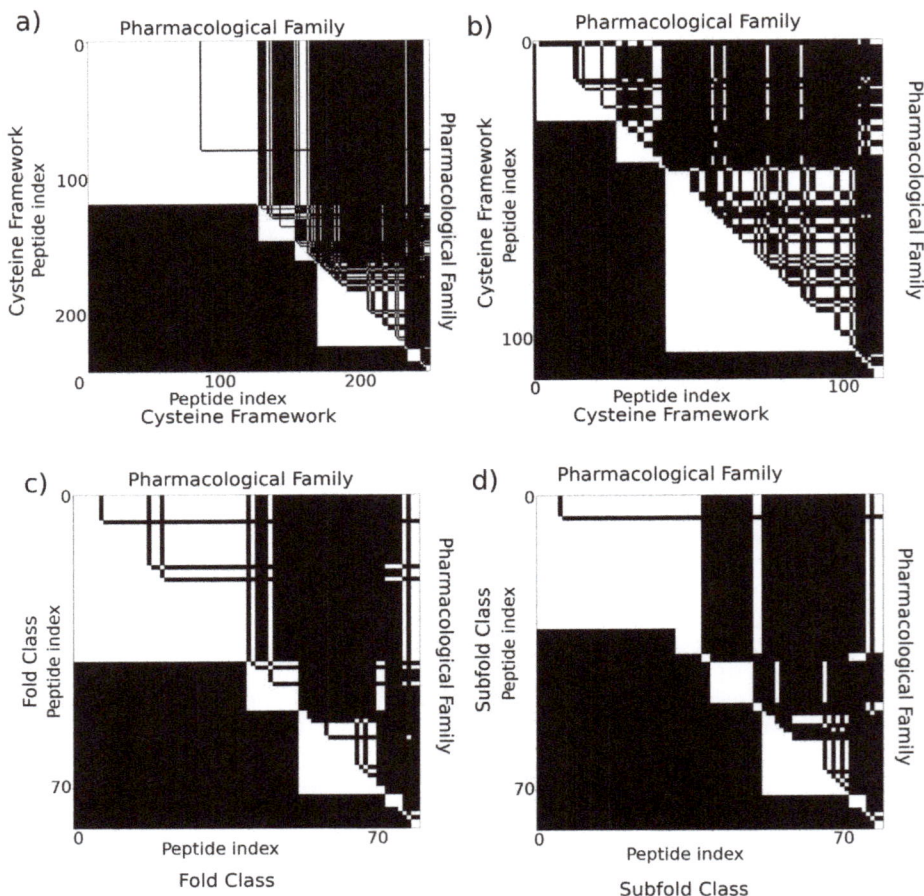

Figure 5. Comparison of different categories with pharmacological family. (**a**) Comparison between cysteine framework and pharmacological target for all pairs of 243 peptides with determined pharmacological targets downloaded from the Conoserver [17,54]. Black indicates that two peptides are assigned different categories, while white indicates the two peptides are assigned the same category. The lower triangular shows cysteine framework; the upper triangular pharmacological target. (**b**) Comparison between cysteine framework and pharmacological target for the subset of 106 sequences with more than four cysteines. In (**c**) and (**d**), we show a comparison between fold and subfold class and pharmacological family for all pairs of 80 peptides with a defined pharmacological target and fold/subfold classes as described in Akondi et al. [3].

In Figure 5c,d, we demonstrate the similarities and differences between conopeptide classification as described by the (c) fold and (d) subfold and pharmacological family categories for a subset of the peptides described in Akondi et al. [3]. We focus only on cysteine-containing peptides that have a known pharmacological family and a defined fold and subfold, which results in a set of 80 peptides comprised of one sequence with two cysteines, 45 sequences with four cysteines, 32 sequences with six cysteines, and two sequences with eight cysteines. We see that there is a relatively large overlap between fold class and pharmacological target: 76% of peptide pairs that are assigned the same fold class have the same pharmacological target, and 89% of peptide pairs that are assigned a different fold class have different targets, while 80% of peptide pairs assigned the same subfold class have the same pharmacological target and 83% of peptide pairs assigned different subfold classes have different targets. It should be noted, however, that this is a small subsample of the vast array of possible conopeptides and that bias in the assessed peptides may lead to artificially high cross-categorical similarity due to high sequence similarity that would not be expected in general, particularly since there are no sequences in the dataset containing more than eight cysteines and most contain six or fewer. Indeed, almost 75% of all conopeptide studies have been performed on the four-cysteine α-conotoxins [78].

In Figure 6, we demonstrate the extent to which loop class can discriminate between the groupings of other categorization schemes, using the 103 cysteine-containing peptides from Akondi et al. [3]. The latter dataset comprises seven sequences with two cysteines, 59 sequences with four cysteines, 35 sequences with six cysteines, and two sequences with eight cysteines. The distance between a pair of points in this plot is a visual indication of the difference between their loop classes, while different colors represent different categories. If loop class is indicative of a category, then points with the same color should be clustered together, whereas if loop class and the other classification type have no relation, then nearby points should appear to be colored randomly. Panel (a) of Figure 6, in which different colors represent different folds, demonstrates several clusters that are primarily one color, with the major sources of overlap between categories being the central cluster of points where folds A, D, and E reside almost on top of one another. Indeed, there are several overlapping points with identical loop classes that have different folds (see also Section 2.2.2).

Panel (b) of Figure 6, in which different colors represent different pharmacological families, also demonstrates some clustering of similar colors, although there are several points that have the same color as their neighbors in panel (a) but different colors in panel (b) (see red arrows for three examples). Thus, there is an overlap between pharmacological family and loop class, but it is somewhat weaker than that of the overlap between fold and loop class, even in this small dataset. This demonstrates that pharmacological family is not solely dictated by three-dimensional structure (see also Section 3.2 for a detailed discussion of molecular mechanisms that control selectivity and binding affinities for target receptors).

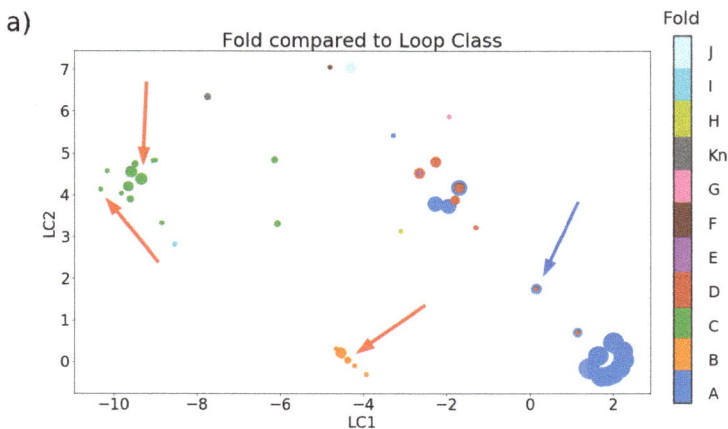

Figure 6. *Cont.*

b)

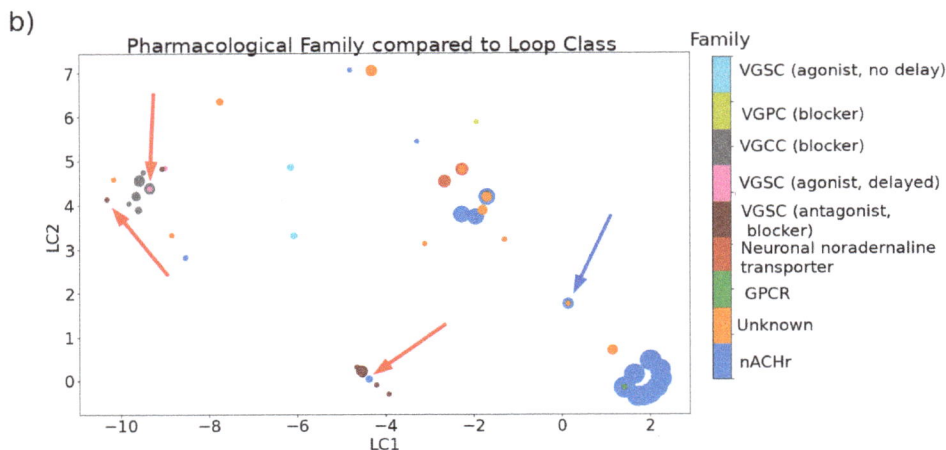

Figure 6. Two-dimensional embedding of loop class, demonstrating its relationship to (a) fold and (b) pharmacological family. Data compiled from Akondi et al. [3], which includes 103 peptides with measured structures, 80 of which had identified pharmacological targets. Loop class was represented as a seven-dimensional vector, with vectors representing classes containing fewer than eight cysteines padded with negative ones for direct comparison. In all images, size of a given marker indicates the number of conopeptides with identical loop class and category, while color indicates category. Red arrows draw the reader's attention to differences in clustering between the two panels. Blue arrows indicate an example of a structural isomer. The embedding was done for visualization purposes employing the t-Distributed Stochastic Neighbor Embedding (t-SNE) algorithm as implemented in Scikit Learn [79,80].

2.2.2. Disulfide Connectivity Determines Fold

Another important point brought up by Figure 6 is the extent to which fold is dictated by disulfide connectivity over detailed sequence. The blue arrows indicate an example where an identical sequence has a very different structural fold and may also have a different target (the isomer's target is often unknown). We elaborate a more specific set of examples in Figure 7a. Conotoxins α-GI [60,81] and α-BuIA [82,83] have a native connectivity between cysteines 1–3 and 2–4 that corresponds to the "globular" motif, but altering this connectivity to cysteines 1–4 and 2–3 forces both to adopt a "ribbon" motif. Interestingly, the disulfide connectivity has also been found to impact the conformational dynamics of the conopeptide. In the case of conotoxin α-GI, the native "globular" conformation was found to have less backbone conformational variability than the induced "ribbon" conformation [81]. The reverse is true, however, for conotoxin α-BuIA, where the induced "ribbon" motif was found to have less backbone conformational variability than the native "globular" motif, even though only the latter motif is capable of inhibiting the function of the target nAChR [83].

Not only do different disulfide connectivities imply different structures irrespective of sequence, but, perhaps more importantly, similar disulfide connectivities imply similar structure irrespective of sequence, as demonstrated in Figure 7b. The conotoxins α-EI (PDB 1K64 [84]) and α-IMI (PDB structure 1G2G [51]), for instance, both adopt a "globular" connectivity with disulfide linkages between cysteines 1-3 and 2-4 (Figure 7b top). However, a sequence alignment between these two conotoxins shows no sequence identity or similarity besides a single proline and the four cysteine residues (Figure 7b bottom). Surprisingly, even diverse sequences with a different number of disulfide bonds have been found to adopt similar structural folds if similar underlying disulfide connectivities exist. For example, the conotoxins ω-MVIIA (PDB 1MVJ [85]) and ι-RXIA (PDB 2P4L [86]), which have six and eight cysteines respectively, have both been found to adopt a cysteine knot. This structural motif is the most commonly observed in small disulfide-rich proteins, occurring in nearly 40% of available structures [55]. It is comprised of a ring formed by two of the disulfide bonds and the interconnecting backbone, with the third disulfide bond passing through this ring [87]. In conotoxin ι-RXIA, which has eight cysteines, the cysteine knot arises from disulfide bond formation between cysteines 1–4, 2–6, and 3–7, with cysteines 6 and 7 taking the place of cysteines 5 and 6 in a six-cysteine conotoxin (see e.g., of conotoxin μ-GS in Figure 4b) [86].

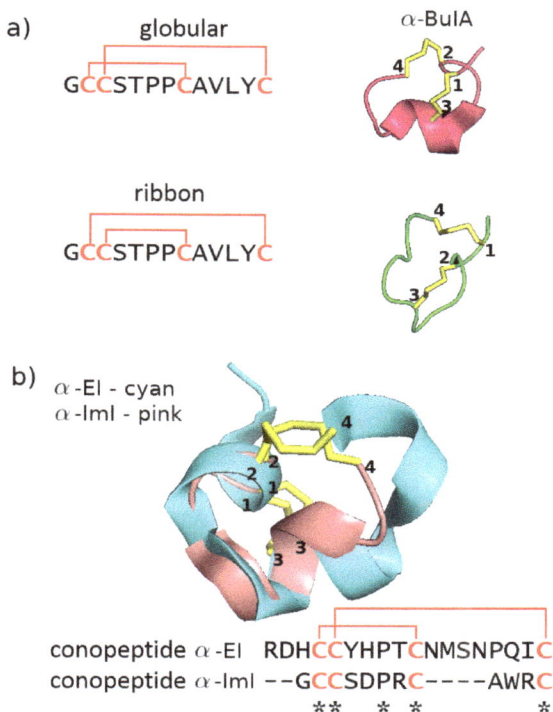

Figure 7. Impact of disulfide connectivity on conotoxin structure. (**a**) The same sequence can adopt different structural folds given different disulfide connectivities [69]. Conotoxin α-BuIA in globular form with connectivity 1-3, 2-4 (top, PDB structure 2I28 [82]) and in ribbon form with connectivity 1-4, 2-3 (bottom, PDB structure 2NS3 [83]). (**b**) Different sequences can adopt similar structural folds given the same disulfide connectivity. Conotoxin α-EI in cyan (PDB structure 1K64 [84]) and conotoxin α-IMI in pink (PDB structure 1G2G [51]), both in globular form with connectivity 1-3, 2-4. All images rendered in Pymol with disulfide bonds represented as yellow sticks [53].

3. Computational Strategies to Understand and Predict Conopeptide Structure and Function

The increased and efficient discovery of new conopeptides has been facilitated by advances in the fields of transcriptomics, proteomics, and bioinformatics and their integration into a new field called venomics, the in-depth study of venoms [88–90]. As we have demonstrated, the understanding of conopeptides is complicated by their diversity along many different axes, making application-specific design a difficult if not intractable problem. In this section, we discuss different ways in which in silico methods have been used to partially address these questions, both in terms of detailed characterization of individual conopeptides and in terms of identification of broad conopeptide trends (see Figure 8 for a visual summary of methologies and Table A1 for a tabulated version of the references cited in this section). We begin by introducing in Section 3.1 the progress that has been made in employing machine learning techniques to predict the pharmacological targets of conopeptides from their sequences. Then, in Section 3.2, we report the ways in which docking studies and molecular dynamics simulations have been used—often in conjunction—to shed light on the structure and function of a number of individual conopeptides and conopeptide pharmacological families. Finally, in Section 3.3, we provide an overview of computationally-driven studies that were used to design conopeptides for specific applications.

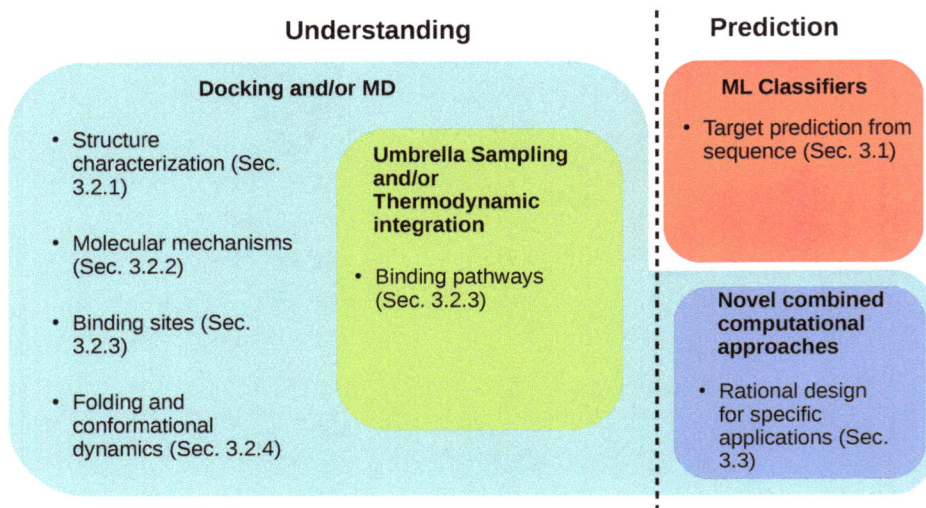

Figure 8. A visual overview of Section 3, with a focus on the different computational techniques employed.

3.1. Predicting Function from Sequence through Machine Learning

Classification via data-mining of a set of training data encompasses a broad set of techniques that have been growing in popularity in recent years, demonstrating utility in such disparate areas as agriculture [91], medical image processing [92], bioinformatics [93], and many others. Attempts have been made to employ such methods to the categorization of the incredibly diverse group that makes up the conopeptides. Indeed, extensive work has been done on developing sequence-based predictors that use machine learning techniques for identifying the target receptor type of a novel conopeptide sequence, achieving predictive accuracies of up to 97% [94], although they are currently limited to discriminating the toxins targeting voltage-gated sodium, calcium, and potassium channels. Additionally, a very recent tool, ConusPipe, has attempted the classification of RNA sequences by employing three different machine learning models, in order to identify potential novel conotoxin sequences within *Conus* transcriptomes without resorting to sequence homology type searches, which may fail due to the high diversity of the sequences in question [95].

A number of different peptide representations and classification algorithms have been experimented with to optimize performance. Innovations include representing conopeptide sequences by their amino acid composition and dipeptide composition [96]—that is, the composition based on neighboring amino acid pairs—or their "pseudo" amino acid composition, which incorporates information about the correlation between physicochemical properties of the compositional amino acids [97]. Dimensionality reduction to identify pertinent features has improved performance: relatively recent feature selection techniques employed include the binomial distribution [98], the relief algorithm [99], the f-score algorithm [97,100], and analysis of variance [96]. Several relatively well-known machine-learning algorithms have demonstrated good performance: support vector machines [96,97,100], radial basis functions [98], and random forests [99]. The best performance was achieved by ICTCPred, with an average accuracy of 0.973, an overall accuracy of 0.957, and a minimum sensitivity of 0.919 for correctly discriminating between the possible targets of voltage-gated sodium, potassium, or calcium channel on a testing dataset of 70 conopeptides [99] (It should be noted that a manual investigation of the training set for this study suggests it was not properly pruned, as several ion channel sequences were erroneously included and labeled as conopeptides; however, this minor error did not appear to have a strong impact on the results, as the testing set did not include any such errors.). For a more detailed explanation, we refer the interested reader to a comprehensive review by Dao et al. [94] of recent machine learning techniques as applied to the conopeptides.

Despite the availability of algorithms that can accurately predict target receptors based on conopeptide sequence [94,99,101] with high accuracy, these methods are still subject to a number of limitations. The size of current benchmarks for the conopeptides is not large enough to imply generalizability over the entire family. For example, we found 243 conopeptides in the Conoserver with identified pharmacological targets, out of a total of 6254 identified sequences [17,54], while most predictor studies have used training sets on the order of about 100–150 sequences to eliminate redundancy and reserve data for testing [94]. The high variability of conopeptide sequence, in addition to the possibility of synthetic analogues, suggests that this is not sufficient to create a classifier that would be accurate for a general sequence. Furthermore, these methods do not provide details on the mechanisms of how conopeptides function upon binding to their targets. Such details can be elucidated mainly through modeling and analysis of conopeptide structures, which can allow for the estimation of folding free energies and binding affinities. In addition, the relative toxicity of a conopeptide in different target animals can be more reliably assessed from a structural perspective. Finally, understanding how rational modifications in engineered conopeptides can alter their toxicity in specific animals, including humans, necessitates a more mechanistic approach, which is the focus of the next few sections.

3.2. Docking Studies and Molecular Dynamics Simulations for Understanding of Conopeptide Structure and Binding

Docking studies and molecular dynamics (MD) simulations are complementary computational techniques used to study proteins and peptides in molecular-level detail. Docking studies provide an in silico representation of the binding between a receptor and its ligand, which may be used for high-throughput screening and prediction of binding energies and affinities [45]. The overall procedure consists of a search through the conformational space of the "docked" complex followed by scoring of the possible configurations thus identified. Although there are still some outstanding questions in the field, including the optimal method for handling solvation, how to model flexibility of the target binding site, and how to correctly assess protein-protein interactions when the ligands are not small molecules, docking studies nonetheless boast a rich history of profitable application in a number of areas [102]. Molecular dynamics simulations, which typically consist of solving Newton's laws of motion over a number of time steps, can complement docking for the understanding and prediction of molecular mechanisms, as well as being a sophisticated technique in their own right. They can better handle conformational entropy and predict dynamical fluctuations at the cost of significantly higher computational expense. In a sense, if docking studies provide breadth of understanding of protein systems, MD simulations provide depth. For example, an attractive procedure for designing compounds to interact with a particular target is to perform docking to identify an initial set of potential compounds followed by performing MD for their detailed characterization [103,104].

With respect to the conopeptides, docking studies and/or MD simulations have been used to (i) complement nuclear magnetic resonance (NMR) and X-ray crystallography experiments to characterize the three-dimensional structure of conopeptides and receptor/toxin complexes, (ii) investigate the importance of structure, electrostatics, and hydrophobicity for receptor/toxin binding and identify key residues contributing to binding, (iii) identify and characterize molecular mechanisms of binding and binding/unbinding pathways, and in a few cases (iv) to characterize thermodynamics, kinetics, and environmental effects on conopeptide folding.

3.2.1. Conopeptide and Receptor Structural Characterization

Structure is an important predictor of function: conopeptides are, broadly speaking, either steric pore blockers or "lock-and-key" (ant)agonists that bind to and alter the functional properties of their target proteins [3]. Furthermore, since it is generally easier to determine the structures of small peptides with high accuracy than those of large proteins, conopeptides themselves can help determine the structures of the ion channels to which they bind with remarkable selectivity. For this reason, efforts have been devoted to characterizing the structures of a number of different conopeptides.

At the time of this article, there are 161 defined three-dimensional conopeptide structures in the PDB database [56], a number of which were refined with the help of docking and molecular dynamics. For example, MD simulations were used to refine the three-dimensional structures predicted from NMR data of conotoxin BtIIIA [105], α conotoxin MI [106], α conotoxin EIVA [107] and conantokin G in complex with calcium atoms [15]. Furthermore, by also using homology modeling based on a conotoxin with a known three-dimensional structure, ι-RXIA, Aguilar et al. [108] refined the structure of a new conotoxin, sr11a, a pore blocker in certain mammalian potassium channels. From a more ab initio perspective, Li et al. [109] and Platt et al. [110] used structure prediction algorithms followed by MD simulations to determine and assess three-dimensional structures for two different conopeptide systems, namely Vt3.1 and a subset of the conantokins, which can inhibit neuronal N-methyl-D-aspartate (NMDA) receptors in the brain.

As previously indicated, a number of computational studies have been performed demonstrating the use of conopeptides to aid in the structural determination of ion channels. For example, the comparison of a combined docking and MD simulation study with prior experimental data demonstrated the validity of an in silico approach for making microscopic predictions about complexes and the relevant microscopic forces controlling their interactions [111]. Molecular simulation refinement of a homology model of the complex of α conotoxin LvIA and the $\alpha_3\beta_2$ subtype of the nicotinic acetylcholine receptor (nAChR) based on the crystal structure of LvIA in complex with the acetylcholine-binding protein (AchBP) revealed important structural interactions between them [112]. Docking simulations of μ conotoxins demonstrated the validity of homology models for voltage-gated eukaryotic sodium channels, difficult to characterize experimentally, based on prokaryotic ones [113]. A more in-depth comparison of bacterial and mammalian sodium channel binding by μ-GIIIA, employing docking and biased and unbiased MD simulations, showed deeper insertion of the conotoxin into bacterial channels, which explained a corresponding loss of functionality of certain μ conotoxins when binding to the mammalian channels [114]. Finally, the α conotoxin family was used as a testing ground for a new docking algorithm called ToxDock, which employs ensemble docking to predict the structure of large receptor complexes bound to smaller peptide ligands [115].

3.2.2. Molecular Mechanisms of Selectivity and Binding

Beyond shedding light on the detailed three-dimensional structures of conopeptides and receptor/toxin complexes, docking and MD have been employed to assess the relative importance of conopeptide structure, electrostatic distribution, and hydrophobicity to their interactions with ion channel receptors, as well as to identify the key residues within the structures that are responsible for the high pharmacological selectivity of conopeptides for specific receptor subtypes. For instance, MD and docking, both in conjunction with experimental data and from first principles, have shown how electrostatic effects contribute to pore-blocking the voltage-gated potassium and sodium channels and how they control selectivity for receptors. Specifically, docking studies were used to elucidate the importance of a positively-charged ring around the center of the conopeptides that bind to various subtypes of the voltage-gated potassium channels and similarly to elucidate the how certain basic residues of conopeptides interact with the negatively charged ring in the outer vestibule of different isoforms of the voltage-gated sodium channel [77,116,117]. In addition, to assess the contributions of various effects, Beissner et al. [118] used docking studies and MD simulations to calculate binding enthalpies to support their conclusion that charge is more important than steric contributions in controlling the selectivity of α conotoxins for the $\alpha_3\beta_2$ nAChR subtype over the $\alpha_4\beta_2$ subtype. Using a similar approach involving a computational scan and the calculation of binding energies for single point mutants of the α conotoxin ImI in complex with the α_7 nAChR, Yu et al. [119] showed that dispersion and desolvation forces control its binding affinity to nAChRs, while electrostatic forces influence selectivity. Kwon et al. [120] employed MD simulations to probe the conformations and hydrogen-bonding networks of native and cyclic κ-PVIIA and explain the loss of interaction with the Shaker potassium channel occurring upon cyclization, which they demonstrated to be primarily due to loss of electrostatic interactions with the N terminus, but also noted that certain hydrogen bonds formed by the native toxin might contribute to its stability. The microscopic forces that govern the changing electrostatics themselves have also been probed from an in silico perspective: Lúcio and Mazzoni [121] used a detailed quantum/classical approach to reveal structural and electronic changes occurring upon a single point mutation of ω-MVIIA and ω-MVIIC and to determine how changing electronic structure can predict changing hydrogen-bonding patterns; McDougal et al. [122] used constant pH MD simulations to probe the effects of pH upon the protonation state of key residues of α-MII.

Several studies have also identified overall hydrophobic and structural components to receptor/ligand interactions. Docking studies performed by Hopping et al. [123] rationalized, at a molecular level, the strong effect of hydrophobicity on selectivity of α-[A10L]PnIA for the α_7 over the $\alpha_3\beta_2$ nAChR subtype; MD simulations performed by Cuny et al. [124] revealed that receptor side chain length is responsible for the experimentally determined affinities of α-RegIIA for human $\alpha_3\beta_2$ and $\alpha_3\beta_4$ nAChRs; and MD simulations performed by Chhabra et al. [125] demonstrated that a loss of key contacts of a cis-[2,8]-dicarba mutant of α-RgIA compared to the native form in complex with the nAChR $\alpha_9\alpha_{10}$ subtype was responsible for its lower binding affinities to the receptor. Pucci et al. [126] used a combination of MD and docking to elucidate the key interactions of the α-PIA N-terminal tripeptide tail with the $\alpha_6\beta_2$ nAChR subtype, while Lee et al. [127] employed a similar approach to demonstrate that the differences in the binding of α-GIC to the $\alpha_3\beta_2$ and $\alpha_3\beta_4$ nAChR subtypes are due to differing receptor side chain orientations (*cf.* Figure 9 for an image of α-GIC in complex with a receptor).

Finally, a number of studies have probed the underlying molecular mechanisms of pharmacological selectivity via identification and analysis of the key residues involved in receptor/toxin binding, which often differ from peptide to peptide. Lin et al. [128] used homology modeling and docking studies to supplement analysis of the X-ray crystal structure of α-GIC with AchBP to show that His-5 in the conotoxin primarily contributes to binding to the $\alpha_3\beta_2$ and $\alpha_3\beta_4$ nAChR subtypes, whereas Gln-13 in the conotoxin primarily controls its selectivity for the $\alpha_3\beta_2$ subtype (see Figure 9). Kim and McIntosh [129] employed MD simulations as part of a demonstration that the mechanism of selectivity of α-BuIA for the $\alpha_6\beta_2$ nAChR subtype compared to the $\alpha_4\beta_2$ subtype is due to nonlocal interactions of the conotoxin with three key residues of the $\alpha_6\beta_2$ receptor: Lys-185, Thr-187, and Ile-188. Similarly, Kompella et al. [130] pinpointed a single residue difference between the rat and human nAChR $\alpha_3\beta_2$ subtypes–Glu-198 in the rat–that leads to lower binding affinity for α-RegIIA in the human receptor due to steric hindrance. Dutertre et al. [131] employed docking studies and binding energy calculations to verify their experimental hypothesis that the most important interaction controlling α conotoxin affinity for the $\alpha_3\beta_2$ nAChR subtype in general is a conserved proline interacting with residue Leu-119 in the receptor. Pérez et al. [132] used combined docking and MD to identify that Arg-7 and Arg-9 in α-RgIA control affinity and selectivity for the $\alpha_9\alpha_{10}$ nAChR subtype via interactions with Glu-195 and Asp-114 on the receptor. Grishin et al. [133] used MD and homology modeling to demonstrate that Phe-9 of α-AuIB determines key binding interactions of that toxin with the $\alpha_3\beta_4$ nAChR. Finally, Yu et al. [134] and Wu et al. [135] used positional scanning in α-TxID to demonstrate that Ser-9 is responsible for the selectivity of that conotoxin for the $\alpha_3\beta_4$ nAChR subtype; they then used MD simulations to identify the cause of the selectivity as attributable to minor steric changes in the binding pocket between different nAChR subtypes and to supplement design of a mutated analogue with greater affinity for $\alpha_3\beta_4$ due to putative disruption of a single hydrogen bond. In addition, a simulation and docking study identified a key methionine residue responsible for the toxicity of ω-MVIIA, information that may be particularly impactful as it has the potential to aid in studies designed to reduce the severe side effects in the analgesic ziconotide that limit its usefulness [136].

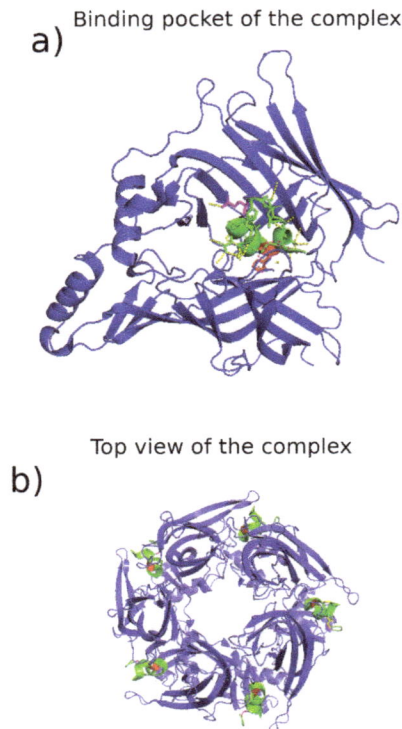

Figure 9. Illustration of binding modes and key residues. Figure shows conotoxin α-GIC in complex with the acetylcholine binding protein (AchBP) from *Aplysia californica*, often employed for homology modeling of nAChRs. Structure downloaded from the PDB server (code 5CO5). We highlight the key residues for selectivity identified by the study that also characterized the crystal structure through a combination of experimental and computational techniques [128]—in red, His-5, and in magenta, Gln-13, shown to control binding affinity and selectivity, respectively, for the $\alpha_3\beta_2$ nACHr subtype. (**a**) shows a zoom in of one of the binding pockets, with hydrogen bonds represented as yellow dotted lines, while (**b**) shows a top view. In both panels, the main body of the conotoxins are colored green and AchBP is colored blue. Images rendered with Pymol [53].

3.2.3. Identification of Binding Sites, Complexes, and Pathways

In addition to probing the effects underlying conopeptide selectivity for receptor type and subtype, docking and molecular dynamics have been employed to characterize the actual binding modes: to identify binding sites and expected binding orientations and to qualitatively and quantitatively study binding and unbinding pathways.

As it is not always obvious what the actual binding site or orientation of binding of a ligand in a receptor is, and only a few receptor/toxin complexes have been crystallized, computational approaches have been invaluable in identifying and characterizing specific binding sites, as well as raising intriguing questions about the apparent multitargeting ability of certain conopeptides. For example, Ellison et al. [137] used docking studies of α-ImI to explain the respective affinities of it and α-ImII for different nAChR binding sites, and McArthur et al. [138] verified and explained the proposed binding orientation of μ-PIIIA in the voltage-gated sodium channel via experiment combined with MD simulation and Poisson-Boltzmann calculations. In addition, Cortez et al. [139] used docking studies to identify two different modes of binding of α-MI for binding sites on the α/δ interface of the *Torpedo marmorata* nAChR, and Grishin et al. [71] showed that two different structural isomers of α-AuIB bind to completely different sites on the $\alpha_3\beta_4$ nAChR subtype, despite both demonstrating affinity for the receptor and having identical sequences. Finally, Yu et al. [140] employed a combination of MD simulations and binding free energy calculations in conjunction with experiment to identify the binding site of α-Vc1.1 to the $\alpha_9\alpha_{10}$ nAChR subtype.

Once the binding sites have been identified, the dynamics of interaction between receptors and toxins can be examined, as has been done in several studies. Lin et al. [141] calculated binding free energies from MD to determine different metal-binding models for conantokin-T and conantokin-G, while Armishaw et al. [142] used docking refined with MD to investigate the binding interactions of α-ImI analogs produced from a large synthetic combinatorial library. Docking approaches have also been profitably employed by themselves: Luo et al. [143] elucidated the microscopic underpinnings of rapid unbinding of α-LtIA with the $\alpha_3\beta_2$ nAChR as part of the characterization of the overall complex and the identification of its novel binding mode and Dutertre et al. [144] highlighted the differences between conotoxin binding and snake toxin binding to the nAChR. Meanwhile Tietze et al. [145] performed an in-depth docking and MD analysis, including a model of the full toxin binding site, to probe the molecular basis of binding between δ-EVIA and voltage-gated sodium channels. Finally, Mahdavi and Kuyucak [146] undertook a systematic analysis of binding modes of different μ conotoxins to the Na$_V$1.4 sodium channel subtype through both docking and MD, and Chen et al. [147] used a comprehensive combination of docking, nonequilibrium MD, and theoretical methods to calculate binding energies and predict the specificity of μ-PIIIA for eight different Na$_V$ subtypes.

In addition to the fluctuations and interactions of the binding modes themselves, it is of interest to characterize binding and unbinding pathways by which conopeptides dynamically associate with their target receptors. Although these pathways are of clear importance in analyzing receptor/toxin interaction, they are somewhat difficult to characterize experimentally. A number of studies, primarily relying on nonequilibrium molecular dynamics approaches, have been performed to probe the kinetics of binding and unbinding. Two popular methods are thermodynamic integration [43] and umbrella sampling [148]. Often such studies are used to characterize free energy changes and potentials of mean force along the pathways. For instance, Chen and Chung [149] used such an approach to characterize multiple binding modes of ω-GVIA in the calcium Ca$_V$2.2 channel subtype and accurately predicted IC50 values for channel inhibition. Chen et al. [150] performed umbrella sampling of the unbinding of μ-PIIIA from the Na$_V$1.4 sodium channel and computed the potential of mean force and dissociation constants for the complex. Yu et al. [151] qualitatively reproduced the experimental binding affinities of α-ImI and α-PnIA[A10L,D14K] to AchBP and demonstrated that a large structural rearrangement of the receptor C-loop is necessary for unbinding, while Suresh and Hung [152] used umbrella sampling to compare the binding of α-[Y4E]GID with the $\alpha_4\beta_2$ nAChR subtype to that with the α_7 subtype. In an example of the use of other nonequilibrium techniques, Yu et al. [153] employed random accelerated molecular dynamics and steered molecular dynamics to characterize multiple unbinding pathways of α-ImI from the α_7 nAChR subtype and computed the potentials of mean force for unbinding using Jarzynski's equation [154]. Meanwhile, Huang et al. [155] took a multiscaled approach by using a combination of atomistic molecular dynamics and coarse-grained Brownian dynamics simulations to model the binding process of κ-PVIIA: they were able to show that approach to the Shaker potassium channel is mediated by long-range electrostatics, while the final deep insertion is the result of a combination of electrostatic interactions from the Lys-7 side chain and hydrogen bonding and hydrophobicity primarily mediated by Phe-9 and Phe-23.

3.2.4. Folding Kinetics and Isolated Conformations of Conopeptides in Solution

A slightly different but equally important question in the study of conopeptides is the study of their folding and dynamical conformations under different environmental conditions, an understanding of which provides a route forward for design of kinetically or thermodynamically controllable structures. Although fewer studies have been performed in this area, the number of such studies has increased in recent years. For example, Jiang and Ma [156] performed folding studies on α-GI with simplified quantum chemical computations and proved their usefulness in rapid simulations of folding/unfolding, while Karayiannis et al. [157] harvested trajectories from long parallel MD simulations of α-AuIB to quantitatively characterize its structural and dynamic properties: the fluctuations of its size and shape and its translational and rotational diffusivities in water. An interesting recent study done by Jain and Pirogova [158] probed the effects of electric field strength on the conformations taken on by MrIIIe in solution. Finally, Sajeevan and Roy performed MD simulations of α-AuIB and α-GI with disconnected disulfide bonds in water and water-ionic-liquid. They showed that the different solvents controlled the conformational landscape of the studied toxins, thus demonstrating that different ensembles of different isomers are thermodynamically favorable under different solvent conditions, potentially providing a route for thermodynamic control of in vitro folding [159,160].

As mentioned in Section 2.2, one of the strongest dictators of final conopeptide structure is disulfide connectivity, and several studies have been performed to probe aspects thereof, with somewhat peptide-dependent results. Paul George et al. [161] explored how the conformations of five different μ-conotoxins changed with successive removal of the native disulfide bonds. By doing so, they demonstrated that the set of conotoxins studied fall in a continuum from hirudin-like folding, in which folding proceeds by creation of intermediates with non-native disulfide connectivities, to BPTI-like folding, in which folding proceeds by progressive connection of native disulfide connectivities, and that the native structures of the studied toxins are retained upon removal of a single disulfide bond, but lost upon removal of two disulfide bonds. Several other simulations demonstrated that the removal of disulfide bonds is non-perturbative to the structure of cyclic conopeptides [162], but that non-cyclic conopeptides suffer greater structural perturbation [163]. Recently, Xu et al. [164] used MD simulations to show that all three disulfide bonds contribute significantly to the binding energies of μ-PIIIA to the Na$_V$1.4 VGSC.

3.2.5. Summary

We have compiled extensive docking and MD-based computational studies categorized under specific topics in a compact manner and summarized in Table A1. These studies have been invaluable in assessing the structures of conopeptides and predicting the structures of the ion channels to which they bind. They have further been of great use in characterizing the precise natures of the binding interactions between conopeptides and their target receptors. However, it is worth noting a few limitations associated with these computational studies. Only a narrow subset of the conopeptides have been explored with docking and MD studies, and the choice of which peptides to explore has been dictated more by interest in specific receptors or similarity to previously studied peptides than by any rational attempt to characterize the conopeptides as a class. Indeed, the majority of the studies have focused on a specific target, the nicotinic acetylcholine receptor. Furthermore, MD-based studies are time-consuming and computationally intensive and lack the high-throughput required for studying a large number of conopeptides. As we discussed in Section 2, out of the over 6000 identified sequences, less than a twentieth have associated characterized structures or targets, which may limit the usefulness of high-throughput analyses such as homology modeling and introduce difficulties in assessing overall trends. We recommend a few fruitful avenues of future inquiries. There is a need to have more iterative studies between experiments and theory that can help to improve the accuracy of computational methods and rationally inform experimental focus. Importantly, we envision the need to design further methodologies to integrate time-consuming, high-accuracy techniques such as ab initio MD with rapid, low-accuracy techniques such as homology modeling in a rational manner, which has the potential to lead to efficient, high-throughput studies that will result in greater understanding of the conopeptides as a whole. As we discuss in the next section, we are beginning to see a focus on novel, high-throughput computational techniques for design of conopeptides for specific applications, but further efforts are certainly called for.

3.3. Computational Design of Conopeptides for Specific Applications

In recent years, as the availability of computational resources has grown and confidence in computational algorithms has increased, there has been a concomitant increase in the number of design studies employing computational approaches in many areas, and the conopeptides are no different. For example, as part of a rational approach to design neurotensin analogues for pharmaceutical applications, Lee et al. [165] employed MD simulations and binding free energy calculations to demonstrate that glycosylation of contulakin-G lowers its affinity for the neurotensin 1 receptor, and as part of designing a methionine-lacking mutant, Ren et al. [166] employed MD simulations to demonstrate the effects of the methionine residue on α-TxID and its interactions with the $\alpha_3\beta_4$ nAChR subtype.

Perhaps more intriguingly, a number of more innovative, computationally-driven approaches have been introduced over the past decade. Through a combination of docking and MD simulations, Younis and Rashid [104] characterized the binding affinities of all available three-dimensional structures of conopeptides in the PDB database with a new target: the lysophosphatidic acid receptor 6 (LPAR6), which is implicated in several aggressive cancers. They identified α-BuIA as strongly binding to LPAR6, making it a good candidate for investigation and refinement as a possible anti-cancer drug. Gao et al. [167] performed a homology search of *Conus betulinus* venoms to identify six sequences similar to α-ImI, of which two were demonstrated to have desirable insecticidal properties, while Barba et al. [168] performed a sequence scan followed by MD simulations as the starting point for the design of an ω-GVIA mutant that strongly binds copper atoms to be used for environmental applications. Using conantokin-G as a starting sequence, Reyes-Guzman et al. [169] employed docking studies to evaluate mutants and guide a search that resulted in two peptides (EAR16 and EAR18) that are capable of reversibly blocking the GluN2B NMDA receptor, which is implicated in neuronal function. Of particular note have been several studies that have developed novel methodologies while also utilizing them for design purposes. In this vein, King et al. [170] used a genetic algorithm approach to perform a search through millions of sequences and designed a mutant of α-MII with more than double its binding affinity for the $\alpha_3\beta_2$ nAChR subtype. Two years later, the same authors used a more mature form of that approach in which they employed α-MII as a starting point for "drug repurposing": searching a set of FDA-approved drugs for ones predicted to have high binding affinity to a new target, in this case once again the $\alpha_3\beta_2$ nAChR subtype [171]. Finally, Kasheverov et al. [172] employed a method they term Protein Surface Topography, which essentially creates a two-dimensional "topographical" map of the electrostatic potential of a ligand, to design an α conotoxin mutant with nanomolar affinity for the α_7 nAChR subtype.

4. Future Outlook

As the study of proteins and peptides has matured, so too has the study of the conopeptides. A great deal of progress has been made on understanding their structures and functions, which in turn has shed valuable light on the structures and functions of ion channels and has improved methods for targeting those ion channels therapeutically. Computational approaches have helped to probe many different aspects of these inquiries: (i) machine learning predictors classify conopeptide targets with high accuracy on the basis of sequence; (ii) docking studies and molecular dynamics simulations reveal microscopic aspects of structure, binding, and dynamical conformations; and (iii) integrated computational approaches demonstrate their value for the rational design of conopeptides as therapeutic agents.

Many questions remain unanswered in the field of conopeptides. Identification of the three-dimensional structure of a new conopeptide is still a time-consuming process that often requires a combination of experimental techniques, such as X-ray crystallography and NMR, with docking and molecular dynamics, or computationally expensive ab initio folding. There are currently relatively few conopeptides for which pharmacological families have been determined, and, although classifiers with high accuracy exist, their generalizability to the full highly-diverse family of conopeptide sequences remains in question. Even fewer conopeptides are associated with verified three-dimensional structures, which makes knowledge-based prediction of targets or modes of action a difficult problem. In the remainder of this section, we discuss some of the challenges with overcoming these limitations.

The accurate prediction of the 3D structure of a protein from its sequence remains one of the "holy grails" of computational biology [39]. Ab initio (also called de novo) modeling approaches for obtaining protein structure predictions are very challenging and expensive except for small proteins such as "Trp-cage" (20 residues) [173], villin headpiece (35 residues) [174], NTL9 (39 residues) [175], and gpW (62 residues) [176]. Currently, ROSETTA is an actively used tool for de novo structure prediction from sequence, which is able to predict structures of single domain proteins up to a few hundred residues in length [177]. Structure prediction for a query sequence becomes more tractable when related sequences have available experimentally-resolved structures; this is referred to as homology modeling [178]. For typical proteins (at least 100 amino acids long), a general rule for building a homology model of a protein with unknown structure using another protein as the structural template is that both proteins should share at least 25% sequence identity; below this is considered an uncertain "twilight zone" [179–182]. Homology modeling has already been applied in a few cases to predict conopeptide three-dimensional structures [108,183–185]; however, applying it to an arbitrary conopeptide still suffers from notable difficulties. The majority of conopeptides do not reach the "typical" protein length of 100 amino acids and would therefore require a higher sequence identity cutoff for identification of an appropriate template for homology modeling, which in turn implies that such a template may not exist due to the high sequence variability of the mature toxins and the small number of determined three-dimensional structures [185]. Although their short lengths makes them more tractable for ab initio approaches, the large number of conopeptide sequences renders this approach of limited use for the characterization of the family itself.

As discussed in Section 2.2, the three-dimensional structure of the cysteine-rich peptides that comprise the bulk of the known conopeptides is largely determined by their disulfide connectivity. Indeed, in the few cases where homology modeling of conopeptides has been successfully applied, the appropriate disulfide connectivity for cysteine-containing conopeptides was known or assumed a priori [108,183,184]. In theory, prediction of the connectivity should allow the construction of a reasonable three-dimensional structure for any cysteine-rich conopeptide by analogy with another three-dimensional structure harboring the same connectivity. In practice, however, this is not straightforward. The number of possible connectivities grows extremely rapidly: in a protein with n cysteines the total number of possible connectivities is [186],

$$\frac{n!}{\left(\frac{n}{2}\right)!2^{n/2}},$$ (1)

which is a tractable three connectivities for a four-cysteine framework, but grows to fifteen for a six-cysteine framework, and over a hundred for an eight-cysteine framework. Indeed, the prediction of disulfide connectivity in general is still an active area of research, although state-of-the-art methods are beginning to reach over 80% accuracy in general [187–190].

Although most currently characterized conopeptides with a particular cysteine framework are claimed to have the same native disulfide connectivity, it is not obvious to what extent sequence similarity among the relatively small subset of conopeptides with known three-dimensional structures is responsible for this, which calls into question the generalizability of this trend. More intriguingly, there is evidence that different connectivities, observed experimentally, can bind to different receptor subtypes with reasonable affinity [71] and that different connectivities can represent metastable, kinetically-trapped states under certain conditions [160,191]. Some evidence even points to the existence of a thermodynamic ensemble of different structural isomers that can be affected by environmental factors [161]. Even if only one native isomer exists in vivo, kinetic rather than thermodynamic control in vitro could be a possible avenue for design of conopeptides with novel action. In vitro studies often have difficulty in correctly forming "native" disulfide connectivities [192], but from the perspective of isomeric design this might be turned into an advantage.

5. Conclusions

The series of venoms produced by the family of cone snails provides a diverse wealth of short disulfide-rich peptides with potential pharmaceutical value due to their high affinities for specific ion channel receptors. In this review, we have discussed the various efforts that have been made from a computational perspective to classify and characterize many of the different conopeptides. We have described the difficulties associated with drawing general conclusions about a set of such short, sequentially diverse peptides in the context of potential areas of future research. As the impact of computational approaches continues to grow, we hope to see an increase in the number of large-scale and high-throughput computational studies of the conopeptides, supported by a continuous increase in available structural data from experiment, with a concomitant increase in their value as novel ion-channel targeting drugs.

Author Contributions: Conceptualization, R.A.M., T.T. and S.G.; formal analysis, R.A.M.; investigation, R.A.M. and T.T.; data curation, R.A.M. and T.T.; writing—original draft preparation, R.A.M. and T.T.; writing—review and editing, R.A.M., T.T., B.H.M., J.M.F. and S.G.; supervision, S.G.; project administration, S.G.; funding acquisition, B.H.M., J.M.F. and S.G.

Funding: T.T., B.H.M., J.M.F., and S.G. were supported by the Functional Genomic and Computational Assessment of Threats (Fun-GCAT) program of the Intelligence Advanced Research Projects Activity (IARPA) agency within the Office of the Director of National Intelligence. T.T. was also partially supported by the Center for Nonlinear Studies (CNLS) at LANL. Triad National Security, LLC (Los Alamos, NM, USA) operator of the Los Alamos National Laboratory under Contract No. 89233218CNA000001 with the U.S. Department of Energy. R.A.M. was supported by a Los Alamos National Laboratory Director's Postdoctoral Fellowship.

Acknowledgments: We thank Amy Migliori and Srirupa Chakraborty for fruitful discussions.

Conflicts of Interest: The authors declare no conflict of interest.

Abbreviations

The following abbreviations are used in this manuscript:

AchBP	Acetylcholine binding protein
GPCR	G protein-coupled receptor
h-bonding	hydrogen bonding
MD	Molecular dynamics
ML	Machine learning
nAChR	Nicotinic acetylcholine receptor
NMR	Nuclear magnetic resonance
NMDA	N-methyl-D-aspartate receptor
PDB	Protein Data Bank
VGCC	Voltage-gated calcium channel
VGSC	Voltage-gated sodium channel
VGPC	Voltage-gated potassium channel

Appendix A

Table A1. Summary of work cited in Section 3. For each study, we note the broad goal and related subsection, the toxins involved, the methods employed, and a brief description of the results. Studies are listed in the order they are mentioned in the main text.

Goal	Toxin(s)	Methods	Results/Citations
Train ML classifier (Section 3.1)	toxins targeting VGSC, VGCC, VGPC	Support vector machines (SVMs)	Predictor of sequence to target with average accuracy 90.3% [100]
		SVMs	Predictor of sequence to target with average accuracy 95.3% [97]
		SVMs	Predictor of sequence to target with average accuracy 94.2% [96]
		Radial basis function network	Predictor of sequence to target with average accuracy 89.7% [98]
		Random forests	Predictor of sequence to target with average accuracy 97.3% [99]
	RNA sequences from ten species	Logit, Label spreading, Perceptron	ConusPipe identifies potential conotoxins from sequence [95]
Structure prediction (Section 3.2.1)	BtIIIA	MD simulation	Structure refinement [105]
	α-MI	MD simulation	Structure refinement [106]
	α-EIVA	MD simulation	Structure refinement [107]
	conantokin G	MD simulation	Structure refinement in complex with calcium [15]
	sr11a, ι-RXIA	MD, homology modeling	Structure refinement of sr11a [108]
	Vt3.1	MD, secondary structure predictors	Structure determination [109]
	conantokins conBk-A, conBk-B, conBk-C	MD, secondary structure predictors	Structure determination [110]
	α-GI	Docking, MD	Validation of in silico predictions [111]
	α-LvIA	Homology modeling, MD	Revealed molecular interactions between toxin and nAChR [112]
	μ-GIIIA, μ-PIIIA, μ-KIIIA	Docking	Validation of homology models for eukaryotic sodium channels [113]
	μ-GIIIA	Docking, biased MD, unbiased MD	Characterization of insertion into mammalian and bacterial channels [114]
	α-GID and analogues	Docking	Testing of ToxDock algorithm [115]
Molecular mechanisms (Section 3.2.2)	κ-RIIIK	Docking	Identification of charged ring interaction with Shaker VGPC [116]
	α/κ-PIXIVA	Docking	Identification of charged ring interaction with Shaker VGPC [77]
	μ-GIIIA	Docking	Identification of charged ring interaction with VGSC [117]
	α-MII, α-TxIA, α-[A10L]TxIA	Docking, MD	Charge more important than steric for selectivity for $\alpha_3\beta_2$ nAChR [118]
	α-ImI and mutants	Docking, MD	Binding versus selectivity to nAChR subtypes [119]
	ω-MVIIA, ω-MVIIC, mutants	Quantum and classical MD	Find electronic changes from mutation and relate to h-bonding [121]
	α-MII	Constant-pH MD	Probe pH effects on protonation [122]
	cyclic κ-PVIIA	MD simulation	Cyclization effects on interaction with VGPC [120]
	α-[A10L]PnIA	Docking	Hydrophobic effect on α_7, $\alpha_3\beta_2$ nAChR selectivity [123]
	α-RegIIA	MD simulation	Receptor side chain length relation to affinity for $\alpha_3\beta_2$, $\alpha_3\beta_4$ nAChR [124]
	α-RgIA	MD simulation	Effect of dicarba instead of disulfide bridges on $\alpha_9\beta_{10}$ nAChR binding [125]

Table A1. *Cont.*

Goal	Toxin(s)	Methods	Results/Citations
	α-PIA	Docking, MD	Tripeptide tail interaction with $\alpha_6\beta_2$ nAChR [126]
	α-GIC	Docking, MD	Receptor side chain orientation effects on binding to $\alpha_3\beta_2$, $\alpha_3\beta_4$ nAChR [127]
	α-GIC	Homology modeling, Docking	His-5, Gln-13 key residues control $\alpha_3\beta_2$, $\alpha_3\beta_4$ nAChR interaction [128]
	α-BuIA	MD simulation	Mechanism of selectivity for $\alpha_6\beta_2$ over $\alpha_4\beta_2$ nAChR [129]
	α-RegIIA	MD simulation	Residue Glu-198 controls affinity for rat over human $\alpha_3\beta_2$ nAChR [130]
	α-MII, α-PnIA, α-GID	Docking	Conserved proline controls affinity with $\alpha_3\beta_2$ nAChR [131]
	α-RgIA	Docking, MD	Arg-7, Arg-9 controls affinity and selectivity for $\alpha_9\alpha_{10}$ nAChR [132]
	α-AuIB	Homology modeling, MD	Phe-9 controls binding with $\alpha_3\beta_4$ nAChR [133]
	α-TxID	MD simulation	Selectivity for $\alpha_3\beta_4$ nAChR due to steric changes in binding pocket [134]
	α-TxID	MD simulation	Selectivity for $\alpha_3\beta_4$ nAChR due to steric changes in binding pocket, design of mutated analogue [135]
	ω-MVIIA	Docking, MD	Key methionine residue responsible for toxicity [136]
Binding site and pathway characterization (Section 3.2.3)	α-ImI, α-ImII	Docking	Affinities for different nAChR binding sites [137]
	μ-PIIIA	MD simulation	Verified and explained proposed binding orientation in VGSC [138]
	α-MI	Docking	Identification of two different nAChR binding modes [139]
	α-AuIB	Docking	Structural isomers bind to different sites on $\alpha_3\beta_4$ nAChR [71]
	α-Vc1.1	MD, binding energy calculations	Identify binding site to $\alpha_9\alpha_{10}$ nAChR [140]
	conantokin-T, conantokin-G	MD simulation	Determined metal-binding models [141]
	α-LtIA	Docking	Microscopic interactions of rapid unbinding from $\alpha_3\beta_2$ nAChR [143]
	α-ImI, α-PnIB, α-PnIA, α-MII	Docking	Differences between conotoxin and snake toxin binding at nAChR [144]
	α-ImI, analogues	Docking, MD	Binding interaction investigation [142]
	δ-EVIA	Docking, MD	Molecular basis of binding to VGSC [145]
	μ-PIIIA, μ-KIIIA, μ-BuIIIB	Docking, MD	Systematic analysis of binding modes to $Na_V1.4$ sodium channel [146]
	μ-PIIIA	Docking, MD, umbrella sampling	Predict specificity for 8 different Na_V subtypes [147]
	ω-GVIA	Umbrella sampling	Predict IC50 values for $Ca_V2.2$ channel inhibition [149]
	μ-PIIIA	Umbrella sampling	Dissociation constants from $Na_V1.4$ sodium channel [150]
	α-Imi, α-PnIA variants	Umbrella sampling	Binding pathway characterization [151]
	α-GID mutant	Umbrella sampling	Identification of multiple pathways in binding to $\alpha_4\beta_2$ and α_7 nAChRs [152]
	α-ImI	Random accelerated MD, Steered MD	Characterize multiple unbinding pathways from α_7 nAChR [153]
	κ-PVIIA	MD, coarse-grained Brownian dynamics	Contribution of long-range electrostatics, h-bonding, hydrophobicity to approach and insertion into VGPC [155]

Table A1. *Cont.*

Goal	Toxin(s)	Methods	Results/Citations
Folding and conformational dynamics (Section 3.2.4)	α-GI	Simplified quantum chemical calculations	Rapid simulations of folding/unfolding [156]
	α-AuIB	MD simulation	Size/shape fluctuations, translational and rotational diffusivity determination [157]
	MrIIIe	MD simulation	Effects of electric field strength [158]
	α-AuIB, α-GI	MD simulation	Ensembles of different isomers thermodynamically favorable under different solvent conditions [159,160]
	μ-GIIIA, μ-KIIIA, μ-PIIIA, μ-SIIIA, μ-SmIIIA	MD simulation	Effects of removal of successive disulfide bonds and characterization of folding types [161]
	cyclic α-Vc1.1	MD simulation	Removal of disulfide bonds does not perturb structure [162]
	α-Vc1.1, α-BuIA, α-ImI, α-AuIB	MD simulation	Removal of disulfide bonds perturbs non-cyclic structures [163]
Rational design (Section 3.3)	contulakin-G	MD simulation, binding free energy calculations	Design of neurotensin analogues [165]
	α-TxID	MD simulation	Design of methionine-lacking mutant [166]
	148 conopeptides with 3D structures in PDB [56]	Docking, MD	Design of conotoxin targeting LPAR6 [104]
	Conus betulinus venoms	Homology search	Find sequences with insecticidal properties [167]
	ω-GVIA and mutants	MD simulation	Find strong copper-binding conopeptides to remove metals from environment [168]
	conantokin-G and mutants	Docking	Design of EAR16, EAR18 that reversibly block GluN2B NMDA receptor [169]
	α-MII and mutants	Docking, genetic algorithms	Design mutant with double the binding affinity for $α_3β_2$ nAChR [170]
	α-MII and a set of FDA-approved drugs	Docking, genetic algorithms	Drug repurposing algorithm [171]
	α-PnIA and analogues	Docking, Protein Surface Topography	Design mutant with nanomolar affinity for $α_7$ nAChR [172]
	μ-PIIIA	MD, binding energy calculation	Assess importance of different disulfide bonds to binding with VGSC [164]

References

1. Robinson, S.D.; Norton, R.S. Conotoxin Gene Superfamilies. *Mar. Drugs* **2014**, *12*, 6058–6101. [CrossRef] [PubMed]
2. Lewis, R.J.; Dutertre, S.; Vetter, I.; Christie, M.J. Conus venom peptide pharmacology. *Pharmacol. Rev.* **2012**, *64*, 259–298. [CrossRef] [PubMed]
3. Akondi, K.B.; Muttenthaler, M.; Dutertre, S.; Kaas, Q.; Craik, D.J.; Lewis, R.J.; Alewood, P.F. Discovery, Synthesis, and Structure–Activity Relationships of Conotoxins. *Chem. Rev.* **2014**, *114*, 5815–5847. [CrossRef] [PubMed]
4. Davis, J.; Jones, A.; Lewis, R.J. Remarkable inter- and intra-species complexity of conotoxins revealed by LC/MS. *Peptides* **2009**, *30*, 1222–1227. [CrossRef] [PubMed]
5. Jones, R.M.; Bulaj, G. Conus peptides—Combinatorial chemistry at a cone snail's pace. *Curr. Opin. Drug Discov. Dev.* **2000**, *3*, 141–154.

6. Buczek, O.; Bulaj, G.; Olivera, B.M. Conotoxins and the posttranslational modification of secreted gene products. *Cell. Mol. Life Sci.* **2005**, *62*, 3067–3079. [CrossRef] [PubMed]
7. Puillandre, N.; Koua, D.; Favreau, P.; Olivera, B.M.; Stöcklin, R. Molecular Phylogeny, Classification and Evolution of Conopeptides. *J. Mol. Evol.* **2012**, *74*, 297–309. [CrossRef] [PubMed]
8. Lebbe, E.K.M.; Tytgat, J. In the picture: Disulfide-poor conopeptides, a class of pharmacologically interesting compounds. *J. Venom. Anim. Toxins Incl. Trop. Dis.* **2016**, *22*, 30. [CrossRef] [PubMed]
9. Olivera, B.M. Conus Venom Peptides: Reflections from the Biology of Clades and Species. *Annu. Rev. Ecol. Evol. Syst.* **2002**, *33*, 25–47. [CrossRef]
10. Craig, A.G.; Bandyopadhyay, P.; Olivera, B.M. Post-translationally modified neuropeptides from Conus venoms. *Eur. J. Biochem.* **1999**, *264*, 271–275. [CrossRef] [PubMed]
11. Cruz, L.J.; Gray, W.R.; Olivera, B.M.; Zeikus, R.D.; Kerr, L.; Yoshikami, D.; Moczydlowski, E. Conus geographus toxins that discriminate between neuronal and muscle sodium channels. *J. Biol. Chem.* **1985**, *260*, 9280–9288. [PubMed]
12. Loughnan, M.; Bond, T.; Atkins, A.; Cuevas, J.; Adams, D.J.; Broxton, N.M.; Livett, B.G.; Down, J.G.; Jones, A.; Alewood, P.F.; et al. alpha-conotoxin EpI, a novel sulfated peptide from Conus episcopatus that selectively targets neuronal nicotinic acetylcholine receptors. *J. Biol. Chem.* **1998**, *273*, 15667–15674. [CrossRef] [PubMed]
13. McIntosh, M.; Cruz, L.; Hunkapiller, M.; Gray, W.; Olivera, B. Isolation and structure of a peptide toxin from the marine snail Conus magus. *Arch. Biochem. Biophys.* **1982**, *218*, 329–334. [CrossRef]
14. Craig, A.G.; Zafaralla, G.; Cruz, L.J.; Santos, A.D.; Hillyard, D.R.; Dykert, J.; Rivier, J.E.; Gray, W.R.; Imperial, J.; DelaCruz, R.G.; et al. An O-Glycosylated Neuroexcitatory Conus Peptide. *Biochemistry* **1998**, *37*, 16019–16025. [CrossRef] [PubMed]
15. Rigby, A.C.; Baleja, J.D.; Li, L.; Pedersen, L.G.; Furie, B.C.; Furie, B. Role of γ-Carboxyglutamic Acid in the Calcium-Induced Structural Transition of Conantokin G, a Conotoxin from the Marine Snail Conus geographus. *Biochemistry* **1997**, *36*, 15677–15684. [CrossRef] [PubMed]
16. Gao, B.; Peng, C.; Yang, J.; Yi, Y.; Zhang, J.; Shi, Q. Cone snails: A big store of conotoxins for novel drug discovery. *Toxins* **2017**, *9*, 397. [CrossRef] [PubMed]
17. Kaas, Q.; Westermann, J.C.; Halai, R.; Wang, C.K.L.; Craik, D.J. ConoServer, a database for conopeptide sequences and structures. *Bioinformatics* **2008**, *24*, 445–446. [CrossRef] [PubMed]
18. Becker, S.; Terlau, H. Toxins from cone snails: properties, applications and biotechnological production. *Appl. Microbiol. Biotechnol.* **2008**, *79*, 1–9. [CrossRef] [PubMed]
19. Mir, R.; Karim, S.; Amjad Kamal, M.; Wilson, C.; Mirza, Z. Conotoxins: Structure, Therapeutic Potential and Pharmacological Applications. *Curr. Pharm. Des.* **2016**, *22*, 582–589. [CrossRef] [PubMed]
20. Mohammadi, S.A.; Christie, M.J. Conotoxin Interactions with $\alpha 9\alpha 10$-nAChRs: Is the $\alpha 9\alpha 10$-Nicotinic Acetylcholine Receptor an Important Therapeutic Target for Pain Management? *Toxins* **2015**, *7*, 3916–3932. [CrossRef] [PubMed]
21. Wilson, M.J.; Yoshikami, D.; Azam, L.; Gajewiak, J.; Olivera, B.M.; Bulaj, G.; Zhang, M.M. μ-Conotoxins that differentially block sodium channels NaV1.1 through 1.8 identify those responsible for action potentials in sciatic nerve. *Proc. Natl. Acad. Sci. USA* **2011**, *108*, 10302–10307. [CrossRef] [PubMed]
22. Zhao, R.; Dai, H.; Mendelman, N.; Cuello, L.G.; Chill, J.H.; Goldstein, S.A.N. Designer and natural peptide toxin blockers of the KcsA potassium channel identified by phage display. *Proc. Natl. Acad. Sci. USA* **2015**, *112*, 7013–7021. [CrossRef] [PubMed]
23. Zamponi, G.W. Targeting voltage-gated calcium channels in neurological and psychiatric diseases. *Nat. Rev. Drug. Discov.* **2016**, *15*, 19–34. [CrossRef] [PubMed]
24. Sadeghi, M.; McArthur, J.R.; Finol-Urdaneta, R.K. Analgesic conopeptides targeting G protein-coupled receptors reduce excitability of sensory neurons. *Neuropharmacology* **2017**, *127*, 116–123. [CrossRef] [PubMed]
25. Olivera, B.M.; Teichert, R.W. Diversity of the neurotoxic Conus peptides: A model for concerted pharmacological discovery. *Mol. Interv.* **2007**, *7*, 251–260. [CrossRef] [PubMed]
26. Terlau, H.; Olivera, B.M. Conus Venoms: A Rich Source of Novel Ion Channel-Targeted Peptides. *Physiol. Rev.* **2004**, *84*, 41–68. [CrossRef] [PubMed]
27. Anderson, P.D.; Bokor, G. Conotoxins: Potential Weapons from the Sea. *J. Bioterror. Biodef.* **2012**, *3*, 2157–2526.
28. Dutertre, S.; Jin, A.H.; Alewood, P.F.; Lewis, R.J. Intraspecific variations in Conus geographus defence-evoked venom and estimation of the human lethal dose. *Toxicon* **2014**, *91*, 135–144. [CrossRef] [PubMed]

29. Thapa, P.; Espiritu, M.J.; Cabalteja, C.C.; Bingham, J.P. Conotoxins and their regulatory considerations. *Regul. Toxicol. Pharmacol.* **2014**, *70*, 197–202. [CrossRef] [PubMed]
30. Armishaw, C.; Alewood, P. Conotoxins as Research Tools and Drug Leads. *Curr. Protein Pept. Sci.* **2005**, *6*, 221–240. [CrossRef] [PubMed]
31. Ramírez, D.; Gonzalez, W.; Fissore, R.; Carvacho, I. Conotoxins as Tools to Understand the Physiological Function of Voltage-Gated Calcium (CaV) Channels. *Mar. Drugs* **2017**, *15*, 313. [CrossRef] [PubMed]
32. Netirojjanakul, C.; Miranda, L.P. Progress and challenges in the optimization of toxin peptides for development as pain therapeutics. *Curr. Opin. Chem. Biol.* **2017**, *38*, 70–79. [CrossRef] [PubMed]
33. Olivera, B.M. Conus peptides: biodiversity-based discovery and exogenomics. *J. Biol. Chem.* **2006**, *281*, 31173–31177. [CrossRef] [PubMed]
34. Clark, R.; Jensen, J.; Nevin, S.; Callaghan, B.; Adams, D.; Craik, D. The Engineering of an Orally Active Conotoxin for the Treatment of Neuropathic Pain. *Angew. Chem. Int. Ed.* **2010**, *49*, 6545–6548. [CrossRef] [PubMed]
35. Obata, H.; Conklin, D.; Eisenach, J.C. Spinal noradrenaline transporter inhibition by reboxetine and Xen2174 reduces tactile hypersensitivity after surgery in rats. *Pain* **2005**, *113*, 271–276. [CrossRef] [PubMed]
36. Brust, A.; Palant, E.; Croker, D.E.; Colless, B.; Drinkwater, R.; Patterson, B.; Schroeder, C.I.; Wilson, D.; Nielsen, C.K.; Smith, M.T.; et al. χ-Conopeptide Pharmacophore Development: Toward a Novel Class of Norepinephrine Transporter Inhibitor (Xen2174) for Pain. *J. Med. Chem.* **2009**, *52*, 6991–7002. [CrossRef] [PubMed]
37. Miljanich, G. Ziconotide: Neuronal Calcium Channel Blocker for Treating Severe Chronic Pain. *Curr. Med. Chem.* **2004**, *11*, 3029–3040. [CrossRef] [PubMed]
38. Pope, J.E.; Deer, T.R. Ziconotide: A clinical update and pharmacologic review. *Expert Opin. Pharmacother.* **2013**, *14*, 957–966. [CrossRef] [PubMed]
39. Huang, P.S.; Boyken, S.E.; Baker, D. The coming of age of de novo protein design. *Nature* **2016**, *537*, 320–327. [CrossRef] [PubMed]
40. Rosenfeld, L.; Heyne, M.; Shifman, J.M.; Papo, N. Protein Engineering by Combined Computational and In Vitro Evolution Approaches. *Trends Biochem. Sci.* **2016**, *41*, 421–433. [CrossRef] [PubMed]
41. Hachmann, J.; Afzal, M.A.F.; Haghighatlari, M.; Pal, Y. Building and deploying a cyberinfrastructure for the data-driven design of chemical systems and the exploration of chemical space. *Mol. Simul.* **2018**, *44*, 921–929. [CrossRef]
42. Karplus, M.; McCammon, J.A. Molecular dynamics simulations of biomolecules. *Nat. Struct. Biol.* **2002**, *9*, 646–652. [CrossRef] [PubMed]
43. Frenkel, D.; Smit, B. *Understanding Molecular Simulation: From Algorithms to Applications*, 2nd ed.; Academic Press: San Diego, CA, USA, 2001.
44. Van Gunsteren, W.F.; Daura, X.; Hansen, N.; Mark, A.E.; Oostenbrink, C.; Riniker, S.; Smith, L.J. Validation of Molecular Simulation: An Overview of Issues. *Angew. Chem. Int. Ed.* **2018**, *57*, 884–902. [CrossRef] [PubMed]
45. Moreira, I.S.; Fernandes, P.A.; Ramos, M.J. Protein-protein docking dealing with the unknown. *J. Comput. Chem.* **2009**, *31*, 317–342. [CrossRef] [PubMed]
46. Chen, P.C.; Kuyucak, S. Developing a comparative docking protocol for the prediction of peptide selectivity profiles: investigation of potassium channel toxins. *Toxins* **2012**, *4*, 110–138. [CrossRef] [PubMed]
47. Gómez-Bombarelli, R.; Wei, J.N.; Duvenaud, D.; Hernández-Lobato, J.M.; Sánchez-Lengeling, B.; Sheberla, D.; Aguilera-Iparraguirre, J.; Hirzel, T.D.; Adams, R.P.; Aspuru-Guzik, A. Automatic Chemical Design Using a Data-Driven Continuous Representation of Molecules. *ACS Cent. Sci.* **2018**, *4*. [CrossRef] [PubMed]
48. Lee, E.Y.; Wong, G.C.; Ferguson, A.L. Machine learning-enabled discovery and design of membrane-active peptides. *Bioorg. Med. Chem.* **2018**, *26*, 2708–2718. [CrossRef] [PubMed]
49. Curtarolo, S.; Hart, G.L.W.; Nardelli, M.B.; Mingo, N.; Sanvito, S.; Levy, O. The high-throughput highway to computational materials design. *Nat. Mater.* **2013**, *12*, 191–201. [CrossRef] [PubMed]
50. Kaas, Q.; Westermann, J.C.; Craik, D.J. Conopeptide characterization and classifications: An analysis using ConoServer. *Toxicon* **2010**, *55*, 1491–1509. [CrossRef] [PubMed]
51. Lamthanh, H.; Jegou-Matheron, C.; Servent, D.; Menez, A.; Lancelin, J.M. Minimal conformation of the alpha-conotoxin ImI for the alpha7 neuronal nicotinic acetylcholine receptor recognition: correlated CD, NMR and binding studies. *FEBS Lett.* **1999**, *454*, 293–298. [PubMed]

52. Kavanaugh, J.S.; Rogers, P.H.; Arnone, A. Crystallographic Evidence for a New Ensemble of Ligand-Induced Allosteric Transitions in Hemoglobin: The T-to-THigh Quaternary Transitions. *Biochemistry* **2005**, *44*, 6101–6121. [CrossRef] [PubMed]

53. Schrödinger LLC. *The PyMOL Molecular Graphics System, Version 1.8*; Technical Report; Schrödinger LLC: New York, NY, USA, 2015.

54. Kaas, Q.; Yu, R.; Jin, A.H.; Dutertre, S.; Craik, D.J. ConoServer: Updated content, knowledge, and discovery tools in the conopeptide database. *Nucleic Acids Res.* **2012**, *40*, D325–D330. [CrossRef] [PubMed]

55. Cheek, S.; Krishna, S.S.; Grishin, N.V. Structural Classification of Small, Disulfide-rich Protein Domains. *J. Mol. Biol.* **2006**, *359*, 215–237. [CrossRef] [PubMed]

56. Berman, H.M.; Westbrook, J.; Feng, Z.; Gilliland, G.; Bhat, T.N.; Weissig, H.; Shindyalov, I.N.; Bourne, P.E. The Protein Data Bank. *Nucleic Acids Res.* **2000**, *28*, 235–242. [CrossRef] [PubMed]

57. Ellison, M.; Feng, Z.P.; Park, A.J.; Zhang, X.; Olivera, B.M.; McIntosh, J.M.; Norton, R.S. α-RgIA, a Novel Conotoxin That Blocks the α9α10 nAChR: Structure and Identification of Key Receptor-Binding Residues. *J. Mol. Biol.* **2008**, *377*, 1216–1227. [CrossRef] [PubMed]

58. Favreau, P.; Benoit, E.; Hocking, H.G.; Carlier, L.; D'hoedt, D.; Leipold, E.; Markgraf, R.; Schlumberger, S.; Córdova, M.A.; Gaertner, H.; et al. A novel μ-conopeptide, CnIIIC, exerts potent and preferential inhibition of NaV1.2/1.4 channels and blocks neuronal nicotinic acetylcholine receptors. *Br. J. Pharmacol.* **2012**, *166*, 1654–1668. [CrossRef] [PubMed]

59. Volpon, L.; Lamthanh, H.; Barbier, J.; Gilles, N.; Molgó, J.; Ménez, A.; Lancelin, J.M. NMR solution structures of δ-conotoxin EVIA from Conus ermineus that selectively acts on vertebrate neuronal Na+ channels. *J. Biol. Chem.* **2004**, *279*, 21356–21366. [CrossRef] [PubMed]

60. Gehrmann, J.; Alewood, P.F.; Craik, D.J. Structure determination of the three disulfide bond isomers of α-conotoxin GI: A model for the role of disulfide bonds in structural stability. *J. Mol. Biol.* **1998**, *278*, 401–415. [CrossRef] [PubMed]

61. Kang, T.S.; Jois, S.D.; Kini, R.M. Solution structures of two structural isoforms of CMrVIA χ/λ-conotoxin. *Biomacromolecules* **2006**, *7*, 2337–2346. [CrossRef] [PubMed]

62. Imperial, J.S.; Bansal, P.S.; Alewood, P.F.; Daly, N.L.; Craik, D.J.; Sporning, A.; Terlau, H.; López-Vera, E.; Bandyopadhyay, P.K.; Olivera, B.M. A novel conotoxin inhibitor of Kv1.6 channel and nAChR subtypes defines a new superfamily of conotoxins. *Biochemistry* **2006**, *45*, 8331–8340. [CrossRef] [PubMed]

63. Korukottu, J.; Bayrhuber, M.; Montaville, P.; Vijayan, V.; Jung, Y.S.; Becker, S.; Zweckstetter, M. Fast High-Resolution Protein Structure Determination by Using Unassigned NMR Data. *Angew. Chem. Int. Ed.* **2007**, *46*, 1176–1179. [CrossRef] [PubMed]

64. Du, W.H.; Han, Y.H.; Huang, F.J.; Li, J.; Chi, C.W.; Fang, W.H. Solution structure of an M-1 conotoxin with a novel disulfide linkage. *FEBS J.* **2007**, *274*, 2596–2602. [CrossRef] [PubMed]

65. Han, K.H.; Hwang, K.J.; Kim, S.M.; Kim, S.K.; Gray, W.R.; Olivera, B.M.; Rivier, J.; Shon, K.J. NMR structure determination of a novel conotoxin,[Pro 7, 13] αA-conotoxin PIVA. *Biochemistry* **1997**, *36*, 1669–1677. [CrossRef] [PubMed]

66. Eliseo, T.; Cicero, D.O.; Romeo, C.; Schininà, M.E.; Massilia, G.R.; Polticelli, F.; Ascenzi, P.; Paci, M. Solution structure of the cyclic peptide contryphan-Vn, a Ca2+-dependent K+ channel modulator. *Biopolymers* **2004**, *74*, 189–198. [CrossRef] [PubMed]

67. Han, Y.; Huang, F.; Jiang, H.; Liu, L.; Wang, Q.; Wang, Y.; Shao, X.; Chi, C.; Du, W.; Wang, C. Purification and structural characterization of a d-amino acid-containing conopeptide, conomarphin, from Conus marmoreus. *FEBS J.* **2008**, *275*, 1976–1987. [CrossRef] [PubMed]

68. Zhang, B.; Huang, F.; Du, W. Solution structure of a novel α-conotoxin with a distinctive loop spacing pattern. *Amino Acids* **2012**, *43*, 389–396. [CrossRef] [PubMed]

69. Daly, N.L.; Craik, D.J. Structural studies of conotoxins. *IUBMB Life* **2009**, *61*, 144–150. [CrossRef] [PubMed]

70. Han, T.; Zhang, M.M.; Walewska, A.; Gruszczynski, P.; Robertson, C.; Cheatham, T.; Yoshikami, D.; Olivera, B.; Bulaj, G. Structurally Minimized μ-Conotoxin Analogues as Sodium Channel Blockers: Implications for Designing Conopeptide-Based Therapeutics. *ChemMedChem* **2009**, *4*, 406–414. [CrossRef] [PubMed]

71. Grishin, A.A.; Wang, C.I.A.; Muttenthaler, M.; Alewood, P.F.; Lewis, R.J.; Adams, D.J. Alpha-conotoxin AuIB isomers exhibit distinct inhibitory mechanisms and differential sensitivity to stoichiometry of alpha3beta4 nicotinic acetylcholine receptors. *J. Biol. Chem.* **2010**, *285*, 22254–22263. [CrossRef] [PubMed]

72. Hu, S.H.; Gehrmann, J.; W Guddat, L.; Alewood, P.F.; Craik, D.J.; Martin, J.L. The 1.1 å crystal structure of the neuronal acetylcholine receptor antagonist, α-conotoxin PnIA from Conus pennaceus. *Structure* **1996**, *4*, 417–423. [CrossRef]

73. Nilsson, K.P.R.; Lovelace, E.S.; Caesar, C.E.; Tynngård, N.; Alewood, P.F.; Johansson, H.M.; Sharpe, I.A.; Lewis, R.J.; Daly, N.L.; Craik, D.J. Solution structure of χ-conopeptide MrIA, a modulator of the human norepinephrine transporter. *Biopolymers* **2005**, *80*, 815–823. [CrossRef] [PubMed]

74. Hill, J.M.; Alewood, P.F.; Craik, D.J. Solution structure of the sodium channel antagonist conotoxin GS: A new molecular caliper for probing sodium channel geometry. *Structure* **1997**, *5*, 571–583. [CrossRef]

75. The UniProt Consortium. UniProt: The universal protein knowledgebase. *Nucleic Acids Res.* **2017**, *45*, D158–D169. [CrossRef] [PubMed]

76. Kudryavtsev, D.S.; Shelukhina, I.V.; Son, L.V.; Ojomoko, L.O.; Kryukova, E.V.; Lyukmanova, E.N.; Zhmak, M.N.; Dolgikh, D.A.; Ivanov, I.A.; Kasheverov, I.E.; et al. Neurotoxins from snake venoms and α-conotoxin ImI inhibit functionally active ionotropic γ-aminobutyric acid (GABA) receptors. *J. Biol. Chem.* **2015**, *290*, 22747–58. [CrossRef] [PubMed]

77. Mondal, S.; Babu, R.M.; Bhavna, R.; Ramakumar, S. In silico detection of binding mode of J-superfamily conotoxin pl14a with Kv1.6 channel. *In Silico Biol.* **2007**, *7*, 175–186. [PubMed]

78. Turner, M.W.; Cort, J.R.; McDougal, O.M. α-Conotoxin Decontamination Protocol Evaluation: What Works and What Doesn't. *Toxins* **2017**, *9*, 281. [CrossRef] [PubMed]

79. Maaten, L.v.d.; Hinton, G. Visualizing Data using t-SNE. *J. Mach. Learn. Res.* **2008**, *9*, 2579–2605.

80. Pedregosa, F.; Varoquaux, G.; Gramfort, A.; Michel, V.; Thirion, B.; Grisel, O.; Blondel, M.; Prettenhofer, P.; Weiss, R.; Dubourg, V.; et al. Scikit-learn: Machine Learning in Python. *J. Mach. Learn. Res.* **2011**, *12*, 2825–2830.

81. Guddat, L.W.; Martin, J.A.; Shan, L.; Edmundson, A.B.; Gray, W.R. Three-Dimensional Structure of the α-Conotoxin GI at 1.2 Å Resolution. *Biochemistry* **1996**, *35*, 11329–11335. [CrossRef] [PubMed]

82. Chi, S.W.; Kim, D.H.; Olivera, B.M.; McIntosh, J.M.; Han, K.H. NMR structure determination of α-conotoxin BuIA, a novel neuronal nicotinic acetylcholine receptor antagonist with an unusual 4/4 disulfide scaffold. *Biochem. Biophys. Res. Commun.* **2006**, *349*, 1228–1234. [CrossRef] [PubMed]

83. Jin, A.H.; Brandstaetter, H.; Nevin, S.T.; Tan, C.; Clark, R.J.; Adams, D.J.; Alewood, P.F.; Craik, D.J.; Daly, N.L. Structure of α-conotoxin BuIA: influences of disulfide connectivity on structural dynamics. *BMC Struct. Biol.* **2007**, *7*, 28. [CrossRef] [PubMed]

84. Park, K.H.; Suk, J.E.; Jacobsen, R.; Gray, W.R.; McIntosh, J.M.; Han, K.H. Solution conformation of alpha-conotoxin EI, a neuromuscular toxin specific for the alpha 1/delta subunit interface of torpedo nicotinic acetylcholine receptor. *J. Biol. Chem.* **2001**, *276*, 49028–49033. [CrossRef] [PubMed]

85. Nielsen, K.J.; Thomas, L.; Lewis, R.J.; Alewood, P.F.; Craik, D.J. A Consensus Structure for ω-Conotoxins with Different Selectivities for Voltage-sensitive Calcium Channel Subtypes: Comparison of MVIIA, SVIB and SNX-202. *J. Mol. Biol.* **1996**, *263*, 297–310. [CrossRef] [PubMed]

86. Buczek, O.; Wei, D.; Babon, J.J.; Yang, X.; Fiedler, B.; Chen, P.; Yoshikami, D.; Olivera, B.M.; Bulaj, G.; Norton, R.S. Structure and Sodium Channel Activity of an Excitatory I1-Superfamily Conotoxin. *Biochemistry* **2007**, *46*, 9929–9940. [CrossRef] [PubMed]

87. Norton, R.S.; Pallaghy, P.K. The cystine knot structure of ion channel toxins and related polypeptides. *Toxicon* **1998**, *36*, 1573–1583. [CrossRef]

88. Xie, B.; Huang, Y.; Baumann, K.; Fry, B.; Shi, Q. From Marine Venoms to Drugs: Efficiently Supported by a Combination of Transcriptomics and Proteomics. *Mar. Drugs* **2017**, *15*, 103. [CrossRef] [PubMed]

89. Kaas, Q.; Craik, D.J. Bioinformatics-Aided Venomics. *Toxins* **2015**, *7*, 2159–2187. [CrossRef] [PubMed]

90. Prashanth, J.R.; Lewis, R.J.; Dutertre, S. Towards an integrated venomics approach for accelerated conopeptide discovery. *Toxicon* **2012**, *60*, 470–477. [CrossRef] [PubMed]

91. Kamilaris, A.; Prenafeta-Boldú, F.X. Deep learning in agriculture: A survey. *Comput. Electron. Agric.* **2018**, *147*, 70–90. [CrossRef]

92. Shen, D.; Wu, G.; Suk, H.I. Deep Learning in Medical Image Analysis. *Annu. Rev. Biomed. Eng.* **2017**, *19*, 221–248. [CrossRef] [PubMed]

93. Min, S.; Lee, B.; Yoon, S. Deep learning in bioinformatics. *Brief. Bioinform.* **2016**, *18*, bbw068. [CrossRef] [PubMed]

94. Dao, F.Y.; Yang, H.; Su, Z.D.; Yang, W.; Wu, Y.; Hui, D.; Chen, W.; Tang, H.; Lin, H. Recent Advances in Conotoxin Classification by Using Machine Learning Methods. *Molecules* **2017**, *22*, 1057. [CrossRef] [PubMed]

95. Li, Q.; Watkins, M.; Robinson, S.; Safavi-Hemami, H.; Yandell, M. Discovery of Novel Conotoxin Candidates Using Machine Learning. *Toxins* **2018**, *10*, 503. [CrossRef] [PubMed]

96. Xianfang, W.; Junmei, W.; Xiaolei, W.; Yue, Z. Predicting the Types of Ion Channel-Targeted Conotoxins Based on AVC-SVM Model. *BioMed. Res. Int.* **2017**, *2017*, 1–8. [CrossRef] [PubMed]

97. Wu, Y.; Zheng, Y.; Tang, H. Identifying the Types of Ion Channel-Targeted Conotoxins by Incorporating New Properties of Residues into Pseudo Amino Acid Composition. *BioMed. Res. Int.* **2016**, *2016*, 1–5. [CrossRef] [PubMed]

98. Yuan, L.F.; Ding, C.; Guo, S.H.; Ding, H.; Chen, W.; Lin, H. Prediction of the types of ion channel-targeted conotoxins based on radial basis function network. *Toxicol. In Vitro* **2013**, *27*, 852–856. [CrossRef] [PubMed]

99. Zhang, L.; Zhang, C.; Gao, R.; Yang, R.; Song, Q. Using the SMOTE technique and hybrid features to predict the types of ion channel-targeted conotoxins. *J. Theor. Biol.* **2016**, *403*, 75–84. [CrossRef] [PubMed]

100. Ding, H.; Deng, E.Z.; Yuan, L.F.; Liu, L.; Lin, H.; Chen, W.; Chou, K.C. iCTX-type: A sequence-based predictor for identifying the types of conotoxins in targeting ion channels. *BioMed. Res. Int.* **2014**, *2014*, 286419. [CrossRef] [PubMed]

101. Fan, Y.X.; Song, J.; Kong, X.; Shen, H.B. PredCSF: An Integrated Feature-Based Approach for Predicting Conotoxin Superfamily. *Protein Pept. Lett.* **2011**, *18*, 261–267. [CrossRef] [PubMed]

102. Ferreira, L.G.; Dos Santos, R.N.; Oliva, G.; Andricopulo, A.D. Molecular Docking and Structure-Based Drug Design Strategies. *Molecules* **2015**, *20*, 13384–13421. [CrossRef] [PubMed]

103. Śledź, P.; Caflisch, A. Protein structure-based drug design: from docking to molecular dynamics. *Curr. Opin. Struct. Biol.* **2018**, *48*, 93–102. [CrossRef] [PubMed]

104. Younis, S.; Rashid, S. Alpha conotoxin-BuIA globular isomer is a competitive antagonist for oleoyl-L-alpha-lysophosphatidic acid binding to LPAR6; A molecular dynamics study. *PLoS ONE* **2017**, *12*, e0189154. [CrossRef] [PubMed]

105. Akcan, M.; Cao, Y.; Chongxu, F.; Craik, D.J. The three-dimensional solution structure of mini-M conotoxin BtIIIA reveals a disconnection between disulfide connectivity and peptide fold. *Bioorg. Med. Chem.* **2013**, *21*, 3590–3596. [CrossRef] [PubMed]

106. Gouda, H.; Yamazaki, K.i.; Hasegawa, J.; Kobayashi, Y.; Nishiuchi, Y.; Sakakibara, S.; Hirono, S. Solution structure of α-conotoxin MI determined by 1H-NMR spectroscopy and molecular dynamics simulation with the explicit solvent water. *BBA Protein Struct. Mol. Enzymol.* **1997**, *1343*, 327–334. [CrossRef]

107. Chi, S.W.; Park, K.H.; Suk, J.E.; Olivera, B.M.; McIntosh, J.M.; Han, K.H. Solution conformation of alphaA-conotoxin EIVA, a potent neuromuscular nicotinic acetylcholine receptor antagonist from Conus ermineus. *J. Biol. Chem.* **2003**, *278*, 42208–42213. [CrossRef] [PubMed]

108. Aguilar, M.B.; Pérez-Reyes, L.I.; López, Z.; de la Cotera, E.P.H.; Falcón, A.; Ayala, C.; Galván, M.; Salvador, C.; Escobar, L.I. Peptide sr11a from Conus spurius is a novel peptide blocker for Kv1 potassium channels. *Peptides* **2010**, *31*, 1287–1291. [CrossRef] [PubMed]

109. Li, M.; Chang, S.; Yang, L.; Shi, J.; McFarland, K.; Yang, X.; Moller, A.; Wang, C.; Zou, X.; Chi, C.; et al. Conopeptide Vt3.1 preferentially inhibits BK potassium channels containing β4 subunits via electrostatic interactions. *J. Biol. Chem.* **2014**, *289*, 4735–4742. [CrossRef] [PubMed]

110. Platt, R.J.; Curtice, K.J.; Twede, V.D.; Watkins, M.; Gruszczyński, P.; Bulaj, G.; Horvath, M.P.; Olivera, B.M. From molecular phylogeny towards differentiating pharmacology for NMDA receptor subtypes. *Toxicon* **2014**, *81*, 67–79. [CrossRef] [PubMed]

111. Nasiripourdori, A.; Ranjbar, B.; Naderi-Manesh, H. Binding of long-chain alpha-neurotoxin would stabilize the resting state of nAChR: a comparative study with alpha-conotoxin. *Theor. Biol. Med. Model.* **2009**, *6*, 3. [CrossRef] [PubMed]

112. Zhangsun, D.; Zhu, X.; Wu, Y.; Hu, Y.; Kaas, Q.; Craik, D.J.; McIntosh, J.M.; Luo, S. Key residues in the nicotinic acetylcholine receptor β2 subunit contribute to α-conotoxin LvIA binding. *J. Biol. Chem.* **2015**, *290*, 9855–9862. [CrossRef] [PubMed]

113. Korkosh, V.S.; Zhorov, B.S.; Tikhonov, D.B. Folding similarity of the outer pore region in prokaryotic and eukaryotic sodium channels revealed by docking of conotoxins GIIIA, PIIIA, and KIIIA in a NavAb-based model of Nav1.4. *J. Gen. Physiol.* **2014**, *144*, 231–244. [CrossRef] [PubMed]

114. Patel, D.; Mahdavi, S.; Kuyucak, S. Computational Study of Binding of μ-Conotoxin GIIIA to Bacterial Sodium Channels NaVAb and NaVRh. *Biochemistry* **2016**, *55*, 1929–1938. [CrossRef] [PubMed]

115. Leffler, A.E.; Kuryatov, A.; Zebroski, H.A.; Powell, S.R.; Filipenko, P.; Hussein, A.K.; Gorson, J.; Heizmann, A.; Lyskov, S.; Tsien, R.W.; et al. Discovery of peptide ligands through docking and virtual screening at nicotinic acetylcholine receptor homology models. *Proc. Natl. Acad. Sci. USA* **2017**, *114*, E8100–E8109. [CrossRef] [PubMed]

116. Verdier, L.; Al-Sabi, A.; Rivier, J.E.F.; Olivera, B.M.; Terlau, H.; Carlomagno, T. Identification of a novel pharmacophore for peptide toxins interacting with K+ channels. *J. Biol. Chem.* **2005**, *280*, 21246–21255. [CrossRef] [PubMed]

117. Choudhary, G.; Aliste, M.P.; Tieleman, D.P.; French, R.J.; Dudley, S.C., Jr. Docking of μ-Conotoxin GIIIA in the Sodium Channel Outer Vestibule. *Channels* **2007**, *1*, 344–352. [CrossRef] [PubMed]

118. Beissner, M.; Dutertre, S.; Schemm, R.; Danker, T.; Sporning, A.; Grubmuller, H.; Nicke, A. Efficient Binding of 4/7 α-Conotoxins to Nicotinic α4β2 Receptors Is Prevented by Arg185 and Pro195 in the α4 Subunit. *Mol. Pharmacol.* **2012**, *82*, 711–718. [CrossRef] [PubMed]

119. Yu, R.; Craik, D.J.; Kaas, Q. Blockade of Neuronal α7-nAChR by α-Conotoxin ImI Explained by Computational Scanning and Energy Calculations. *PLoS Comput. Biol.* **2011**, *7*, e1002011. [CrossRef] [PubMed]

120. Kwon, S.; Bosmans, F.; Kaas, Q.; Cheneval, O.; Conibear, A.C.; Rosengren, K.J.; Wang, C.K.; Schroeder, C.I.; Craik, D.J. Efficient enzymatic cyclization of an inhibitory cystine knot-containing peptide. *Biotechnol. Bioeng.* **2016**, *113*, 2202–2212. [CrossRef] [PubMed]

121. Lúcio, A.D.; Mazzoni, M.S. Toxins by first-principles: Electronic structure mapping structural changes. *J. Mol. Struc-Theochem* **2008**, *853*, 58–61. [CrossRef]

122. McDougal, O.M.; Granum, D.M.; Swartz, M.; Rohleder, C.; Maupin, C.M. pKa Determination of Histidine Residues in α-Conotoxin MII Peptides by 1H NMR and Constant pH Molecular Dynamics Simulation. *J. Phys. Chem. B* **2013**, *117*, 2653–2661. [CrossRef] [PubMed]

123. Hopping, G.; Wang, C.I.A.; Hogg, R.C.; Nevin, S.T.; Lewis, R.J.; Adams, D.J.; Alewood, P.F. Hydrophobic residues at position 10 of α-conotoxin PnIA influence subtype selectivity between α7 and α3β2 neuronal nicotinic acetylcholine receptors. *Biochem. Pharmacol.* **2014**, *91*, 534–542. [CrossRef] [PubMed]

124. Cuny, H.; Kompella, S.N.; Tae, H.S.; Yu, R.; Adams, D.J. Key Structural Determinants in the Agonist Binding Loops of Human β2 and β4 Nicotinic Acetylcholine Receptor Subunits Contribute to α3β4 Subtype Selectivity of α-Conotoxins. *J. Biol. Chem.* **2016**, *291*, 23779–23792. [CrossRef] [PubMed]

125. Chhabra, S.; Belgi, A.; Bartels, P.; van Lierop, B.J.; Robinson, S.D.; Kompella, S.N.; Hung, A.; Callaghan, B.P.; Adams, D.J.; Robinson, A.J.; et al. Dicarba Analogues of α-Conotoxin RgIA. Structure, Stability, and Activity at Potential Pain Targets. *J. Med. Chem.* **2014**, *57*, 9933–9944. [CrossRef] [PubMed]

126. Pucci, L.; Grazioso, G.; Dallanoce, C.; Rizzi, L.; De Micheli, C.; Clementi, F.; Bertrand, S.; Bertrand, D.; Longhi, R.; De Amici, M.; et al. Engineering of α-conotoxin MII-derived peptides with increased selectivity for native α6β2* nicotinic acetylcholine receptors. *FASEB J.* **2011**, *25*, 3775–3789. [CrossRef] [PubMed]

127. Lee, C.; Lee, S.H.; Kim, D.H.; Han, K.H. Molecular docking study on the α3β2 neuronal nicotinic acetylcholine receptor complexed with α-Conotoxin GIC. *BMB Rep.* **2012**, *45*, 275–280. [CrossRef] [PubMed]

128. Lin, B.; Xu, M.; Zhu, X.; Wu, Y.; Liu, X.; Zhangsun, D.; Hu, Y.; Xiang, S.H.; Kasheverov, I.E.; Tsetlin, V.I.; et al. From crystal structure of α-conotoxin GIC in complex with Ac-AChBP to molecular determinants of its high selectivity for α3β2 nAChR. *Sci. Rep.* **2016**, *6*, 22349. [CrossRef] [PubMed]

129. Kim, H.W.; McIntosh, J.M. α6 nAChR subunit residues that confer α-conotoxin BuIA selectivity. *FASEB J.* **2012**, *26*, 4102–4110. [CrossRef] [PubMed]

130. Kompella, S.N.; Cuny, H.; Hung, A.; Adams, D.J. Molecular Basis for Differential Sensitivity of α-Conotoxin RegIIA at Rat and Human Neuronal Nicotinic Acetylcholine Receptors. *Mol. Pharmacol.* **2015**, *88*, 993–1001. [CrossRef] [PubMed]

131. Dutertre, S.; Nicke, A.; Lewis, R.J. Beta2 subunit contribution to 4/7 alpha-conotoxin binding to the nicotinic acetylcholine receptor. *J. Biol. Chem.* **2005**, *280*, 30460–30468. [CrossRef] [PubMed]

132. Pérez, E.G.; Cassels, B.K.; Zapata-Torres, G. Molecular modeling of the α9α10 nicotinic acetylcholine receptor subtype. *Bioorg. Med. Chem. Lett.* **2009**, *19*, 251–254. [CrossRef] [PubMed]

133. Grishin, A.A.; Cuny, H.; Hung, A.; Clark, R.J.; Brust, A.; Akondi, K.; Alewood, P.F.; Craik, D.J.; Adams, D.J. Identifying key amino acid residues that affect α-conotoxin AuIB inhibition of α3β4 nicotinic acetylcholine receptors. *J. Biol. Chem.* **2013**, *288*, 34428–34442. [CrossRef] [PubMed]

134. Yu, J.; Zhu, X.; Harvey, P.J.; Kaas, Q.; Zhangsun, D.; Craik, D.J.; Luo, S. Single Amino Acid Substitution in α-Conotoxin TxID Reveals a Specific α3β4 Nicotinic Acetylcholine Receptor Antagonist. *J. Med. Chem.* **2018**, *61*, 9256–9265. [CrossRef] [PubMed]

135. Wu, Y.; Zhangsun, D.; Zhu, X.; Kaas, Q.; Zhangsun, M.; Harvey, P.J.; Craik, D.J.; McIntosh, J.M.; Luo, S. α-Conotoxin [S9A]TxID Potently Discriminates between α3β4 and α6/α3β4 Nicotinic Acetylcholine Receptors. *J. Med. Chem.* **2017**, *60*, 5826–5833. [CrossRef] [PubMed]

136. Wang, F.; Yan, Z.; Liu, Z.; Wang, S.; Wu, Q.; Yu, S.; Ding, J.; Dai, Q. Molecular basis of toxicity of N-type calcium channel inhibitor MVIIA. *Neuropharmacology* **2016**, *101*, 137–145. [CrossRef] [PubMed]

137. Ellison, M.; Gao, F.; Wang, H.L.W.; Sine, S.M.; McIntosh, J.M.; Olivera, B.M. α-Conotoxins ImI and ImII Target Distinct Regions of the Human α7 Nicotinic Acetylcholine Receptor and Distinguish Human Nicotinic Receptor Subtypes. *Biochemistry* **2004**, *43*, 16019–16026. [CrossRef] [PubMed]

138. McArthur, J.R.; Singh, G.; O'Mara, M.L.; McMaster, D.; Ostroumov, V.; Tieleman, D.P.; French, R.J. Orientation of μ-Conotoxin PIIIA in a Sodium Channel Vestibule, Based on Voltage Dependence of Its Binding. *Mol. Pharmacol.* **2011**, *80*, 219–227. [CrossRef] [PubMed]

139. Cortez, L.; Marino-Buslje, C.; de Jiménez Bonino, M.B.; Hellman, U. Interactions between α-conotoxin MI and the Torpedo marmorata receptor α–δ interface. *Biochem. Biophys. Res. Commun.* **2007**, *355*, 275–279. [CrossRef] [PubMed]

140. Yu, R.; Kompella, S.N.; Adams, D.J.; Craik, D.J.; Kaas, Q. Determination of the α-Conotoxin Vc1.1 Binding Site on the α9α10 Nicotinic Acetylcholine Receptor. *J. Med. Chem.* **2013**, *56*, 3557–3567. [CrossRef] [PubMed]

141. Lin, C.; Chan, F.; Hwang, J.; Lyu, P. Calcium binding mode of γ-carboxyglutamic acids in conantokins. *Protein Eng. Des. Sel.* **1999**, *12*, 589–595. [CrossRef]

142. Armishaw, C.J.; Singh, N.; Medina-Franco, J.L.; Clark, R.J.; Scott, K.C.M.; Houghten, R.A.; Jensen, A.A. A synthetic combinatorial strategy for developing alpha-conotoxin analogs as potent alpha7 nicotinic acetylcholine receptor antagonists. *J. Biol. Chem.* **2010**, *285*, 1809–1821. [CrossRef] [PubMed]

143. Luo, S.; Akondi, K.B.; Zhangsun, D.; Wu, Y.; Zhu, X.; Hu, Y.; Christensen, S.; Dowell, C.; Daly, N.L.; Craik, D.J.; Wang, C.I.A.; Lewis, R.J.; Alewood, P.F.; McIntosh, J.M. Atypical alpha-conotoxin LtIA from Conus litteratus targets a novel microsite of the alpha3beta2 nicotinic receptor. *J. Biol. Chem.* **2010**, *285*, 12355–12366. [CrossRef] [PubMed]

144. Dutertre, S.; Nicke, A.; Tyndall, J.D.A.; Lewis, R.J. Determination of α-conotoxin binding modes on neuronal nicotinic acetylcholine receptors. *J. Mol. Recognit.* **2004**, *17*, 339–347. [CrossRef] [PubMed]

145. Tietze, D.; Leipold, E.; Heimer, P.; Böhm, M.; Winschel, W.; Imhof, D.; Heinemann, S.H.; Tietze, A.A. Molecular interaction of δ-conopeptide EVIA with voltage-gated Na+ channels. *BBA—Gen. Subjects* **2016**, *1860*, 2053–2063. [CrossRef] [PubMed]

146. Mahdavi, S.; Kuyucak, S. Systematic study of binding of μ-conotoxins to the sodium channel NaV1.4. *Toxins* **2014**, *6*, 3454–3470. [CrossRef] [PubMed]

147. Chen, F.; Huang, W.; Jiang, T.; Yu, R. Determination of the μ-Conotoxin PIIIA Specificity Against Voltage-Gated Sodium Channels from Binding Energy Calculations. *Mar. Drugs* **2018**, *16*, 153. [CrossRef] [PubMed]

148. Torrie, G.; Valleau, J. Nonphysical sampling distributions in Monte Carlo free-energy estimation: Umbrella sampling. *J. Comput. Phys.* **1977**, *23*, 187–199. [CrossRef]

149. Chen, R.; Chung, S.H. Complex Structures between the N-Type Calcium Channel (CaV 2.2) and ω-Conotoxin GVIA Predicted via Molecular Dynamics. *Biochemistry* **2013**, *52*, 3765–3772. [CrossRef] [PubMed]

150. Chen, R.; Robinson, A.; Chung, S.H. Mechanism of μ-Conotoxin PIIIA Binding to the Voltage-Gated Na+ Channel NaV1.4. *PLoS ONE* **2014**, *9*, e93267. [CrossRef] [PubMed]

151. Yu, R.; Tabassum, N.; Jiang, T. Investigation of α-conotoxin unbinding using umbrella sampling. *Bioorg. Med. Chem. Lett.* **2016**, *26*, 1296–1300. [CrossRef] [PubMed]

152. Suresh, A.; Hung, A. Molecular Simulation study of the unbinding of α-conotoxin [Y4E]GID at the α7 and α4β2 neuronal nicotinic acetylcholine receptors. *J. Mol. Graph. Model.* **2016**, *70*, 109–121. [CrossRef] [PubMed]

153. Yu, R.; Kaas, Q.; Craik, D.J. Delineation of the Unbinding Pathway of α-Conotoxin ImI from the α7 Nicotinic Acetylcholine Receptor. *J. Phys. Chem. B* **2012**, *116*, 6097–6105. [CrossRef] [PubMed]

154. Jarzynski, C. Nonequilibrium equality for free energy differences. *Phys. Rev. Lett.* **1997**, *78*, 2690. [CrossRef]

155. Huang, X.; Dong, F.; Zhou, H.X. Electrostatic Recognition and Induced Fit in the κ-PVIIA Toxin Binding to Shaker Potassium Channel. *J. Am. Chem. Soc.* **2005**, *127*, 6836–6849. [CrossRef] [PubMed]

156. Jiang, N.; Ma, J. Conformational Simulations of Aqueous Solvated α-Conotoxin GI and Its Single Disulfide Analogues Using a Polarizable Force Field Model. *J. Phys. Chem. A* **2008**, *112*, 9854–9867. [CrossRef] [PubMed]

157. Karayiannis, N.C.; Laso, M.; Kroger, M. Detailed Atomistic Molecular Dynamics Simulations of α-Conotoxin AuIB in Water. *J. Phys. Chem. B* **2009**, *113*, 5016–5024. [CrossRef] [PubMed]

158. Jain, S.; Pirogova, E. Static electric fields induce conformational changes in alpha conotoxin: A molecular dyanamics simulation study. In Proceedings of the 2017 Progress in Electromagnetics Research Symposium—Fall (PIERS— FALL), Singapore, 19–22 November 2017; pp. 1273–1277.

159. Sajeevan, K.A.; Roy, D. Aqueous ionic liquids influence the disulfide bond isoform equilibrium in conotoxin AuIB: A consequence of the Hofmeister effect? *Biophys. Rev.* **2018**, *10*, 769–780. [CrossRef] [PubMed]

160. Sajeevan, K.A.; Roy, D. Peptide Sequence and Solvent as Levers to Control Disulfide Connectivity in Multiple Cysteine Containing Venom Toxins. *J. Phys. Chem. B* **2018**, *122*, 5776–5789. [CrossRef] [PubMed]

161. Paul George, A.A.; Heimer, P.; Maaß, A.; Hamaekers, J.; Hofmann-Apitius, M.; Biswas, A.; Imhof, D. Insights into the Folding of Disulfide-Rich μ-Conotoxins. *ACS Omega* **2018**, *3*, 12330–12340. [CrossRef] [PubMed]

162. Yu, R.; Seymour, V.A.L.; Berecki, G.; Jia, X.; Akcan, M.; Adams, D.J.; Kaas, Q.; Craik, D.J. Less is More: Design of a Highly Stable Disulfide-Deleted Mutant of Analgesic Cyclic α-Conotoxin Vc1.1. *Sci. Rep.* **2015**, *5*, 13264. [CrossRef] [PubMed]

163. Tabassum, N.; Tae, H.S.; Jia, X.; Kaas, Q.; Jiang, T.; Adams, D.J.; Yu, R. Role of Cys I–Cys III Disulfide Bond on the Structure and Activity of α-Conotoxins at Human Neuronal Nicotinic Acetylcholine Receptors. *ACS Omega* **2017**, *2*, 4621–4631. [CrossRef] [PubMed]

164. Xu, X.; Xu, Q.; Chen, F.; Shi, J.; Liu, Y.; Chu, Y.; Wan, S.; Jiang, T.; Yu, R. Role of the disulfide bond on the structure and activity of μ-conotoxin PIIIA in the inhibition of NaV1.4. *RSC Adv.* **2019**, *9*, 668–674. [CrossRef]

165. Lee, H.K.; Zhang, L.; Smith, M.D.; Walewska, A.; Vellore, N.A.; Baron, R.; McIntosh, J.M.; White, H.S.; Olivera, B.M.; Bulaj, G. A marine analgesic peptide, Contulakin-G, and neurotensin are distinct agonists for neurotensin receptors: uncovering structural determinants of desensitization properties. *Front. Pharmacol.* **2015**, *6*, 11. [CrossRef] [PubMed]

166. Ren, J.; Li, R.; Ning, J.; Zhu, X.; Zhangsun, D.; Wu, Y.; Luo, S. Effect of Methionine Oxidation and Substitution of α-Conotoxin TxID on α3β4 Nicotinic Acetylcholine Receptor. *Mar. Drugs* **2018**, *16*, 215. [CrossRef] [PubMed]

167. Gao, B.; Peng, C.; Lin, B.; Chen, Q.; Zhang, J.; Shi, Q. Screening and Validation of Highly-Efficient Insecticidal Conotoxins from a Transcriptome-Based Dataset of Chinese Tubular Cone Snail. *Toxins* **2017**, *9*, 214. [CrossRef] [PubMed]

168. Barba, M.; Sobolev, A.P.; Zobnina, V.; Bonaccorsi di Patti, M.C.; Cervoni, L.; Spiezia, M.C.; Schininà, M.E.; Pietraforte, D.; Mannina, L.; Musci, G.; et al. Cupricyclins, Novel Redox-Active Metallopeptides Based on Conotoxins Scaffold. *PLoS ONE* **2012**, *7*, e30739. [CrossRef] [PubMed]

169. Reyes-Guzman, E.A.; Vega-Castro, N.; Reyes-Montaño, E.A.; Recio-Pinto, E. Antagonistic action on NMDA/GluN2B mediated currents of two peptides that were conantokin-G structure-based designed. *BMC Neurosci.* **2017**, *18*, 44. [CrossRef] [PubMed]

170. King, M.D.; Long, T.; Andersen, T.; McDougal, O.M. Genetic Algorithm Managed Peptide Mutant Screening: Optimizing Peptide Ligands for Targeted Receptor Binding. *J. Chem. Inf. Model.* **2016**, *56*, 2378–2387. [CrossRef] [PubMed]

171. King, M.D.; Long, T.; Pfalmer, D.L.; Andersen, T.L.; McDougal, O.M. SPIDR: small-molecule peptide-influenced drug repurposing. *BMC Bioinform.* **2018**, *19*, 138. [CrossRef] [PubMed]

172. Kasheverov, I.E.; Chugunov, A.O.; Kudryavtsev, D.S.; Ivanov, I.A.; Zhmak, M.N.; Shelukhina, I.V.; Spirova, E.N.; Tabakmakher, V.M.; Zelepuga, E.A.; Efremov, R.G.; et al. High-Affinity α-Conotoxin PnIA Analogs Designed on the Basis of the Protein Surface Topography Method. *Sci. Rep.* **2016**, *6*, 36848. [CrossRef] [PubMed]

173. Pitera, J.W.; Swope, W. Understanding folding and design: replica-exchange simulations of "Trp-cage" miniproteins. *Proc. Natl. Acad. Sci. USA* **2003**, *100*, 7587–7592. [CrossRef] [PubMed]

174. Ensign, D.L.; Kasson, P.M.; Pande, V.S. Heterogeneity Even at the Speed Limit of Folding: Large-scale Molecular Dynamics Study of a Fast-folding Variant of the Villin Headpiece. *J. Mol. Biol.* **2007**, *374*, 806–816. [CrossRef] [PubMed]

175. Voelz, V.A.; Bowman, G.R.; Beauchamp, K.; Pande, V.S. Molecular Simulation of ab Initio Protein Folding for a Millisecond Folder NTL9(1-39). *J. Am. Chem. Soc.* **2010**, *132*, 1526–1528. [CrossRef] [PubMed]

176. Sborgi, L.; Verma, A.; Piana, S.; Lindorff-Larsen, K.; Cerminara, M.; Santiveri, C.M.; Shaw, D.E.; de Alba, E.; Muñoz, V. Interaction Networks in Protein Folding via Atomic-Resolution Experiments and Long-Time-Scale Molecular Dynamics Simulations. *J. Am. Chem. Soc.* **2015**, *137*, 6506–6516. [CrossRef] [PubMed]

177. Rohl, C.A.; Strauss, C.E.; Misura, K.M.; Baker, D. Protein structure prediction using Rosetta. In *Methods in Enzymology*; Elsevier: Amsterdam, The Netherlands, 2004; Volume 383, pp. 66–93.

178. Dill, K.A.; MacCallum, J.L. The protein-folding problem, 50 years on. *Science* **2012**, *338*, 1042–1046. [CrossRef] [PubMed]

179. Baker, D.; Sali, A. Protein structure prediction and structural genomics. *Science* **2001**, *294*, 93–96. [CrossRef] [PubMed]

180. Xiang, Z. Advances in Homology Protein Structure Modeling. *Curr. Protein Pept. Sci.* **2006**, *7*, 217–227. [CrossRef] [PubMed]

181. Krieger, E.; Nabuurs, S.B.; Vriend, G. Homology modeling. *Methods Biochem. Anal.* **2003**, *44*, 509–523. [PubMed]

182. Rost, B. Twilight zone of protein sequence alignments. *Protein Eng. Des. Sel.* **1999**, *12*, 85–94. [CrossRef]

183. Everhart, D.; Cartier, G.E.; Malhotra, A.; Gomes, A.V.; McIntosh, J.M.; Luetje, C.W. Determinants of Potency on α-Conotoxin MII, a Peptide Antagonist of Neuronal Nicotinic Receptors. *Biochemistry* **2004**, *43*, 2732–2737. [CrossRef] [PubMed]

184. Mondal, S.; Vijayan, R.; Shichina, K.; Babu, R.M.; Ramakumar, S. I-Superfamily Conotoxins: Sequence and Structure Analysis. *In Silico Biol.* **2005**, *5*, 557–571. [PubMed]

185. Twede, V.D.; Teichert, R.W.; Walker, C.S.; Gruszczynski, P.; Kazmierkiewicz, R.; Bulaj, G.; Olivera, B.M. Conantokin-Br from Conus brettinghami and Selectivity Determinants for the NR2D Subunit of the NMDA Receptor. *Biochemistry* **2009**, *48*, 4063–4073. [CrossRef] [PubMed]

186. Verdes, A.; Anand, P.; Gorson, J.; Jannetti, S.; Kelly, P.; Leffler, A.; Simpson, D.; Ramrattan, G.; Holford, M. From Mollusks to Medicine: A Venomics Approach for the Discovery and Characterization of Therapeutics from Terebridae Peptide Toxins. *Toxins* **2016**, *8*, 117. [CrossRef] [PubMed]

187. Heimer, P.; Tietze, A.A.; Bäuml, C.A.; Resemann, A.; Mayer, F.J.; Suckau, D.; Ohlenschläger, O.; Tietze, D.; Imhof, D. Conformational μ-Conotoxin PIIIA Isomers Revisited: Impact of Cysteine Pairing on Disulfide-Bond Assignment and Structure Elucidation. *Anal. Chem.* **2018**, *90*, 3321–3327. [CrossRef] [PubMed]

188. Lin, H.H.; Tseng, L.Y. DBCP: A web server for disulfide bonding connectivity pattern prediction without the prior knowledge of the bonding state of cysteines. *Nucleic Acids Res.* **2010**, *38*, W503–W507. [CrossRef] [PubMed]

189. Yang, J.; He, B.J.; Jang, R.; Zhang, Y.; Shen, H.B. Accurate disulfide-bonding network predictions improve ab initio structure prediction of cysteine-rich proteins. *Bioinformatics* **2015**, *31*, btv459. [CrossRef] [PubMed]

190. Jiang, J.; Zou, S.; Sun, Y.; Zhang, S. GL-BLSTM: A novel structure of bidirectional long-short term memory for disulfide bonding state prediction. *arXiv* **2018**, arXiv:1808.03745.

191. Espiritu, M.J. Disulfide Bond and Topological Isomerization of the Conopeptide PnID: Disulfide Bonds with a Twist. Ph.D. Thesis, University of Hawai'i at Manoa, Honolulu, HI, USA, 2017.

192. Steiner, A.M.; Bulaj, G. Optimization of oxidative folding methods for cysteine-rich peptides: A study of conotoxins containing three disulfide bridges. *J. Pept. Sci.* **2011**, *17*, 1–7. [CrossRef] [PubMed]

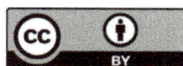

Article

Redesigning Arenicin-1, an Antimicrobial Peptide from the Marine Polychaeta *Arenicola marina*, by Strand Rearrangement or Branching, Substitution of Specific Residues, and Backbone Linearization or Cyclization

Dmitriy S. Orlov [1,†], Olga V. Shamova [1,†,*], Igor E. Eliseev [2], Maria S. Zharkova [1], Oleg B. Chakchir [2], Nikolinka Antcheva [3], Sotir Zachariev [4], Pavel V. Panteleev [5], Vladimir N. Kokryakov [1], Tatiana V. Ovchinnikova [5,6] and Alessandro Tossi [3]

[1]   Institute of Experimental Medicine, 12 Academic Pavlov str., St. Petersburg 197376, Russia;
      ds-orlov@yandex.ru (D.S.O.); manyvel@mail.ru (M.S.Z.); kokryak@yandex.ru (V.N.K.)
[2]   St. Petersburg Academic University, 8/3 Khlopina str., St. Petersburg 194021, Russia;
      eliseev@spbau.ru (I.E.E.); chakchir@spbau.ru (O.B.C.)
[3]   Department of Life Sciences, University of Trieste, Building Q, Via Giorgieri 5, 34127 Trieste, Italy;
      nantcheva@gmail.com (N.A.); atossi@units.it (A.T.)
[4]   International Centre for Genetic Engineering and Biotechnology, AREA Science Park, Padriciano 99,
      34149 Trieste, Italy; sotir@icgeb.org
[5]   M.M. Shemyakin & Yu.A. Ovchinnikov Institute of Bioorganic Chemistry, the Russian Academy of Sciences,
      Mikhluho-Maklaya str. 16/10, Moscow 117997, Russia; alarm14@gmail.com (P.V.P.); ovch@ibch.ru (T.V.O.)
[6]   Department of Biotechnology, I.M. Sechenov First Moscow State Medical University, Moscow 119991, Russia
*   Correspondence: oshamova@yandex.ru; Tel.: +7-911-253-0929
†   These authors contributed equally to this work.

Received: 20 May 2019; Accepted: 21 June 2019; Published: 23 June 2019

Abstract: Arenicin-1, a β-sheet antimicrobial peptide isolated from the marine polychaeta *Arenicola marina* coelomocytes, has a potent, broad-spectrum microbicidal activity and also shows significant toxicity towards mammalian cells. Several variants were rationally designed to elucidate the role of structural features such as cyclization, a certain symmetry of the residue arrangement, or the presence of specific residues in the sequence, in its membranolytic activity and the consequent effect on microbicidal efficacy and toxicity. The effect of variations on the structure was probed using molecular dynamics simulations, which indicated a significant stability of the β-hairpin scaffold and showed that modifying residue symmetry and β-strand arrangement affected both the twist and the kink present in the native structure. In vitro assays against a panel of Gram-negative and Gram-positive bacteria, including drug-resistant clinical isolates, showed that inversion of the residue arrangement improved the activity against Gram-negative strains but decreased it towards Gram-positive ones. Variants with increased symmetry were somewhat less active, whereas both backbone-cyclized and linear versions of the peptides, as well as variants with R→K and W→F replacement, showed antimicrobial activity comparable with that of the native peptide. All these variants permeabilized both the outer and the inner membranes of *Escherichia coli*, suggesting that a membranolytic mechanism of action was maintained. Our results indicate that the arenicin scaffold can support a considerable degree of variation while maintaining useful biological properties and can thus serve as a template for the elaboration of novel anti-infective agents.

Keywords: marine peptides; arenicin-1; molecular symmetry; structure–activity relationship; antibacterial; cytotoxic; chemical synthesis; molecular dynamics

---

1. Introduction

The growing resistance of pathogenic bacteria to currently used drugs dictates an urgent search for novel antibiotics. The antimicrobial peptides produced by the innate immune system of animals or plants are considered as potential new agents to combat drug-resistant bacteria, since they have a potent and rapid antimicrobial action and act via a multi-target mode of action. The innate immune system plays a vital role in the host defense of invertebrates, in particular, as their adaptive immunity is poorly developed, so that they have evolved a wide range of antimicrobial peptides (AMPs). Those of marine invertebrates can be considered as one of the most promising sources of new and effective antibiotics, especially AMPs from species inhabiting coastal zones, which are environments teeming with microbes, where the peptides are vital to help them avoid infection.

The subject of our study is a cationic antimicrobial peptide, arenicin-1, from the coelomocytes of one such invertebrate animal—the lugworm *Arenicola marina* [1]. This peptide adopts a β-hairpin structure [2–4] and possesses a potent microbicidal activity towards a broad spectrum of Gram-negative and Gram-positive bacteria (including drug-resistant clinical isolates), as well as towards fungi. However, it also displays a substantial cytotoxicity towards mammalian cells [1–3]. The mechanism of antimicrobial action of arenicin-1 is associated with a distinctive membranolytic activity [5–12]. Its potent antibiotic activity makes this peptide a fascinating lead for designing variants to test which features determine the antimicrobial and/or cytotoxic capacities and to disclose if they can be in some way extricated.

Though some of the structural characteristics of arenicins have already been explored, the significance of an intriguing feature of this molecule—its pseudosymmetric residue arrangement—remains unexplored (Figure 1).

The β-hairpin structures of arenicins show marked right-handed twist and kink in aqueous solution, as revealed by NMR spectroscopy [2,4] as well as by molecular dynamics simulation [6]. These features effectively allow the side chains of hydrophobic residues to be screened in an aqueous environment, thus reducing the overall amphiphilicity of the peptide. In more anisotropic, membrane-mimicking environments, arenicins form dimers stabilized by hydrogen bonds between parallel N-terminal β-strands in two neighboring molecules [5]. Dimerization occurs at the membrane surface and induces a substantial conformational change, so that the molecules adopt almost planar amphipathic β-sheet structures [8,13]. This more regular conformation appears conducive to subsequent oligomerization and membrane disruption and therefore appears to be a relevant feature for antibacterial activity. Conformational regularity might be favored by an increased symmetry in residue arrangement.

The present study aimed to probe for a possible biological significance of the apparent residue symmetry displayed by arenicin-1 molecules and to determine whether altering or increasing this symmetry could result in improved antimicrobial characteristics, also in view of their potential as leads for novel anti-infective agents. We furthermore wanted to test how an increased rigidity of the β-hairpin could affect the biological properties as well as the roles played by specific residues.

Several variants of arenicin-1 were therefore elaborated for a structure–activity relationship study to analyze the role of sequence symmetry, residue content, and conformational rigidity in microbicidal efficacy, membranolytic activity, and cytotoxicity towards mammalian cells. We constructed a set of peptides with a varying degree of symmetrization of the amino acid sequence and speculated that this could result in a more planar arrangement of the peptide hairpin, with a reduction of the kink and twist observed in the strands of the native peptide's structure. To test this, we performed extensive molecular dynamics simulations of the peptides, using different initial conformations, and analyzed their folding capacity, stability, secondary structural features such as kink and twist angles, and hydrogen bonding patterns.

Additional variants were also studied, in which key residues, such as the arginines that provide the peptide's charge or the tryptophan residues that flank the β-hairpin, were respectively replaced with lysine and phenylalanine. We furthermore prepared a linear variant of arenicin-1 with reduced and alkylated (iodoacetamidated) cysteine residues to probe the significance of the β-hairpin scaffold and, finally, a backbone-cyclized arenicin-1 analogue to explore if the increased rigidity that is likely to result from this type of cyclization could affect activity and/or toxicity towards mammalian cells.

2. Results

Arenicin-1 (AR) adopts a characteristic β-hairpin structure stabilized by the presence of a disulfide bridge and displays a peculiar symmetry in residue arrangement along the two strands (Figure 1). It is a fascinating scaffold for designing variants to test features that may affect the molecule's antimicrobial and/or cytotoxic capacities.

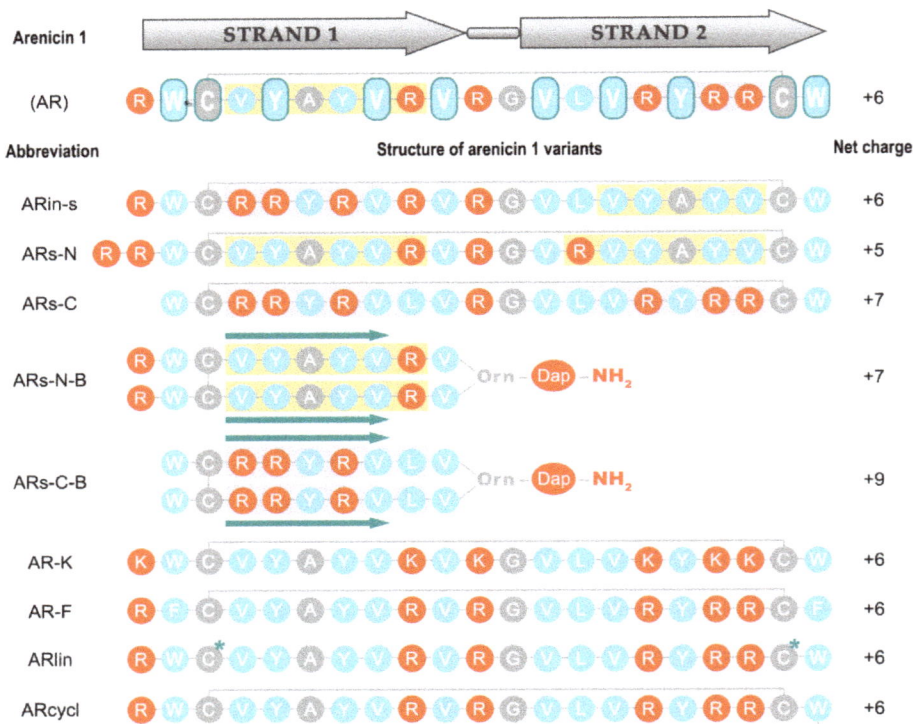

Figure 1. Pseudosymmetric sequence of the arenicin-1 molecule and structure of its designed analogues. The hydrophobic residues are marked in blue, the polar residues are in red, and the palindromic arrangement of the WCxxYxxVxVxxVxVxYxxCW motif in the initial arenicin-1 sequence is indicated with rounded boxes. The VYYAYV(R) and (L)VRYRR motifs present in strands 1 and 2 of arenecin-1 are, respectively, highlighted by yellow and blue-grey boxes and were swapped (ARin-s), placed symmetrically with inversion (ARs-N and -C), or branched from a central residue (ARsin-N-B and ARs-C-B) in variants designed to test the role of the residue symmetry. Asterisks (*) in the linear version of arenicin-1 (ARlin) mark the sites of Cys alkylation with iodoacetamide. Green arrows accentuate the parallel arrangement of the strands in ARs-N-B and ARs-C-B peptides, obtained by linking the "branches" of the hairpin to the α and δ amines of an ornithine residue (Orn), in turn coupled to an amidated diaminopropionic acid (Dap) group at the C-terminus (Figure 7).

2.1. AR Variants Design

ARin-s was designed to alter the sequence symmetry by inverting the VYAYV and VRYRR motifs, respectively present in the N- and C-terminal strands of wild-type AR (Figure 1). ARs-N had increased symmetry based on only the VYAYVR motif of the N-terminal strand; an additional Arg residue was added to offset the decrease in overall charge that this entails. ARs-C, instead, had increased symmetry based on the VRYRR motif of the C-terminal strand. To increase symmetry even further, two non-proteinogenic variants—ARs-N-B and ARs-C-B—were constructed by branching either the VYAYVRV sequence of strand 1 or the VLVRYRR sequence of strand 2 (fragments 1–10 and 13–21, respectively, Figure 1) from the α and δ amines of an ornithine (Orn) residue. This resulted in a parallel arrangement of the hairpin strands, so that the obtained peptides had two N-termini. The branching Orn residue was linked to an amidated diaminopropionic acid (Dap) residue at the peptide's C-terminus, in an attempt to maintain a structure of the branching site as far as possible isosteric with the Arg residue normally present in the turn region (see Figure 7 in the Methods section).

We also constructed a backbone-cyclized version of AR (ARcycl) by linking the N-terminus to the C-terminus using an innovative native chemical ligation (NCL) protocol. It has been reported that the introduction of a second disulfide bridge in arenicin increases its rigidity and that this has beneficial effects on both antimicrobial activity and toxicity [14]. However, this required replacing internal residues (namely, Val^8 and Val^{13}) with Cys, while backbone cyclization of the N- and C-termini, that are spatially close in the peptide β-hairpin, should be less invasive.

Additional variants were prepared with substitution of key residues. In AR-K, all Arg residues were substituted with Lys to probe the relevance of these charged residues; analogously, in the AR-F variant, Trp was replaced with Phe to probe the relevance of the flanking tryptophan residues. Finally, we also prepared a linear variant of arenicin-1 with reduced and carboxamidomethylated (iodoacetamidated) cysteine residues (RCM-Cys).

2.2. Assessing the Structure Using Molecular Dynamics Simulations

In our computational analysis of arenicin-1 analogues, we first developed a quantitative measure of sequence symmetry by aligning the original and the inverted primary structures. As can be appreciated from their sequences (Figure 1), the "branched" peptides ARs-N-B and ARs-C-B are ideal palindromes, having not only identical sequences of both strands but also the same orientation.

We then performed an extensive molecular dynamics (MD) simulation of the peptides in an aqueous environment to analyze their structure and dynamics. The peptides were modelled with different starting conformations, in the presence or absence of the disulfide bonds. The linearized version of the original arenicin-1, as well as the variant with reduced, carboxamidomethylated cysteines (ARlin) and the linearized versions of the ARin-s and ARs-C variants, all demonstrated the ability to fold rapidly from a fully extended linear conformation to a well-defined β-hairpin structure, which was relatively stable even without the disulfide bond. The process of peptide folding was monitored by measuring both the distance from the initial structure and the appearance of secondary structure elements. The folding of ARs-C, with rapid emergence of the characteristic β-strands connected by a turn, is shown in Figure S1. ARin-s and ARs-C were also modelled from more natural β-hairpin starting structures, obtained using replica-exchange Monte Carlo simulations in the *Quark* program, which also confirmed a high stability of this conformation even in the absence of the disulfide bond.

The ARs-N-B and ARs-C-B variants, instead, failed to fold from an initial extended linear conformation, in the timescales used for our simulations. Therefore, we used a manually constructed β-sheet structure with a disulfide bond to perform simulated annealing experiments. These resulted in the formation of relatively flat β-sheet structures, which were further equilibrated by an additional MD simulation. The resulting average structures obtained for all modelled peptides are shown in Figure 2a, in which it can be clearly seen that the β-hairpin structures of ARin-s and ARs-C show the same characteristic kink as AR, while the parallel β-hairpin of ARs-N-B and ARs-C-B are flatter and less twisted.

(a) *Average equilibrium structures* **(b)** *Alignment with AR (2JSB)*

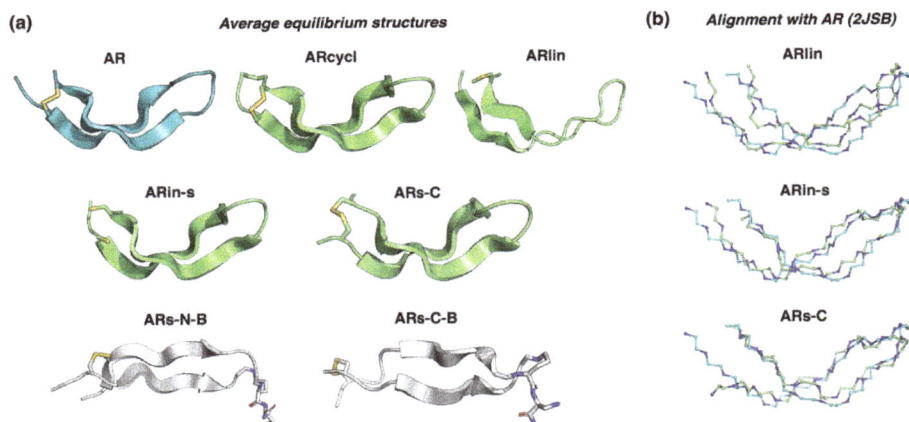

Figure 2. Average equilibrium structures obtained for all studied peptides by molecular dynamics (MD) simulations. (**a**) Schematic ribbon representation, parallel and antiparallel β-strands are based on secondary structure assignment by the STRIDE algorithm. (**b**) Structural alignment of ARlin, ARin-s, and Ars-C with experimental arenicin-1 structure 2JSB. Only backbone atoms are shown, the coloring matches panel (**a**).

The increase in sequence symmetry in the parallel β-stranded branched peptides made their planar spatial structures the most distant from that of the original arenicin-1. Data on the structural distance from the experimental arenicin-1 structure (root-mean-square deviation, RMSD), secondary structure content, and average number of mainchain hydrogen bonds for each peptide are provided in Table 1. These show that the linearized version with reduced, carboxyamidomethylated cysteines (ARlin) formed a more distorted β-hairpin, with lower secondary structure content and greater distance from the experimental structure than the other antiparallel β-hairpin structures. On the other hand, the cyclic variant (ARcycl) and ARin-s were almost indistinguishable from the original arenicin-1, as shown in the structural alignments in Figure 2b, so that the rearrangement of residues in the two strands or backbone cyclization did not seem to greatly affect the overall conformation. It is interesting to note that the backbone cyclization can accommodate quite a tight cycle based on only five residues (CWRWC), even though the three central residues are bulky, so that the motif could be quite rigid.

Table 1. Structural analysis of the resulting peptide models.

Peptide	[a] C^α RMSD with 2JSB (Å)	[b] Average N° of H-Bonds (±SD)	[c] Average 2^y Structure Content
AR	1.37	8.3 ± 1.2	14/21
ARin-s	1.67	8.3 ± 1.2	16/21
ARs-C	1.90	6.4 ± 1.1	14/20
ARs-N-B	4.29	7.1 ± 1.3	13/22
ARs-C-B	3.30	6.2 ± 1.1	10/20
ARlin	3.13	5.4 ± 1.2	9/21
ARcycl	1.57	7.1 ± 1.2	16/21

[a] Root-mean-square deviation (RMSD) of the coordinates of C^α atoms in variant structures of the experimental arenicin-1 NMR structure. [b] Average number (N°) of mainchain H-bonds calculated from the equilibrium parts of the MD trajectories. [c] Ratio of residues in antiparallel or parallel β-sheet conformation assigned by the STRIDE algorithm to the total N° of residues. 2JSB: Protein Data Bank (PDB) ID of arenicin-1.

The parallel, branched β-hairpin peptides ARs-N-B and ARs-C-B were structurally the most distant from the original conformation, with RMSD > 4 Å for ARs-N-B. Moreover, although the average number of intramolecular main-chain hydrogen bonds was similar for all peptides, AR, ARin-s, ARs-C

Mar. Drugs **2019**, *17*, 376

displayed the standard hydrogen bonding pattern of an antiparallel β-sheet (Figure 3), while ARs-N-B and ARs-C-B showed a bonding pattern characteristic of a parallel β-sheet. Supposedly, this difference in intramolecular hydrogen bonding could affect also intermolecular H-bonding and so alter the mechanism of dimerization and oligomerization on the membrane surface.

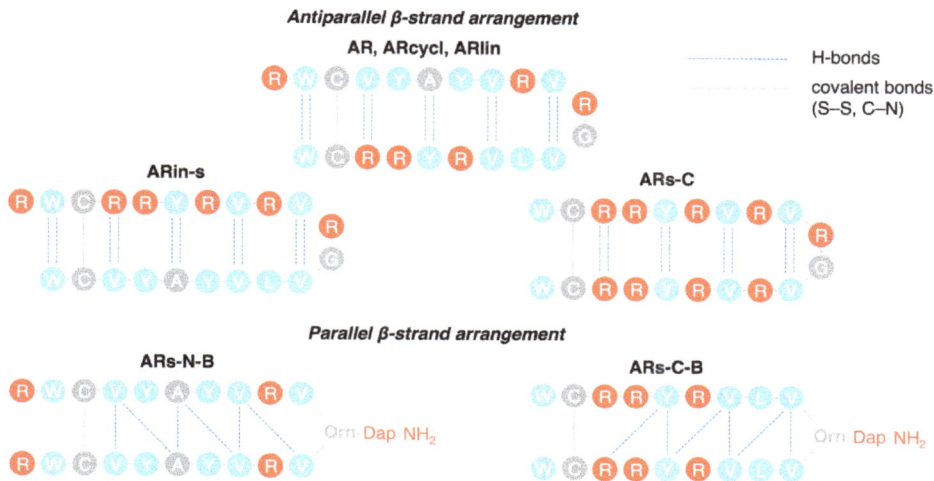

Figure 3. Different hydrogen bonding patterns observed for arenicin variants. AR, ARin-s, and ARs-C show the same H-bonding pattern (dotted blue lines) typical of antiparallel β-strands (two H-bonds connect the α-amine and α-carboxyl groups of an amino acid on one side of the hairpin with the α-amine and α-carboxyl groups of an amino acid on the other side of the hairpin). ARs-N-B and ARs-C-B instead show the pattern typical of parallel β-strands (two H-bonds connect the α-amine and α-carboxyl groups of an amino acid on one side of the hairpin with the α-amine and α-carboxyl groups of two different amino acids on the other side). The disulfide bond is indicated by a solid grey line, as well as branching from the ornithine residue α- and δ-amines (Figure 7).

The structural stability of the peptides was analyzed by calculating the fluctuations (root-mean-square fluctuations, RMSF) of the backbone C^α atoms at equilibrium. All peptides demonstrated a fluctuation pattern typical of a β-sheet with a higher mobility at the termini and near the turn connecting the two β-strands (Figure S2a). The peptide ARs-C-B exhibited a remarkably high structural stability, with low fluctuations even on the β-strand termini. This behavior could be attributed to an additional stabilization due to stacking of two N-terminal tryptophan residues, which is shown in Figure S2b.

Finally, we analyzed the effect of sequence symmetry on the overall geometry of the peptide. For each peptide, we determined the average twist and kink angles from the equilibrium parts of the MD trajectories. We then plotted the twist and kink angles versus sequence symmetry for each peptide, as shown in Figure 4. As expected, and in agreement with the MD simulations, the more symmetrical sequences of ARs-N-B and ARs-C-B resulted in significantly lower twist and kink of the peptides, which both had nearly planar parallel β-hairpin structures, quite distant from the original arenicin-1 structure and rather uncommon for β-hairpin peptides, which cannot by, definition, have symmetric, parallel β-strands.

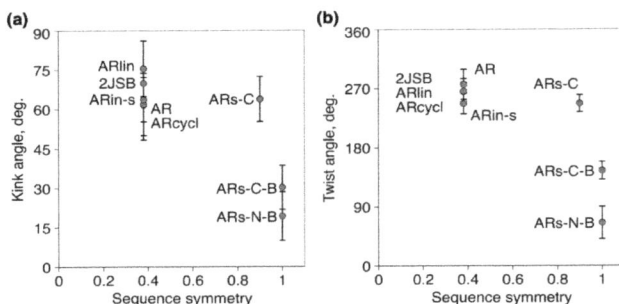

Figure 4. Average kink (**a**) and twist (**b**) angles for the peptides as a function of their sequence symmetry. Sequence symmetrization in ARs-N-B and ARs-C-B results in significantly lower kink and twist.

2.3. Antimicrobial Activity

We tested the antimicrobial activity of the peptides against a set of Gram-negative and Gram-positive bacteria, including drug-resistant clinical isolates. As shown using the broth microdilution assay (Table 2), the peptide with inverted symmetry (ARin-s) had a reduced activity against Gram-negative strains and lost activity against Gram-positive ones. This may be due to the replacement of the VYAYV motif in the N-terminal strand, which is reported to be important for oligomerization, with the inverted C-terminal motif RRYRVL. However, the fact that the variant with a symmetrically placed RRYRVL motif in both strands (ARs-C) maintained a substantial activity, while the one with a symmetrically placed VYAYV motif lost activity, suggests that this type of oligomerization is only one of the factors determining activity and that the C-terminal strand may also have a significant role. ARs-C (+7) may act as a monomer for which the higher charge is beneficial, and while we attempted to maintain a reasonable cationicity (+5) for ARs-N by adding an Arg residue at the N-terminus, it was still reduced with respect to arenicin-1 (+6). It is interesting that the same trend was observed for the "branched" variants, where ARs-C-B (+9), based on the RRYRVL motif of the C-terminal strand, was more active than ARs-N-B (+7), based on the VYAYV motif of the N-terminal strand, but the latter becomes significantly more active than the less cationic ARs-N peptide based on a canonical antiparallel β-hairpin.

The backbone-cyclized and linear versions of arenicin-1, as well as the peptides with Arg replaced with Lys (AR-K) and Trp replaced with Phe (AR-F), showed an antimicrobial activity comparable with that of the native peptide. However, it was not possible to determine from the minimal inhibitory concentrations (MIC) values alone if and how the mechanism of action had changed. One may simply suggest that it continued to involve an initial interaction with the membrane determined by electrostatic interactions and that the subsequent insertion into the membrane was due to the presence of hydrophobic residues, but the mechanism of the subsequent membrane permeabilization (which involves peptide oligomerization) could be affected. Our MD simulations would in any case suggest that the β-hairpin structure was maintained in all these variants, even the linear one, with a strong propensity for the scaffold to fold into this conformation. It is interesting to note that, while altering the symmetry reduced the antimicrobial activity against drug-resistant clinical isolates in particular, backbone cyclization of arenicin-1 resulted in improved activity towards these isolates.

To obtain a global assessment of the effect on antimicrobial activity, the geometric mean of the MIC (G-MIC) was calculated, and from this, the overall improvement or impoverishment with respect to arenicin-1. In general, inverting the symmetry or decreasing the charge had detrimental effects. Turning the peptide into a parallel β-hairpin also did not improve activity. Linearizing the peptide did not seem to significantly affect its activity, while substituting Lys for Arg and Phe for Trp seemed to slightly improve it. Taken together, these results suggest that these modifications did not markedly improve the already potent antibacterial activity of the parent peptide but rather subtly alter its activity spectrum.

Table 2. Antimicrobial activity of the arenicin-1 variants (broth microdilution assay).

	Minimal Inhibitory Concentrations (MIC) [a], µM									
	AR	ARin-s	ARs-N	ARs-C	ARs-N-B	ARs-C-B	AR K	AR F	ARlin	ARcycl
Gram-negative laboratory strains										
Escherichia coli ML35p	1–2	4–8	16	1	4	1–2	1	1	1–2	1–2
E. coli ATCC 25922	2	8	>16	2	8	4	2	1	2	2
E. coli M15	2	8	>16	2	4	8	1	1	2	2
Pseudomonas aeruginosa ATCC 27853	2	4–8	>16	1	2	1	1–2	1	2	1
Gram-positive laboratory strains										
Listeria monocytogenes EGD	1–2	2	8	1	2–4	2	2	2	2	2
Staphylococcus aureus 710A	2	16	>16	2–4	8	4	2	2	2	2
S. aureus ATCC 25923	2	16	>16	4	8	4	2	2	2	2
MRSA ATCC 33591	4	>16	>16	4–8	8	8	2	2	4	4
Clinical isolates										
P. aeruginosa c.i.	4	>16	>16	16	16	16	2–4	2	4–8	2
Acinetobacter baumanii c.i.	4	16	>16	2	4	8–16	1	2	4	4
Staphylococcus intermidius	8	>16	>16	8	8	4	4	4	8	4
S. aureus c.i.	4	>16	>16	16	8	4–8	4	4	8–16	4
Overall statistics										
G-MIC [b]	2.7	≥12.8	≥26.9	3.2	5.9	4.4	1.9	1.8	3.1	2.3
G-MIC improvement ratio in comparison with AR [c]	1.0	≤0.2	≤0.1	0.8	0.5	0.6	1.4 *	1.5 *	0.9	1.2 *

[a] Minimal inhibitory concentrations (MIC) values were derived from 3–5 experiments which were performed in triplicates. [b] Geometric mean of the MIC (G-MIC) is the geometric mean of all determined MICs; the median values of MICs were used for calculation. In the case of MIC > 16 µM, the next concentration in the series of two-fold dilutions (32 µM) was used for G-MIC assessment. [c] As the lower MIC corresponds to the higher activity, MIC improvement was calculated as a ratio of G-MIC of native arenicin (AR) to G-MIC of the peptide of interest. *: higher overall activity, compared to AR.

2.4. Effect of Arenicin Variants on Bacterial Membrane Integrity

The *Escherichia coli* ML35p strain expresses a plasmid-encoded periplasmic β-lactamase and is constitutive for cytoplasmic β-galactosidase, while lacking lactose permease [15]. This makes it very useful to monitor the permeabilization of both its outer and inner membranes, using real-time assays. From Figure 5, it can be seen that the outer membrane became fully permeable to nitrocefin, a β-lactamase substrate, ~30 min after adding most arenicin-1 analogs. However, all variants with a modified symmetry demonstrated a decreased ability to permeabilize the inner membrane of *E. coli* ML35p, suggesting a reduced membranolytic activity.

It is interesting to note that, whereas some variants did show an improved capacity to permeabilize the outer membrane with respect to arenicin-1 (e.g., AR-K and ARcycl), none of the variants (with the possible exception of AR-F) showed an improved capacity to permeabilize the cytoplasmic membrane.

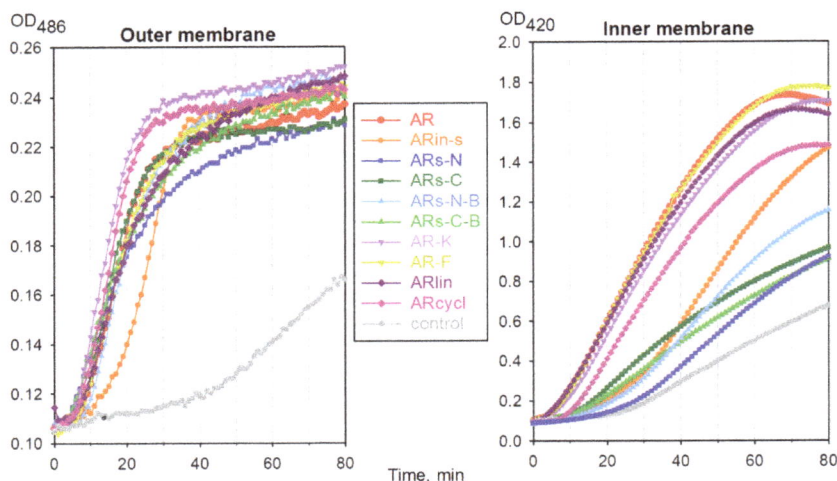

Figure 5. Permeabilizing effect of arenicin-1 variants on *E. coli* ML35p outer and cytoplasmic membranes. The incubation wells contained 10mM sodium phosphate buffer, 100 mM NaCl, 2.5×10^7 colony-forming units (CFU) of washed, stationary-phase *E. coli* ML35p, and the peptides of interest at a concentration equivalent to $2 \times$ MIC, or an equivalent volume of acidified water (controls).

2.5. Cytotoxicity of Arenicin-1 Variants towards Mammalian Cells

The toxicity of arenicin peptide variants towards eukaryotic cells was tested using the MTT assay on the human erythroleukemia cell line (K-562). The arenicin variants with Arg-to-Lys (AR-K) and Trp-to-Phe (AR-F) substitutions, which exerted a slightly improved antimicrobial activity compared to the native peptide (see Table 2), were also found to be somewhat more cytotoxic, the half-maximal inhibitory concentration (IC_{50}) decreasing by a factor of 2 (Table 3). This is quite typical of membranolytic AMPs, for which a higher antibacterial activity is often accompanied by an increased toxicity to host cells [16,17].

The cytotoxic activity of the backbone-cyclized variant ARcycl and of variants modified to increase the symmetry in an antiparallel β-sheet structure (ARs-N and ARs-C) was comparable (ARcycl, ARs-N) or only moderately increased (ARs-C), with respect to that of the original peptide. On the other hand, both of the "branched" symmetrical variants (ARs-N-B and ARs-C-B) and the linearized arenicin (ARlin) showed at least a two-fold reduction of cytotoxicity. The same was observed for ARin-s with inverted symmetry, but in this case, it was accompanied by a significantly lower antibacterial activity.

The impact of the peptides on eukaryotic membranes was also analyzed using the hemolysis assay, with peptide concentrations up to 80 μM (Figure 6). None of the modifications completely abolished the relatively high hemolytic activity of wild-type arenicin, although the branched variant based on the C-terminal motif (ARs-C-B), which was moderately active on bacteria, demonstrated a significantly lowered ability to lyse the erythrocytes. On the other hand, other variants with improved antimicrobial activity (e.g., AR-F and AR-K) did not show a significantly increased hemolytic activity, based on the HC_{50} value.

Table 3. Cytotoxic effects of arenicin-1 variants towards human erythroleukemia K-562 cells and human erythrocytes.

	Effects of the Peptides									
	AR	ARin-s	ARs-N	ARs-C	ARs-N-B	ARs-C-B	AR-K	AR-F	ARlin	ARcyclic
Cytotoxicity towards K-562 cell line (human erythroleukemia cells)										
IC_{50}[a], μM (MTT-assay)	17.9	37.7	18.0	11.6	35.1	39.0	7.7	9.3	>40	16.2
SI_1 assessment IC_{50}/G-MIC	6.6	≤2.9	≤0.7	3.6	6.0	8.8	4.0	5.2	>12.8	7.0
SI_1 improvement ratio in comparison with AR[b]	1.0	≤0.4	≤0.1	0.5	0.9	1.3 *	0.6	0.8	>1.9 *	1.1
Hemolysis of human red blood cells										
HC_{50}[c], μM	66.3	>80	>80	66.0	>80	>80	63.0	60.5	>80	65.5
SI_2 assessment HC_{50}/G-MIC	24.6	-	-	20.6	>13.7	>18.1	33.1	34.0	>25.6	28.2
SI_2 improvement ratio in comparison with AR[b]	1.0	-	-	0.8	>0.6	>0.7	1.3	1.4	>1.0	1.1
HC_{15}[c], μM	10.3	17.2	23.5	11.8	12.4	56.4	10.1	10.6	29.9	14.0
SI_3 assessment HC_{15}/G-MIC	3.8	≤1.3	≤0.9	3.7	2.1	12.7	5.3	6.0	9.5	6.0
SI_3 improvement ratio in comparison with AR[b]	1.0	≤0.4	≤0.2	1.0	0.6	3.3 *	1.4	1.6	2.5 *	1.6

[a] Half-maximal inhibitory concentration (IC_{50}) was calculated using Sigma Plot Standard Curve Analysis based on 3–4 independent experiments. [b] Selectivity index (SI) improvement was calculated as a ratio of the SI of the peptide of interest to the SI of native AR. The peptides with the highest SI values are the least cytotoxic. [c] Half-maximal hemolytic concentration (HC_{50}) and 15% maximal hemolytic concentration (HC_{15}) were calculated using Sigma Plot Standard Curve Analysis based on 3–8 independent experiments. *: variants with the most significant reduction of toxicity in both hemolysis and MTT-test, compared to AR.

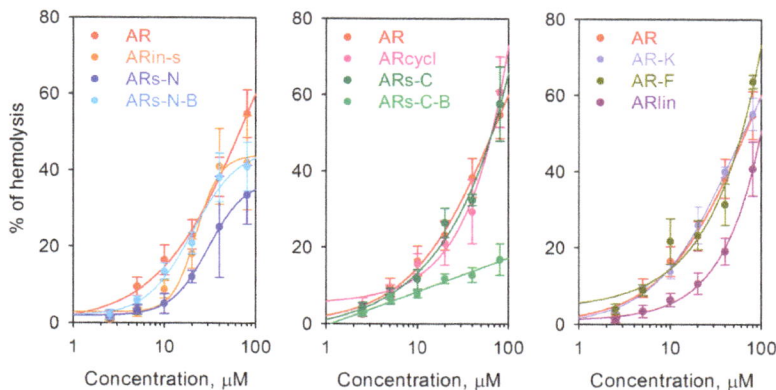

Figure 6. The hemolytic activity of arenicin-1 variants towards human red blood cells (RBC). All values are means ± SD and were derived from 3–8 experiments which were performed in triplicates.

We used both the MTT and hemolysis data to make an in vitro estimate of selectivity indices (SI) of the peptides (see Table 3), as these help characterize the width of the 'therapeutic window' of a compound and thus its suitability for possible therapeutic application. We used the G-MIC as a measure of the overall antimicrobial activity of the peptides (see Table 2) and the half-maximal MTT inhibitory concentration (IC_{50}) or half-maximal hemolytic concentration (HC_{50}) as a measure of their toxicity. In the case of hemolytic activity, only 5 of the 10 investigated variants reached their HC_{50} at a concentration of 80 μM, which somewhat limited the SI assessment. For a more precise comparison of the SI, we therefore calculated the HC_{15}, a hemolysis level which could be reliably calculated for all tested peptides on the basis of the experimental data (Figure 6). Both hemolysis- and MTT-derived selectivity index estimates (SI_1 and SI_3, see Table 3) indicated that the branched symmetrical arenicin-1 variant based on the C-terminal motif (ARs-C-B) and the linearized arenicin (ARlin) possessed the best combination of antibacterial and cytotoxic properties, amongst the tested arenicin-1 analogues.

ARs-C-B showed over a three-fold improvement in SI_3 compared with native arenicin. The variants with the poorest SI characteristics were the one with inversed symmetry (ARin-s: low antimicrobial activity but relatively high cytotoxicity) and the N-terminal motif-based symmetrical arenicin ARs-N.

3. Discussion

Marine animals are recognized as a rich source of potentially useful novel bioactive substances, including new anti-infective drugs. Several AMPs from marine invertebrates have been described to date, such as the penaeidins from shrimp [18], mytilins from mussels [19], aurelin from jellyfish [20], tachyplesins from the horse-shoe crab [21], arasin from the spider crab [22], and several others. One of the most potent AMPs is arenicin-1, from the lugworm *A. marina* [1]. However, to be suitable as a lead compound for drug development, this highly active peptide requires optimization, as it is also significantly hemolytic.

We observed that this peptide possesses a rather unique pseudosymmetric structure and explored the significance of this feature with respect to its antimicrobial activity as well as its cytotoxicity for mammalian cells. This peptide presents two Trp residues at each terminus and three Tyr residues distributed along the β-strands. A study of other tryptophan-rich peptides, such as the bovine, cathelicidin-derived peptides tritrpticin and indolicidin, has shown that sequence symmetrization can result in improvement of the antimicrobial activity, accompanied by a decreased hemolytic action [23]. A zipper-like symmetric arrangement of aromatic residues along the strands can also increase the stability of β-hairpin AMPs, increasing their activity [24]. Furthermore, synthetic, disulfide-stabilized, β-hairpin peptides based on symmetric sequences of a VR motif also provide an appreciable, broad-spectrum antimicrobial activity with a membranolytic mechanism [25].

For these reasons, several arenicin-1 variants with increased or modified symmetry, as well as with changes in other primary structural features, have been designed (Figure 1), chemically synthesized, and investigated. Molecular dynamics simulations allowed us to predict possible effects on the structures of these variants and to analyze their conformational stability and dynamics. A linearized version of arenicin-1, as well as two variants with β-strand permutations, ARin-s and ARs-C, showed a rapid and robust folding into a well-defined β-hairpin structure that showed a remarkable similarity with the experimentally determined structure of the parent peptide arenicin-1. The RMSD was relatively low (1.6–1.9 Å, Figure 2b), and the hydrogen bonding pattern between the flanking β-strands was the same (Figure 3), so that the overall geometric parameters, twist and kink angles, were virtually indistinguishable from those of arenicin-1. These simulations suggested that permutations of whole β-strands, including palindromic symmetrization, did not significantly affect the characteristic β-hairpin structure of the scaffold, although switching the VYAYV and RRYRVL motifs between N- and C-terminal strands (as in ARs-in), might affect the mechanism of self-association in a membrane environment, which is reported to involve the N-terminal strand of the native peptide.

On the other hand, MD simulations on peptides with a non-canonical, branched, parallel β-hairpin arrangement achieved by chemical synthesis supported our hypothesis that an increased symmetry in the primary structure would translate into a more symmetrical β-structure, with reduced twist and kink angles. For the two highly symmetric analogues of this type (ARs-N-B and ARs-C-B), the β-hairpin became almost flat, and the hydrogen bonding pattern between the strands was altered (Figure 3). This would result in a different pattern of vacant hydrogen donor/acceptors on the other side of the peptide's β-strands, also affecting intermolecular contacts. Considering that native arenicin molecules form dimers by a parallel association of the N-terminal β-strands [5,11], the branched variants could have an altered oligomerization propensity and, therefore, a modified pore-forming activity. Their biological activity might be reduced.

In effect, the structure–antimicrobial activity relationship of arenicin-1 turned out to be rather robust, with all studied variants, except ARin-s (with an inverted strand arrangement) and the symmetrical variant ARs-N (with reduced charge), maintaining an appreciable activity against both Gram-negative and Gram-positive bacteria, including drug-resistant strains. The charge dependence of the activity for ARs-N (+5) was also suggested by the fact that the activity was partly re-established for the parallel-stranded analog ARs-N-B (+7), which is supported by similar observations for other AMPs [26,27]. The activity loss in ARin-s is significant, and as the secondary structure was modelled to be very similar to that of the parent peptide, could be due either to the altered residue arrangement or to a reduced propensity of the altered N-terminal strand to dimerize in the membrane.

The cytotoxic action of arenicin-1 variants towards mammalian cells was less sensitive to the molecule's charge and more sensitive to its symmetry and three-dimensional organization. The flatter, symmetrically branched peptides ARs-N-B and ARs-C-B were less toxic to K-562 cells by a factor of two than the native peptide, whereas ARs-N and ARs-C—with a more pseudo-symmetric but antiparallel β-hairpin conformation—showed a comparable or slightly increased cytotoxicity. When native arenicin-1 dimerizes by the parallel association of its N-terminal strands, it adopts a more planar conformation [5,11]. The intrinsically more planar conformations of ARs-N-B and ARs-C-B might thus be expected to favor oligomerization, and in line with several studies, an increased propensity for self-association in solution should correlate with increased cytotoxicity [23,28,29]. The fact that these analogs showed both a reduced bacterial membrane permeability (Figure 5) and host cell cytotoxicity, compared to the parent peptide, suggests that this was not the case. Possibly, the different intramolecular H-bonding patterns of the parallel branches in the modified peptides affected their capacity to form the intermolecular H-bonds.

Analysis of other variants revealed that an improvement of the in vitro antimicrobial activity could be obtained by Arg-to-Lys (AR-K) or Trp-to-Phe (AR-F) substitutions, but at the expense of an even more prominently increased toxicity towards mammalian cells. Interestingly, other reports on Arg-to-Lys substitutions in AMPs [30,31] suggest that the arginine side chain can form more hydrogen bonds and thus interact more strongly with phospholipid components of bacterial membranes, with respect to lysine, which should enhance the activity of Arg-rich AMPs with respect to the Lys-rich analogues [31,32]. Previously published data on an arenicin-1 analogue with Arg-to-Lys substitutions indicated that the activity of this peptide is comparable to that of the parent AR, but in a salt-, medium- and bacterial species-dependent manner [7].

The replacement of Trp with Phe may favor the insertion of the AR-F peptide into membranes but it does not seem to discriminate between bacterial and eukaryotic membranes. Furthermore, it is reported that the kinked arenicin-1 hairpin becomes significantly flatter upon membrane contact and oligomerization [5]. Molecular dynamics simulations with ARs-C-B indicated that Trp stacking in parallel strands may contribute to stabilizing the flattened conformation.

The backbone-cyclized analogue of arenicin-1 acted similarly to the parent peptide towards both bacterial and mammalian cells, while the linear variant showed a higher selectivity for the bacterial cells. The macro-cyclization of AMPs has been reported to reduce the toxicity of some AMPs towards host cells (e.g., protegrin 1, tachyplesin 1, and gomesin AMPs [33–35]), but in the case of arenicin, it did not substantially alter the biological activity. In fact, as it occurs close to the disulphide bridge, it results in a rather tight, five-residue cycle (CWRWC), which could be quite rigid considering the steric bulk of the central residues. MD simulations with the linear AR variant showed that it has a strong propensity to fold to a β-hairpin even in the absence of a disulphide bridge, which suggests that backbone cyclization could replace disulphide bridging to stabilize the peptide, freeing the positions of the Cys residues for variations that may improve its activity. This has been observed for macrocyclic antimicrobial conotoxin analogues with replaced cysteines [36].

With respect to the linearized arenicin, a variant with the replacement of cysteine residues with serine has previously been reported and was shown to have a 2–4-fold decreased antimicrobial activity [3,7]. Our linearized analogue, with alkylated cysteine residues, instead substantially maintained the antimicrobial activity. As MD simulations suggested, it also displays a substantial propensity to fold to a β-hairpin conformation, albeit with a reduced stability with respect to the parent peptide; it may also maintain some of its capacity to oligomerize and permeabilize bacterial membranes. In any case, studies on other linearized β-hairpin AMPs with reduced Cys or Cys replaced with Ser (e.g., bovine cyclic dodecapeptide [37] and porcine protegrin 1 [38]) indicate that, while activity may be reduced to some extent, it is not entirely abrogated. In fact, some linearized analogues of bovine dodecapeptide (bactenecin 1) demonstrated a potent antibacterial action and higher selectivity for bacterial cells than the parent peptide [39]. Studies with cyclic, linear, or dimeric (parallel and antiparallel) cyclic dodecapeptide suggest that the antimicrobial activity is quite robust and retained to some extent by all these forms, even though characteristics such as the salt-dependence of the activity can vary [40].

4. Materials and Methods

4.1. Peptide Synthesis

4.1.1. Antiparallel β-Hairpins

Solid-phase peptide synthesis of most variants was performed on a microwave-enhanced CEM Liberty synthesizer (Charlotte, NC, USA), loaded with Trp-substituted, 2-chlorotrityl chloride resin (substitution of 0.2 mmol/g). Insertion of the C-terminal Trp was performed manually according to the instructions provided in the synthesis notes section (section 2.17) of the Novabiochem catalogue. Double coupling was affected at all positions, with a four-fold excess of fluoren-9-dymethoxycarbonyl amino acid/HATU/diisopropylethylamine (1:1:1.7, by vol.) at 70 °C. For couplings involving Cys, the temperature was limited to 50 °C. Branched peptides (ARs-N-B and ARs-C-B) were synthesized as amides, using the NovaPEG Rink Amide resin (substitution 0.22 mmol/g). Diamminopropionic acid (Fmoc-DAP(Boc)-OH) was loaded as the C-terminal residue, followed by (Fmoc-Orn(Fmoc)-OH) and then branching from the Orn residue. Peptides were cleaved from the resin and deprotected using a cocktail consisting of trifluoroacetic acid (TFA), water, ethanedithiol, triisopropylsilane mixture (94:2.5:2.5:1, by vol.). The free peptides were precipitated and washed with t-butyl methyl ether and dried under nitrogen.

4.1.2. Branched, Parallel Hairpins, and Simulation of the Turn Region

While the primary structure of the native peptide imposed an antiparallel arrangement of the strands in the β-hairpin [2], the synthetic variants with the parallel prongs of the hairpin were designed to achieve a more symmetric arrangement of the peptide molecule. In the design of these "branched" peptides, it was attempted to maintain a structure of the branching site as far as possible isosteric with the Arg residue normally present in the turn (Figure 7), by branching from an ornithine (Fmoc-Orn(Fmoc)-OH) coupled to a C-terminal Dap amide (Fmoc-Dap(Boc)-OH) coupled to a Rink amide resin]. The synthesis and cleavage were carried out in the same conditions as for the β-hairpin peptides. ARs-N-B and ARs-C-B have identical co-directional prongs in the two parallel strands of the branched peptide, based, respectively, on the N- or C- terminal strands of arenicin.

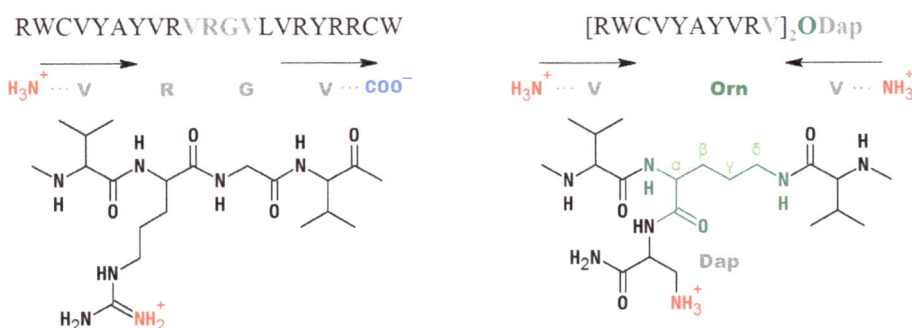

Figure 7. Sequence of the turn region of native arenicin (–VRGV–) and simulated turn region of the "branched" arenicin 1 variants (–VOrn(δ)V–) where the Orn α-amine is coupled to amidated Dap.

4.1.3. Backbone-Cyclized Arenicin

The cyclic variant (ARcycl) was synthesized using the same Trp-substituted, 2-chlorotrityl chloride resin (substitution of 0.2 mmol/g), but with the sequence Boc–CVYAYVRVRGVLVRYRRCW, to provide an N-terminal Cys residue for native chemical ligation. The methodology has been described previously for native ligation of two peptide fragments [41] and was adapted for backbone cyclization. Briefly, the fully protected peptide carboxylic acid (including Boc-protected N-terminus) was cleaved from the resin with hexafluoroisopropanol (HFIP) in dichloromethane (DCM), and the product was esterified to the corresponding 4-acetamidophenyl-thioester, according to a published procedure [42,43]. After acid deprotection of this peptide thioaryl ester with a thiol free cleavage mixture, it was suspended to a concentration of 30 mM in a solution of 6 M guanidinium hydrochloride, 100 mM sodium acetate, 2 mM EDTA in the presence of 10 eq. of tris(2-carboxyethyl)phosphine (TCEP) to ensure the Cys residues were reduced, and left for 1 h. The backbone-cyclized peptide was then purified by RP-HPLC and resuspended in folding buffer (pH 8.5), and the disulphide bridge was formed as described below.

4.1.4. Disulphide Bond Formation

Disulphide bonds in the arenicin variants were formed by adding the peptides to a freshly prepared N_2-saturated aqueous buffer (1 M guanidinium chloride/0.1 M ammonium acetate/2 mM EDTA, pH 8.5) in the presence of 1 mM cysteine and 0.1 mM cystine. The final peptide concentration was kept below 10 μM to avoid dimer formation, and oxidation was carried out overnight. The linear variant of arenicin-1 was obtained by means of reduction of the parent AR followed by alkylation of the reduced peptide with iodacetamide using a standard protocol.

Folding was monitored by analytical RP-HPLC (GE Life Sciences Äkta FPLC 900 Pittsburg, PA, USA) using a Waters Symmetry®C18 column (3.5 μm, 100 Å, 4.6 mm × 50 mm), and after completion, the final desalting and purification were carried out using a Waters Delta-Pak®C18 column (15 μm, 300 Å, 25 mm × 100 mm). Gradients were typically 5%–55% acetonitrile in H_2O (0.05% trifluoroacetic acid) for 30 min. The correct structure and purity were confirmed by ESI–MS using a Bruker Daltonics Esquire 4000 mass spectrometer (Billerica, MA, USA), working in positive mode, directly on the eluate fractions.

4.2. Molecular Modeling

4.2.1. Molecular Dynamics Simulations

All MD simulations were performed with the *Gromacs-4.5.4* software package [44] with *GROMOS 43a2* forcefield [45]. Two types of initial conformations were used to simulate the folding and dynamics of the peptides: an extended linear conformation and a β-sheet structure. The preparation of the initial conformations is described in Supplementary materials. The topologies for ornithine and diaminopropionic acid in ARs-N-B and ARs-C-B were constructed manually, analogously to a lysine residue. The linearized version of arenicin-1 (ARlin) had reduced, carboxamidomethylated cysteines (RCM-Cys), and the cyclic variant (ARcycl) had an additional peptide bond between the terminal residues. All calculations utilized periodic boundary conditions. Long-range electrostatic interactions were computed by the particle-mesh Ewald (PME) method. The cut-off for non-bonded van der Waals interactions was set to 1.2 nm. Each system was first energy-minimized by 5000 steps of steepest descent. Energy minimization was followed by two 100 ps equilibration runs using NVT and NPT ensembles during which the positions of peptide atoms were restrained by a harmonic potential with a force constant of 1000 $kJ·mol^{-1}·nm^{-2}$. The equilibration was followed by 50–120 ns production MD runs integrated with a 2 fs timestep. During the MD simulations, temperature was maintained at 300–315 K by a Nose–Hoover thermostat with a time coupling constant 0.5 ps, and pressure was maintained at 1 atm by a Parrinello–Rahman barostat with a time coupling constant 2.0 ps. In the case of the peptides ARs-N-B and ARs-C-B, we also performed a periodic simulated annealing with temperatures at 300–365 K. The coordinates were written to an output trajectory file every 2 ps for further analysis. The resulting MD trajectories and the corresponding simulation parameters are summarized in Table S1.

4.2.2. Analysis of the Simulation Results

The analysis of the MD trajectories was done using various utilities in the *Gromacs* package. To monitor the folding process, we calculated the RMSD of C^α carbon atoms from their initial positions. The evolution of the secondary structure was followed using the *DSSP* structure assignment program [46]. The stability and dynamics of the peptides were accessed by calculating RMSF of C^α carbon atoms and the average number of hydrogen bonds at the tail of a MD trajectory, where the system reached equilibrium. The same equilibrium parts of the trajectories were used to clusterize the conformations and determine the mean peptide structures. These mean structures were used to estimate the structural similarity with arenicin-1 by calculating the RMSD with experimental NMR structure PDB: 2JSB and to determine the secondary structure content by the STRIDE algorithm [47]. The kink and twist angles were analyzed analogously to a previous work on molecular dynamics simulation of arenicin-2 [6]; the details of the analysis methodology are given in Supplementary materials (Supplementary Chapter S1, [4,48–50]). The figures of the peptides were prepared using PyMol [49].

4.3. Antibacterial Assays

4.3.1. Bacterial Strains

E. coli ML35p, *Listeria monocytogenes* EGD, methicillin-resistant *Staphylococcus aureus* (MRSA) ATCC 33591 were kindly provided by Prof. Robert Lehrer (University of California, Los Angeles, CA, USA); *E. coli* ATCC 25922, *E. coli* M15, *Pseudomonas aeruginosa* ATCC 27853, *S. aureus* ATCC 25923 were provided by Dr. Elena Ermolenko (Institute of Experimental Medicine, St-Petersburg, Russia); drug-resistant clinical isolates were provided by Prof. Gennadiy Afinogenov (Saint Petersburg State University, Russia); *S. aureus* 710A has been described previously [51]. The following clinical isolates of bacteria were used: *P.s aeruginosa* resistant to aztreonam, ceftazidime, cefotaxime (obtained from the urine of a patient with cystitis), *Acinetobacter baumannii* resistant to meropenem (from an infected wound); *Staphylococcus intermedius* (from an infected wound caused by a dog bite) resistant to ciprofloxacin, cefuroxime, clindamycin, erythromycin, rifampin, gentamicin, benzylpenicillin, oxacillin.

4.3.2. Broth Microdilution Assay

This assay was applied to determine the MIC, according to the guidelines of the Clinical and Laboratory Standards Institute, using Mueller Hinton (MH) Broth. We prepared 2x stocks of peptides and serially diluted them in sterile PBS instead of Mueller Hinton Broth, so that the treatment of the bacteria with the peptides was carried out in a medium containing 50% of MH and 50% of PBS, as described [52]. The overnight cultures of each strain were transferred to fresh MH media and further incubated to obtain a mid-logarithmic-growth-phase culture of bacteria. The absorbance of each bacterial suspension was measured at 620 nm, and bacteria were then diluted to approximately 2×10^5 CFU/mL. Then, 50 µL of the suspensions were mixed with 50 µL of the peptide dilutions in the wells of a microtiter plate (pre-treated for 1 h at 37 °C with 0.2% bovine serum albumin (BSA) in water, sterilized by filtration, to diminish the non-specific binding of the peptides to the plastic surfaces).

After incubation for 18 h at 37 °C, the MIC was read as the lowest concentration of antimicrobial agent resulting in the complete inhibition of visible growth; results were obtained from 3–5 independent determinations and are shown as medians.

The overall activity against a set of tested bacterial strains was determined by way of the commonly used geometric mean of measured MIC values [29,53,54]. Unlike the arithmetic mean, this parameter is less sensitive to positive outbursts (extreme values) [55], so that possible isolated cases of bacterial resistance do not dramatically outweigh all other MIC values. At the same time, the geometric mean can still discriminate antimicrobial agents showing minor variations in activity; in other words, it has a better "resolution" than the median MIC (MIC_{50}) [54]. Some mathematical basics for choosing the geometric mean for antimicrobial activity comparison are further discussed in the Supplementary Chapter S3.

4.3.3. Membrane Permeabilization Assay

The *E. coli* ML35p outer membrane permeability was assessed by monitoring hydrolysis of the chromogenic β-lactamase substrate nitrocefin (3-(2,4-dinitrostyryl)-(6R,7R)-7-(2-thienyl acetamido)ceph-3-em-4-carboxylic acid) (Calbiochem-Novabiochem, San-Diego, CA, USA) by detection of the hydrolysis product at 486 nm. Inner membrane permeability was monitored by measuring the hydrolysis of *o*-nitrophenyl-β-D-galactoside (ONPG, Sigma, La Jolla, CA, USA) at 420 nm [15]. The *E. coli* ML35p strain expresses a plasmid-encoded periplasmic β-lactamase; it constitutively expresses cytoplasmic β-galactosidase and lacks lactose permease [15]. *E. coli* ML35p was maintained on trypticase soy agar plates containing 100 mg of ampicillin per mL. The bacteria used for antimicrobial testing or membrane permeability assays were picked from a single colony, incubated in 50 mL of sterile Trypticase soy broth for 16 h at 37 °C, washed three times with 10 mM sodium phosphate buffer (pH 7.4), adjusted to an optical density at 620 nm of 1 (2.5×10^8 CFU/mL), and kept on ice until use. The assays were performed in 96-well microtiter plates that were monitored every minute with a SpectraMax 250 Microplate Spectrophotometer (Molecular Devices, Sunnyvale, CA, USA) using the SOFTmax PRO software supplied by the manufacturer. The final incubation medium contained 10 mM sodium phosphate buffer, 100 mM NaCl, pH 7.4. Incubation wells (final volume of 100 µL) also contained either 2.5 mM of ONPG or 20 µM of nitrocefin, 2.5×10^7 CFU/mL of washed, stationary-phase *E. coli* ML35p cells, and the peptide of interest at a concentration equal to 2× MIC or an equivalent volume of acidified water (negative controls). Assays were run at 37 °C, with 5 s of shaking every minute. The reactions were started by adding the bacteria. The data were processed using the Sigma Plot 11 software; the results of a typical experiment are presented at the Figure 5.

4.4. Cytotoxicity Assays

4.4.1. Hemolytic Activity

Hemolysis assays were carried out on human red blood cells according to the ethical principles of the Declaration of Helsinki. Peripheral blood was drawn from healthy donors (written informed consent was obtained from all volunteers) into vacutainers containing EDTA under aseptic conditions and washed twice with an ice-cold phosphate buffered saline (PBS). The supernatant was discarded, and the pellet was resuspended in PBS. Hemolytic action was tested by incubating increasing concentrations of peptides with a suspension (2.5% v/v) of washed red blood cells in PBS. After 30 min at 37 °C, the tubes were centrifuged for 3 min at 10,000 g. Hemoglobin release was monitored at 540 nm using the SpectraMax 250 Microplate Spectrophotometer (Molecular Devices, Sunnyvale, CA, USA). Total lysis (100% hemolysis) was determined by adding 1% (v/v) Triton X-100, and the negative control value was determined by incubating red blood cells in buffer only. The percentage of hemolysis was calculated as:

$$\% \text{ Hemolysis} = ((A_{\text{exper}} - A_{\text{control}})/(A_{\text{total}} - A_{\text{control}})) \times 100, \tag{1}$$

where A_{exper} and A_{control} signify the absorbance values of the supernatants from treated and untreated red blood cells, and A_{total} is the supernatant of the cells treated with 1% Triton X-100. All evaluations were repeated in 3–6 separate experiments, carried out in triplicates.

4.4.2. MTT Test

The standard MTT ((3-(4,5-Dimethylthiazol-2-yl)-2,5-diphenyltetrazolium bromide) test was used for the examination of the cytotoxic activity of AMPs [56] towards human erithroleukemia cells K-562. The cells were purchased from Biolot (Saint Petersburg, Russia) and were grown in RPMI 1640 medium

(Biolot, Saint Petersburg, Russia) supplemented with glutamine and 10% FCS. Before the experiment, the culturing medium was replaced with serum-free RPMI 1640. Serial dilutions of the peptides in RPMI were plated in sterile 96-well microplates, and the target cells were dispensed to the microplates (10^5 cells/well in RPMI 1640). The plates were incubated for 24 h at 37 °C under 5% CO_2. Cell-free media and cells incubated without peptides served as controls. Four hours before the incubation ended, MTT in PBS (5 mg/mL) was added to each well. After the incubation was stopped by adding isopropanol/ 0.04 M HCl, the optical density was measured at 540 nm, subtracting the background absorbance at 690 nm. Toxicity was determined by nonlinear regression analysis of the corresponding dose–response curves using the Sigma Plot 11 program to calculate the IC_{50} values (the concentration of the test substance that reduced the OD_{540} capacity by 50%).

5. Conclusions

Antibiotic substances from marine invertebrates, and in particular antimicrobial peptides, are a promising source of novel anti-infective drugs. Among these, arenicin-1 isolated from the lugworm *A. marina* coelomocytes, is one of the most potent. It exerts a marked microbicidal activity towards a variety of Gram-negative and Gram-positive bacteria (including drug-resistant clinical isolates) and also possesses significant toxicity towards mammalian cells. An intriguing feature of this peptide is a markedly symmetric arrangement of some residues in its sequence. Several variants have been elaborated to elucidate the role of this sequence symmetry in the peptides' function and mode of action, to determine the effect of structural variations such as backbone cyclization or linearization, and to probe the importance of key residues for microbicidal efficacy, membranolytic activity, and toxicity towards mammalian cells.

The results of this work allow us to make the following considerations:

- Stand inversion or palyndromic symmetrization of the arenicin scaffold does not greatly affect its twisted and kinked antiparallel β-sheet conformation, whereas symmetrization by artificially branching strands results in a flattened and more regular parallel β-hairpin;
- Inverting the strand residue arrangement of the native peptide causes a decrease in activity. This may be due to decreased capacity to oligomerize via the inverted N-terminal strand;
- A more symmetric, palindromic strand arrangement did not improve the activity and decreased it if accompanied by a reduced net charge;
- Increasing symmetry by artificially "branching" strands in a parallel hairpin arrangement allowed to recover the antimicrobial activity while reducing the cytotoxic activity;
- All variants with a modified symmetry demonstrated a reduced capacity to permeabilize the inner membrane of *E. coli* ML35, possibly pointing to a reduced capacity for oligomerization and/or pore formation.
- The backbone cyclization of the arenicin-1 molecule resulted in improved activity towards drug-resistant clinical isolates but did not markedly affect cytotoxicity.
- Linearization of the peptide somewhat increased selectivity, while not greatly altering antimicrobial activity.

These findings suggest that the residue layout of the arenicin-1 molecule plays a significant role in its biological activity, although the contribution of the peculiar, pseudo-symmetric arrangement of some residues is still unclear. Furthermore, several other characteristics of the peptides (charge, hydrophobicity, residues involved in oligomerization) must also be taken in account. We suggest that recent developments in the computational design of AMPs employing pattern discovery [57] and deep learning [58], trained also using data from this type of study, may allow for an efficient optimization of these entangled parameters. Our results indicate that this molecule from a marine animal can serve as a robust template for the elaboration of novel therapeutic agents and they add to a plethora of other studies showing that it is arduous to redesign synthetic antimicrobial peptides from natural ones, improving both efficacy and selectivity.

Supplementary Materials: The following are available online at http://www.mdpi.com/1660-3397/17/6/376/s1, Chapter S1: Molecular dynamics simulation protocol; Chapter S2: Analysis of the simulation results; Chapter S3: Why use geometric mean of MIC as an assessment of overall antimicrobial activity?

Author Contributions: D.S.O., O.V.S., M.S.Z. – investigation (biological activity testing), data analysis or curation, writing—original draft preparation; I.E.E. and O.B.C. – investigation (molecular modeling), formal analysis, funding acquisition; N.A. and S.Z. – peptide synthesis; V.N.K., P.V.P. – investigation (biological activity testing); T.V.O. – data analysis, validation, writing—review and editing; A.T. – peptides design, supervision, writing—review and editing.

Funding: The work was supported by the Ministry of Science and Higher Education of the Russian Federation (project 0557-2019-0010 – D.S.O., O.V.S., M.S.Z., V.N.K. and project 16.9790.2017 – I.E.E. and O.B.C.).

Acknowledgments: We acknowledge Anna Kakesnik and Alexander Artamonov for the technical support, Robert Lehrer, Gennadiy Afinogenov, Elena Ermolenko for the kind donation of the bacterial strains used for the experiments.

Conflicts of Interest: The authors declare no conflict of interest.

References

1. Ovchinnikova, T.V.; Aleshina, G.M.; Balandin, S.V.; Krasnosdembskaya, A.D.; Markelov, M.L.; Frolova, E.I.; Leonova, Y.F.; Tagaev, A.A.; Krasnodembsky, E.G.; Kokryakov, V.N. Purification and primary structure of two isoforms of arenicin, a novel antimicrobial peptide from marine polychaeta *Arenicola marina*. *FEBS Lett.* **2004**, *577*, 209–214. [CrossRef] [PubMed]

2. Ovchinnikova, T.V.; Shenkarev, Z.O.; Nadezhdin, K.D.; Balandin, S.V.; Zhmak, M.N.; Kudelina, I.A.; Finkina, E.I.; Kokryakov, V.N.; Arseniev, A.S. Recombinant expression, synthesis, purification, and solution structure of arenicin. *Biochem. Biophys. Res. Commun.* **2007**, *360*, 156–162. [CrossRef] [PubMed]

3. Lee, J.U.; Kang, D.I.; Zhu, W.L.; Shin, S.Y.; Hahm, K.S.; Kim, Y. Solution structures and biological functions of the antimicrobial peptide, arenicin-1, and its linear derivative. *Biopolymers* **2007**, *88*, 208–216. [CrossRef] [PubMed]

4. Andrä, J.; Jakovkin, I.; Grötzinger, J.; Hecht, O.; Krasnodembskaya, A.D.; Goldmann, T.; Gutsmann, T.; Leippe, M. Structure and mode of action of the antimicrobial peptide arenicin. *Biochem. J.* **2008**, *410*, 113–122. [CrossRef]

5. Ovchinnikova, T.V.; Shenkarev, Z.O.; Balandin, S.V.; Nadezhdin, K.D.; Paramonov, A.S.; Kokryakov, V.N.; Arseniev, A.S. Molecular insight into mechanism of antimicrobial action of the β-hairpin peptide arenicin: Specific oligomerization in detergent micelles. *Biopolymers* **2008**, *89*, 455–464. [CrossRef] [PubMed]

6. Stavrakoudis, A.; Tsoulos, I.G.; Shenkarev, Z.O.; Ovchinnikova, T.V. Molecular dynamics simulation of antimicrobial peptide arenicin-2: Beta-hairpin stabilization by noncovalent interactions. *Biopolymers* **2009**, *92*, 143–155. [CrossRef] [PubMed]

7. Andrä, J.; Hammer, M.U.; Grötzinger, J.; Jakovkin, I.; Lindner, B.; Vollmer, E.; Fedders, H.; Leippe, M.; Gutsmann, T. Significance of the cyclic structure and of arginine residues for the antibacterial activity of arenicin-1 and its interaction with phospholipid and lipopolysaccharide model membranes. *Biol. Chem.* **2009**, *390*, 337–349. [CrossRef]

8. Salnikov, E.S.; Aisenbrey, C.; Balandin, S.V.; Zhmak, M.N.; Ovchinnikova, T.V.; Bechinger, B. Structure and alignment of the membrane-associated antimicrobial peptide arenicin by oriented solid-state NMR spectroscopy. *Biochemistry* **2011**, *50*, 3784–3795. [CrossRef]

9. Cho, J.; Lee, D.G. The characteristic region of arenicin-1 involved with a bacterial membrane targeting mechanism. *Biochem. Biophys. Res. Commun.* **2011**, *405*, 422–427. [CrossRef]

10. Park, C.; Cho, J.; Lee, J.; Lee, D.G. Membranolytic antifungal activity of arenicin-1 requires the N-terminal tryptophan and the beta-turn arginine. *Biotechnol. Lett.* **2011**, *33*, 185–189. [CrossRef]

11. Panteleev, P.V.; Bolosov, I.A.; Ovchinnikova, T.V. Bioengineering and functional characterization of arenicin shortened analogs with enhanced antibacterial activity and cell selectivity. *J. Pept. Sci.* **2016**, *22*, 82–91. [CrossRef] [PubMed]

12. Panteleev, P.V.; Myshkin, M.Y.; Shenkarev, Z.O.; Ovchinnikova, T.V. Dimerization of the antimicrobial peptide arenicin plays a key role in the cytotoxicity but not in the antibacterial activity. *Biochem. Biophys. Res. Commun.* **2017**, *482*, 1320–1326. [CrossRef] [PubMed]

13. Shenkarev, Z.O.; Balandin, S.V.; Trunov, K.I.; Paramonov, A.S.; Sukhanov, S.V.; Barsukov, L.I.; Arseniev, A.S.; Ovchinnikova, T.V. Molecular mechanism of action of β-hairpin antimicrobial peptide arenicin: Oligomeric structure in dodecylphosphocholine micelles and pore formation in planar lipid bilayers. *Biochemistry* **2011**, *50*, 6255–6265. [CrossRef] [PubMed]

14. Lee, J.U.; Park, K.H.; Lee, J.Y.; Kim, J.; Shin, S.Y.; Park, Y.; Hahm, K.S.; Kim, Y. Cell Selectivity of Arenicin-1 and Its Derivative with Two Disulfide Bonds. *Bull. Korean Chem. Soc.* **2008**, *29*, 1190–1194. [CrossRef]

15. Lehrer, R.I.; Barton, A.; Ganz, T. Concurrent assessment of inner and outer membrane permeabilization and bacteriolysis in *E. coli* by multiple-wavelength spectrophotometry. *J. Immunol. Methods* **1988**, *108*, 153–158. [CrossRef]

16. Edwards, I.A.; Elliott, A.G.; Kavanagh, A.M.; Zuegg, J.; Blaskovich, M.A.; Cooper, M.A. Contribution of Amphipathicity and Hydrophobicity to the Antimicrobial Activity and Cytotoxicity of β-Hairpin Peptides. *ACS Infect. Dis.* **2016**, *2*, 442–450. [CrossRef] [PubMed]

17. Jindal, H.M.; Le, C.F.; Yusof, M.Y.M.; Velayuthan, R.D.; Lee, V.S.; Zain, S.M.; Isa, D.M.; Sekaran, S.D. Antimicrobial Activity of Novel Synthetic Peptides Derived from Indolicidin and Ranalexin against *Streptococcus pneumoniae*. *PLoS ONE* **2015**, *10*, e0128532. [CrossRef] [PubMed]

18. Tassanakajon, A.; Amparyup, P.; Somboonwiwat, K.; Supungul, P. Cationic antimicrobial peptides in penaeid shrimp. *Mar. Biotechnol.* **2010**, *12*, 487–505. [CrossRef]

19. Charlet, M.; Chernysh, S.; Philippe, H.; Hetru, C.; Hoffmann, J.A.; Bulet, P. Innate immunity. Isolation of several cystein-rich antimicrobial peptides from the blood of a mollusc, *Mytilus edulis. J. Biol. Chem.* **1996**, *271*, 21808–21813. [CrossRef]

20. Ovchinnikova, T.V.; Balandin, S.V.; Aleshina, G.M.; Tagaev, A.A.; Leonova, Y.F.; Krasnodembsky, E.D.; Men'shenin, A.V.; Kokryakov, V.N. Aurelin, a novel antimicrobial peptide from jellyfish *Aurelia aurita* with structural features of defensins and channel-blocking toxins. *Biochem. Biophys. Res. Commun.* **2006**, *348*, 514–523. [CrossRef]

21. Nakamura, T.; Furunaka, H.; Miyata, T.; Tokunaga, F.; Muta, T.; Iwanaga, S.; Niwa, M.; Takao, T.; Shimonishi, Y. Tachyplesin, a class of antimicrobial peptide from the hemocytes of the horseshoe crab (*Tachypleus tridentatus*). Isolation and chemical structure. *J. Biol. Chem.* **1988**, *263*, 16709–16713. [PubMed]

22. Stensvåg, K.; Haug, T.; Sperstad, S.V.; Rekdal, O.; Indrevoll, B.; Styrvold, O.B. Arasin 1, a prolinearginine-rich antimicrobial peptide isolated from the spider crab, *Hyas araneus. Dev. Comp. Immunol.* **2008**, *32*, 275–285. [CrossRef] [PubMed]

23. Yang, S.T.; Shin, S.Y.; Hahm, K.S.; Kim, J.I. Design of perfectly symmetric Trp-rich peptides with potent and broad-spectrum antimicrobial activities. *Int. J. Antimicrob. Agents* **2006**, *27*, 325–330. [CrossRef] [PubMed]

24. Xu, L.; Chou, S.; Wang, J.; Shao, C.; Li, W.; Zhu, X.; Shan, A. Antimicrobial activity and membrane-active mechanism of tryptophan zipper-like β-hairpin antimicrobial peptides. *Amino Acids* **2015**, *47*, 2385–2397. [CrossRef] [PubMed]

25. Dong, N.; Ma, Q.; Shan, A.; Lv, Y.; Hu, W.; Gu, Y.; Li, Y. Strand length-dependent antimicrobial activity and membrane-active mechanism of arginine- and valine-rich β-hairpin-like antimicrobial peptides. *Antimicrob. Agents Chemother.* **2012**, *56*, 2994–3003. [CrossRef] [PubMed]

26. Takahashi, D.; Shukla, S.K.; Prakash, O.; Zhang, G. Structural determinants of host defense peptides for antimicrobial activity and target cell selectivity. *Biochimie* **2010**, *92*, 1236–1241. [CrossRef]

27. Teixeira, V.; Feio, M.J.; Bastos, M. Role of lipids in the interaction of antimicrobial peptides with membranes. *Prog. Lipid Res.* **2012**, *51*, 149–177. [CrossRef]

28. Feder, R.; Dagan, A.; Mor, A. Structure-activity relationship study of antimicrobial dermaseptin S4 showing the consequences of peptide oligomerization on selective cytotoxicity. *J. Biol. Chem.* **2000**, *275*, 4230–4238. [CrossRef]

29. Jiang, Z.; Vasil, A.I.; Vasil, M.L.; Hodges, R.S. "Specificity Determinants" Improve Therapeutic Indices of Two Antimicrobial Peptides Piscidin 1 and Dermaseptin S4 against the Gram-Negative Pathogens *Acinetobacter baumannii* and *Pseudomonas aeruginosa. Pharmaceuticals* **2014**, *7*, 366–391. [CrossRef]

30. Arias, M.; Piga, K.B.; Hyndman, M.E.; Vogel, H.J. Improving the Activity of Trp-Rich Antimicrobial Peptides by Arg/Lys Substitutions and Changing the Length of Cationic Residues. *Biomolecules* **2018**, *8*, 19. [CrossRef]

31. Chan, D.I.; Prenner, E.J.; Vogel, H.J. Tryptophan- and arginine-rich antimicrobial peptides: Structures and mechanisms of action. *Biochim. Biophys. Acta* **2006**, *1758*, 1184–1202. [CrossRef] [PubMed]

32. Schmidt, N.W.; Wong, G.C. Antimicrobial peptides and induced membrane curvature: Geometry, coordination chemistry, and molecular engineering. *Curr. Opin. Solid State Mater. Sci.* **2013**, *17*, 151–163. [CrossRef] [PubMed]

33. Tam, J.; Wu, C.; Yang, J.-L. Membranolytic selectivity of cystine-stabilized cyclic protegrins. *Eur. J. Biochem.* **2000**, *267*, 3289–3300. [CrossRef] [PubMed]

34. Tam, J.; Lu, Y.-A.; Yang, J.-L. Marked Increase in Membranolytic Selectivity of Novel Cyclic Tachyplesins Constrained with an Antiparallel Two-β Strand Cystine Knot Framework. *Biochem. Biophys. Res. Commun.* **2000**, *267*, 783–790. [CrossRef] [PubMed]

35. Chan, L.Y.; Zhang, V.M.; Huang, Y.H.; Waters, N.C.; Bansal, P.S.; Craik, D.J.; Daly, N.L. Cyclization of the antimicrobial peptide gomesin with native chemical ligation: Influences on stability and bioactivity. *ChemBioChem* **2013**, *14*, 617–624. [CrossRef] [PubMed]

36. Hemu, X.; Tam, J.P. Macrocyclic Antimicrobial Peptides Engineered from ω-Conotoxin. *Curr. Pharm. Des.* **2017**, *23*, 2131–2138. [CrossRef]

37. Wu, M.; Hancock, R.E. Interaction of the cyclic antimicrobial cationic peptide bactenecin with the outer and cytoplasmic membrane. *J. Biol. Chem.* **1999**, *274*, 29–35. [CrossRef]

38. Lai, J.R.; Huck, B.R.; Weisblum, B.; Gellman, S.H. Design of non-cysteine-containing antimicrobial beta-hairpins: Structure-activity relationship studies with linear protegrin-1 analogues. *Biochemistry* **2002**, *41*, 12835–12842. [CrossRef]

39. Hai Nan, Y.; Jacob, B.; Kim, Y.; Yub Shin, S. Linear bactenecin analogs with cell selectivity and anti-endotoxic activity. *J. Pept. Sci.* **2012**, *18*, 740–747. [CrossRef]

40. Lee, J.Y.; Yang, S.T.; Lee, S.K.; Jung, H.H.; Shin, S.Y.; Hahm, K.S.; Kim, J.I. Salt-resistant homodimeric bactenecin, a cathelicidin-derived antimicrobial peptide. *FEBS J.* **2008**, *275*, 3911–3920. [CrossRef]

41. Mosco, A.; Zlatev, V.; Guarnaccia, C.; Pongor, S.; Campanella, A.; Zahariev, S.; Giulianini, P.G. Novel protocol for the chemical synthesis of crustacean hyperglycemic hormone analogues—An efficient experimental tool for studying their functions. *PLoS ONE* **2012**, *7*, e30052. [CrossRef] [PubMed]

42. Benincasa, M.; Zahariev, S.; Pelillo, C.; Milan, A.; Gennaro, R.; Scocchi, M. PEGylation of the peptide Bac7(1-35) reduces renal clearance while retaining antibacterial activity and bacterial cell penetration capacity. *Eur. J. Med. Chem.* **2015**, *95*, 210–219. [CrossRef] [PubMed]

43. von Eggelkraut-Gottanka, R.; Klose, A.; Beck-Sickinger, A.G.; Beyermann, M. Peptide $^\alpha$thioester formation using standard Fmoc-chemistry. *Tetrahedron Lett.* **2003**, *44*, 3551–3554. [CrossRef]

44. Pronk, S.; Páll, S.; Schulz, R.; Larsson, P.; Bjelkmar, P.; Apostolov, R.; Shirts, M.R.; Smith, J.C.; Kasson, P.M.; van der Spoel, D.; et al. GROMACS 4.5: A high-throughput and highly parallel open source molecular simulation toolkit. *Bioinformatics* **2013**, *29*, 845–854. [CrossRef]

45. van Gunsteren, W.F.; Billeter, S.R.; Eising, A.A.; Hünenberger, P.H.; Krüger, P.K.H.C.; Mark, A.E.; Scott, W.R.P.; Tironi, I.G. *Biomolecular Simulation: The GROMOS96 Manual and User Guide*; Vdf Hochschulverlag AG an der ETH Zürich: Zürich, Switzerland, 1996; ISBN 9783728124227.

46. Kabsch, W.; Sander, C. Dictionary of protein secondary structure: Pattern recognition of hydrogen-bonded and geometrical features. *Biopolymers* **1983**, *22*, 2577–2637. [CrossRef] [PubMed]

47. Frishman, D.; Argos, P. Knowledge-based protein secondary structure assignment. *Proteins* **1995**, *23*, 566–579. [CrossRef] [PubMed]

48. Needleman, S.B.; Wunsch, C.D. A general method applicable to the search for similarities in the amino acid sequence of two proteins. *J. Mol. Biol.* **1970**, *48*, 443–453. [CrossRef]

49. Schrödinger, LLC. *The PyMOL Molecular Graphics System*; Version 2.2.0; Schrödinger, LLC: New York, NY, USA, 2018.

50. Xu, D.; Zhang, Y. Ab initio protein structure assembly using continuous structure fragments and optimized knowledge-based force field. *Proteins* **2012**, *80*, 1715–1735. [CrossRef]

51. Giangaspero, A.; Sandri, L.; Tossi, A. Amphipathic alpha helical antimicrobial peptides. *Eur. J. Biochem.* **2001**, *268*, 5589–5600. [CrossRef]

52. Tossi, A.; Scocchi, M.; Zanetti, M.; Gennaro, R.; Storici, P.; Romeo, D. An Approach Combining Rapid cDNA Amplification and Chemical Synthesis for the Identification of Novel, Cathelicidin-Derived, Antimicrobial Peptides. In *Antibacterial Peptide Protocols. Methods in Molecular Biology™*; Shafer, W.M., Ed.; Humana Press: Totowa, NJ, USA, 1997; Volume 78, pp. 133–151. ISBN 978-0-89603-408-2.

53. Lyu, Y.; Yang, Y.; Lyu, X.; Dong, N.; Shan, A. Antimicrobial activity, improved cell selectivity and mode of action of short PMAP-36-derived peptides against bacteria and *Candida*. *Sci. Rep.* **2016**, *6*, 27258. [CrossRef]

54. Davies, B.I. The importance of the geometric mean MIC. *J. Antimicrob. Chemother.* **1990**, *25*, 471–472. [CrossRef] [PubMed]

55. Manikandan, S. Measures of central tendency: The mean. *J. Pharmacol. Pharmacother.* **2011**, *2*, 140–142. [CrossRef] [PubMed]

56. Mosmann, T. Rapid colorimetric assay for cellular growth and survival: Application to proliferation and cytotoxicity assays. *J. Immunol. Methods* **1983**, *65*, 55–63. [CrossRef]

57. Eliseev, I.E.; Terterov, I.N.; Yudenko, A.N.; Shamova, O.V. Linking sequence patterns and functionality of alpha-helical antimicrobial peptides. *Bioinformatics* **2018**. [CrossRef] [PubMed]

58. Veltri, D.; Kamath, U.; Shehu, A. Deep learning improves antimicrobial peptide recognition. *Bioinformatics* **2018**, *34*, 2740–2747. [CrossRef]

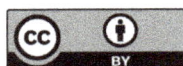

marine drugs

MDPI

Article

Modulation of Human Complement System by Antimicrobial Peptide Arenicin-1 from *Arenicola marina*

Ekaterina S. Umnyakova [1], Nikolay P. Gorbunov [1,2], Alexander V. Zhakhov [2], Ilia A. Krenev [3], Tatiana V. Ovchinnikova [4], Vladimir N. Kokryakov [1,3] and Mikhail N. Berlov [1,*]

[1] Institute of Experimental Medicine, Acad. Pavlov Str. 12, Saint Petersburg 197376, Russia;
    umka-biolog@mail.ru (E.S.U.); kokryak@yandex.ru (V.N.K.)
[2] Research Institute of Highly Pure Biopreparations, Pudozhskaya Str., 7, Saint Petersburg 197110, Russia;
    n.p.gorbynov@hpb.spb.ru (N.P.G.); a.v.zachov@hpb.spb.ru (A.V.Z.)
[3] Department of Biochemistry, Saint-Petersburg State University, Universitetskaya Embankment, 7/9,
    Saint-Petersburg 199034, Russia; il.krenevv13@yandex.ru
[4] M.M. Shemyakin and Yu. A. Ovchinnikov Institute of Bioorganic Chemistry, Russian Academy of Sciences,
    Miklukho-Maklaya Str., 16/10, Moscow 117997, Russia; ovch@ibch.ru
*   Correspondence: berlov@yandex.ru; Tel.: +7-911-936-9839

Received: 17 October 2018; Accepted: 27 November 2018; Published: 1 December 2018

Abstract: Antimicrobial peptides from marine invertebrates are known not only to act like cytotoxic agents, but they also can display some additional activities in mammalian organisms. In particular, these peptides can modulate the complement system as was described for tachyplesin, a peptide from the horseshoe crab. In this work, we investigated the influence on complement activation of the antimicrobial peptide arenicin-1 from the marine polychaete *Arenicola marina*. To study effects of arenicin on complement activation in human blood serum, we used hemolytic assays of two types, with antibody sensitized sheep erythrocytes and rabbit erythrocytes. Complement activation was also assessed, by the level of C3a production that was measured by ELISA. We found that the effect of arenicin depends on its concentration. At relatively low concentrations the peptide stimulates complement activation and lysis of target erythrocytes, whereas at higher concentrations arenicin acts as a complement inhibitor. A hypothetical mechanism of peptide action is proposed, suggesting its interaction with two complement proteins, C1q and C3. The results lead to the possibility of the development of new approaches for therapy of diseases connected with complement dysregulation, using peptide regulators derived from natural antimicrobial peptides of invertebrates.

Keywords: *Arenicola marina*; antimicrobial peptides; arenicin; complement; C3a

---

1. Introduction

The biologically active compounds derived from marine organisms are known to be unique, and can be used as a pattern for the development of new, effective pharmacological agents for treatment of different diseases [1]. Antimicrobial peptides named arenicins are found in coelomocytes of the marine polychaete *Arenicola marina*. Three isoforms of arenicins have been described: arenicin-1, -2 [2] and -3 [3]. These cationic peptides consist of 21 amino acid residues, and have the structure of a β-hairpin [4,5] stabilized by one (for arenicins-1 and -2) or two (for arenicin-3) intramolecular disulfide bonds. Arenicins have also been detected in epithelia of the body wall and gut of *A. marina* [6]. At micromolar concentrations, these peptides demonstrate significant antimicrobial activity towards a wide range of Gram-positive and Gram-negative bacteria, as well as of fungi [2,3,7–9], and they seem to play a significant role in host defense of this polychaete. The mechanism of antimicrobial activity is realized by the action of peptide molecules on the microbial cytoplasmic membrane forming transmembrane pores [7,9,10]. Several attempts have been made to design a structure of peptide antibiotics derived from arenicins [11–14]. As potential medical drug prototypes, arenicins should be tested for their biological effects beyond direct antimicrobial activity.

Arenicins have similar amino acid sequence and spatial structure to another group of antimicrobial peptides, tachyplesins, which have been isolated earlier from the horseshoe crab *Tachypleus trindentatus*, and polyphemusins from *Limulus polyphemus*, which are related to tachyplesins [15,16] (Figure 1). Tachyplesins, like arenicins, have a β-hairpin structure that is stabilized by two intramolecular disulfide bonds. This similarity indicates that these peptides may belong to a common family of antimicrobial peptides [17]. On the other hand, the structures of arenicins' and tachyplesins' precursors, and their posttranslational processing, are quite different [2,18]. Thus, the evolutionary relationship between these peptides remains questionable.

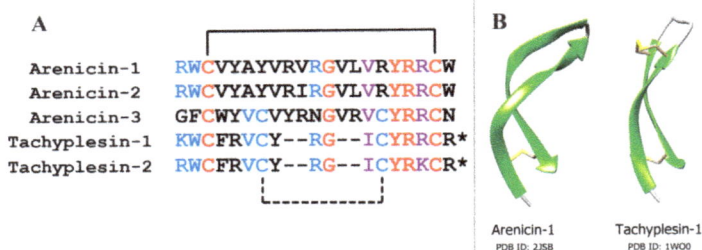

Figure 1. Structural similarities between arenicins and tachyplesins. (**A**) Multiple sequence alignment of three arenicins and two tachyplesins. Identical and highly similar residues in the same positions for all five peptides are colored with red and violet, respectively. Identical or highly similar residues shared by one or two arenicins and two tachyplesins are colored with blue. Black lines indicate cysteine pairing, the disulfide bond absent in arenicins-1 and -2 shown as a dashed line. Asterisks indicate amidated arginine residues. (**B**) Spatial structures of arenicins-1 and tachyplesin-1; images were generated with Chimera 1.11 software.

It has been shown that tachyplesin-1 is capable of forming a complex with human C1q complement protein that leads to antibody-independent complement classical pathway activation in human blood serum. In particular, tachyplesin can bind to the surface of TSU human prostate carcinoma cells, making these cells a target for complement action [19]. It was determined that the interaction of tachyplesin with C1q requires the integrity of peptide spatial structure, since the reduction and alkylation of disulfide bonds lead to a weaker binding to C1q.

The complement system is a part of the immune defense in mammals, represented by a network of serum proteins (complement components) [20,21]. Complement activation leads to opsonization of target cells, or their lysis by the membrane attack complex (MAC). The latter event is usually restricted to Gram-negative bacteria, however host cells, especially erythrocytes, may also be lysed by MAC. There are three main pathways of complement activation, named the classical, alternative, and lectin pathways. All of them converge on proteolytic cleavage of C3 component to C3a and C3b by so-called C3-convertases. After the cleavage, C3b is able to bind covalently to hydroxyl-containing molecules via its intrinsic thioester bond. This can mediate its accumulation on the surface of target cells, normally microbes or apoptotic cells. C3b is incorporated into C3-convertases, changing their specificity for C5 component cleavage, which initiates MAC assembly.

According to the structural similarity between arenicins and tachyplesins, we assumed that arenicin could also interact with C1q and that this might influence the complement activation. In a previous paper, we demonstrated that arenicin-1 really forms a stable complex with human C1q [22].

In this paper, we studied the effects of arenicin-1 on complement activation and target cell lysis in two hemolytic models in vitro. We also used an ELISA test for C3a to confirm the complement activation in these models. We found that the effect of arenicin on the complement system depends on the concentration of the peptide. At relatively low concentrations, arenicin stimulates complement activation and/or target erythrocyte lysis. However, at higher concentrations arenicin behaves as a complement system inhibitor. Though it was not demonstrated directly, our results provide strong evidence about the interaction of arenicin with the C3 complement protein, in addition to the previously established interaction with C1q.

2. Results

In the hemolytic assay with antibody sensitized sheep erythrocytes (E^{sh}), which is the model for the classical pathway of complement activation, we observed more than twice the baseline level of E^{sh} lysis by 1% normal human serum (NHS) in the presence of arenicin-1 at concentrations 10 and 20 μg/mL, compared with control (samples without peptide) (Figure 2A). However, at higher concentrations (80 μg/mL), arenicin displayed a reverse effect and almost totally abolished complement-mediated hemolysis. In all concentrations tested, arenicin itself revealed no hemolytic activity in experimental conditions, because in samples with active serum replaced for heat-inactivated serum there was no lysis above background level (data not shown).

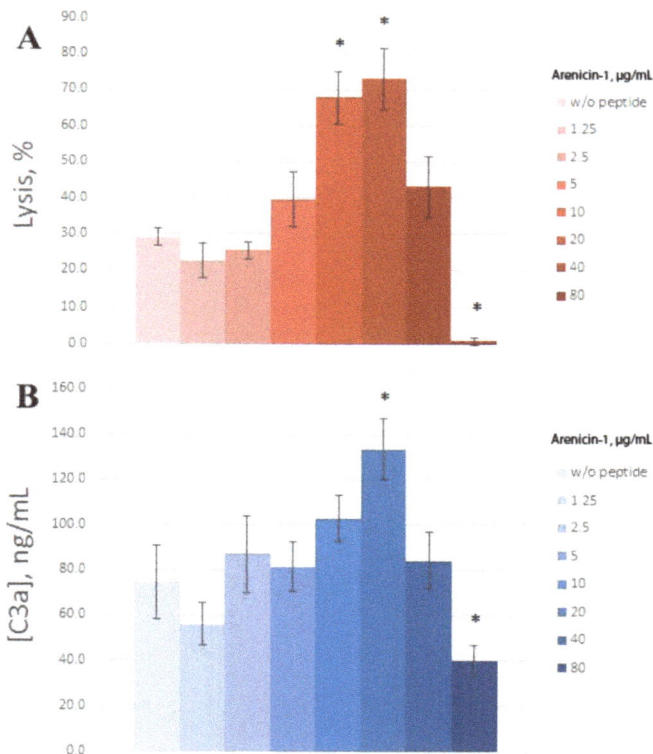

Figure 2. The action of arenicin-1 on complement activation and lysis of antibody sensitized sheep erythrocytes (E^{sh}). Data are represented as mean ± SD ($n = 5$). * $p < 0.05$ vs. control (samples without peptide). (**A**) E^{sh} lysis level, %; (**B**) C3a concentration in samples, ng/mL.

To assess whether E^{sh} lysis level differences reflect different complement activation levels, we developed an ELISA system for human C3a, a derivative of the complement protein C3, which is produced on complement activation. The test system was suitable for detection of C3a in the range 25–500 ng/mL, with no cross-reactivity to the uncleaved C3 protein.

After hemolytic assay, the same samples were used for C3a determination (Figure 2B). Both increased and decreased lysis levels were accompanied by concerted alterations in C3a production, though these alterations were less prominent compared with lysis. In fact, the enhanced value of C3a differed significantly from the control one only for 20 µg/mL of arenicin. The relationship between E^{sh} lysis and C3a production is illustrated in Figure 3. Pearson correlation coefficient was calculated as 0.93, which is significant for $p < 0.05$.

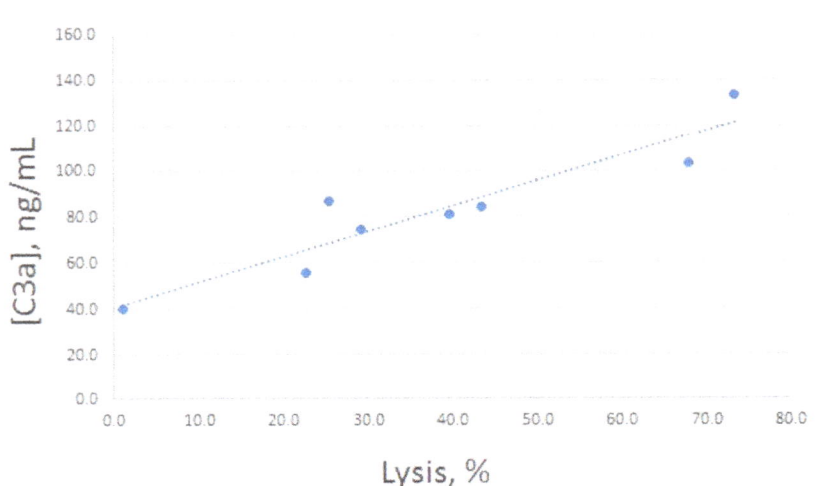

Figure 3. Correlation between percentages of antibody sensitized sheep erythrocytes lysed by human serum at different concentrations of arenicin-1 and C3a production in these samples. Pearson correlation coefficient was calculated as 0.93.

As a model of complement activation via the alternative pathway, a hemolytic assay with rabbit erythrocytes (E^{rab}) is widely used. We utilized this assay to study arenicin action on the complement system as well. Since we used 4% serum in this model, we took a broader concentration range of arenicin. We found that in this model, arenicin retained its inhibitory action at high concentrations (80 and 160 µg/mL), essentially decreasing hemolysis level (Figure 4A). No significant effect was observed for lower concentrations of the peptide. Similar to the previous model, arenicin did not induce E^{rab} lysis itself in heat-inactivated serum (data not shown).

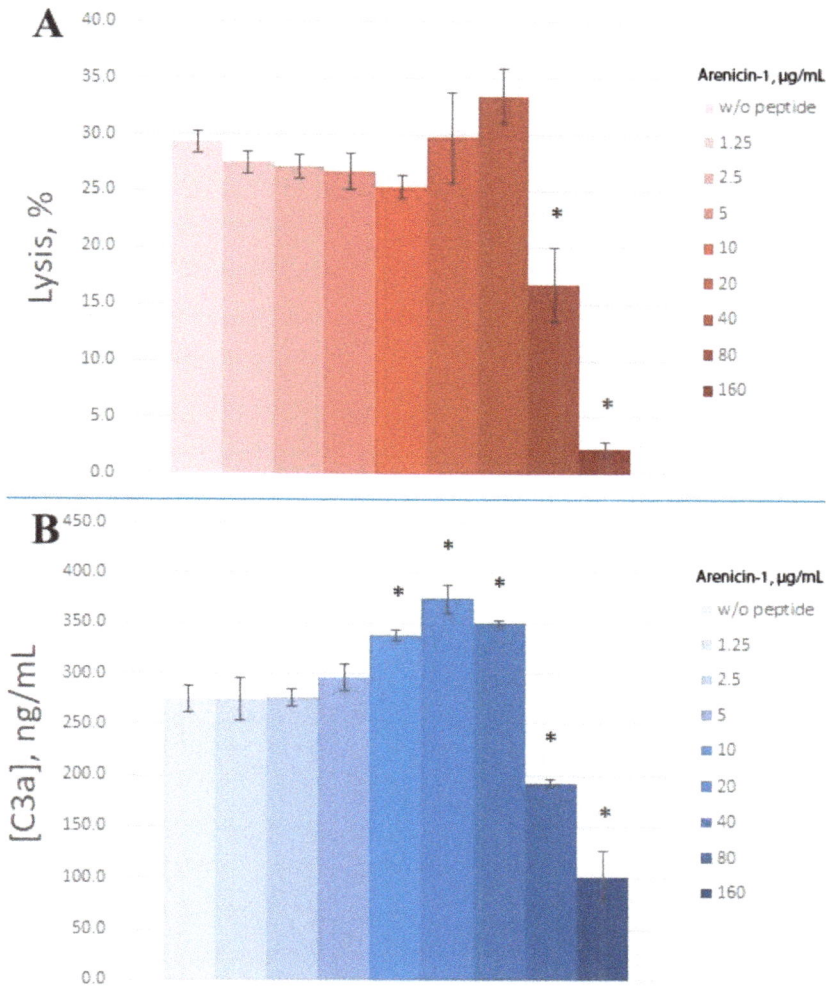

Figure 4. The action of arenicin-1 on complement activation and lysis of rabbit erythrocytes (E^{rab}). Data are represented as mean $\pm$ SD ($n = 5$). * $p < 0.05$ vs. control (samples without peptide). (**A**) E^{rab} lysis level, %; (**B**) C3a concentration in samples, ng/mL.

Inhibitory action of arenicin on E^{rab} lysis by NHS was confirmed to reflect its influence on complement activation, since C3a levels in the samples with high arenicin concentrations (80 and 160 µg/mL) were significantly diminished (Figure 4B). Unexpectedly, we found that in the presence of arenicin at 10–40 µg/mL, a modest but reproducible increase in C3a production was observed in the E^{rab} model. While this did not lead to enhanced E^{rab} lysis, the Pearson correlation coefficient for this model was 0.88, which is significant for $p < 0.05$. Correlation between E^{rab} lysis and C3a generation is shown in Figure 5.

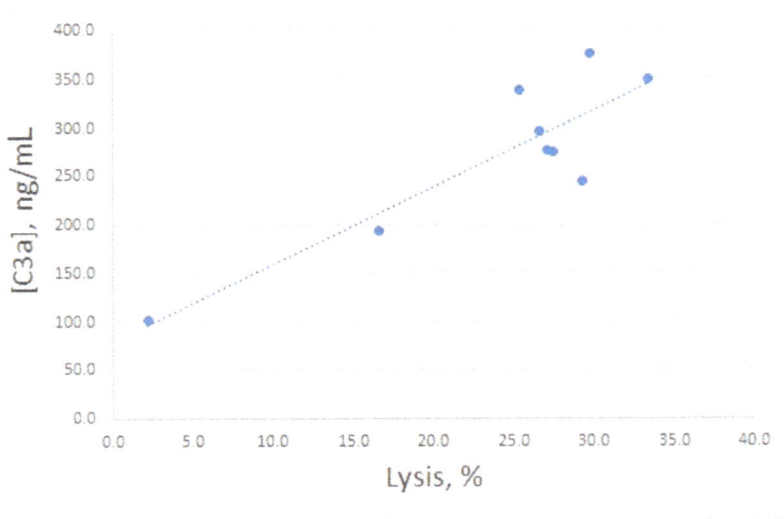

Figure 5. Correlation between percentages of rabbit erythrocytes lysed by human serum at different concentrations of arenicin-1 and C3a production in these samples. Pearson correlation coefficient was calculated as 0.88.

To sum up, complement activation stimulated by different types of erythrocytes was of an approximately equal level. Differences between C3a concentrations for control samples (Figures 2 and 4) are due to different serum dilution in these models (1:100 for E^{sh} and 1:25 for E^{rab}). In both models, arenicin revealed both activating and inhibitory effects depending on its concentration.

3. Discussion

Previously, it has been demonstrated that the antimicrobial peptide tachyplesin interacts with C1q protein and activates the classical complement pathway. Generally, the classical pathway is initiated as a consequence of recognition by C1q of IgGs or IgMs in complex with their antigens. However, tachyplesin seems to activate the complement system independently of antibodies [19]. Since arenicin structurally resembles tachyplesin and interacts with C1q [22], a similar action of this peptide on the complement system was expected.

It is commonly accepted that antibody sensitized E^{sh} stimulates the classical pathway of the complement system and activation via the alternative pathway is insignificant, whereas E^{rab} hemolysis is a model for alternative pathway investigations. However, we observed a stimulating action of arenicin-1 in both hemolytic models, though it was expressed mainly in lysis level in the case of E^{sh}, and in C3a production in the case of E^{rab}. Unexpectedly, at high doses (80–160 μg/mL) arenicin displayed reverse effects, essentially diminishing lysis level and C3a generation, in both experimental systems. Apparently, high doses of arenicin inhibit both the classical and alternative pathways, and the latter cannot be explained by the interaction of arenicin with C1q. Instead, the inhibitory effect of arenicin must be related to the action on the common point of both pathways, i.e., C3 cleavage. Most likely, this is the interaction of arenicin with C3 protein leading to its protection from cleavage, although interactions of arenicin with C3-convertases are also possible.

There are three types of C3-convertases: C4b2a, a common C3-convertase of classical and lectin pathways; C3(H$_2$O)Bb generated at spontaneous 'tick-over' activation of the complement cascade by the alternative pathway; C3bBb, a convertase of the 'amplification loop' of the complement system, also usually considered as part of the alternative pathway. The tick-over C3-convertase is an exclusively fluid phase enzyme, while the other two could be covalently bound to the surface of a target cell [23]. Our results imply that arenicin-1 is able to inhibit C3 cleavage by all these convertases.

It is more difficult to explain stimulating effects of arenicin on the complement system at relatively low concentrations. It could be assumed that interaction of arenicin with C1q can lead both to antibody-independent classical pathway activation (as it was described for tachyplesin [19]) and to accelerated antibody-dependent complement activation. These two types of action could be reflected in experiments with E^{rab} (not treated with antibodies) and sensitized E^{sh}, respectively. In the case of using E^{sh}, arenicin interacts with C1q near the cell surface because C1q is bound to antibodies to surface antigens. On the other hand, C1q remains in the fluid phase in the E^{rab} model, and most C3b generated by classical pathway C3-convertase will not be attached to the erythrocyte surface. Thus, both classical pathway and amplification loop C3-convertases locate mainly in a fluid phase where they are highly unstable [21,23], and do not turn to C5-convertases. This could be a reason why there is no visible effect on lysis. However, this interpretation is in contradiction with use of Ca^{2+}-free buffer for E^{rab} hemolysis, which is not compatible with the classical pathway activation. Thus, stimulating effects of arenicin on the complement system remain enigmatic, at least for E^{rab} hemolysis assay.

While the antimicrobial peptide tachyplesin-1 was shown to activate the classical complement pathway [19], we described here that structurally similar arenicin-1 is able to activate or inhibit the complement system at different doses in two experimental models, corresponding to classical and alternative pathways of complement system activation. It is not clear whether these differences in mode of action reflect structural differences of the two peptides, or if they could be explained by different assay types. Further experiments are required to compare the effects of arenicin and tachyplesin directly.

The ability of arenicin-1 to act as a potent complement system inhibitor makes it a prospective molecular source for the design of novel therapeutics directed to the complement system. Currently, the almost complete lack of therapeutic agents that regulate the level of complement activation is a serious medical problem. When hyperactivated, the complement system is perhaps the most dangerous pro-inflammatory and cytotoxic machinery in the human body. The complement system plays a significant role in the pathogenesis of a number of diseases, including age-related macular degeneration, paroxysmal nocturnal hemoglobinuria, hereditary angioedema, and some kidney diseases such as atypical hemolytic uremic syndrome and membranoproliferative glomerulonephritis type II [24–27]. In addition, the complement system and its components are involved in the development and course of autoimmune pathological processes such as systemic lupus erythematosus, rheumatoid arthritis, autoimmune hemolytic anemia; neurodegenerative and neoplastic diseases; and also complications after heart attacks, strokes and transplantations. Existing therapy for diseases connected with complement dysregulation is very expensive, and unavailable for the majority of patients.

Our results indicate that at low concentrations arenicin-1 acts differently on the complement system, depending on the presence of antibodies detecting target cells. Although we described this action as complement activation in both cases, fluid phase C3 conversion could be regarded as a kind of complement inhibition, since the C3 pool becomes depleted (C3 consumption). However, the host cells could also be targets of the complement system, for example in the case of autoimmune disorders. Moreover, C3a, a moderate anaphylatoxin, is produced due to fluid phase C3 conversion, which can induce some proinflammatory effects [28,29]. If one would like to escape these side-effects and obtain a "pure" complement inhibitor based on arenicin, there is a need for an arenicin derivative devoid of its stimulating activity on C3 conversion at low doses, but retaining the ability to protect C3 from cleavage at higher doses.

Arenicin-1 is known as a hemolytic peptide for human erythrocytes [8]. It could be expected to be a complication when using hemolytic assays for studying arenicin action on the complement system. However, as it was described above, no direct hemolytic action of arenicin was observed in our experiments. As we observed in human erythrocytes, supplementing buffer with gelatin is enough to reduce significantly the hemolytic activity of arenicin-1 (unpublished data). Presumably, gelatin presence is also the reason for the resistance of sheep and rabbit erythrocytes to arenicin in our experiments. Alternatively, serum components could protect erythrocytes from the lytic action of arenicin. It cannot be excluded that complement proteins are those serum components inhibiting the hemolytic action of arenicin, and thus, the complement system in turn can modulate the activity of arenicin. In any case, we cannot exclude the interaction of arenicin with erythrocyte membrane, which can influence the rate of erythrocyte lysis by MAC.

In conclusion, we revealed that arenicin-1 is able to both activate and inhibit the complement system in utilized test models in vitro. Our results imply that arenicin can be considered as the basis for the development of a new therapeutic drug for complement system modulation. In addition, the ability of arenicin to interact with the complement system should be taken into account in attempts to create novel antibiotic drugs derived from its structure. The presented observations should be treated as initial results due to the application of relatively simple methods of analysis of the complement system activation. The assays were conducted only with diluted serum, which is not physiologically relevant. In vivo tests on an animal model were not conducted. Further investigations are required to clarify mechanisms of arenicin action on the complement system, and its feasibility under in vivo conditions.

4. Materials and Methods

4.1. Peptides

Arenicin-1 was synthesized based on the standard 9-fluorenylmethoxycarbonyl (Fmoc) protocol with the *O*-(benzotriazol-1-yl)-*N,N,N′,N′*-tetramethyluronium tetrafluoroborate/*N,N*-diisopropylethylamine (TBTU/DIEA) activation, using Wang-resin as the solid-phase and triphenylmethyl protecting groups for cysteines, as described previously [7]. Human C3a was kindly provided by Dr. A.M. Ischenko (Research Institute of Highly Pure Biopreparations, Saint Petersburg, Russia).

4.2. Serum and Erythrocytes

Normal human serum (NHS) was collected by medical staff (Laboratory of Viral Infections Diagnostics, Department of Clinical Microbiology, Pavlov First Saint Petersburg State Medical University) from more than 20 healthy volunteers, pooled, aliquoted, and stored at $-70\,^{\circ}$C no longer than two months. Serum aliquots were thawed at $4\,^{\circ}$C in the day of the experiment, kept in ice baths before introducing to test tubes, and were not used repetitively. To obtain serum with an inactivated complement system, it was incubated at $56\,^{\circ}$C for an hour immediately before the experiment.

Animal erythrocytes were purified from whole blood of rabbit and sheep. They were stored in Alsever's solution at $4\,^{\circ}$C for no more than 5 days. Before use, they were washed with an appropriate buffer: DGVB^{++} (dextrose gelatin veronal buffer with Ca^{2+} and Mg^{2+}) for sheep erythrocytes (E^{sh}), and GVB$^+$ (gelatin veronal buffer with Mg^{2+}) for rabbit erythrocytes (E^{rab}). DGVB^{++} is a 2.5 mM sodium barbital buffer containing 71 mM NaCl, 150 mM glucose, 1 mM MgCl$_2$, 0.15 mM CaCl$_2$, 0.05% gelatin; pH 7.35. GVB$^+$ is a 2.5 mM sodium barbital buffer containing 150 mM NaCl, 10 mM Mg-EGTA, 0.05% gelatin; pH 7.35. Before experiments, sheep erythrocytes were sensitized with antibodies (anti-sheep red blood cell stroma antibodies produced in rabbits, S1389, Sigma, St. Louis, MO, USA); we used a 1:1600 dilution of these antibodies and incubated sheep red blood cells for 30 min at $37\,^{\circ}$C.

4.3. Hemolytic Assays

Hemolytic functional assays were performed utilizing erythrocytes (E^{sh} and E^{rab}) as target cells as described elsewhere [30], with some modifications. Sensitized sheep erythrocytes were used for evaluation of complement activation via the classical pathway; to measure the activity of alternative pathway, rabbit erythrocytes were used.

Experimental samples contained erythrocytes, diluted NHS as a source of complement proteins, and arenicin at different concentrations. For the classical pathway assay, E^{sh} were introduced to a final concentration of 5×10^8 cells per mL, serum was diluted to 1%, and DGVB^{++} was used to dilute all the components. For the alternative pathway assay, there were 2.5×10^8 cells per mL of E^{rab}, 4% NHS, and GVB^+. Some samples contained no serum and were used further as a blank. Inactivated serum was also used to control the effect of arenicin on erythrocytes in the absence of an active complement system.

The incubation was carried out for half an hour at 37 °C. After the incubation, the lysis of the erythrocytes was stopped by the addition of PBS (phosphate buffered saline, pH 7.4) in a ratio of 1:7.5. To some test tubes, distilled water was added instead of buffer, and thus samples were obtained with 100% lysis. Samples were centrifuged at $500 \times g$ for 5 min at room temperature, and then hemoglobin was determined in supernatants by measuring the optical density at 414 nm (OD_{414}) in a microplate reader (Multiskan MS, Labsystems, Vantaa, Finland). After measurement, the samples were used for C3a determination by ELISA.

4.4. C3a Determination by ELISA

4.4.1. Monoclonal Antibodies for C3a

For the immunization of F2-hybrid mice, 0.5 mg of C3a peptide in 1 mL of PBS was mixed with equal volume of Freund's complete adjuvant (or Freund's incomplete adjuvant for reimmunization). The reimmunization was carried out after 30 days; 12 days after that, the lymphocytes from the inguinal, peritoneal and axillary lymph nodes were collected for hybridization with Sp2/0 myeloma cells in the ratio 2:1. Cell hybridization was performed in PEG/DMSO (Sigma), using serial dilution with culture media [31]. The hybrids were transferred to 96-well culture plates, and cultivated for 12–16 days in RPMI-1640 medium (Sigma) containing 20% fetal calf serum. The HAT supplement (Sigma) was added to the culture medium solution for selection of hybridomas.

Clone screening was performed using ELISA in a 96-well microplate. Briefly, 50 µL of culture media was added to wells precoated with C3a antigen, and after incubation for 1 h, peroxidase-conjugated goat anti-mouse IgGs were added. Detection was performed with 3,3′,5,5′-tetramethylbenzidine (TMB) substrate solution.

For C3a ELISA development, two monoclonal murine antibodies to C3a, with different epitope specificities designated as CC3a-5 and CC3a-1, were selected. CC3a-5 was immobilized on a solid phase as a capture antibody, while CC3a-1 was conjugated with horseradish peroxidase and was used as a detection antibody.

4.4.2. ELISA System for C3a

ELISA for C3a was performed in 96-well microplates. Wells of a microplate were coated with capture antibodies and blocked by 1% BSA in PBS, pH 7.2. The same BSA solution was used as diluent on subsequent steps. Ten-fold diluted experimental samples and calibration samples were introduced to the wells, after which the plates were incubated for 1 h at 37 °C. Then, 100 µL of peroxidase-conjugated detection antibodies were added to each well. After incubation for 1 h at 37 °C, the TMB substrate solution (Xema Co. Ltd., Moscow, Russia) was added. After 15–20 min, the reaction was stopped by adding sulfuric acid, and the absorbance at 450 nm was measured in a microplate reader (Multiscan MS, Labsystems).

4.5. Statistical Analysis

Statistical significance of the values was evaluated by paired *t*-test using the software package STATISTICA (version 7.0, TIBCO Software Inc., Palo Alto, CA, USA). All of the experiments were repeated five times. All data are presented as mean $\pm$ standard deviation (SD). Pearson coefficients were calculated and used for evaluation of the correlation level between C3a concentration and percentage of lysed cells. For both tests, *p*-values of less than 0.05 were considered statistically significant.

Author Contributions: M.N.B. conceived and designed this study; N.P.G. and A.V.Z. developed the ELISA system for C3a; E.S.U. and I.A.K. performed the experiments; M.N.B. and E.S.U. analyzed the data and wrote the paper; T.V.O. and V.N.K. analyzed all the experimental data, revised the manuscript critically, and prepared it for publication.

Funding: This work was supported by the Russian Science Foundation (Project No. 14-50-00131).

Acknowledgments: We thank A.M. Ischenko (Research Institute of Highly Pure Biopreparations, Saint Petersburg) for providing C3a peptide, and colleagues from the Laboratory of Viral Infections Diagnostics, Department of Clinical Microbiology, Pavlov First Saint Petersburg State Medical University, for assistance in human serum collecting.

Conflicts of Interest: The authors declare no conflicts of interest.

References

1. Lazcano-Pérez, F.; Román-González, S.A.; Sánchez-Puig, N.; Arreguin-Espinosa, R. Bioactive peptides from marine organisms: A short overview. *Prot. Pept. Lett.* **2012**, *19*, 700–707. [CrossRef]
2. Ovchinnikova, T.V.; Aleshina, G.M.; Balandin, S.V.; Krasnosdembskaya, A.D.; Markelov, M.L.; Frolova, E.I.; Leonova, Y.F.; Tagaev, A.A.; Krasnodembsky, E.G.; Kokryakov, V.N. Purification and primary structure of two isoforms of arenicin, a novel antimicrobial peptide from marine polychaeta *Arenicola marina*. *FEBS Lett.* **2004**, *577*, 209–214. [CrossRef] [PubMed]
3. Sandvang, D.; Kristensen, H.-H.; Neve, S. Arenicin-3: A novel antimicrobial peptide showing potent in vitro activity against gram-negative multi-resistant clinical isolates. In Proceedings of the 46th Annual Meeting Infectious Diseases Society of America, Washington, DC, USA, 24–28 October 2008; p. F1-3986.
4. Andrä, J.; Jakovkin, I.; Grötzinger, J.; Hecht, O.; Krasnosdembskaya, A.D.; Goldmann, T.; Gutsmann, T.; Leippe, M. Structure and mode of action of the antimicrobial peptide arenicin. *Biochem. J.* **2008**, *410*, 113–122. [CrossRef] [PubMed]
5. Ovchinnikova, T.V.; Shenkarev, Z.O.; Balandin, S.V.; Nadezhdin, K.D.; Paramonov, A.S.; Kokryakov, V.N.; Arseniev, A.S. Molecular insight into mechanism of antimicrobial action of the β-hairpin peptide arenicin: Specific oligomerization in detergent micelles. *Biopolymers* **2008**, *89*, 455–464. [CrossRef] [PubMed]
6. Maltseva, A.L.; Kotenko, O.N.; Kokryakov, V.N.; Starunov, V.V.; Krasnodembskaya, A.D. Expression pattern of arenicins—The antimicrobial peptides of polychaete *Arenicola marina*. *Front. Physiol.* **2014**, *5*, 497–503. [CrossRef]
7. Ovchinnikova, T.V.; Shenkarev, Z.O.; Nadezhdin, K.D.; Balandin, S.V.; Zhmak, M.N.; Kudelina, I.A.; Finkina, E.I.; Kokryakov, V.N.; Arseniev, A.S. Recombinant expression, synthesis, purification, and solution structure of arenicin. *Biochem. Biophys. Res. Commun.* **2007**, *360*, 156–162. [CrossRef] [PubMed]
8. Lee, J.U.; Kang, D.I.; Zhu, W.L.; Shin, S.Y.; Hahm, K.S.; Kim, Y. Solution structures and biological functions of the antimicrobial peptide, arenicin-1, and its linear derivative. *Pept. Sci.* **2007**, *88*, 208–216. [CrossRef]
9. Andrä, J.; Hammer, M.U.; Grötzinger, J.; Jakovkin, I.; Lindner, B.; Vollmer, E.; Fedders, H.; Leippe, M.; Gutsmann, T. Significance of the cyclic structure and of arginine residues for the antibacterial activity of arenicin-1 and its interaction with phospholipid and lipopolysaccharide model membranes. *Biol. Chem.* **2009**, *390*, 337–349. [CrossRef]
10. Shenkarev, Z.O.; Balandin, S.V.; Trunov, K.I.; Paramonov, A.S.; Sukhanov, S.V.; Barsukov, L.I.; Arseniev, A.S.; Ovchinnikova, T.V. Molecular mechanism of action of β-hairpin antimicrobial peptide arenicin: Oligomeric structure in dodecylphosphocholine micelles and pore formation in planar lipid bilayers. *Biochemistry* **2011**, *50*, 6255–6265. [CrossRef]
11. Panteleev, P.V.; Bolosov, I.A.; Balandin, S.V.; Ovchinnikova, T.V. Design of antimicrobial peptide arenicin analogs with improved therapeutic indices. *J. Pept. Sci.* **2015**, *21*, 105–113. [CrossRef]
12. Panteleev, P.V.; Bolosov, I.A.; Ovchinnikova, T.V. Bioengineering and functional characterization of arenicin shortened analogs with enhanced antibacterial activity and cell selectivity. *J. Pept. Sci.* **2016**, *22*, 82–91. [CrossRef]
13. Wang, X.; Wang, X.; Teng, D.; Zhang, Y.; Mao, R.; Xi, D.; Wang, J. Candidacidal mechanism of the arenicin-3-derived peptide NZ17074 from *Arenicola marina*. *Appl. Microbiol. Biotechnol.* **2014**, *98*, 7387–7398. [CrossRef]
14. Yang, N.; Liu, X.; Ten, D.; Li, Z.; Wang, X.; Mao, R.; Wang, X.; Hao, Y.; Wang, J. Antibacterial and detoxifying activity of NZ17074 analogues with multi-layers of selective antimicrobial actions against *Escherichia coli* and *Salmonella enteritidis*. *Sci. Rep.* **2017**, *7*, 3392. [CrossRef]

15. Nakamura, T.; Furunaka, H.; Miyata, T.; Tokunaga, F.; Muta, T.; Iwanaga, S.; Niwa, M.; Takao, T.; Shimonishi, Y. Tachyplesin, a class of antimicrobial peptide from the hemocytes of the horseshoe crab (*Tachypleus tridentatus*). Isolation and chemical structure. *J. Biol. Chem.* **1988**, *263*, 16709–16713.

16. Miyata, T.; Tokunaga, F.; Yoneya, T.; Yoshikawa, K.; Iwanaga, S.; Niwa, M.; Takao, T.; Shimonishi, Y. Antimicrobial peptides, isolated from horseshoe crab hemocytes, tachyplesin II, and polyphemusins I and II: Chemical structures and biological activity. *J. Biochem.* **1989**, *106*, 663–668. [CrossRef]

17. Berlov, M.N.; Maltseva, A.L. Immunity of the lugworm *Arenicola marina*: Cells and molecules. *Invertebr. Surviv. J.* **2016**, *13*, 247–256.

18. Shigenaga, T.; Muta, T.; Toh, Y.; Tokunaga, F.; Iwanaga, S. Antimicrobial tachyplesin peptide precursor. cDNA cloning and cellular localization in the horseshoe crab (*Tachypleus tridentatus*). *J. Biol. Chem.* **1990**, *265*, 21350–21354.

19. Chen, J.; Xu, X.M.; Underhill, C.B.; Yang, S.; Wang, L.; Chen, Y.; Hong, S.; Creswell, K.; Zhang, L. Tachyplesin activates the classic complement pathway to kill tumor cells. *Cancer Res.* **2005**, *65*, 4614–4622. [CrossRef]

20. Ricklin, D.; Hajishengallis, G.; Yang, K.; Lambris, J.D. Complement: A key system for immune surveillance and homeostasis. *Nat. Immunol.* **2010**, *11*, 785–797. [CrossRef]

21. Merle, N.S.; Church, S.E.; Fremeaux-Bacchi, V.; Roumenina, L.T. Complement system part I—Molecular mechanisms of activation and regulation. *Front. Immunol.* **2015**, *6*, 262. [CrossRef]

22. Berlov, M.N.; Umnyakova, E.S.; Leonova, T.S.; Milman, B.L.; Krasnodembskaya, A.D.; Ovchinnikova, T.V.; Kokryakov, V.N. Interaction of arenicin-1 with C1q protein. *Russ. J. Bioorg. Chem.* **2015**, *41*, 597–601. [CrossRef]

23. Ricklin, D.; Reis, E.S.; Mastellos, D.C.; Gros, P.; Lambris, J.D. Complement component C3—The "Swiss Army Knife" of innate immunity and host defense. *Immunol. Rev.* **2016**, *274*, 33–58. [CrossRef]

24. Zipfel, P.F. Complement and immune defense: From innate immunity to human diseases. *Immunol. Lett.* **2009**, *126*, 1–7. [CrossRef]

25. Ricklin, D.; Lambris, J.D. Complement in immune and inflammatory disorders: Pathophysiological mechanisms. *J. Immunol.* **2013**, *190*, 3831–3838. [CrossRef]

26. Liszewski, M.K.; Java, A.; Schramm, E.C.; Atkinson, J.P. Complement dysregulation and disease: Insights from contemporary genetics. *Annu. Rev. Pathol.* **2017**, *12*, 25–52. [CrossRef]

27. Wong, E.K.S.; Kavanagh, D. Diseases of complement dysregulation—An overview. *Semin. Immunopathol.* **2018**, *40*, 49–64. [CrossRef]

28. Klos, A.; Tenner, A.J.; Johswich, K.O.; Ager, R.R.; Reis, E.S.; Köhl, J. The role of the anaphylatoxins in health and disease. *Mol. Immunol.* **2009**, *46*, 2753–2766. [CrossRef]

29. Sacks, S.H. Complement fragments C3a and C5a: The salt and pepper of the immune response. *Eur. J. Immunol.* **2010**, *40*, 668–670. [CrossRef]

30. Roos, A.; Nauta, A.J.; Broers, D.; Faber-Krol, M.C.; Trouw, L.A.; Drijfhout, J.W.; Daha, M.R. Specific inhibition of the classical complement pathway by C1q-binding peptides. *J. Immunol.* **2001**, *167*, 7052–7059. [CrossRef]

31. Kohler, G.; Milstein, C. Continuous cultures of fused cells secreting antibody of predefined specificity. *Nature* **1975**, *256*, 495–497. [CrossRef]

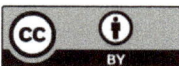

marine drugs

MDPI

Article

Novel Antimicrobial Peptides from the Arctic Polychaeta *Nicomache minor* Provide New Molecular Insight into Biological Role of the BRICHOS Domain

Pavel V. Panteleev *, Andrey V. Tsarev, Ilia A. Bolosov, Alexander S. Paramonov, Mariana B. Marggraf, Sergey V. Sychev, Zakhar O. Shenkarev and Tatiana V. Ovchinnikova

M.M. Shemyakin & Yu.A. Ovchinnikov Institute of Bioorganic Chemistry, the Russian Academy of Sciences, Miklukho-Maklaya str. 16/10, 117997 Moscow, Russia; 79175492709@yandex.ru (A.V.T.); b_off2@mail.ru (I.A.B.); apar@nmr.ru (A.S.P.); thpcb92@mail.ru (M.B.M.); svs@ibch.ru (S.V.S.); zakhar-shenkarev@yandex.ru (Z.O.S.); ovch@ibch.ru (T.V.O.)
* Correspondence: alarm14@gmail.com; Tel.: +7-495-335-09-00

Received: 30 September 2018; Accepted: 20 October 2018; Published: 23 October 2018

Abstract: Endogenous antimicrobial peptides (AMPs) are among the earliest molecular factors in the evolution of animal innate immunity. In this study, novel AMPs named nicomicins were identified in the small marine polychaeta *Nicomache minor* in the Maldanidae family. Full-length mRNA sequences encoded 239-residue prepropeptides consisting of a putative signal sequence region, the BRICHOS domain within an acidic proregion, and 33-residue mature cationic peptides. Nicomicin-1 was expressed in the bacterial system, and its spatial structure was analyzed by circular dichroism and nuclear magnetic resonance spectroscopy. Nicomicins are unique among polychaeta AMPs scaffolds, combining an amphipathic *N*-terminal α-helix and *C*-terminal extended part with a six-residue loop stabilized by a disulfide bridge. This structural arrangement resembles the Rana-box motif observed in the α-helical host-defense peptides isolated from frog skin. Nicomicin-1 exhibited strong in vitro antimicrobial activity against Gram-positive bacteria at submicromolar concentrations. The main mechanism of nicomicin-1 action is based on membrane damage but not on the inhibition of bacterial translation. The peptide possessed cytotoxicity against cancer and normal adherent cells as well as toward human erythrocytes.

Keywords: antimicrobial peptide; polychaeta; innate immunity; BRICHOS domain; recombinant peptide; α-helix; Rana-box; nuclear magnetic resonance (NMR)

1. Introduction

Endogenous antimicrobial peptides (AMPs), also known as host-defense peptides (HDPs), are among the most ancient molecular components of the innate immunity system that contribute to the first line of defense against pathogens of most life forms [1]. The complex membrane-targeting mechanism of their antimicrobial action and the ability to rapidly kill pathogens prevent the evolution of resistance to AMPs. Some AMPs inhibit a number of metabolic processes via interaction with intracellular targets [2]. Marine invertebrate animals have no acquired immunity and lack a system of antibody diversification. They live in a microbe-laden environment and use AMP-based defense against potential pathogens. Polychaeta is a largely unexplored class of invertebrates in the context of discovery of new AMPs. The large majority of polychaeta species are marine animals that inhabit all places, from the Arctic to the Antarctic, and from the littoral zone to the deepest depths of the oceans. They are considered the most primitive annelids, based on morphology, physiology, and development [3]. To date, AMPs have been identified in several species of polychaetes: 21-residue β-hairpin arenicins from *Arenicola marina* [4,5], 51-residue perinerin from *Perinereis aibuhitensis* [6], 22-residue α-helical hedistin from *Nereis diversicolor* [7], and 22-residue β-hairpin alvinellacin from *Alvinella pompejana* [8]. These AMPs are predominantly expressed in coelomocytes and therefore actively participate in cellular immunity. Notably, all the peptides were directly isolated from comparatively large polychaeta. Also, a putative β-hairpin antimicrobial peptide, designated capitellacin, was predicted based on the genome data of polychaeta *Capitella teleta* [8].

Here, we report novel AMPs, named nicomicin-1 and -2, found in the small polychaeta *Nicomache minor* (the Maldanidae family, Figure S1). The peptides were found under the project aimed at searching for novel AMPs from marine animals that dwell in the White Sea, a part of Arctic Ocean. *N. minor* is a benthic polychaeta widespread in the North Atlantic, North Pacific, and Arctic regions at depths of up to 100 m. *N. minor* permanently lives in cold water in massive hard tubes attached to stones [9], which is fundamentally different from the Arenicolidae and Capitellidae families that have borrowing and mobile lifestyles and thermotolerant *Alvinella pompejana* that dwells in active deep-sea hydrothermal vents. Nicomicin-1 has a unique spatial structure compared to other polychaeta AMPs. The peptide adopts an *N*-terminal α-helix and *C*-terminal extended part, bearing a loop stabilized by a disulfide bridge. Surprisingly, this structure resembles those of amphibian host-defense peptides having the Rana-box motif. The propiece of nicomicin precursor includes the BRICHOS domain, which is known to participate in the complex post-translational processing of proteins and possesses anti-amyloid chaperone activity [10]. The BRICHOS domain has been described in polychaeta only as precursor of β-hairpin AMPs. Therefore, the obtained results reveal that the BRICHOS domain could participate in the biosynthesis of different structural types of polychaeta AMPs. The identification procedure, structural organization of the precursor protein, spatial structure, biological activities, and structure-functional analysis of nicomicin-1 are described in this paper.

2. Results and Discussion

2.1. Nicomicin Is a Novel BRICHOS Domain-Related AMP

There are a number of methods for searching for novel AMPs: direct peptide isolation from tissues and cells, whole genome and/or transcriptome sequencing followed by bioinformatic analysis, cloning of cDNA amplified by primers targeting for conserved regions. The latter, in particular, is used to identify novel cathelicidins due to the high homology of cathelin-like domains (CLDs) among vertebrate species [11]. Direct peptide isolation of AMPs is a challenge due to the labor-consuming process of catching small solitary animals. A weak sequence homology between known polychaeta AMPs makes it difficult to identify novel peptides by sequence similarity-based methods. The BRICHOS domain is found in precursor proteins of β-hairpin antimicrobial peptides of polychaetes. So far, this domain has been reported for precursors of five AMPs: arenicin-1 and -2 [4], arenicin-3 also known as NZ17000 [12], alvinellacin [8], and capitellacin [8]. In contrast with the CLD, the sequence homology of the BRICHOS domain is quite low among polychaetes. The high variability of the BRICHOS domain sequences, even within a single species, may be associated with an adaptation mechanism enabling the correct biosynthesis of β-hairpin peptides in certain environments [13].

In this study, the rapid amplification of cDNA ends (RACE) approach was implemented to identify novel BRICHOS-related peptides using *N. minor* cDNA and degenerate gene-specific primers (GSP, Table 1) that anneal to sequences with the highest primary structure homology among the BRICHOS domains of precursors of polychaeta AMPs (arenicin-1, arenicin-3, capitellacin, alvinellacin), specifically to sequences within two regions near conservative Cys residues (Figure 1A and Figure S2). One-round 3′RACE with any degenerate GSP and the universal adaptor-specific mix (step-out primer mix) failed to amplify fragments of interest. Therefore, two-round nested PCR was performed. Cloning and sequencing of 3′RACE products (Figure 1B), approximately 800 bp in length, revealed the sequence coding for the *C*-terminus of the BRICHOS domain, a putative mature AMP, and the 3′ untranslated region (3′UTR) of its cDNA. The 3′UTR length was found to be similar in several analyzed clones. Notably, two tandem repeats were found within the 3′UTR. This information was considered when designing 5′RACE GSPs. A 5′RACE (Figure 1C) using antisense GSPs annealing 3′UTR and adaptor primers provided sequence data extending to the 5′-end of the transcript.

Table 1. Oligonucleotide primer sequences.

Primer Name	Sequence 5′→3′
3′-GSP1	GTGTTACGTCATGGGTGG(G,C)(G,C)T(G,T)GAC
3′-GSP2	GAGTGCTAC(T,C)TG(A,G)TCGG(A,C)GG
3′-GSP3	TGC(G,T,C)AGGG(A,C)AA(A,G)CCTGT(C,T)TTCTGG(A,C)T
5′-GSP1	GTGGTCAATGAATATCTGCAATACA
5′-GSP2	GAGCTTATACCCATAGGGCTTCCTTATAC
5′-GSP3	ATTAAGAACGTTGTCCAAAGCGTAATG
AP	GTTGATCCGACAGTCGCTTGC

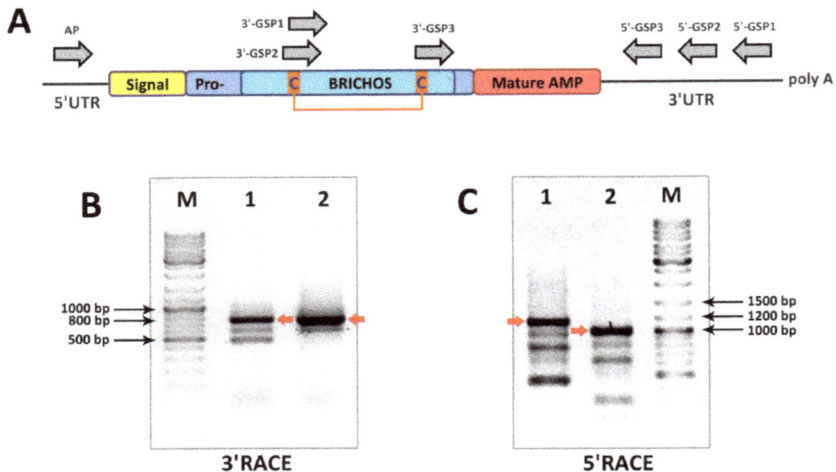

Figure 1. Rapid amplification of cDNA ends (RACE) analysis and identification of BRICHOS-related peptides in cDNA of *Nicomache minor*. (**A**) Scheme of prepronicomicin mRNA and primer annealing sites. Two rounds of step-out polymerase chain reaction (PCR) using nested gene-specific primers (GSP) were performed for both 3′RACE and 5′RACE. First round of 3′RACE was performed separately using 3′-GSP1 or 3′-GSP2 and step-out primer mix1. Then, diluted products were used in the second round with 3′-GSP3 and step-out primer mix2. The PCR products of the second round of 3′RACE were visualized by agarose gel electrophoresis: (**B**) M—marker; 1—3′-GSP1/3′-GSP3 product; and 2—3′-GSP2/3′-GSP3 product. The target bands are marked with red arrows. The first round of 5′RACE was performed with 5′-GSP1 and step-out primer mix1. Then diluted products were used in the second round using 5′-GSP2 or 5′-GSP3 and step-out primer mix2. The PCR products of the second round of 5′RACE were visualized by agarose gel electrophoresis: (**C**) M—marker; 1—5′-GSP1/5′-GSP2 product; 2—5′-GSP1/5′-GSP3 product. The one-round amplification of whole prepronicomicin coding sequence was then performed using AP and 5′-GSP2 primers.

The full-length mRNA sequence included a 720-bp open reading frame encoding a 239-residue prepropeptide consisting of a putative 22-residue signal sequence region, a proregion with the dibasic propeptide cleavage site, and the last 33 residues constituting the mature cationic peptide (Figure S3). Sequence analysis with the use of SignalP 4.1 (Figure 2) pointed out the Gly22-Leu23 bond as the most probable cleavage site for eukaryotic signal peptidase. The Glu-Lys-Lys motif preceding a putative propeptide cleavage site of nicomicin indicated that a precursor is probably activated by a subtilisin-like proprotein convertase [14]. More specifically, the kexin/furin family of proteases recognizes such dibasic sites—typically Arg-Arg or Lys-Arg and less frequently Arg-Lys, Lys-Lys, or Arg-X-X-Arg.

This is a common feature for other BRICHOS-related AMPs (Figure 2). The Glu-Lys-Lys site was found to be a specific substrate for serine protease ASP, a putative virulence factor of the Gram-negative facultative anaerobic bacterium *Aeromonas sobria* [15]. This bacterium is known to cause infections of marine animals, and the nicomicin propeptide cleavage by proteases of invading pathogens (or epibionts) cannot be excluded.

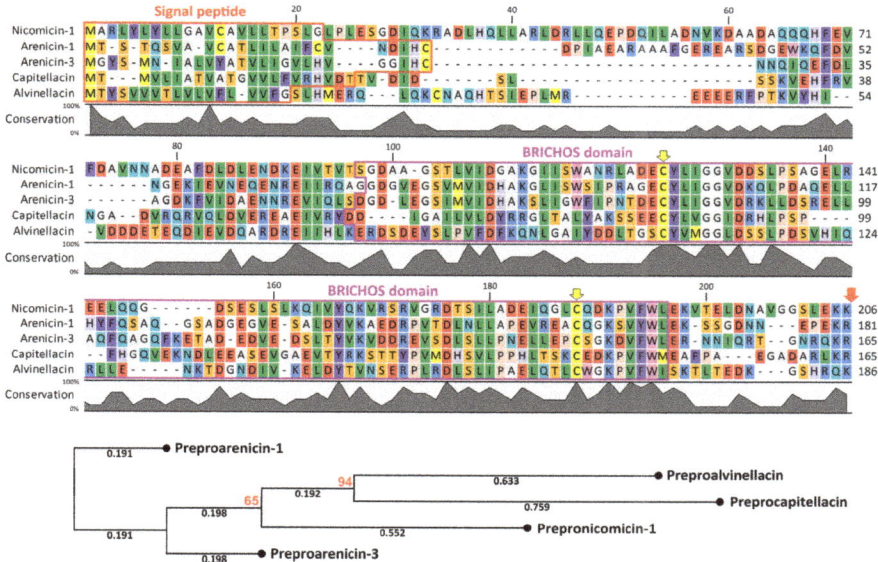

Figure 2. Amino acid sequence alignment and a neighbor-joining phylogenetic tree of the precursors without mature peptides of nicomicin-1, arenicin-1, arenicin-3, capitellacin, and alvinellacin. The alignment and phylogenetic tree were constructed using CLC Sequence Viewer software (version 8.0). Bootstrap values >50 are presented at the nodes and marked in red. The values were obtained from 1000 replicates. Signal peptide sequence identified with SignalP 4.1 (http://www.cbs.dtu.dk/services/SignalP/) and BRICHOS domain sequence identified with MyHits Motif Scan (https://myhits.isb-sib.ch/cgi-bin/motif_scan) are highlighted with red and purple boxes, respectively. The conservative cysteine residues in BRICHOS domain are marked with yellow arrows. Putative post-translational processing sites are marked with a red arrow.

A number of clones were analyzed after one-round amplification of the whole prepronicomicin nucleotide sequence with the use of 5′-GSP2 and the designed AP primer annealing to the 5′UTR. As the result, the 5′-terminal part of cDNA coding for the second isoform (named nicomicin-2) was found. This isoform has a single amino acid substitution, K19R. The precursor of nicomicin-2 bears three amino acid substitutions (V71E, D99G, and K191N), whereas the 5′UTR has a 6-bp deletion (GTTACA). At the same time, several different transcripts coding nicomicin-1 were identified, and polymorphisms were detected both in the signal sequence and in the propiece. The sequences coding prepronicomicins have been deposited in GenBank with the accession IDs MH898866–MH898867. Similar to known polychaeta AMPs arenicins, alvinellacin, and capitellacin, nicomicins are processed from a larger precursor molecule containing a signal peptide and an anionic proregion that includes the BRICHOS domain. This domain was found in many evolutionary distant animals and performs different functions [16,17]. It is characterized by low amino acid sequence conservation with only two Cys and one Asp residue, which are strictly conserved in all representatives of the BRICHOS superfamily [18]. The BRICHOS domain is known to be a part of proteins associated with different human diseases such as dementia, chondrosarcoma, and respiratory distress syndrome [19]. It participates in the complex post-translational processing of proteins and possesses anti-amyloid chaperone activity [10]. In this study, for the first time, the BRICHOS domain was shown to be a part of a precursor of AMP with a structure different from β-hairpin (Figure 3). Therefore, the BRICHOS domain might be a universal prodomain that participates in the biosynthesis of different types of AMPs in polychaeta, like the cathelin-like domain (CLD) does in vertebrates.

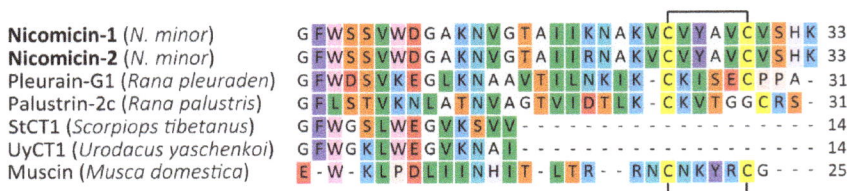

Nicomicin-1 (*N. minor*)	G F W S S V W D G A K N V G T A I I K N A K V C V Y A V C V S H K	33
Nicomicin-2 (*N. minor*)	G F W S S V W D G A K N V G T A I I R N A K V C V Y A V C V S H K	33
Pleurain-G1 (*Rana pleuraden*)	G F W D S V K E G L K N A A V T I L N K I K - C K I S E C P P A -	31
Palustrin-2c (*Rana palustris*)	G F L S T V K N L A T N V A G T V I D T L K - C K V T G G C R S -	31
StCT1 (*Scorpiops tibetanus*)	G F W G S L W E G V K S V V - - - - - - - - - - - - - - - - - - -	14
UyCT1 (*Urodacus yaschenkoi*)	G F W G K L W E G V K N A I - - - - - - - - - - - - - - - - - - -	14
Muscin (*Musca domestica*)	E - W - K L P D L I I N H I T - L T R - - R N C N K Y R C G - - -	25

Figure 3. Amino acid sequence alignment of mature nicomicins with known antimicrobial peptides. The disulfide bonds are marked with square brackets.

2.2. Nicomicin Is Unique Among Polychaeta AMPs but Shares Structural Similarities with Other Animal Host-Defense Peptides

Nicomicin-1 is composed of 33 amino acid residues including four basic Lys, one acidic Asp, and two Cys, forming a disulfide bridge (Figure 3). The nicomicin-1 amphipathic structure (see corresponding section below), as well as amino acid composition with a net positive charge and plenty of hydrophobic residues, suggest antimicrobial potential. A number of invertebrate AMPs containing a single disulfide bond are known: arenicin-1 and -2 from the lugworm *Arenicola marina* [4], thanatin from the spined soldier bug *Podisus maculiventris* [20], muscin from the house fly *Musca domestica* [21], and scarabaecin from the coconut rhinoceros beetle *Oryctes rhinoceros* [22]. Bioinformatic analysis revealed that the mature nicomicins do not share similarity higher than ~43% with any known AMPs listed in different AMP databases. The peptides exhibit the highest homology with amphibian AMPs (Figure 3), in particular, pleurain-G1 from skin secretions of the frog *Rana pleuraden* [23] and palustrin-2c from skin secretions of *Rana palustris* [24]. Despite the weak sequence homology, nicomicins and amphibian AMPs have similar structure organization, including an *N*-terminal amphipathic α-helix and a *C*-terminal extended region containing a disulfide-stabilized loop. This *C*-terminal, motif known as 'Rana-box' (6- or 7-residue loop), has been found in many amphibian AMP families: esculentins, gaegurins, ranalexins, and others [25]. At the same time, nicomicins have fundamentally different molecular organization of AMP precursors [23].

Several peptides of different origins are characterized by the presence of the *N*-terminal loop stabilized by a single disulfide bridge and followed by an α-helix: toxin Oxt 4a from the lynx spider *Oxyopes takobius* [26], bacterial pediocin-like antimicrobial peptides [27], and islet amyloid polypeptides (IAPP, also known as amylin) from vertebrates [28]. Aggregation of IAPP into amyloid fibrils in islets of Langerhans is associated with type 2 diabetes. Interaction of the peptide with the lipid membrane is of particular interest as it increases the rate of peptide aggregation, which can in turn result in membrane disruption [29]. Human IAPP has been shown to possess antibacterial activity with potency dependent on its aggregation states [30]. Notably, the BRICHOS domain of the precursor of the integral membrane protein 2B (Bri2), a transmembrane protein expressed in several peripheral tissues and in the brain, effectively inhibits human IAPP fibril formation in vitro [31]. Therefore, the nicomicin propiece containing the BRICHOS domain could be considered as a polypeptide-binding IAPP. Finally, the *N*-terminal part of nicomicin is significantly homologous with the short α-helical AMPs StCT1 [32] and UyCT1 [33] from venom of the scorpions *Scorpiops tibetanus* and *Urodacus yaschenkoi*, respectively (Figure 3).

2.3. Recombinant Expression and Purification of Nicomicin-1 and Its Fragments

Nicomicin-1 is a hydrophobic peptide (51% of hydrophobic residues) stabilized by one disulfide bridge. Heterologous expression in the bacterial system of the peptide fused with a highly soluble carrier protein was applied for its production. To analyze the antimicrobial potential of the *N*-terminal amphipathic α-helix and the C-terminal extended region containing a disulfide-stabilized loop, the corresponding fragments of nicomicin-1, designated as Nico(1-17) and Nico(18-33), were obtained. In this study, modified thioredoxin A was used as a fusion partner that promoted the correct disulfide bond formation and masked the toxic effects of AMPs. Previously, several frog AMPs bearing Rana-box were obtained in the heterologous *Escherichia coli* expression system [34–36]. A high proportion of a fusion protein in reference to total cell protein was achieved with the use of thioredoxin A or glutathione S-transferase (GST). A final concentration of a fusion protein amounted to at least 1 mg/L. In this study, all the fusion proteins are expressed in *E. coli* BL21 (DE3) cells, and the obtained total cell lysates were fractionated by affinity chromatography. After purification and cleavage of the fusion proteins, reverse-phase high performance liquid chromatography (RP-HPLC) was used to obtain mature recombinant nicomicin-1 and its fragments (Figure 4A).

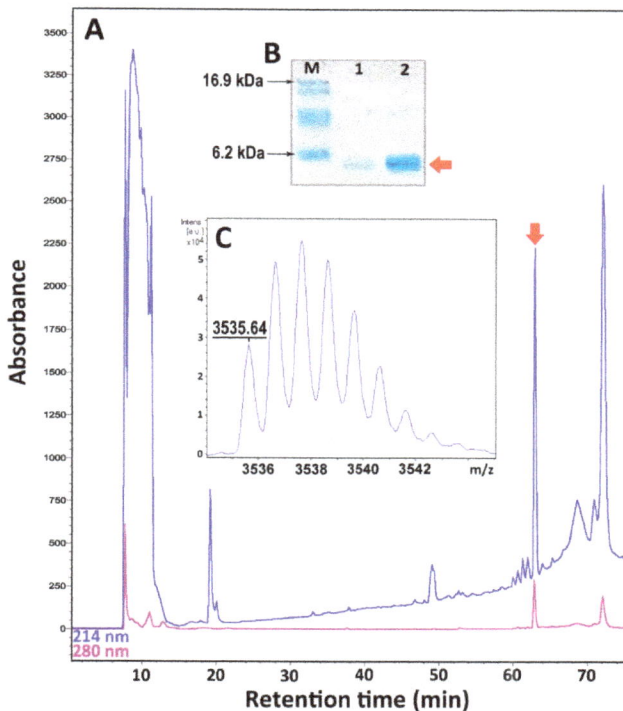

Figure 4. (**A**) Reverse-phase high-performance liquid chromatography (RP-HPLC) purification of the recombinant nicomicin-1. The fraction of recombinant nicomicin-1 is marked with a red arrow. (**B**) Tricine-SDS-polyacrylamide gel electrophoresis (Tricine-SDS-PAGE) of the recombinant nicomicin-1: M—molecular mass marker; 1—recombinant nicomicin-1 (3 µg); 2—recombinant nicomicin-1 (3 µg) boiled with 2-mercaptoethanol. (**C**) MALDI-TOF mass spectrometry analysis of the recombinant nicomicin-1. The experimental [M + H]$^+$ monoisotopic mass is presented in the picture.

Tricine-SDS-polyacrylamide gel electrophoresis (Tricine-SDS-PAGE) revealed that the purified mature nicomicin-1 was expressed as a monomer (Figure 4B). Reduction of the disulfide bond with 2-mercaptoethanol did not alter electrophoretic mobility of the peptide but increased its interaction with Coomassie dye. The peptides were then analyzed by MALDI-TOF mass spectrometry. The calculated $[M + H]^+$ monoisotopic molecular mass corresponding to the amino acid sequence of nicomicin-1 (3537.8 Da) exceeded the measured value (*m/z* 3535.6) by ~2 Da indicating formation of the disulfide bond between Cys24 and Cys29 and the absence of any other modifications (Figure 4C). The experimentally measured *m/z* values of the nicomicin-1 fragments matched the calculated molecular masses (Table 2). The final yields of the fragments were several-fold higher than for wild-type nicomicin-1 (0.9 mg per 1 L of the culture). Notably, induction of nicomicin-1 biosynthesis by isopropyl β-D-1-thiogalactopyranoside (IPTG) resulted in inhibition of *E. coli* BL21 (DE3) growth with a final optical density (OD_{600}) value similar to that at the induction time point. In contrast, four hours after the fragments expression was IPTG-induced, the final OD_{600} increased at least three-fold, which is common for most AMPs according to our observations.

Table 2. Properties of nicomicin-1 and its fragments.

Peptide	RP-HPLC Retention Time [1] (min)	Calculated $[M + H]^+$ Monoisotopic Mass (Da)	Measured Monoisotopic *m/z* Value [2]	Recombinant Peptide Final Yield (mg/L)
Nicomicin-1	63	3535.81 *	3535.64	0.9
Nico(1-17)	56	1794.87	1794.84	6.2
Nico(18-33)	42.5	1759.94 *	1759.97	4.3

[1] Retention times of the peptides on semi-preparative reverse-phase high performance liquid chromatography (HPLC); [2] Molecular masses were determined using MALDI-TOF MS; * assuming two Cys residues form cystine.

Both nicomicin-1 and its fragment Nico(1-17) were extremely hydrophobic, illustrated by the RP-HPLC retention times of 63 and 56 min, respectively. In comparison, the retention time of recombinant tachyplesin-1 (47% of hydrophobic residues) in the same system was 43 min. Both peptides were poorly soluble in water: nicomicin-1 formed visible aggregates at concentrations above 2 mg/mL, whereas Nico(1-17) formed a gel structure at a concentration of 2 mg/mL (Figure S4). Nicomicin-1 did not form oligomers on SDS-PAGE in contrast to arenicins [37]. Gel formation was reported for a range of classical amyloids or amyloid-like polypeptides, in particular for the above-mentioned IAPP [38]. In addition, the amyloid fibril-forming properties were shown for 17-residue α-helical AMP uperin 3.5 isolated from the skin secretions of the Australian toadlet *Uperoleia mjobergii* [39]. The presence of the C-terminal domain in the structure of nicomicin probably reduced the ability of the N-terminal α-helix to aggregate, but did not abolish it.

2.4. Nicomicin-1 Is Disordered in Aqueous Solution but Forms an α-Helical Structure in a Membrane-Mimicking Environment

The structures of nicomicin-1 and its fragments were studied by circular dichroism (CD) spectroscopy. To observe the peptide structure changes upon interaction with lipid bilayers, we used anionic sodium dodecyl sulfate (SDS) and zwitterionic dodecylphosphocholine (DPC) micelles as a membrane-mimicking environment. Similar to lipid bilayers, the micelles have anisotropic properties, and hydrophobic regions of fatty tails are segregated from the polar water solution [40]. In contrast to isotropic mixtures of trifluoroethanol (TFE)/water or chloroform/methanol, the detergent micelles have a lower propensity to distort spatial structures of solubilized proteins or peptides and do not induce the formation of artificial helical structures [41]. As shown in Figure 5, the CD spectra of Nico(18-33) dissolved in water showed a negative peak at 200 nm, which indicated that the peptide mainly adopted a random coil conformation. The addition of micelles resulted in slight structuring of the peptide with the appearance of a weak positive peak at 190 nm. In contrast, the CD spectra of nicomicin-1 and Nico(1-17) in the membrane-mimicking environment showed a strong positive peak at 195 nm, and two negative peaks at 208 and 220 nm, which indicated that the peptides mainly adopted α-helix conformation.

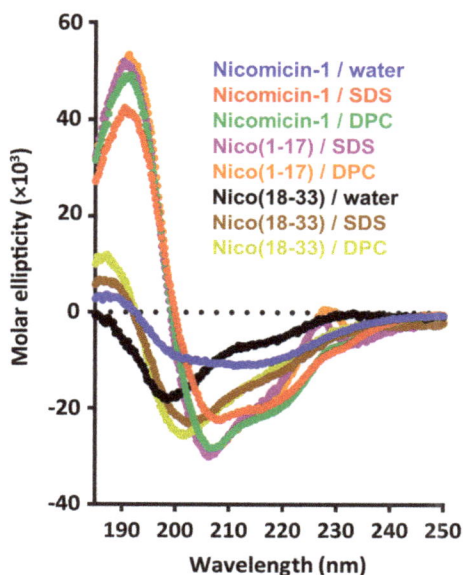

Figure 5. Circular dichroism (CD) spectra of nicomicin-1 and its fragments in water, 30 mM sodium dodecyl sulfate (SDS) micelles, and 30 mM dodecylphosphocholine (DPC) micelles. The spectrum of Nico(1-17) in water was not obtained in this study.

For a detailed investigation of the nicomicin-1 structure, we employed the standard nuclear magnetic resonance (NMR) spectroscopy methods [42]. Complete ^{1}H and partial ^{13}C resonance assignments of the peptide in water were obtained at pH 4.0 and 30 °C. A summary of the obtained NMR data is shown in Figure 6A. The ^{13}C$^\beta$ chemical shifts of Cys24 and Cys29 residues were observed at 37.2 and 40.2 ppm, respectively, which are characteristic for oxidized Cys residues forming a disulfide bond. The small values of the secondary chemical shifts of ^{1}H$^\alpha$ nuclei (-0.07 ppm on average) and lack of medium- and long-range nuclear Overhauser effect (NOE) contacts (data not shown) revealed the absence of defined secondary structure elements in the peptide molecule. This could be the consequence of the enhanced intramolecular mobility of nicomicin-1 in aqueous solution. The measured values of the $^3J_{H^N H^\alpha}$ coupling constants (~7 Hz, Figure 6A) are in agreement with the dynamic switching of the peptide backbone between α- and β-structural conformations. Thus, nicomicin-1 in a water environment adopts a disordered random structure.

It is generally assumed that micelles of anionic detergents, compared to zwitterionic ones, better mimic the negatively charged bacterial membranes. Some of the anionic detergents (e.g., SDS) are well known as harsh denaturing agent, that are able to disrupt tertiary and secondary structures of proteins. The CD data obtained in SDS and DPC solutions revealed that nicomicin-1 is less structured in the SDS micelles (Figure 5, red and green traces, respectively). Therefore, to investigate the spatial structure of nicomicin-1 in a membrane-mimicking environment, we used the zwitterionic DPC micelles solution. An extreme broadening of the nicomicin-1 resonances was observed upon titration of the peptide sample with DPC. The majority of cross-peaks in the amide region of two-dimensional (2D) Total Correlation Spectroscopy (TOCSY) and Nuclear Overhauser effect spectroscopy (NOESY) spectra were broadened beyond the detection limit at detergent to peptide molar ratios (D:P) from 5:1 to 75:1. Further increase in DPC concentration to D:P of 100:1 resulted in the narrowing of the amide proton signals, and cross-peaks in the 2D spectra became visible. The observed resonance broadening is the consequence of the peptide exchange between bulk aqueous phase and the micelles. To minimize the influence of this exchange process, we used a D:P ratio of 200:1 for the structural study. We assumed that at these conditions almost all peptide molecules were in the micelle-bound form. The conditions of NMR measurements were further optimized by varying sample pH and temperature. As a result, we obtained almost complete ^{1}H and partial ^{13}C resonance assignments of the peptide in DPC solution at pH 3.15 and 45 °C. Only one residue (Lys11) remained unassigned; its signals were not identified in the spectra. A summary of the measured NMR data is shown in Figure 6B.

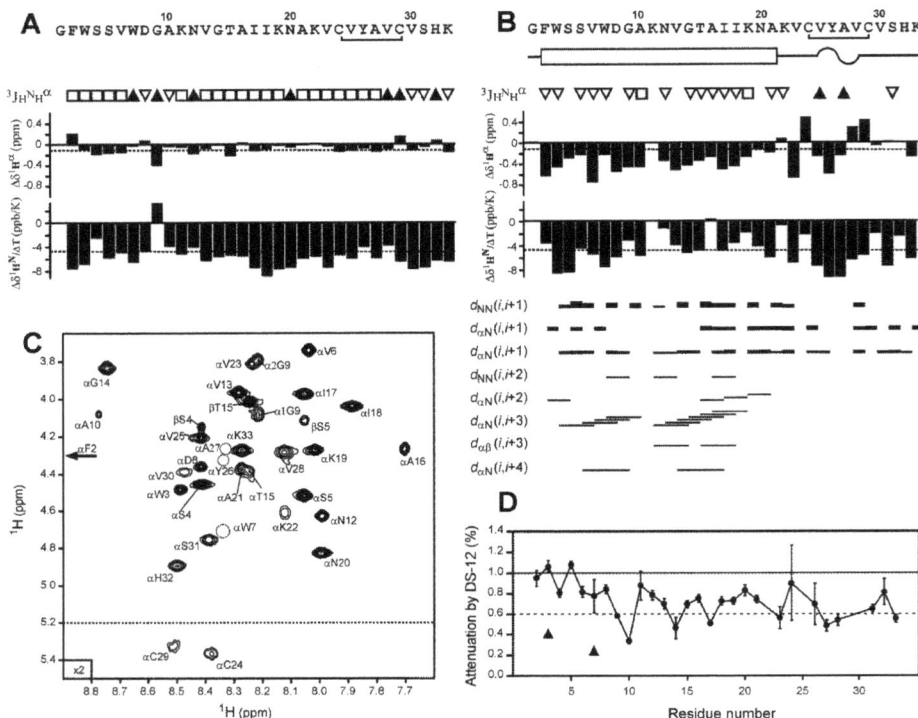

Figure 6. NMR data define the secondary structure of nicomicin-1 and topology of the peptide interaction with the dodecylphosphocholine (DPC) micelles. (**A,B**) Overview of NMR data collected for nicomicin-1 in H$_2$O (pH 4.0, 30 °C) or DPC (pH 3.15, 45 °C, D:P ratio of 200:1) solutions, respectively. The resonances of Lys11 were not identified in the spectra and the residue remains unassigned. (From top to bottom) Secondary structure (helix—bar, β-turns—wavy line) of nicomicin-1 in the DPC micelles environment. Large (>8 Hz), small (<6 Hz), and medium (others) $^3J_{H^NH}{}^\alpha$ couplings are indicated by the filled triangles, open triangles, and open squares, respectively. The positive and negative values of the secondary $^1H^\alpha$ chemical shifts ($\Delta\delta^1H^\alpha$) correspond to β-structure and α-helix, respectively. The −0.1 ppm threshold value for helical secondary structure is shown by a dashed line. Amide protons demonstrating temperature gradients ($\Delta\delta^1H^N/\Delta T$) with amplitude <4.5 ppb/K could participate in hydrogen bond formation. NOE connectivities observed in the 100 ms two-dimensional (2D) NOESY spectrum for the peptide in DPC micelles are additionally shown in the panel (**B**). (**C**) The fragment of the 2D TOCSY spectrum of nicomicin-1/DPC sample (0.25/50 mM, pH 3.15, 45 °C). The resonance assignment is shown. The broadened signals that are below the drawing threshold are shown by dashed circles. (**D**) Attenuation of intensities of H^N-H$^\alpha$ and H^N-H$^\beta$ cross-peaks in the 100 ms NOESY spectrum of the nicomicin-1/DPC sample by the paramagnetic probe (1 mM of lipid soluble 12-doxylstearate). The 0.6 threshold line subdivides data points in two groups: the residues situated inside or outside the micelle. The attenuation observed for $^1H^\varepsilon$ resonances of the Trp3 and Trp7 side chains is shown by triangles.

Negative values of $^1H^\alpha$ secondary chemical shifts (-0.44 ppm on average), $^3J_{H^NH^\alpha}$ couplings with amplitude <6 Hz, and observed ($i,i + 3$) and ($i,i + 4$) H^α-H^N NOE contacts (Figure 6B) revealed formation of an α-helix at the *N*-terminal region (Gly1-Ala21) of the peptide. Thus, interaction with the DPC micelles induces formation of a secondary structure in the nicomicin-1 molecule. At the same time, the temperature coefficients of the amide protons ($\Delta\delta^1H^N/\Delta T$) pointed to the low stability of this structure. Stable hydrogen bonds (characterized by $|\Delta\delta^1H^N/\Delta T| < 4.5$ ppb/K) were observed only on one side of the *N*-terminal helix. The $^1H^N$ protons of Ser5, Gly9, Asn12, Val13, Ala16, and Ile18-Asn20 residues could participate in hydrogen bond formation. In the *C*-terminal part (Lys22-Lys33) of the peptide, only four stable hydrogen bonds can be formed. Together with the observed $^3J_{H^NH^\alpha}$ values, this indicates the absence of α-helix or β-structure in this region of the nicomicin-1 molecule.

Analysis of the fingerprint region in the 2D TOCSY spectrum (Figure 6C) revealed unequal line-widths and intensities of the $^1H^N$ resonances. In the *N*-terminal fragment, significant broadening was observed for the amide proton of Trp7 and the resonances of Lys11 were probably broadened beyond the detection limit. Contrarily, 6 of 11 residues of the *C*-terminal region (Lys22, Cys24, Tyr26, Ala27, Cys29, and Val30) were significantly broadened. This indicated the presence of μs time-scale conformational exchange process(es), which are more pronounced in the *C*-terminal part of micelle-bound nicomicin-1.

The set of 20 nicomicin-1 structures (Figure 7A) was calculated in the CYANA program using experimentally derived distance and torsion angle restraints, and additional restraints that maintain closed backbone-backbone hydrogen bonds and disulfide (Table S1). We found that the peptide molecule consisted of two structurally independent domains connected by the hinge at the Lys22 residue. The *N*-terminal domain contains a prolonged α-helix (Phe2-Ala21) and its structure was precisely defined by NMR data (backbone root mean square deviation (RMSD) of 0.24 Å). In contrast, the *C*-terminal domain (Lys22-Lys33) adopts an extended conformation and accommodates two consecutive β-turns (Val25-Val30 residues) and a Cys24-Cys29 disulfide bond. Due to signal broadening and lack of experimental data, the structure of the *C*-terminal domain was less precisely defined (backbone RMSD of 0.69 Å).

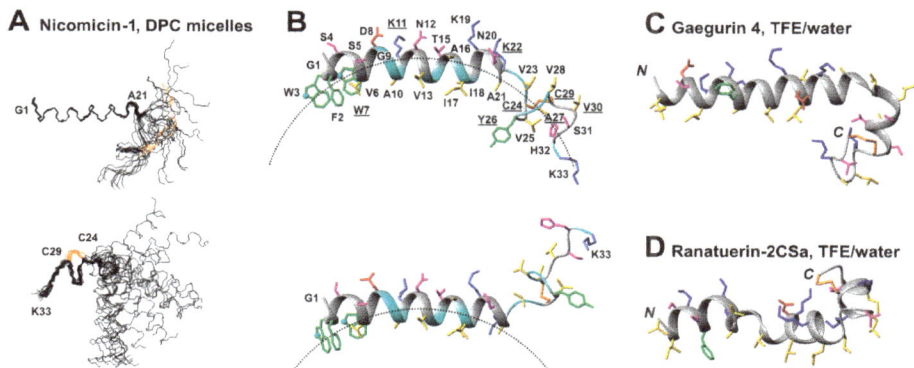

Figure 7. Spatial structure of nicomicin-1 in complex with dodecylphosphocholine (DPC) micelle. (**A**) The ensemble of 20 calculated nicomicin-1 structures is superimposed by the backbone atoms of *N*-terminal (Gly1-Ala21) and *C*-terminal (Lys22-Lys33) domains. The Cys24-Cys29 disulfide bond is shown in orange. (**B**) The representative conformers of nicomicin-1 in ribbon representation. The disulfide bond, positively charged, negatively charged, hydrophobic, aromatic, and polar residues are colored in orange, blue, red, yellow, green, and magenta, respectively. The approximate micelle surface (R ~24Å) is shown as a dashed line. The peptide ribbon is colored according to 12-doxylstearate paramagnetic relaxation enhancement data (presented on the Figure 6D). The residues located inside the micelle are colored in cyan. The N$^\varepsilon$ atoms of the Trp3 and Trp7 side chains are shown by spheres. (**C,D**) Spatial structure of amphibian peptides gaegurin 4 and ranatuerin-2CSa, PDB codes 2G9L and 2K10, respectively.

2.5. Topology of Nicomicin-Micelle Interaction

The nicomicin-1 molecule in the DPC environment demonstrates a pronounced amphipathicity. The polar and charged residues are segregated at one face of the *N*-terminal α-helix and in the *C*-terminal Ser31-Lys33 region (Figure 7B). The other face of the α-helix and the region around the Cys24-Cys29 disulfide bond contains only aromatic and hydrophobic residues.

To elucidate the location of the nicomicin-1 molecule in the DPC micelle, we used a 12-doxylstearate relaxation probe. The nitroxide moiety of this probe is located in the hydrophobic region of the micelle [43]. Specific broadening of the nicomicin-1 proton signals was monitored using NOESY spectra at a DPC/probe molar ratio of 50:1 (i.e., about one relaxation probe per micelle). To characterize the effect of the relaxation probe on the nicomicin-1 protons, we compared the amplitudes of selected intraresidual cross-peaks with and without the probe (Figure 6D). The data indicated that two parts of the molecule were in contact with the hydrophobic region of the micelle. Significant cross-peak attenuation was observed for the residues located at the hydrophobic side of the α-helix in its central part (Gly9-Ile17), and in the region around the Cys24-Cys29 disulfide (Figure 6D). The *N*-terminal part of the α-helix (Gly1-Asp8) probably contacts the micelle only by aromatic side chain groups. Significant attenuation was observed for the signals of $H^{\epsilon 1}$ protons of Trp3 and Trp7 side chains (Figure 6D, triangles).

The observed pattern of signal attenuation is consistent with the binding of the nicomicin-1 molecule to the surface of the DPC micelle by the *N*-terminal α-helix (Figure 7B). Due to significant scatter in the determined structures, the *C*-terminal domain could span different locations from being buried into the micelle to fully protruded into aqueous phase. Figure 7B illustrates this variability. The observed distribution of µs-timescale motions in the nicomicin-1 molecule (Figure 7B, underlined residues) indicated that the *C*-terminal domain underwent significant structural fluctuations. These fluctuations could be connected with the changes in the surrounding environment. We assume that the hinge-like motions around the Lys22 residue resulted in the dynamic partition of the *C*-terminal domain into the micelle. However, µs-timescale motions observed at Trp7-Lys11 residues forming one turn of the α-helix suggest the presence of another hinge region in the *N*-terminal domain.

To confirm incorporation of nicomicin-1 into DPC micelles, we measured the intrinsic fluorescence of Trp residues, which are known to be sensitive to the polarity of an environment [44]. Nicomicin-1 has two Trp residues (Trp3 and Trp7), and their fluorescence can be exploited to estimate the location of the peptide *N*-terminus in the micelle. A blue shift of emission maximum (353 → 332 nm) was observed upon transfer of nicomicin-1 from water to DPC micelles. This indicated that the Trp aromatic rings are in contact with the hydrophobic core of the micelle. The nicomicin-1 structure was also studied in water and in DPC micelles by fluorescence quenching experiments. Strict compliance with the Stern-Volmer equation was observed. Therefore, Trp3 and Trp7 are equally accessible for the quencher. Surprisingly, the transfer of nicomicin-1 from water to micelles only slightly decreased the Stern-Volmer constant from 9.2 to 8.5 M^{-1}. The Trp side chains in the micelle-bound peptide probably experience an intensive dynamic (collisional) quenching. This may be caused by the presence of a positively charged group, which increases the concentration of the negative iodide (I^-) quencher in the vicinity of Trp side chain within ~10 Å [44,45]. According to the determined spatial structure of nicomicin-1 (Figure 7B), presumably the *N*-terminal amino group (NH_3^+-) is responsible for the observed effect. In addition, the quencher can effectively reach the Trp side chains, which may prove that they are located at the interface between the polar and hydrophobic region of the micelle. This location agrees well with the NMR data and proposed model of nicomicin-1/micelle complex (Figure 7B).

2.6. Comparison of Spacial Structures of Nicomicin-1 and Amphibian Peptides Containing 'Rana-Box' Motif

The α-helix in the nicomicin-1 molecule is terminated by the fragment containing several β-turns stabilized by a Cys24-Cys29 disulfide bond. This structural arrangement resembles the Rana-box motif found in helical antimicrobial peptides isolated from frog skin [25]. The spatial structures of several peptides from this family were previously determined by NMR spectroscopy, but only two structures (gaegurin 4 [46] and ranatuerin-2CSa [47]) are available in the PDB database (Figure 7C,D). Similar to nicomicin-1, both peptides contain prolonged amphipathic helical regions, whereas the C-termini of the molecules are capped by positively charged disulfide-stabilized Rana-box motifs. In contrast to amphibian peptides, the Rana-box in nicomicin-1 does not contain positively charged residues and demonstrates significant hydrophobicity. Notably, nicomicin-1 possesses the additional four-residue fragment after the Rana-box. This region of the molecule is relatively polar and contains basic Lys33 residue.

2.7. Antibacterial Activity and Mechanism of Action

The antibacterial activity of nicomicin-1 and its fragments was determined using a two-fold serial dilution assay in lysogeny broth (LB) medium with or without NaCl. Minimum inhibitory concentrations (MICs) of the peptides against Gram-positive and Gram-negative bacteria are presented in Table 3. Melittin, known as a potent cytolytic and bactericidal agent, was used as a positive control. Nicomicin-1 exhibited a pronounced antimicrobial effect against Gram-positive bacteria, similar to that of α-helical cationic peptide melittin. The activity against Gram-negative microorganisms was modest and at least two- to four-fold lower than that of melittin. Interestingly, the α-helix peptide hedistin from *Nereis diversicolor* was also inactive against a set of Gram-negative microorganisms, except the marine bacterium *Vibrio alginolyticus*, which is a causative agent of infections of marine invertebrates [7]. Surprisingly, none of the peptides inhibited growth of *Bacillus megaterium* at concentrations up to 16 μM. Previous structure–activity relationship (SAR) studies of Rana-box amphibian AMPs revealed that the cyclic C-terminal part of these peptides does not influence the antibacterial activity, whereas the N-terminal α-helix is responsible for membrane disruption [25]. The α-helical peptide Nico(1-17) did not show any antibacterial activity at concentrations of 16 μM or higher. Notably, the net charge of the entire Nico(1-17) was zero and its most homologous AMP, 14-residue StCT1 from scorpion *Scorpiops tibetanus*, displayed poor antibacterial properties [32]. Weak activity of Nico(18-33) was detected only against several Gram-positive bacteria in a salt-free medium.

Table 3. Antibacterial activity of the peptides.

Bacteria	Minimum Inhibitory Concentration (μM)							
	Melittin		Nicomicin-1		Nico(1-17)		Nico(18-33)	
	Without Salt	+NaCl	Without Salt	+NaCl	Without Salt	+NaCl	Without Salt	+NaCl
Gram-positive								
Micrococcus luteus	0.25	0.25	0.125	0.25	>16	>16	16	>16
Bacillus subtilis	0.5	0.5	0.062	0.25	>16	>16	16	>16
B. licheniformis	0.25	0.25	0.125	0.25	>16	>16	8	>128
B. megaterium	>16	>16	>16	>16	>16	>16	>16	>16
Staphylococcus aureus 209P	2	32	2	32	>16	>16	>16	>16
S. aureus ATCC 29213	1	1	2	16	>16	>16	>128	>128
Rhodococcus sp.	0.5	0.25	0.125	0.25	>16	>16	>16	>16
Gram-negative								
E. coli BL21 (DE3)	2	4	2	32	>64	>64	>64	>64
E. coli ML-35p	8	16	16	>32	>64	>64	>64	>64
E. coli C600	4	8	32	>32	>64	>64	>64	>64
Acinetobacter baumanii	8	32	32	>32	>64	>64	>64	>64
Pseudomonas aeruginosa PAO1	>32	32	32	>32	>64	>64	>128	>128

Cationic AMPs realize their antibacterial function by damaging membrane integrity and/or specifically inhibiting intracellular processes [2]. In this study, an effect of the peptides on bacterial cytoplasmic membrane integrity was analyzed with the use of *E. coli* ML-35p, a strain lacking the functional lactose permease necessary for the uptake of o-nitrophenyl-β-D-galactoside (ONPG) and constitutively expressing β-galactosidase. The latter produces o-nitrophenol, a chromogenic product with absorbance at 405 nm. Both nicomicin-1 and melittin effectively damaged membranes in a salt-free environment (Figure 8A). However, the addition of 150 mM NaCl markedly reduced the activity of nicomicin-1 (Figure 8B), which could explain the weak antibacterial effect of the peptide against *E. coli* in the presence of salt (Table 3). Salt probably both promotes peptide aggregation in a test medium and affects primary electrostatic attraction, thus impairing nicomicin-1 interaction with the bacterial membrane. This salt inhibiting effect is quite surprising in light of the marine origin of the host. Notably, both fragments of nicomicin-1 had a negligible ability to damage the membrane integrity of *E. coli* ML-35p, which was comparable to that of the negative control (data not shown). Therefore, the α-helical amphipathic part of nicomicin-1 cannot effectively interact with the membrane bilayer without the C-terminal fragment of the peptide and vice versa.

On the other hand, the ability of nicomicin-1 to inhibit its own biosynthesis in the *E. coli* expression system suggests a more complicated mechanism of action of the peptide against Gram-negative bacteria, which may differ from direct membrane destruction. Induction of nicomicin-1 biosynthesis resulted in inhibition of *E. coli* BL21 (DE3) growth (Section 2.3). Similarly, Pro-rich ribosome-targeting AMP apidaecin fused to a large carrier protein effectively inhibited growth of bacterial cells during heterologous expression in *E. coli* [48]. Therefore, we tested an ability of nicomicin-1 and other antimicrobial compounds to inhibit protein biosynthesis in vitro. The obtained results indicated a slight inhibition of the biosynthesis process. Nicomicin-1 caused only a 20% inhibition of enhanced green fluorescent protein (EGFP) expression at a concentration of 64 µM (Figure 8C). The observed effect was similar neither to streptomycin—a specific ribosome-targeting inhibitor of bacterial translation (IC_{50} 0.2 µM)—nor to tachyplesin-1 that effectively binds nucleic acids [49]. Therefore, the major mechanism of nicomicin-1 antibacterial action did not seem to be related to the inhibition of bacterial translation.

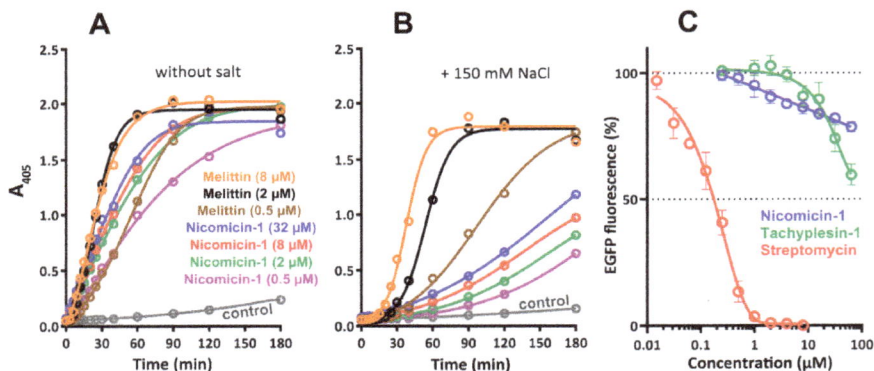

Figure 8. Analysis of nicomicin-1 antibacterial mechanism of action. *Escherichia coli* ML-35p cytoplasmic membrane permeabilization by nicomicin-1 at various concentrations from 0.5 to 32 µM, highlighted with colors (**A**) in the absence or (**B**) in the presence of NaCl. The cytolytic peptide melittin was used as the positive control from 0.5 to 8 µM, highlighted with colors. Three independent experiments were performed, and the curve pattern was similar for all three series. (**C**) Effects of nicomicin-1, tachyplesin-1, and streptomycin on the fluorescence resulting from the in vitro translation of EGFP using *E. coli* BL21 (DE3) Star cell extract. The data are presented as the mean ± SD of three independent experiments.

The question about the localization of the peptide in host tissues remains open. Polychaeta species are strictly dependent on epithelial barrier continuity and efficacy of the innate immune system, which are vitally important for their protection against pathogenic microorganisms. The BRICHOS-related peptides, arenicins and alvinellacin, are constitutively expressed both in coelomocytes and in the tegument of hosts, thus indicating involvement of the peptides in both systemic and local epithelial immunity [8,50]. Localization of the nicomicins needs further elucidation with the use of immunohistochemistry approaches.

2.8. Nicomicin-1 Possesses Cytotoxicity Against Mammalian Cells

Considering the ability of nicomicin-1 and Nico(1-17) to aggregate and potentially form fibrils in aqueous solutions, we analyzed the cytotoxic effects of nicomicin-1 and its fragments against adherent cell lines of human embryonic fibroblasts (HEF) and cervix adenocarcinoma cells (HeLa) as well as toward human red blood cells (hRBC). Nicomicin-1 and Nico(18-33) had similar hemolysis profiles with a half maximal hemolysis concentration (HC$_{50}$) of about 64 and 128 µM, respectively (Figure 9A). In contrast, Nico(1-17) almost lacked hemolytic activity and lysed only 1% of red blood cells at a concentration of 128 µM. This is in agreement with data on antibacterial activity of Nico(1-17). Therefore, the *C*-terminal part of nicomicin-1 plays a key role in its hemolyticity. Cytotoxicity of nicomicin-1 toward HeLa cells was shown to be dose-dependent and attained a value of 85% of dead cells at the peptide concentration of 32 µM (Figure 9B). Nicomicin-1 possesses selectivity toward cancer cells. In contrast to hemolytic and antibacterial activities, the peptide fragment Nico(1-17) was cytotoxic toward adherent mammalian cells. Notably, the peptide Nico(1-17) showed a dose-independent cytostatic effect against both HeLa and HEF cells at a concentration range from 0.25 to 32 µM. The molecular mechanism of nicomicin-1 or Nico(1-17) cytotoxicity at submicromolar concentrations is still obscure. The above-mentioned amyloid fibril-forming amphibian AMP uperin 3.5 possessed a similar cytotoxic activity profile against pheochromocytoma cells [39]. Gel formation by amyloids within or outside cells as well as peptides adsorption could perturb membrane integrity, interfere with cell motility and signaling pathways, and alter the collagen gel network of the extracellular matrix [38]. Therefore, the activity of nicomicin-1 may also result from peptide aggregation.

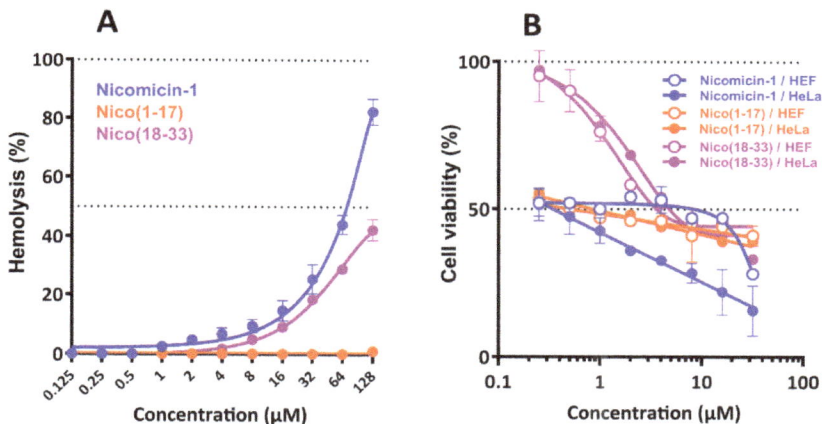

Figure 9.   (**A**) Hemolytic activity of nicomicin-1 and its fragments after 1.5 h incubation (hemoglobin release assay). (**B**) Cytotoxicity of nicomicin-1 and its fragments against human embryonic fibroblasts (HEF) and cervix adenocarcinoma cells (HeLa) after 24 h incubation (3-(4,5-dimethylthiazol-2-yl)-2,5-diphenyltetrazolium bromide (MTT) dye reduction assay). The data are presented as the mean ± SD of three independent experiments.

3. Materials and Methods

3.1. Animal Collection

Nicomache minor (Arwidsson, 1906) tubeworms (Figure S1) were collected in June near the Nikolai Pertsov White Sea Biological Station (WSBS, Republic of Karelia, Russia) in the White Sea at depths of 5–35 m on silty sediments with stones using an ocean 0.1 m^2 grab and diving technique. Several specimens of *N. minor* were cleaned with distilled water, cut, submerged in RNAlater solution

(Thermo Fisher Scientific, Waltham, MA, USA) to preserve RNA before total RNA isolation, and stored at −20 °C until used.

3.2. Total RNA Isolation, RT-PCR, RACE Amplification

The tissue samples were thawed, removed from the solution, and homogenized in liquid nitrogen. Intact total RNA was isolated by using SV Total RNA Isolation System (Promega, Fitchburg, WI, USA). The RNA was quantified at 260 nm using a Ultrospec 3300 Pro spectrophotometer (Amersham Biosciences, Amersham, UK), and reverse transcribed into cDNA using a Mint RACE cDNA amplification kit (Evrogen, Moscow, Russia) according to manufacturer's protocols. The obtained cDNA was analyzed by PCR amplification, cloning, and sequencing of the Folmer fragment of cytochrome oxidase subunit I (COI) gene. COI is adopted as the standard 'taxon barcode' for most animal groups [51]. Amplification of the 517-bp fragment was performed with two designed gene-specific primers: 5′-GGCACCTCTATAAGACTCCT-3′ and 5′-GAACTGGGAGGGAGAGAAGAA-3′. The analyzed sequence was shown to be identical to that of coding COI from *N. minor* isolate SPM11 (GenBank accession ID MG975588.1).

To determine the sequence of the 3′ and 5′ ends of cDNA coding a putative BRICHOS-related peptide, the RACE strategy was used. Two rounds of step-out PCR with the use of nested gene-specific primers (Table 1) were performed for both 3′ and 5′RACE (Figure 1). The 3′RACE was performed using degenerate GSPs that anneal to sequences encoding the two most conservative protein regions (Figure S2) in the BRICHOS domains of the precursors of polychaeta AMPs (arenicin-1, arenicin-3, capitellacin, and alvinellacin). The first round of 3′RACE was performed separately using 3′-GSP1 (outer) or 3′-GSP2 (outer) and adaptor primers—step-out primer mix1 supplied in the kit. Then 1000-fold diluted products were used in the second round with 3′-GSP3 (inner) and step-out primer mix2. Both rounds of nested PCR were performed using the same step-down technique with the following parameters: 95 °C for 60 s, 30 cycles of 94 °C for 30 s, annealing at 66→55 °C for 40 s (66-2, 62-3, 59-4, 57-5, 55-16 cycles) and extension at 72 °C for 60 s, and a final elongation step at 72 °C for 10 min. 5′RACE was performed as a nested PCR with GSPs complementary to the 3′UTR. The first round of 5′RACE was performed with 5′-GSP1 (outer) and step-out primer mix1. Then, 1000-fold diluted products were used in the second round using 5′-GSP2 (inner) or 5′-GSP3 (inner) and step-out primer mix2. Both rounds were performed using the same technique with the following parameters: 95 °C for 60 s; 30 cycles of 94 °C for 30 s, annealing at 62→55 °C for 40 s (62-3, 59-3, 57-4, 55-20 cycles) and extension at 72 °C for 90 s; and a final elongation step at 72 °C for 10 min. The one-round amplification of the whole coding sequence was performed using AP primer complementary to the 5′UTR and 5′-GSP2 with the following parameters: 95 °C for 60 s; 40 cycles of 94 °C for 30 s, annealing at 64→56 °C for 40 s (64-2, 62-3, 60-4, 58-5, 55-26 cycles) and extension at 72 °C for 60 s; and a final elongation step at 72 °C for 10 min. The products were separated by electrophoresis on 1.5% agarose gel and visualized on an ultraviolet (UV) transilluminator. The PCR products were purified from agarose gel and inserted into a pGEM-T vector (Promega, Fitchburg, WI, USA). The ligation products were transformed into the chemically competent *E. coli* DH10B cells. Plasmid DNA was isolated from white colonies on LB agar plates supplemented with ampicillin (100 µg/mL) using Plasmid Miniprep kit (Evrogen, Moscow, Russia). The plasmids were sequenced on both strands using the ABI PRISM 3100-Avant automatic sequencer (Applied Biosystems, Foster City, CA, USA).

3.3. Expression and Purification of the Antimicrobial Peptides

The recombinant plasmids for expression of nicomicin-1, as well as its fragments Nico(1-17) and Nico(18-33), were constructed with the use of pET-based vector as described previously [52]. The expression cassette included the T7 promoter, ribosome binding site (RBS), and the sequence encoding the recombinant protein that included an 8× His tag, the carrier protein (*E. coli* thioredoxin A with the Met37Leu mutation), a methionine residue, and a target peptide. *E. coli* BL21 (DE3) cells were transformed with the constructed plasmids and grown up to OD_{600} 1.0–1.5 at 37 °C in rich medium containing tryptone (15 g/L), yeast extract (17.5 g/L), NaCl (10 g/L), 20 mM glucose, 1 mM $MgSO_4$, 0.1 mM $CaCl_2$, 0.01 mM $FeCl_3$, and 100 µg/mL of ampicillin, and then were induced with IPTG at a final concentration of 0.4 mM. The induction was performed at 30 °C for 4 h under shaking culture conditions at a speed of 220 rpm. The cells were sonicated in the 100 mM phosphate buffer (pH 7.8) containing 20 mM imidazole and 6 M guanidine hydrochloride to fully solubilize the fusion protein. Purification of the peptides involved immobilized metal affinity chromatography (IMAC) of cell lysate with the use of Ni Sepharose (GE Healthcare, Chicago, IL, USA), CNBr cleavage of the fusion protein, and RP-HPLC as described previously [53]. The recombinant peptides were characterized by Tricine-SDS-PAGE according to [54] and MALDI-MS (Bruker Daltonics, Bremen, Germany). Melittin and tachyplesin-1 used in this study were obtained as described earlier [52,55]. The peptides concentrations were estimated using UV absorbance.

3.4. Circular Dichroism Spectroscopy

Secondary structures of the peptides were analyzed by circular dichroism (CD) spectroscopy with the use of Jasco J-810 instrument (Jasco, Tokyo, Japan). Experiments were performed at 25 °C in water, in 30 mM DPC (Anatrace, Maumee, OH, USA) micelles, and in 30 mM SDS (Sigma, St. Louis, MO, USA) micelles. Final concentrations of peptides were of 150 µM. Four consecutive scans were performed and averaged, followed by subtraction of the blank spectrum of the solvent.

3.5. NMR Spectroscopy

[-20]For the NMR study in water and in DPC micelles environment, 0.4 and 0.25 mM samples of the recombinant nicomicin-1 were used, respectively. d38-DPC (CIL, Andover, MA, USA) was added to the NM sample in water using concentrated stock solution. The final DPC concentration was 50 mM. The pH of the samples were adjusted to 4.0 (water) or 3.15 (DPC) using concentrated HCl or NaOH solutions and 5% D_2O was added. NMR spectra were measured at 30 °C (water) or at 45 °C (DPC) on an AVANCE-III 600 spectrometer (Bruker, Karlsruhe, Germany) equipped with cryogenically cooled probe (Bruker, Karlsruhe, Germany). 12-doxylstearate (Sigma, St. Louis, MO, USA) was added to the nicomicin-1/DPC sample (0.25/50 mM) using lyophilized aliquots of stock solution in methanol. NOESY spectra (τ_m = 100 ms) were measured at zero and 1 mM 12-doxylstearate concentrations at pH 3.15.

The protein resonance assignment was performed using a standard approach [42] using a combination of 2D ^{1}H-TOCSY (τ_m = 80 ms), ^{1}H-NOESY (τ_m = 60, 80 and 100 ms), and ^{13}C-Heteronuclear Single Quantum Coherence spectroscopy (HSQC) spectra in the CARA (version 1.84, Zurich, Switzerland) program. The $^3J_{H^NH^\alpha}$ coupling constants were determined from line shape analysis of NOESY and TOCSY cross peaks in the Mathematica program (version 8.0, Wolfram Research, Champaign, IL, USA). The $^3J_{H^\alpha H^\beta}$ coupling constants were estimated from the multiplet patterns in 2D TOCSY spectrum. The spatial structure calculations were performed in the CYANA (version 3.97) program [56]. Upper interproton distance constraints were derived from NOESY cross-peaks (τ_m = 100 ms) via a "$1/r^6$" calibration. Torsion angle restraints and stereospecific assignments were obtained from J coupling constants and NOE intensities. Hydrogen bonds were introduced using temperature coefficients of amide protons ($\Delta\delta^1 H^N/\Delta T$) measured in the range of 20 to 45 °C in the TOCSY or NOESY spectra. Additional upper/lower restraints were applied to close the Cys24-Cys29 disulfide and backbone-backbone hydrogen bonds.

3.6. PDB and BMRB Accession Codes

The ^{1}H and ^{13}C chemical shifts of nicomicin-1 in H_2O and DPC were deposited into the BioMagnetic Resonance Bank (BMRB, www.bmrb.wisc.edu, accession code 27611 and 34313, respectively). NMR constraints and derived atomic coordinates (20 models) for nicomicin-1 in complex with DPC micelle were deposited into the RCSB Protein Data Bank (PDB, https://www.rcsb.org, accession code 6HN9). Before PDB deposition, the obtained nicomicin-1 structure was checked by the internal PDB validation tool. Validation revealed good quality of the obtained structure with 81% of residues located in favored regions and 10% of residues in allowed regions on the Ramachandran plot (Table S1). The full report is available on the PDB website.

3.7. Tryptophan Fluorescence and Quenching

Tryptophan fluorescence was measured by means of Hitachi F-4000 (Hitachi, Tokyo, Japan) fluorescence spectrophotometer using 1×0.4 cm quartz cuvettes (Hellma Analytics, Müllheim/Baden, Germany). Emission and excitation slits were 5 nm wide. The excitation wavelength was 280 nm. Peptide concentration was 10 µM. The DPC to peptide molar ratio was of 200:1. The pH of the samples was of 4.0. Fluorescence was quenched by addition of increasing amounts of 4 M potassium iodide.

3.8. Antimicrobial Assay

The bacteria *Bacillus subtilis* B-886, *Micrococcus luteus* B-1314, and *Bacillus megaterium* VKM41 were obtained from All-Russian Collection of Microorganisms (Pushchino, Russia). *Rhodococcus* sp. SS1 was obtained from Institute of Biochemistry and Physiology of Microorganisms (Pushchino, Russia). *Bacillus licheniformis* VK21 was obtained from the Branch of M.M. Shemyakin & Yu.A. Ovchinnikov Institute of Bioorganic Chemistry (Pushchino, Russia). The extensively drug resistant clinical isolate of *Acinetobacter baumanii* was obtained from Sechenov First Moscow State Medical University hospital. Other strains were obtained from ATCC (Manassas, VA, USA). Bacterial test cultures were grown in LB medium (10 g/L tryptone, 5 g/L yeast extract, 10 g/L NaCl) at 37 °C to mid-log phase and then diluted with the same medium containing or lacking NaCl to reach a final cell concentration of 2×10^5 CFU/mL. Then, 50 µL of the obtained bacterial suspension were added to 50 µL aquilots of the peptide solutions serially diluted with sterilized 0.1% bovine serum albumin (BSA) in 96-well flat-bottom polystyrene microplates (Eppendorf #0030730011, Hamburg, Germany). To avoid the adsorption of AMPs to plastic surfaces, an addition of BSA was used [57]. After incubation for 20 h at 30 °C and 900 rpm on a plate thermoshaker (Biosan, Riga, Latvia), the minimum inhibitory concentrations (MICs) were determined as the lowest peptide concentrations that prevented growth of test microorganisms observed as visible turbidity. In most cases, no significant divergence of MIC values was observed (within ± 1 dilution step). The results are expressed as the median values determined on the basis of at least three independent experiments performed in triplicate.

3.9. Bacterial Membranes Permeability Assay

To examine an ability of the peptides to permeabilize the cytoplasmic bacterial membrane, a colorimetric assay with o-nitrophenyl-β-D-galactoside (ONPG, AppliChem, Darmstadt, Germany) and *E. coli* ML-35p strain was performed as previously described [58] with some modifications. The final concentration of ONPG and *E. coli* ML-35p cells were 2.5 mM and 2×10^7 CFU/mL, respectively. Peptide samples were placed in a 96-well plate with a non-binding surface (NBS, Corning #3641, Corning, NY, USA), and an optical density of the solution was measured at 405 nm using the Multiskan EX microplate reader (Thermo Fisher Scientific, Waltham, MA, USA). The assay was performed in 10 mM sodium phosphate buffer with or without 150 mM NaCl at 30 °C under stirring at 300 rpm. Control experiments were performed under the same conditions without the addition of a peptide. Three independent experiments were performed, and the curve patterns were similar for all three series.

3.10. Cell-Free Protein Expression Assay

The cell lysate required for the translation inhibition assay was prepared using *E. coli* BL21 Star (DE3) cell culture grown at 30 °C in $2\times$ YTPG liquid medium (1.6% tryptone, 1% yeast extract, 0.5% NaCl, 22 mM NaH_2PO_4, 40 mM Na_2HPO_4, 0.1 M glucose). The chromosome of DE3 strains contains a gene encoding T7 RNA polymerase under control of the lacUV5 promoter. The bacterial culture was grown to OD_{600} 0.8–1.0, then the T7 RNA polymerase gene was induced by addition of 0.2 mM

IPTG. Bacteria were harvested at OD_{600} 5.0–6.0 by centrifugation ($3000\times g$, 30 min, 4 °C). The bacterial pellet was washed three times by suspending it in four volumes of wash buffer (10 mM tris-acetate buffer, pH 8.2, 14 mM magnesium acetate, 60 mM potassium glutamate, and 1 mM dithiothreitol), then resuspended in one volume of the same buffer (1 mL per 1 g of wet cell mass) and disrupted by sonication at 5–15 °C. The total cell lysate was centrifuged at $15,000\times g$ (30 min, 4 °C). The supernatant was split into aliquots and stored at −70 °C. In order to investigate effects of AMPs on the translation process, the peptides were added to a cell-free protein synthesis (CFPS) reaction mix with a plasmid encoding EGFP variant (F64L, S65T, Q80R, F99S, M153T, V163A) under a control of the T7 promoter. The reaction mix consisted of the following components: 1.2 mM ATP, 0.8 mM UTP, 0.8 mM GTP, 0.8 mM CTP, 2 mM of each of 20 proteinogenic amino acids, 1.5 mM spermidine, 1 mM putrescine dihydrochloride, 0.06647 mM calcium folinate, 170 ng/mL tRNA from the *E. coli* MRE 600 strain, 0.33 mM nicotinamide adenine dinucleotide (NAD), 10 mM ammonium glutamate, 175 mM potassium glutamate, 60 mM glucose, 120 mM HEPES-KOH (pH 8.0), 15 mM magnesium glutamate, 2% PEG 8000, 25% *E. coli* BL21 Star (DE3) cell lysate, and 10 ng/μL plasmid DNA. The reaction volume was 50 μL. The peptides were dissolved in water with the addition of 0.1% BSA. Streptomycin was used in the positive control reactions. Fluorescence of the sample without inhibitor was set to 100%. The reaction proceeded for 60 min in a 96-well clear flat-bottom black polystyrene microplates (Corning #3340, Corning, NY, USA) in a plate shaker (30 °C, 900 rpm). Fluorescence of the synthesized EGFP was measured with a AF2200 microplate reader (Eppendorf, Hamburg, Germany) (λ_{Exc} = 488 nm, λ_{Em} = 510 nm). The experimental data were obtained from at least three independent experiments.

3.11. Hemolysis and Cytotoxicity Assay

The hemolytic activity of the peptides was tested against the fresh suspension of human red blood cells (hRBC) using the hemoglobin release assay as described previously [53]. Three experiments were performed with hRBC from blood samples of independent donors. The quantitative data are represented as average means with standard deviations. The colorimetric 3-(4,5-dimethylthiazol-2-yl)-2,5-diphenyltetrazolium bromide (MTT) dye reduction assay was used to determine the cytotoxicity of the peptides against HeLa (cervix adenocarcinoma cells) and human embryonic fibroblasts (HEF) cell lines as described previously [52,59]. The experimental data were obtained from at least three independent experiments.

4. Conclusions

This study extends the knowledge of the structure and functions of AMPs from marine invertebrates, and in particular from the small polychaeta tubeworm *N. minor*. Overall, nicomicins represent a novel scaffold among polychaeta, AMPs combining an amphipathic N-terminal α-helix and C-terminal extended part with a six-residue loop stabilized by a disulfide bridge. The recombinant nicomicin-1 is structured in a membrane-mimicking environment, exhibits membrane-active properties, and possesses a pronounced activity against Gram-positive bacteria and cancer cells. The peptide shares similarities in both primary and secondary structure with amphibian host-defense peptides, and has a fundamentally different molecular organization of the precursor. The obtained results reveal that the BRICHOS domain does not exclusively participate in biosynthesis of β-hairpin polychaeta AMPs, but could also be a part of precursor of α-helical AMPs, namely nicomicins. Until now, this domain has been described in polychaeta only as a precursor of β-hairpin AMPs. Therefore, the BRICHOS domain might be a universal prodomain that participates in the biosynthesis of different structural types of AMPs in polychaeta by analogy with the cathelin-like domain in vertebrates.

Supplementary Materials: The following are available online at http://www.mdpi.com/1660-3397/16/11/401/s1. Figure S1: Polychaeta Nicomache minor; Figure S2: Design of degenerate gene-specific primers for amplification of the 3′-end of cDNA encoding BRICHOS-related peptides; Figure S3: The nucleotide sequence of mRNA encoding prepronicomicin-1 and its translation; Figure S4: The peptide Nico(1-17) forms gel structure at concentration of 2 mg/mL in water; Table S1: Statistics for the best CYANA structures of nicomicin-1 in DPC solution at pH 3.15.

Author Contributions: P.V.P., A.V.T., I.A.B., A.S.P., M.B.M., S.V.S. performed the experiments; P.V.P., A.V.T., I.A.B., A.S.P., M.B.M., S.V.S., Z.O.S., T.V.O. designed the experiments and analyzed data; P.V.P., A.V.T., S.V.S., Z.O.S., T.V.O. wrote the paper. T.V.O. contributed to the conception of the work and supervised the whole project. All authors read and approved the final manuscript.

Funding: This work was supported by the Russian Science Foundation (the project No. 14-50-00131).

Acknowledgments: The authors thank A.B. Tzetlin and T.D. Shcherbakova (M.V. Lomonosov Moscow State University) for assistance in the collection and photographing of animals. The authors thank S.V. Balandin for critical reading of the manuscript.

Conflicts of Interest: The authors declare no conflict of interest.

References

1. Hancock, R.E.W.; Brown, K.L.; Mookherjee, N. Host defence peptides from invertebrates—Emerging antimicrobial strategies. *Immunobiology* **2006**, *211*, 315–322. [CrossRef] [PubMed]

2. Graf, M.; Mardirossian, M.; Nguyen, F.; Seefeldt, A.C.; Guichard, G.; Scocchi, M.; Innis, C.A.; Wilson, D.N. Proline-rich antimicrobial peptides targeting protein synthesis. *Nat. Prod. Rep.* **2017**, *34*, 702–711. [CrossRef] [PubMed]

3. Tasiemski, A. Antimicrobial peptides in annelids. *Invertebr. Surviv. J.* **2008**, *5*, 75–82.

4. Ovchinnikova, T.V.; Aleshina, G.M.; Balandin, S.V.; Krasnosdembskaya, A.D.; Markelov, M.L.; Frolova, E.I.; Leonova, Y.F.; Tagaev, A.A.; Krasnodembsky, E.G.; Kokryakov, V.N. Purification and primary structure of two isoforms of arenicin, a novel antimicrobial peptide from marine polychaeta *Arenicola marina*. *FEBS Lett.* **2004**, *577*, 209–214. [CrossRef] [PubMed]

5. Ovchinnikova, T.V.; Shenkarev, Z.O.; Nadezhdin, K.D.; Balandin, S.V.; Zhmak, M.N.; Kudelina, I.A.; Finkina, E.I.; Kokryakov, V.N.; Arseniev, A.S. Recombinant expression, synthesis, purification, and solution structure of arenicin. *Biochem. Biophys. Res. Commun.* **2007**, *360*, 156–162. [CrossRef] [PubMed]

6. Pan, W.; Liu, X.; Ge, F.; Han, J.; Zheng, T. Perinerin, a novel antimicrobial peptide purified from the clamworm *Perinereis aibuhitensis* Grube and its partial characterization. *J. Biochem.* **2004**, *135*, 297–304. [CrossRef] [PubMed]

7. Tasiemski, A.; Schikorski, D.; Le Marrec-Croq, F.; Pontoire-Van Camp, C.; Boidin-Wichlacz, C.; Sautière, P.-E. Hedistin: A novel antimicrobial peptide containing bromotryptophan constitutively expressed in the NK cells-like of the marine annelid, *Nereis diversicolor*. *Dev. Comp. Immunol.* **2007**, *31*, 749–762. [CrossRef] [PubMed]

8. Tasiemski, A.; Jung, S.; Boidin-Wichlacz, C.; Jollivet, D.; Cuvillier-Hot, V.; Pradillon, F.; Vetriani, C.; Hecht, O.; Sönnichsen, F.D.; Gelhaus, C.; et al. Characterization and function of the first antibiotic isolated from a vent organism: The extremophile metazoan *Alvinella pompejana*. *PLoS ONE* **2014**, *9*, e95737. [CrossRef] [PubMed]

9. Shcherbakova, T.D.; Tzetlin, A.B.; Mardashova, M.V.; Sokolova, O.S. Fine structure of the tubes of *Maldanidae* (Annelida). *J. Mar. Biol. Assoc. U. K.* **2017**, *97*, 1177–1187. [CrossRef]

10. Chen, G.; Abelein, A.; Nilsson, H.E.; Leppert, A.; Andrade-Talavera, Y.; Tambaro, S.; Hemmingsson, L.; Roshan, F.; Landreh, M.; Biverstål, H.; et al. Bri2 BRICHOS client specificity and chaperone activity are governed by assembly state. *Nat. Commun.* **2017**, *8*. [CrossRef] [PubMed]

11. Leonard, B.C.; Chu, H.; Johns, J.L.; Gallo, R.L.; Moore, P.F.; Marks, S.L.; Bevins, C.L. Expression and activity of a novel cathelicidin from domestic cats. *PLoS ONE* **2011**, *6*, e18756. [CrossRef] [PubMed]

12. Hoegenhaug, H.H.K.; Mygind, P.H.; Kruse, T.; Segura, D.R.; Sandvang, D.; Neve, S. Antimicrobial Peptide Variants and Polynucleotides Encoding Same. US Patent US20110306750A1; PCT/EP2011/059689, 15 December 2011.

13. Papot, C.; Massol, F.; Jollivet, D.; Tasiemski, A. Antagonistic evolution of an antibiotic and its molecular chaperone: How to maintain a vital ectosymbiosis in a highly fluctuating habitat. *Sci. Rep.* **2017**, *7*. [CrossRef]

14. Bergeron, F.; Leduc, R.; Day, R. Subtilase-like pro-protein convertases: From molecular specificity to therapeutic applications. *J. Mol. Endocrinol.* **2000**, *24*, 1–22. [CrossRef] [PubMed]

15. Imamura, T.; Nitta, H.; Wada, Y.; Kobayashi, H.; Okamoto, K. Impaired plasma clottability induction through fibrinogen degradation by ASP, a serine protease released from *Aeromonas sobria*. *FEMS Microbiol. Lett.* **2008**, *284*, 35–42. [CrossRef] [PubMed]

16. Hedlund, J.; Johansson, J.; Persson, B. BRICHOS—A superfamily of multidomain proteins with diverse functions. *BMC Res. Notes* **2009**, *2*, 180. [CrossRef] [PubMed]

17. Moore, A.D.; Bornberg-Bauer, E. The dynamics and evolutionary potential of domain loss and emergence. *Mol. Biol. Evol.* **2012**, *29*, 787–796. [CrossRef] [PubMed]

18. Song, M.; Song, K.; Kim, S.; Lee, J.; Hwang, S.; Han, C. *Caenorhabditis elegans* BRICHOS domain–containing protein C09F5.1 maintains thermotolerance and decreases cytotoxicity of Aβ42 by activating the UPR. *Genes* **2018**, *9*, 160. [CrossRef] [PubMed]

19. Sánchez-Pulido, L.; Devos, D.; Valencia, A. BRICHOS: A conserved domain in proteins associated with dementia, respiratory distress and cancer. *Trends Biochem. Sci.* **2002**, *27*, 329–332. [CrossRef]

20. Fehlbaum, P.; Bulet, P.; Chernysh, S.; Briand, J.P.; Roussel, J.P.; Letellier, L.; Hetru, C.; Hoffmann, J.A. Structure-activity analysis of thanatin, a 21-residue inducible insect defense peptide with sequence homology to frog skin antimicrobial peptides. *Proc. Natl. Acad. Sci. USA* **1996**, *93*, 1221–1225. [CrossRef] [PubMed]

21. Tang, T.; Li, X.; Yang, X.; Yu, X.; Wang, J.; Liu, F.; Huang, D. Transcriptional response of *Musca domestica* larvae to bacterial infection. *PLoS ONE* **2014**, *9*, e104867. [CrossRef] [PubMed]

22. Tomie, T.; Ishibashi, J.; Furukawa, S.; Kobayashi, S.; Sawahata, R.; Asaoka, A.; Tagawa, M.; Yamakawa, M. Scarabaecin, a novel cysteine-containing antifungal peptide from the rhinoceros beetle, *Oryctes rhinoceros*. *Biochem. Biophys. Res. Commun.* **2003**, *307*, 261–266. [CrossRef]

23. Yang, H.; Wang, X.; Liu, X.; Wu, J.; Liu, C.; Gong, W.; Zhao, Z.; Hong, J.; Lin, D.; Wang, Y.; et al. Antioxidant peptidomics reveals novel skin antioxidant system. *Mol. Cell. Proteom.* **2009**, *8*, 571–583. [CrossRef] [PubMed]

24. Basir, Y.J.; Knoop, F.C.; Dulka, J.; Conlon, J.M. Multiple antimicrobial peptides and peptides related to bradykinin and neuromedin N isolated from skin secretions of the pickerel frog, *Rana palustris*. *Biochim. Biophys. Acta* **2000**, *1543*, 95–105. [CrossRef]

25. Haney, E.F.; Hunter, H.N.; Matsuzaki, K.; Vogel, H.J. Solution NMR studies of amphibian antimicrobial peptides: Linking structure to function? *Biochim. Biophys. Acta Biomembr.* **2009**, *1788*, 1639–1655. [CrossRef] [PubMed]

26. Dubovskii, P.V.; Vassilevski, A.A.; Samsonova, O.V.; Egorova, N.S.; Kozlov, S.A.; Feofanov, A.V.; Arseniev, A.S.; Grishin, E.V. Novel lynx spider toxin shares common molecular architecture with defense peptides from frog skin: Spider toxin with a single disulfide bond. *FEBS J.* **2011**, *278*, 4382–4393. [CrossRef] [PubMed]

27. Haugen, H.S.; Fimland, G.; Nissen-Meyer, J.; Kristiansen, P.E. Three-dimensional structure in lipid micelles of the pediocin-like antimicrobial peptide curvacin A. *Biochemistry* **2005**, *44*, 16149–16157. [CrossRef] [PubMed]

28. Patil, S.M.; Xu, S.; Sheftic, S.R.; Alexandrescu, A.T. Dynamic α-helix structure of micelle-bound human amylin. *J. Biol. Chem.* **2009**, *284*, 11982–11991. [CrossRef] [PubMed]

29. Nanga, R.P.R.; Brender, J.R.; Vivekanandan, S.; Ramamoorthy, A. Structure and membrane orientation of IAPP in its natively amidated form at physiological pH in a membrane environment. *Biochim. Biophys. Acta Biomembr.* **2011**, *1808*, 2337–2342. [CrossRef] [PubMed]

30. Wang, L.; Liu, Q.; Chen, J.-C.; Cui, Y.-X.; Zhou, B.; Chen, Y.-X.; Zhao, Y.-F.; Li, Y.-M. Antimicrobial activity of human islet amyloid polypeptides: An insight into amyloid peptides' connection with antimicrobial peptides. *Biol. Chem.* **2012**, *393*. [CrossRef] [PubMed]

31. Oskarsson, M.E.; Hermansson, E.; Wang, Y.; Welsh, N.; Presto, J.; Johansson, J.; Westermark, G.T. BRICHOS domain of Bri2 inhibits islet amyloid polypeptide (IAPP) fibril formation and toxicity in human beta cells. *Proc. Natl. Acad. Sci. USA* **2018**, *115*, E2752–E2761. [CrossRef] [PubMed]

32. Yuan, W.; Cao, L.; Ma, Y.; Mao, P.; Wang, W.; Zhao, R.; Wu, Y.; Cao, Z.; Li, W. Cloning and functional characterization of a new antimicrobial peptide gene StCT1 from the venom of the scorpion *Scorpiops tibetanus*. *Peptides* **2010**, *31*, 22–26. [CrossRef] [PubMed]

33. Luna-Ramírez, K.; Quintero-Hernández, V.; Vargas-Jaimes, L.; Batista, C.V.F.; Winkel, K.D.; Possani, L.D. Characterization of the venom from the Australian scorpion *Urodacus yaschenkoi*: Molecular mass analysis of

components, cDNA sequences and peptides with antimicrobial activity. *Toxicon* **2013**, *63*, 44–54. [CrossRef] [PubMed]

34. Aleinein, R.A.; Hamoud, R.; Schäfer, H.; Wink, M. Molecular cloning and expression of ranalexin, a bioactive antimicrobial peptide from *Rana catesbeiana* in *Escherichia coli* and assessments of its biological activities. *Appl. Microbiol. Biotechnol.* **2013**, *97*, 3535–3543. [CrossRef] [PubMed]

35. Sun, Y.; Li, Q.; Li, Z.; Zhang, Y.; Zhao, J.; Wang, L. Molecular cloning, expression, purification, and functional characterization of palustrin-2CE, an antimicrobial peptide of *Rana chensinensis*. *Biosci. Biotechnol. Biochem.* **2012**, *76*, 157–162. [CrossRef] [PubMed]

36. Zhou, Q.; Li, M.; Li, C. Cloning and expression of a novel insulin-releasing peptide, brevinin-2GU from *Escherichia coli*. *J. Biosci. Bioeng.* **2009**, *107*, 460–463. [CrossRef] [PubMed]

37. Ovchinnikova, T.V.; Shenkarev, Z.O.; Balandin, S.V.; Nadezhdin, K.D.; Paramonov, A.S.; Kokryakov, V.N.; Arseniev, A.S. Molecular insight into mechanism of antimicrobial action of the beta-hairpin peptide arenicin: Specific oligomerization in detergent micelles. *Biopolymers* **2008**, *89*, 455–464. [CrossRef] [PubMed]

38. Jean, L.; Lee, C.F.; Hodder, P.; Hawkins, N.; Vaux, D.J. Dynamics of the formation of a hydrogel by a pathogenic amyloid peptide: Islet amyloid polypeptide. *Sci. Rep.* **2016**, *6*. [CrossRef] [PubMed]

39. Calabrese, A.N.; Liu, Y.; Wang, T.; Musgrave, I.F.; Pukala, T.L.; Tabor, R.F.; Martin, L.L.; Carver, J.A.; Bowie, J.H. The amyloid fibril-forming properties of the amphibian antimicrobial peptide uperin 3.5. *ChemBioChem* **2016**, *17*, 239–246. [CrossRef] [PubMed]

40. Warschawski, D.E.; Arnold, A.A.; Beaugrand, M.; Gravel, A.; Chartrand, É.; Marcotte, I. Choosing membrane mimetics for NMR structural studies of transmembrane proteins. *Biochim. Biophys. Acta Biomembr.* **2011**, *1808*, 1957–1974. [CrossRef] [PubMed]

41. Jayaraman, G.; Kumar, T.K.; Arunkumar, A.I.; Yu, C. 2,2,2-Trifluoroethanol induces helical conformation in an all beta-sheet protein. *Biochem. Biophys. Res. Commun.* **1996**, *222*, 33–37. [CrossRef] [PubMed]

42. Cavanagh, J.; Fairbrother, W.J.; Palmer, A.G., III; Rance, M.; Skelton, N.J. *Protein NMR Spectroscopy*, 2nd ed.; Academic Press: Cambridge, MA, USA, 2006; ISBN 978-0-12164-491-8.

43. Brown, L.R.; Bösch, C.; Wüthrich, K. Location and orientation relative to the micelle surface for glucagon in mixed micelles with dodecylphosphocholine: EPR and NMR studies. *Biochim. Biophys. Acta* **1981**, *642*, 296–312. [CrossRef]

44. Lakowicz, J.R. *Principles of Fluorescence Spectroscopy*, 3rd ed.; Springer: New York, NY, USA, 2006; ISBN 978-0-387-31278-1.

45. Szabo, A.G. Fluorescence principles and measurements. In *Spectrophotometry and Spectrofluorimetry*, 2nd ed.; Gore, M.G., Ed.; Oxford University Press: New York, NY, USA, 2000; pp. 33–67, ISBN 978-0-19963-812-3.

46. Chi, S.-W.; Kim, J.-S.; Kim, D.-H.; Lee, S.-H.; Park, Y.-H.; Han, K.-H. Solution structure and membrane interaction mode of an antimicrobial peptide gaegurin 4. *Biochem. Biophys. Res. Commun.* **2007**, *352*, 592–597. [CrossRef] [PubMed]

47. Subasinghage, A.P.; Conlon, J.M.; Hewage, C.M. Conformational analysis of the broad-spectrum antibacterial peptide, ranatuerin-2CSa: Identification of a full length helix–turn–helix motif. *Biochim. Biophys. Acta Proteins Proteom.* **2008**, *1784*, 924–929. [CrossRef] [PubMed]

48. Taguchi, S.; Nakagawa, K.; Maeno, M.; Momose, H. In vivo monitoring system for structure-function relationship analysis of the antibacterial peptide apidaecin. *Appl. Environ. Microbiol.* **1994**, *60*, 3566–3572. [PubMed]

49. Yonezawa, A.; Kuwahara, J.; Fujii, N.; Sugiura, Y. Binding of tachyplesin I to DNA revealed by footprinting analysis: Significant contribution of secondary structure to DNA binding and implication for biological action. *Biochemistry* **1992**, *31*, 2998–3004. [CrossRef] [PubMed]

50. Maltseva, A.L.; Kotenko, O.N.; Kokryakov, V.N.; Starunov, V.V.; Krasnodembskaya, A.D. Expression pattern of arenicins—The antimicrobial peptides of polychaete *Arenicola marina*. *Front. Physiol.* **2014**, *5*, 497. [CrossRef] [PubMed]

51. Leray, M.; Yang, J.Y.; Meyer, C.P.; Mills, S.C.; Agudelo, N.; Ranwez, V.; Boehm, J.T.; Machida, R.J. A new versatile primer set targeting a short fragment of the mitochondrial COI region for metabarcoding metazoan diversity: Application for characterizing coral reef fish gut contents. *Front. Zool.* **2013**, *10*, 34. [CrossRef] [PubMed]

52. Panteleev, P.V.; Ovchinnikova, T.V. Improved strategy for recombinant production and purification of antimicrobial peptide tachyplesin I and its analogs with high cell selectivity. *Biotechnol. Appl. Biochem.* **2017**, *64*, 35–42. [CrossRef] [PubMed]

53. Panteleev, P.V.; Bolosov, I.A.; Balandin, S.V.; Ovchinnikova, T.V. Design of antimicrobial peptide arenicin analogs with improved therapeutic indices. *J. Pept. Sci. Off. Publ. Eur. Pept. Soc.* **2015**, *21*, 105–113. [CrossRef] [PubMed]

54. Schägger, H. Tricine–SDS-PAGE. *Nat. Protoc.* **2006**, *1*, 16–22. [CrossRef] [PubMed]

55. Panteleev, P.V.; Myshkin, M.Y.; Shenkarev, Z.O.; Ovchinnikova, T.V. Dimerization of the antimicrobial peptide arenicin plays a key role in the cytotoxicity but not in the antibacterial activity. *Biochem. Biophys. Res. Commun.* **2017**, *482*, 1320–1326. [CrossRef] [PubMed]

56. Güntert, P. Automated NMR structure calculation with CYANA. In *Protein NMR Techniques*; Humana Press: Totowa, NJ, USA, 2004; Volume 278, pp. 353–378, ISBN 978-1-59259-809-0.

57. Wiegand, I.; Hilpert, K.; Hancock, R.E.W. Agar and broth dilution methods to determine the minimal inhibitory concentration (MIC) of antimicrobial substances. *Nat. Protoc.* **2008**, *3*, 163–175. [CrossRef] [PubMed]

58. Shamova, O.V.; Orlov, D.S.; Zharkova, M.S.; Balandin, S.V.; Yamschikova, E.V.; Knappe, D.; Hoffmann, R.; Kokryakov, V.N.; Ovchinnikova, T.V. Minibactenecins ChBac7.Nα and ChBac7.Nβ—Antimicrobial peptides from leukocytes of the goat *Capra hircus*. *Acta Nat.* **2016**, *8*, 136–146.

59. Kuzmin, D.V.; Emelianova, A.A.; Kalashnikova, M.B.; Panteleev, P.V.; Balandin, S.V.; Serebrovskaya, E.O.; Belogurova-Ovchinnikova, O.Y.; Ovchinnikova, T.V. Comparative in vitro study on cytotoxicity of recombinant β-hairpin peptides. *Chem. Biol. Drug Des.* **2018**, *91*, 294–303. [CrossRef] [PubMed]

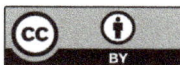

marine drugs

MDPI

Article

Anti-Proliferation Activity of a Decapeptide from *Perinereies aibuhitensis* toward Human Lung Cancer H1299 Cells

Shuoqi Jiang [1], Yinglu Jia [1], Yunping Tang [1,*], Die Zheng [1], Xingbiao Han [1], Fangmiao Yu [1], Yan Chen [1], Fangfang Huang [1], Zuisu Yang [1] and Guofang Ding [1,2,*]

[1] Zhejiang Provincial Engineering Technology Research Center of Marine Biomedical Products, School of Food and Pharmacy, Zhejiang Ocean University, Zhoushan 316022, China; jsq_sxty@163.com (S.J.); lxj19950329@163.com (Y.J.); yangzs87@163.com (D.Z.); 17805805851@163.com (X.H.); fmyu@zjou.edu.cn (F.Y.); cyancy@zjou.edu.cn (Y.C.); gracegang@126.com (F.H.); abc1967@126.com (Z.Y.)

[2] Laboratory of Aquatic Products Processing and Quality Safety, Zhejiang Marine Fisheries Research Institution, Zhoushan 316021, China

* Correspondence: tangyunping1985@zjou.edu.cn (Y.T.); dinggf2007@163.com (G.D.); Tel.: +86-0580-229-9809 (Y.T. & G.D.); Fax: +86-0580-229-9866 (G.D.)

Received: 1 February 2019; Accepted: 15 February 2019; Published: 18 February 2019

Abstract: *Perinereis aibuhitensis* peptide (PAP) is a decapeptide (Ile-Glu-Pro-Gly-Thr-Val-Gly-Met-Met-Phe, IEPGTVGMMF) with anticancer activity that was purified from an enzymatic hydrolysate of *Perinereis aibuhitensis*. In the present study, the anticancer effect of PAP on H1299 cell proliferation was investigated. Our results showed that PAP promoted apoptosis and inhibited the proliferation of H1299 cells in a time- and dose-dependent manner. When the PAP concentration reached 0.92 mM, more than 95% of treated cells died after 72 h of treatment. Changes in cell morphology were further analyzed using an inverted microscope and AO/EB staining and flow cytometry was adopted for detecting apoptosis and cell cycle phase. The results showed that the early and late apoptosis rates of H1299 cells increased significantly after treatment with PAP and the total apoptosis rate was significantly higher than that of the control group. Moreover, after treatment with PAP, the number of cells in the S phase of cells was significantly reduced and the ability for the cells to proliferate was also reduced. H1299 cells were arrested in the G2/M phase and cell cycle progression was inhibited. Furthermore, the results of western blotting showed that nm23-H1 and vascular endothelial growth factor (VEGF) protein levels decreased in a dose-dependent manner, while the pro-apoptotic protein and anti-apoptotic protein ratios and the level of apoptosis-related caspase protein increased in a dose-dependent manner. In conclusion, our results indicated that PAP, as a natural marine bioactive substance, inhibited proliferation and induced apoptosis of human lung cancer H1299 cells. PAP is likely to be exploited as the functional food or adjuvant that may be used for prevention or treatment of human non-small cell lung cancer in the future.

Keywords: *Perinereis aibuhitensis*; decapeptide; lung cancer; cell proliferation; apoptosis

1. Introduction

Primary bronchogenic carcinoma is referred to as lung cancer and can occur at various levels of the bronchial epithelium or glands in the form of a malignant tumor [1]. The incidence and mortality of lung cancer have increased year by year and lung cancer is a disease that seriously threatens human health and life. According to statistics from the United Nations and the European Union, the lung cancer is the most common cause of cancer death, with an estimated 388,000 lung cancer cases resulting in death in Europe in 2018 [2]. In addition, according to the American Cancer Society's 2018 report, the numbers of new cancer diagnoses and cancer deaths in the United States in 2018 are estimated to be

234,030 and 154,050, respectively, with lung cancer having the highest mortality rate in both sexes [3]. According to the pathological morphology, lung cancer generally can be classified into two categories: small-cell lung cancer (SCLC) and non-small-cell lung cancer (NSCLC). NSCLC represents 80% to 85% of all lung cancers and the early diagnosis rate is low. About 85% of patients have distant metastases or inoperable tumors at the time of diagnosis, leaving only comprehensive chemotherapy-based treatment [4]. However, due to the poor sensitivity of NSCLC to chemotherapy and the lack of ideal selective agents, toxicity and drug resistance to existing chemotherapy drugs, the dose of antitumor drugs is limited, the efficacy is affected, and treatment can fail.

Peptides are important natural products in various organisms and their broad spectrum of activities promotes the completion of various complex physiological functions in the body. The requirements for life in the ocean cause marine organisms to produce and accumulate a large number of peptides with unique structures and special biological activities. Extensive research has found that some marine peptides or their derivatives have potential as nutrient supplements or have medicinal value, such as antimicrobial peptides [5], antiviral peptides [6], antitumor/cytotoxic peptides [7], angiotensin-I-converting enzyme (ACE) inhibitory peptides [8], and antioxidant peptides [9,10]. Many of these have been developed as pharmaceutical or dietary supplements. Recently, many polypeptide fractions were isolated from marine organisms with potent anti-proliferative activity against cancer cells. For example, Yu et al. [11] demonstrated that a pentapeptide (Ile-Leu-Tyr-Met-Pro, ILYMP) isolated from *Cyclina sinensis* protein hydrolysate could induce apoptosis in DU-145 prostate cancer cells, whereas Wu et al. [12] reported that an oligopeptide (Tyr-Val-Pro-Gly-Pro, YVPGP) from *Anthopleura anjunae* showed anticancer activity against DU-145 prostate cancer cells. Additionally, Wang and Zhang [13] found an anti-proliferative peptide isolated from the protein hydrolysate of *Spirulina platensis* that exhibited strong inhibition on HT-29 cancer cells with the half maximal inhibitory concentration (IC_{50}) of 99.88 μg/mL. Similarly, Pan et al. [14] purified a hexapeptide (Phe-Ile-Met-Gly-Pro-Tyr, FIMGPY) from the protein hydrolysate of skate (*Raja porosa*) cartilage, which exhibited dose-dependent anti-proliferative activity with an IC_{50} of 4.81 mg/mL against the HeLa cells.

Perinereis aibuhitensis belongs to the *Annelida, Polychaeta, Errantia, Nereidae, Nereis* genus [15]. It is very common in rocky shores, rocks, algal cones and coral reefs or soft sediments in intertidal zones. In recent years, due to the economics of *Perinereis aibuhitensis* rearing, it has provided abundant materials for pharmacological research. It has been reported that Nereis extract shows good insecticidal [16], antithrombotic [17], antihypertensive [18] and antimicrobial [19] activities. However, there are few reports on the inhibitory effects of functional peptides from *Perinereis aibuhitensis* on human lung cancer H1299 cells. *Perinereis aibuhitensis* peptide (PAP) is a decapeptide (Ile-Glu-Pro-Gly-Thr-Val-Gly-Met-Met-Phe, IEPGTVGMMF) with anti-cancer activity that is purified from an enzymatic hydrolysate of *Perinereis aibuhitensis* in our previous study [20]. However, the mechanism of its anticancer activity was not well illustrated. In this study, in vitro cultured human lung cancer H1299 cells were used to observe the effect of PAP on tumor cell proliferation, apoptosis and metastasis, which may lead to another alternative high value-added utilization of *Perinereis aibuhitensis*.

2. Results and Discussion

2.1. Effects of PAP on the Proliferation of H1299 Cells

Normal human cells are tightly regulated, but excessive proliferation of cells and uncontrolled regulation of apoptosis can lead to uncontrolled growth of tumors. The inhibitory effect of PAP on the proliferation of H1299 cells was determined using the CCK-8 method. There was a dose-dependent inhibition of H1299 cell proliferation following PAP treatment (Figure 1). After treatment with 0.23 mM PAP for 24 h, the inhibition rate of H1299 cells was 11.79%. When the concentration of PAP increased to 0.92 mM, the inhibition rate was 67.03% after 24 h treatment. In addition, the inhibition rate of PAP on H1299 cells was also positively correlated with treatment time and the inhibition rate of H1299 cells reached 95% after treatment with 0.92 mM of PAP for 72 h. The inhibitory effect of PAP was significant after 48 h. When the concentration of PAP was between 0.23 and 0.46 mg/mL, significant inhibition on H1299 cells was achieved by increasing the treatment time. The IC_{50} of PAP on H1299 cell proliferation at 24 h, 48 h and 72 h were 0.69 mM, 0.38 mM and 0.27 mM, respectively. Furthermore, PAP has almost no cytotoxic effects on the fibroblast NIH-3T3 cells (data was not shown). Similarly, the marine active peptides Hem and Dol were reported to be cytotoxic to H1299 cells after conjugation with universal BB agonist in a dose-dependent manner (with IC_{50} values of 15 and 25 nM, respectively) [21]. Yu et al. [11] reported that the pentapeptide CSP (ILYMP, with an IC_{50} of 11.25 mM at 72 h) isolated from *Cyclina sinensis* had inhibitory activity against DU-145 cells in a dose-dependent manner. Wu et al. [12] demonstrated that the pentapeptide AAP-H (YVPGP, with IC_{50} values of 9.605 mM, 7.910 mM, and 2.298 mM at 24 h, 48 h, and 72 h, respectively), purified from the sea anemone *Anthopleura anjunae*, also induced apoptosis in a dose- and time-dependent manner. In conclusion, PAP inhibited the proliferation of H1299 cells in a dose- and time-dependent manner, and PAP concentrations below 0.92 mM had no obvious cytotoxicity to the normal cells.

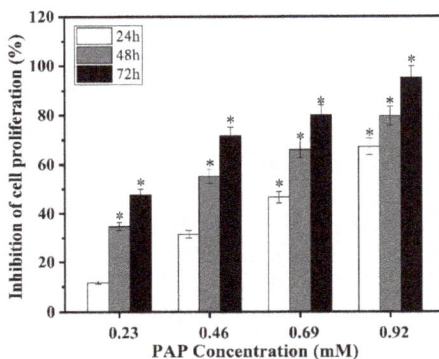

Figure 1. The inhibitory effect of *Perinereis aibuhitensis* peptide (PAP) on the proliferation of H1299 cells. H1299 cells were treated with different concentrations of PAP for 24, 48 and 72 h. All data are presented as the mean ± standard deviation (SD) of three experiments. (*) Results are significantly different from the control ($p < 0.05$).

2.2. Morphological Observations

2.2.1. Inverted Microscope Observations

Viewing the treated cells with an inverted microscope revealed visible damage to H1299 cells caused by PAP, which was enhanced with increasing of PAP concentrations. As shown in Figure 2, the control cells (Figure 2A) adhered to the bottom of the cell culture flasks and the cells grew tightly. When the cells were treated with 0.23 mM PAP, the cells were mostly rounded and dispersed (Figure 2B). When the PAP concentration reached 0.46 mM (Figure 2C), a small number of cells exhibited an irregular shape, while most cells appeared round and bright. When the PAP concentration reached 0.92 mM (Figure 2D), the treated cells became smaller and were longer stuck to the bottle but floated.

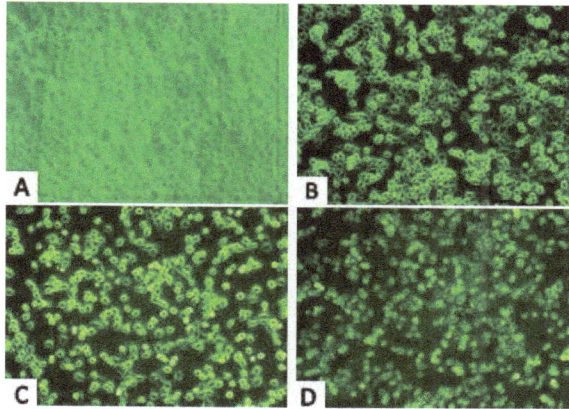

Figure 2. Morphological observation by inverted microscopy (× 200). H1299 cells were untreated (**A**) or treated with 0.23 mM PAP (**B**), 0.46 mM PAP (**C**) and 0.92 mM PAP (**D**). Each experiment was performed in triplicate and the cells exhibited similar morphological features.

2.2.2. AO/EB Fluorescence Staining Results

Acridine orange/ethidium bromide (AO/EB) staining is commonly used for cell morphology and cell cycle analysis. Before the apoptotic rate was calculated by Annexin V-FITC/PI Apoptosis Detection Kit, AO/EB fluorescence staining was used to provide an indication of apoptosis following drug treatment, which can help to determine the appropriate dose and timing of drug intervention. Nuclear chromatin was condensed and distributed along the nuclear membrane in early apoptotic cells. Subsequently, the chromatin further condensed to form apoptotic bodies and the cells entered late apoptosis. The cells in the control group had intact nuclei with uniform green fluorescence and clear cell boundaries observed (Figure 3A). Cells with early apoptotic cell nuclei exhibited yellow-green fluorescence following treatment with 0.23 and 0.46 mM PAP for 24 h, while late-stage apoptotic cells with concentrated and asymmetrically localized nuclear and unclear cyto-membranes were also observed. As the PAP concentration increased to 0.92 mM, apoptotic bodies formed by chromatin condensation or cleavage and the number of late apoptotic cells increased, with necrotic cells showing uneven orange-red fluorescence also observed (Figure 3D). The AO/EB staining results also revealed that the apoptotic characteristics of H1299 cells caused by PAP treatment occurred in a dose-dependent manner.

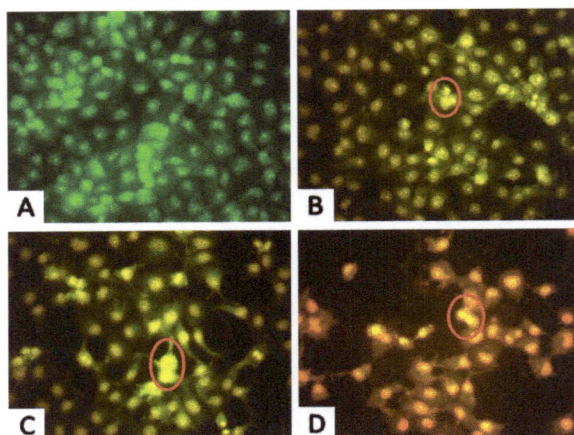

Figure 3. Morphological observation by Acridine orange/ethidium bromide (AO/EB) staining (×
200). H1299 cells were treated with PAP at 0 Mm (**A**), 0.23 mM (**B**), 0.46 mM (**C**), and 0.92 mM (**D**)
for 24 h. The red circles in Figure 3B,C indicate early apoptotic cells, while the red circle in Figure 3D
indicates late apoptotic cells. Each experiment was performed in triplicate and the cells exhibited
similar morphological features.

2.3. Cell Apoptosis Analysis

In the early stages of apoptosis, phosphatidylserine (PS) flips to the surface of the cell membrane
and annexin-V is able to bind PS with high affinity. In addition, propidium iodide (PI) can penetrate
the incomplete cell membrane to stain the nucleus red, which distinguishes between late apoptotic cells
and necrotic cells. The Annexin V-FITC/PI Apoptosis Detection Kit can quantitatively measure the
early apoptotic status of cells. Flow cytometry was used to quantitatively detect the apoptosis rate of
PAP-treated H1299 cells, which is shown in Figure 4, where the upper left quadrant represents necrotic
cells, the lower left quadrant represents normal living cells, the upper right quadrant represents late
apoptotic cells, and the lower right quadrant represents early apoptotic cells. After 24 h of treatment
with PAP, Annexin V-FITC/PI staining showed that PAP increased apoptosis in H1299 cells in a
dose-dependent manner. As shown in Figure 4, the rates of early and late apoptotic stages in H1299
cells without PAP treatment were 4.18% and 3.65%, respectively, with 92.08% of the cells appearing
healthy. As the concentration of PAP increased, the number of late apoptotic cells increased from
2.83% to 10.42% and the percentage of cells in the early stages of apoptosis increased dramatically
from 13.11% to 39.95%.

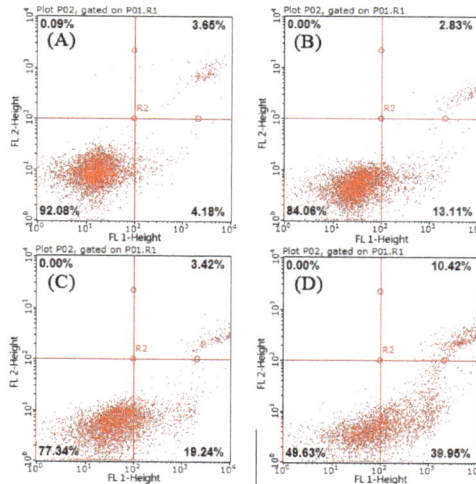

Figure 4. The apoptotic effect of PAP on H1299 cells as determined by flow cytometry. The percentages of early apoptotic cells were 4.18% in the blank control cells (**A**); 13.11% in the 0.23 mM PAP-treated cells (**B**); 19.24% in the 0.46 mM PAP-treated cells (**C**); and 39.95% in the 0.92 mM PAP-treated cells (**D**). One representative apoptosis analysis of three independent experiments was presented.

2.4. Effects of PAP on the Cell Cycle Distribution of H1299 Cells

The cell cycle is the series of events that a cell undergoes from the completion of one division phase to the end of the next. In general, the cell cycle can be divided into interphase (phase I) and mitosis (M phase) and the DNA content of cells is different in different stages. PI, a DNA-binding fluorescent dye, exhibits a fluorescence intensity proportional to the amount of DNA bound to intracellular DNA. Therefore, the distribution of DNA in each phase of the cell cycle is directly reflected by flow cytometry and the proportions of cells in the G0/G1 phase, S phase and G2/M phase can be accurately quantified. In the present study, we determined the cell cycle distribution of H1299 cells treated with PAP. The first peak in Figure 5A represents cells in the G0/G1 phase, the second peak represents cells in the G2/M phase and the valley is cells in the S phase. The proportion of cells in each phase is shown in Figure 5B. After treatment with PAP at 0.23, 0.46 and 0.92 mg/mL for 24 h, the proportion of cells in the S phase in H1299 cells significantly increased from 12.28% to 21.79%. Moreover, there was a decreased proportion of H1299 cells in the S phase (from 42.29% to 16.87%). This result indicated that PAP induced G2/M phase arrest in a dose-dependent manner to arrest the proliferation of tumor cells. Similarly, Huang [22] reported that the oligopeptide (Gln-Pro-Lys, SIO) from *Sepia* ink significantly inhibited the S phase of PC-3 cells and the number of cells in the G0/G1 phase showed a similar increase. SIO arrested PC-3 cells in the G0/G1 phase in a dose-dependent manner. Meanwhile, Yang et al. [23] showed that DU-145 cells treated with a tetrapeptide (Asp-Trp-Pro-His, PROI-1) had a significantly reduced number of cells in the S phase, leading to induction of G2/M phase arrest and apoptosis.

(A)   (B)

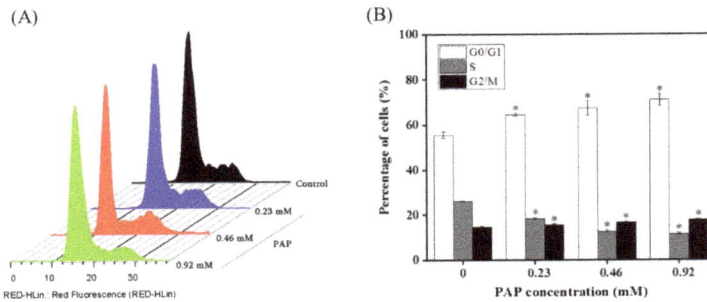

Figure 5. (**A**) Effects of PAP on the cell cycle progression of H1299 cell lines. H1299 cells were treated with PAP at 0, 0.23, 0.46, and 0.92 mM for 24 h. Flow cytometry was used to define the cell cycle distribution in comparison with controls. (**B**) Percentages of H1299 cells in the G0/G1, S and G2/M phases. All data are presented as the mean ± standard deviation (SD) of three experiments. (*) Results are significantly different from the control (*p* < 0.05).

2.5. Western Blotting Results

Apoptosis is a process of programmed cell death that is induced by specific signals produced by various physiological or pathological stimuli. Therefore, the analysis of signaling factors involved in the regulation of apoptosis is useful for elucidating the mechanism of action of the anti-proliferative effects of drugs. To further verify the effects of PAP on H1299 cells and explain the underlying mechanisms, western blotting was used to investigate the expression of apoptosis-related proteins in treated H1299 cells.

Apoptosis is regulated by key regulatory proteins of the Bcl-2 family. Most Bcl-2 family proteins play a role at the mitochondrial level, and excessive apoptosis caused by abnormal changes in the levels of Bcl-2 proteins is a key step in tumor progression [24,25]. Up-regulation of *Bcl-2* gene expression is conducive to the inhibition of apoptosis and anti-apoptotic effect [26]. The *Bax* gene also belongs to the *Bcl-2* gene family and Bax forms a heterodimer with Bcl-2, which inhibits Bcl-2 and promotes apoptosis [27]. A previous study found that the proportional relationship between Bax/Bcl-2 proteins is a key factor in determining the inhibition of apoptosis [24,25]. As shown in Figure 6, PAP showed pro-apoptotic activity against H1299 cells with the Bax/Bcl-2 expression ratios of 1.47%, 2.52% and 6.67%, when the cells treated with 0.23, 0.69 and 0.92 mg/mL of PAP, respectively. Huang [22] reported that SIO induced the death of prostate cancer cells (DU-145, PC-3, and LNCaP) and showed an increase in the Bax/Bcl-2 ratio. Furthermore, Wan et al. [28] found that an oligopeptide (KIKAVLKVLTT) derived from melittin induced the death of thyroid cancer TT cells via upregulation of Bax and down-regulation of Bcl-2. Our results also indicated that PAP induced apoptosis of H1299 cells by up-regulating the Bax/Bcl-2 ratio, which was consistent with previous studies.

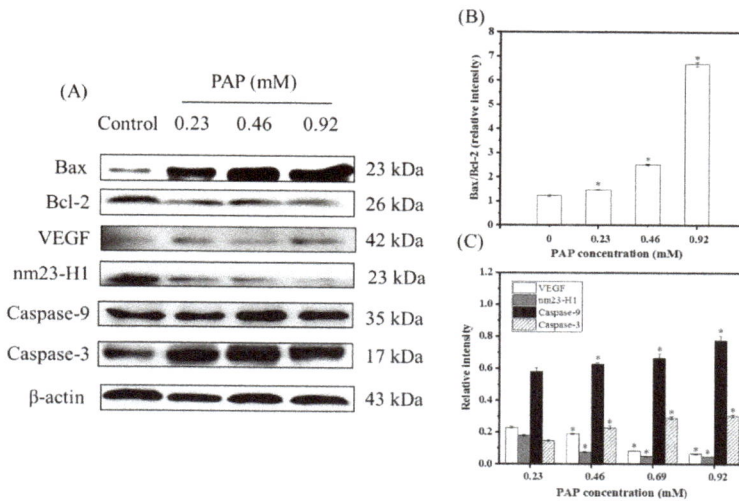

Figure 6. (**A**) Expression of Bax, Bcl-2, VEGF, nm23-H1, Caspase-9, Caspase-3 proteins in H1299 cells treated with different concentrations of PAP (0, 0.23, 0.46 and 0.92 mM) for 24 h. (**B**) The Bax/Bcl-2 ratio expressed in H1299 cells treated with PAP as a function of PAP concentrations for 24 h, where Bax and Bcl-2 were apoptosis-associated. (**C**) VEGF, nm23-H1, Caspase-9, Caspase-3 expression in H1299 cells treated with PAP for 24 h. The blots were detected with β-actin antibody to determine equal sample loading. Each experiment was performed in triplicate. (*) Results are significantly different from the control ($p < 0.05$).

Caspase proteins are proteolytic enzymes that play important roles in programmed cell death. They can be further subdivided into the following two types according to their function in apoptosis: initiator (caspases-9) and effector (caspases-3) caspases [29]. Caspase-9 is activated upon cytochrome c release and acts to activate effector caspase and the pro-apoptotic protein Bid, which ensures that cells with an apoptosome will die without effector caspase. Furthermore, caspase-3 is a major executor of apoptotic death, which makes cell death more effective. PAP significantly up-regulated the expression of caspase-9 and caspase-3. When the PAP concentration ranged from 0 to 0.92 mg/mL, the relative intensities with caspase-9 and caspase-3 increased from 0.58 to 0.78 and 0.15 to 0.30, respectively. This indicated that PAP treatment causes a cascade of reactions in H1299 cells leading to apoptosis.

Nm23-H1 is widely used as an important indictor to determine tumor metastasis. The nm23-H1 protein is highly similar to the α-chain amino acid sequence of the nucleoside diphosphate kinase (NDPK) and has the same activity. It plays a role in cell growth and tumor metastasis by catalyzing the conversion of guanosine triphosphate GTP to guanosine diphosphate (GDP), participating in the polymerization and disintegrating tubulin or by regulating GDP synthesis to participate in G-protein-regulated transmembrane signaling [29]. For example, L9981 cells transfected with nm23-H1 cDNA showed lower expression of nm23-H1 than untransfected cells, and tumor proliferation and invasiveness decreased at the same time [30]. The results of this experiment also showed that the lower the expression of nm23-H1, the lower the degree of tumor differentiation, and the results of the apoptosis experiment were consistent with the western blotting results [31].

VEGF is an essential angiogenic growth factor. High levels of VEGF were found in approximately one-third of NSCLC [32]. VEGF promotes angiogenesis, regulates the apoptosis of vascular endothelial cells and alveolar epithelial cells and increases the permeability of blood vessels, which leads to sustained tumor growth. For example, Xu [33] studied the inhibitory effect of MUC1 on NSCLC cells and the results of western blotting indicated that MUC1 significantly reduced the levels of VEGF and VEGF-C proteins, indicating that MUC1 has an anti-angiogenic effect and can be used as a potential treatment for NSCLC. In the present study, the expression level of VEGF decreased significantly when the PAP concentration increased, indicating that PAP could inhibit tumor angiogenesis and inhibit tumor growth.

3. Materials and Methods

3.1. Materials and Reagents

In a previous study, the peptide PAP (IEPGTVGMMF) was prepared by our laboratory and preserved at $-20°C$ until further use (Figure 7) [20]. The H1299 cell lines and NIH-3T3 cell lines were stored in our laboratory. Cell Counting Kit-8 (CCK-8) and Cell Cycle and Annexin V-FITC/PI Apoptosis Detection Kit were purchased from BestBio Biotechnology (Shanghai, China). The BCA protein detection kit was purchased from Jiancheng Bio-Technology Co., Ltd. (Nanjing, China). Antibodies against β-actin (cat. no. TA-09), Bax (cat. no. 2772S), Bcl-2 (cat. no. 2872S), nm23-H1 (cat. no. bs-1066P), VEGF (cat. no. AF1309), Caspase-3 (cat. no. 9662S), and Caspase-9 (cat. no. 70R-11636) were purchased from ZSGB Biotechnology (Beijing, China). All other reagents used in this study were of analytical grade.

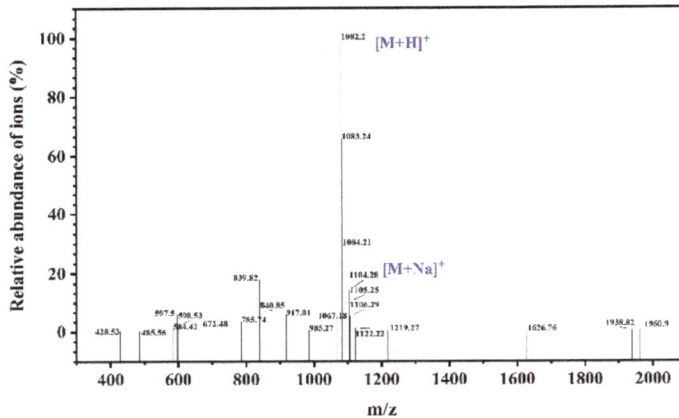

Figure 7. Mass spectrogram of PAP and the sequence of PAP identified as IEPGTVGMMF with a molecular weight of 1081.20 Da.

3.2. Detection of Anti-Proliferation Activity Using CCK-8

The CCK-8 detection kit is a simple and accurate method that is widely used in cell proliferation analysis [22]. The following steps were performed, according to the method of Huang et al. [22] with slight modifications. H1299 cells were adjusted to approximately 1×10^4 cells/100 μL/well in a 96-well tray and incubated overnight in a 5% CO_2 incubator (Forma 3111 CO_2 incubator, Thermo Forma, Waltham, MA, USA) at 37 °C. The cells were then treated with PAP at final concentrations of 0, 0.23, 0.46, 0.69 and 0.92 mM for 24, 48 or 72 h. After the treatment was completed, the culture medium was removed, and 90 μL of phosphate-buffered saline (PBS) and 10 μL CCK-8 were added to each well. Incubation was carried out for 4 h under conventional conditions in a CO_2 incubator and the optical density (OD) value was measured with an automatic microplate reader (SpectraMax M2, Molecular Devices, Sunnyvale, CA, USA) at a detection wavelength of 450 nm. The following equation was used to calculate the relative inhibition rate of cell proliferation:

$$\text{Relative inhibition rate (\%)} = (1 - (OD_{treated}/OD_{control})) \times 100\%.$$

3.3. Cell Morphology Observation Using an Inverted Microscope

H1299 cells (approximately 1×10^5 cells/well) were seeded in a 6-well flat-bottom plate and incubated for 24 h in a 5% CO_2 incubator at 37 °C. The culture medium was then removed and the cells were treated with PAP at a final concentration of 0, 0.23, 0.46 and 0.92 mM. After incubation for another 24 h, morphological changes in the cells were observed using a CKX4 inverted microscope (OLYMPUS, Tokyo, Japan).

3.4. Cell Morphological Analysis by AO/EB Staining

To observe the morphological characteristics of H1299 cells at different stages of apoptosis, cells were stained using AO/EB fluorescence staining as described by Huang et al. [34], with slight modifications. Cleaned coverslips were placed in a 6-well plate (approximately 1×10^5 cells/well) and H1299 cells were seeded as previously described. After the cells were attached, the cells were treated with final concentrations of 0, 0.23, 0.46 and 0.92 mM PAP for 24 h. The coverslips were washed 2 to 3 times with PBS (pH 7.2) and fixed in 95% ethanol for 30 min. Drops containing 50 µL of PBS and 6 µL of AO/EB mixture (0.1 mg/mL AO and EB in PBS, pH = 7.2) were placed on microscope slides, and the side of the coverslip to which the cells had adhered was placed in contact with the AO/EB droplet. Cell morphology was observed by a BX41 fluorescence microscope (OLYMPUS, Tokyo, Japan) and photographed.

3.5. Cell Apoptosis Analysis Using Annexin V FITC/PI

To confirm PAP-induced apoptosis of H1299 cells, flow cytometry was performed as described by Yoon et al. [35]. H1299 cells were seeded in 25-mL culture bottles (approximately 1×10^5 cells/mL). After 24 h incubation, cells were treated with different final concentrations (0, 0.23, 0.46 and 0.92 mM) of PAP and cultured for 24 h. Cells were then harvested following treatment and digested with trypsin. The suspended cells were then collected by centrifugation (1000 rpm, 5 min) and were stained with Annexin V-FITC and PI using the Annexin V-FITC Apoptosis Detection Kit. Finally, apoptosis was immediately detected by flow cytometry (Becton Dickinson, NJ, USA).

3.6. Cell Cycle Analysis by Propidium Iodide Staining

To investigate whether PAP controls the cell cycle to achieve apoptosis, flow cytometry was used to measure the different cell cycle phases of H1299 cells, following the method described by Li et al. [36]. H1299 cells in the logarithmic growth phase were inoculated into a 6-well plate and the cells were cultured for 24 h until they had completely adhered to the bottom of the plate. Different concentrations of PAP (0, 0.23, 0.46 and 0.92 mM) were added to the cells and they were incubated for 24 h. Then cells were trypsinized, harvested and washed twice with pre-cooled PBS. Briefly, RNase A was added to the cells obtained by centrifugation and the mixture was incubated at 37 °C for 30 min. Finally, 350 µL of PI was added, mixed and incubated at 4 °C for 5 min in the dark. The solution was subsequently filtered with a 200 mesh sieve and a cell cycle curve was obtained using flow cytometry.

3.7. Detection of Protein Expression by Western Blotting

To confirm the apoptotic effects of PAP on H1299 cells, we performed western blotting according to the method described by Peng et al. [37]. H1299 cells were seeded in a 6-well plate (approximately 1×10^5 cells/mL) and treated with different final concentrations of PAP (0, 0.23, 0.46 and 0.92 mM). After treatment with PAP for 24 h, cells were harvested and lysed in RIPA lysis buffer. The extracted proteins were quantified by the bicinchoninic acid (BCA) total protein assay kit. SDS-PAGE was used to separate proteins, which were subsequently blotted onto PVDF membranes (Millipore, Billerica, MA, USA). Five percentage of skim milk was used as a blocking solution for 1 h and incubated overnight with the primary antibodies (Bcl-2, Bax, nm23-H1, VEGF, Caspase-3, and Caspase-9) at 4 °C. After washing twice with TBST (10 mL Tris-buffered saline with 20% Tween-20) and once with TBS

(10 mL Tris-Buffered saline), membranes were incubated with the secondary antibodies for 2 h. Finally, membranes were washed as noted above and combined with enhanced chemiluminescence (ECL) reagents and images were captured using an Alpha FluorChem FC3 imaging system (ProteinSimple, San Jose, CA, USA). β-actin was used as an internal control. Image J 1.38 software (NIH, Bethesda, MD, USA) was used to quantify and record the OD.

3.8. Statistical Analysis

All experimental data are expressed as the mean ± standard deviation ($\bar{x} \pm s$, n = 3), and were analyzed using SPSS software version 24.0 (SPSS Inc., Chicago, IL, USA). Statistical significance of the data was compared using one-way analysis of variance (ANOVA). The least significant difference (LSD) was used for post hoc multiple comparisons, and $p < 0.05$ indicates a statistically significant difference.

4. Conclusions

In the present study, PAP (Ile-Glu-Pro-Gly-Thr-Val-Gly-Met-Met-Phe, IEPGTVGMMF) that was purified from an enzymatic hydrolysate of *Perinereis aibuhitensis* showed anti-cancer activity toward H1299 cells. The CCK-8 results showed that PAP inhibited the proliferation of H1299 cells in a time- and dose-dependent manner. The apoptotic status of the cells was also observed with an inverted microscope and AO/EB staining. The results of flow cytometry showed that PAP could induce apoptosis of H1299 cells and the apoptosis rate increased with increasing drug dosage. Therefore, PAP may inhibit the growth of malignant lung cancer cells by inducing G0/G1 phase arrest and tumor cell apoptosis. Furthermore, the results of western blotting showed that the expression of nm23-H1 and VEGF protein decreased in a dose-dependent manner, while the ratio of pro-apoptotic proteins and anti-apoptotic proteins, apoptosis-related caspase proteins increased in a dose-dependent manner. In conclusion, our results indicated that PAP has the potential to be used as the functional or adjuvant food for the prevention or treatment of human NSCLC in the future. However, studies on the structure–activity relationship of PAP and studies on the anticancer activity in vivo of this peptide need to be performed.

Author Contributions: G.D. conceived and designed the experiments. S.J., Y.L., D.Z. and X.H performed the experiments. F.Y., Y.C., F.H. and Z.Y. carried out statistical analysis of the data. S.J. and Y.T. wrote the paper.

Funding: This research was financially supported by the National Natural Science Foundation of China (grant No. 81773629), and the Co-innovation of Zhejiang Science and Technology Program (No. 2016F50039).

Conflicts of Interest: The authors declare no conflict of interest.

References

1. Teh, E.; Belcher, E. Lung cancer: Diagnosis, staging and treatment. *Surgery (Oxford)* **2014**, *32*, 242–248. [CrossRef]
2. Ferlay, J.; Colombet, M.; Soerjomataram, I.; Dyba, T.; Randi, G.; Bettio, M.; Gavin, A.; Visser, O.; Bray, F. Cancer incidence and mortality patterns in Europe: Estimates for 40 countries and 25 major cancers in 2018. *Eur. J. Cancer* **2018**, *103*, 356–387. [CrossRef] [PubMed]
3. Siegel, R.L.; Miller, K.D.; Jemal, A. Cancer statistics, 2018. *CA Cancer J. Clin.* **2018**, *68*, 7–30. [CrossRef] [PubMed]
4. Chirieac, L.R.; Attanoos, R.L. 26—Usual Lung Cancers. In *Pulmonary Pathology*, 2nd ed.; Zander, D.S., Farver, C.F., Eds.; Content Repository Only: Philadelphia, PA, USA, 2018; pp. 534–551.
5. Semreen, M.H.; El-Gamal, M.I.; Abdin, S.; Alkhazraji, H.; Kamal, L.; Hammad, S.; El-Awady, F.; Waleed, D.; Kourbaj, L. Recent updates of marine antimicrobial peptides. *Saudi Pharm. J.* **2018**, *26*, 396–409. [CrossRef] [PubMed]
6. Ma, X.; Nong, X.-H.; Ren, Z.; Wang, J.; Liang, X.; Wang, L.; Qi, S.-H. Antiviral peptides from marine gorgonian-derived fungus *Aspergillus* sp. SCSIO 41501. *Tetrahedron Lett.* **2017**, *58*, 1151–1155. [CrossRef]

7. Lee, Y.; Phat, C.; Hong, S.-C. Structural diversity of marine cyclic peptides and their molecular mechanisms for anticancer, antibacterial, antifungal, and other clinical applications. *Peptides* **2017**, *95*, 94–105. [CrossRef] [PubMed]

8. Lee, S.Y.; Hur, S.J. Antihypertensive peptides from animal products, marine organisms, and plants. *Food Chem.* **2017**, *228*, 506–517. [CrossRef] [PubMed]

9. Gogineni, V.; Hamann, M.T. Marine natural product peptides with therapeutic potential: Chemistry, biosynthesis, and pharmacology. *BBA-Gen Subj.* **2018**, *1862*, 81–196. [CrossRef]

10. Sila, A.; Bougatef, A. Antioxidant peptides from marine by-products: Isolation, identification and application in food systems. A review. *J. Funct. Foods* **2016**, *21*, 10–26. [CrossRef]

11. Yu, F.; Zhang, Y.; Ye, L.; Tang, Y.; Ding, G.; Zhang, X.; Yang, Z. A novel antiproliferative pentapeptide (ILYMP) isolated from *Cyclina sinensis* protein hydrolysate induces apoptosis of DU145 prostate cancer cells. *Mol. Med. Rep.* **2018**, *18*, 771–778.

12. Wu, Z.Z.; Ding, G.F.; Huang, F.F.; Yang, Z.S.; Yu, F.M.; Tang, Y.P.; Jia, Y.L.; Zheng, Y.Y.; Chen, R. Anticancer Activity of *Anthopleura anjunae* Oligopeptides in Prostate Cancer DU-145 Cells. *Mar. Drugs* **2018**, *16*, 125. [CrossRef] [PubMed]

13. Wang, Z.; Zhang, X. Isolation and identification of anti-proliferative peptides from *Spirulina platensis* using three-step hydrolysis. *J. Sci. Food Agric.* **2016**, *97*, 918–922. [CrossRef] [PubMed]

14. Pan, X.; Zhao, Y.-Q.; Hu, F.-Y.; Chi, C.-F.; Wang, B. Anticancer Activity of a Hexapeptide from Skate (*Raja porosa*) Cartilage Protein Hydrolysate in HeLa Cells. *Mar. Drugs* **2016**, *14*, 153. [CrossRef] [PubMed]

15. Sun, R.P. *Fauna Sinica Invertebrata (Vol.33) Annelida Polychaeta II Nereidida*; Science Press: Beijing, China, 2004.

16. Samidurai, K.; Saravanakumar, A. Mosquitocidal properties of nereistoxin against Anopheles stephensi, Aedes aegypti and Culex quinquefasciatus (*Diptera*: *Culicidae*). *Parasitol. Res.* **2011**, *109*, 1107–1112. [CrossRef] [PubMed]

17. Li, Y.; Li, J.; Liu, T.; Wang, Y.; Zhou, Z.; Cheng, F.; Feng, C.; Cheng, X.; Liu, H.; Chen, X. Preparation and antithrombotic activity identification of *Perinereis aibuhitensis* extract: A high temperature and wide pH range stable biological agent. *Food Funct.* **2017**, *8*, 3533–3541. [CrossRef]

18. Chen, L.; Wang, S. Preparation of an ACE-inhibitory peptide from *Perinereis aibuhitensis* protein. *Biotechnol. Biotechnol. Equip.* **2017**, *31*, 1231–1236. [CrossRef]

19. Pan, W.; Liu, X.; Ge, F.; Han, J.; Zheng, T. Perinerin, a novel antimicrobial peptide purified from the clamworm *Perinereis aibuhitensis grube* and its partial characterization. *J. Biochem.* **2004**, *135*, 297–304. [CrossRef] [PubMed]

20. Jia, Y.; Ding, G.; Yang, Z.; Yu, F.; Zheng, Y.; Wu, Z.; Rui, C. Anticancer Activity of a Novel Peptide Derived from Hydrolysates of *Perinereies aibuhitensis* against Lung Cancer A549 Cells. *Food Sci.* **2017**, *38*, 27–35.

21. Moody, T.W.; Pradhan, T.; Mantey, S.A.; Jensen, R.T.; Dyba, M.; Moody, D.; Tarasova, N.I.; Michejda, C.J. Bombesin marine toxin conjugates inhibit the growth of lung cancer cells. *Life Sci.* **2008**, *82*, 855–861. [CrossRef]

22. Huang, F.; Yang, Z.; Yu, D.; Wang, J.; Li, R.; Ding, G. Sepia ink oligopeptide induces apoptosis in prostate cancer cell lines via caspase-3 activation and elevation of Bax/Bcl-2 ratio. *Mar. Drugs* **2012**, *10*, 2153–2165. [CrossRef]

23. Yang, Z.; Zhao, Y.; Yan, H.; Xu, L.; Ding, G.; Yu, D.; Sun, Y. Isolation and purification of oligopeptides from *Ruditapes philippinarum* and its inhibition on the growth of DU145 cells in vitro. *Mol. Med. Rep.* **2015**, *11*, 1063–1068. [CrossRef] [PubMed]

24. Wang, F.Z.; Dai, X.L.; Liu, H.Y. Molecular mechanisms underlying the α-tomatine-directed apoptosis in human malignant glioblastoma cell lines A172 and U-118 MG. *Exp. Ther. Med.* **2017**, *14*, 6183–6192. [CrossRef] [PubMed]

25. Farkas, R.; Pozsgai, E.; Bellyei, S.; Cseke, L.; Szigeti, A.; Vereczkei, A.; Marton, S.; Mangel, L.; Horvath, O.P.; Papp, A. Correlation between tumor-associated proteins and response to neoadjuvant treatment in patients with advanced squamous-cell esophageal cancer. *Anticancer Res.* **2011**, *31*, 1769–1775. [PubMed]

26. Callagy, G.M.; Pharoah, P.D.; Pinder, S.E.; Hsu, F.D.; Nielsen, T.O.; Ragaz, J.; Ellis, I.O.; Huntsman, D.; Caldas, C. Bcl-2 is a prognostic marker in breast cancer independently of the Nottingham Prognostic Index. *Clin. Cancer Res.* **2006**, *12*, 2468–2475. [CrossRef] [PubMed]

27. Gross, A.; Jockel, J.; Wei, M.C.; Korsmeyer, S.J. Enforced dimerization of BAX results in its translocation, mitochondrial dysfunction and apoptosis. *Embo J.* **1998**, *17*, 3878–3885. [CrossRef]

28. Wan, L.; Zhang, D.; Zhang, J.; Ren, L. TT-1, an analog of melittin, triggers apoptosis in human thyroid cancer TT cells via regulating caspase, Bcl-2 and Bax. *Oncol. Lett.* **2018**, *15*, 1271–1278. [CrossRef]
29. Fuentes-Prior, P.; Salvesen, G.S. The protein structures that shape caspase activity, specificity, activation and inhibition. *Biochem. J.* **2004**, *384*, 201–232. [CrossRef]
30. Che, G.; Zhou, Q.; Wang, Y.; Liu, L.; Qin, Y.; Sun, Z.; Sun, Z.; Chen, X. Effect of nm23-H1 on reversing malignant phenotype on human lung cancer cell line L9981. *J. Biomed. Eng.* **2005**, *22*, 530–534.
31. Marino, N.; Marshall, J.-C.; Steeg, P.S. Protein-protein interactions: A mechanism regulating the anti-metastatic properties of Nm23-H1. *N-S Arch. Pharmacol.* **2011**, *384*, 351–362. [CrossRef]
32. O'Byrne, K.J.; Koukourakis, M.I.; Giatromanolaki, A.; Cox, G.; Turley, H.; Steward, W.P.; Gatter, K.; Harris, A.L. Vascular endothelial growth factor, platelet-derived endothelial cell growth factor and angiogenesis in non-small-cell lung cancer. *Br. J. Cancer* **2000**, *82*, 1427–1432. [CrossRef]
33. Xu, T.; Li, D.; Wang, H.; Zheng, T.; Wang, G.; Xin, Y. MUC1 downregulation inhibits non-small cell lung cancer progression in human cell lines. *Exp. Ther. Med.* **2017**, *14*, 4443–4447. [CrossRef] [PubMed]
34. Huang, Y.; Hu, X.; Liu, G.; Liu, H.; Hu, J.; Feng, Z.; Tang, B.; Qian, J.; Wang, Q.; Zhang, Y. A potential anticancer agent 1,2-di (quinazolin-4-yl) diselane induces apoptosis in non-small-cell lung cancer A549 cells. *Med. Chem. Res.* **2015**, *24*, 2085–2096. [CrossRef]
35. Yoon, H.-E.; Kim, S.-A.; Choi, H.-S.; Ahn, M.-Y.; Yoon, J.-H.; Ahn, S.-G. Inhibition of Plk1 and Pin1 by 5′-nitro-indirubinoxime suppresses human lung cancer cells. *Cancer Lett.* **2012**, *316*, 97–104. [CrossRef] [PubMed]
36. Li, X.; Tang, Y.; Yu, F.; Sun, Y.; Huang, F.; Chen, Y.; Yang, Z.; Ding, G. Inhibition of Prostate Cancer DU-145 Cells Proliferation by *Anthopleura anjunae* Oligopeptide (YVPGP) via PI3K/AKT/mTOR Signaling Pathway. *Mar. Drugs* **2018**, *16*, 325. [CrossRef] [PubMed]
37. Peng, Y.; Fu, Z.-Z.; Guo, C.-S.; Zhang, Y.-X.; Di, Y.; Jiang, B.; Li, Q.-W. Effects and Mechanism of Baicalin on Apoptosis of Cervical Cancer HeLa Cells in vitro. *Iran J. Pharm. Res.* **2015**, *14*, 251–261. [PubMed]

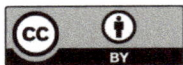

marine drugs

MDPI

Article

Cytotoxic Potential of the Novel Horseshoe Crab Peptide Polyphemusin III

Mariana B. Marggraf [1], Pavel V. Panteleev [1], Anna A. Emelianova [1], Maxim I. Sorokin [2,3], Ilia A. Bolosov [1], Anton A. Buzdin [1,2,3], Denis V. Kuzmin [1] and Tatiana V. Ovchinnikova [1,3,*]

[1]   M.M. Shemyakin & Yu.A. Ovchinnikov Institute of Bioorganic Chemistry, the Russian Academy of Sciences, Mikhluho-Maklaya str. 16/10, Moscow 117997, Russia; thpcb92@mail.ru (M.B.M.); alarm14@gmail.com (P.V.P.); annaemelyan@gmail.com (A.A.E.); b_off2@mail.ru (I.A.B.); buzdin@oncobox.com (A.A.B.); denisk@list.ru (D.V.K.)

[2]   Department of Bioinformatics and Molecular Networks, Omicsway Corp., Walnut, CA 91789, USA; sorokin@oncobox.com

[3]   Department of Biotechnology, I.M. Sechenov First Moscow State Medical University (Sechenov University), Moscow 119991, Russia

*   Correspondence: ovch@ibch.ru; Tel.: +7-495-336-44-44

Received: 3 November 2018; Accepted: 20 November 2018; Published: 26 November 2018

Abstract: Biological activity of the new antimicrobial peptide polyphemusin III from the horseshoe crab *Limulus polyphemus* was examined against bacterial strains and human cancer, transformed, and normal cell cultures. Polyphemusin III has the amino acid sequence RRGCFRVCYRGFCFQRCR and is homologous to other β-hairpin peptides from the horseshoe crab. Antimicrobial activity of the peptide was evaluated and MIC (minimal inhibitory concentration) values were determined. IC_{50} (half-maximal inhibitory concentration) values measured toward human cells revealed that polyphemusin III showed a potent cytotoxic activity at concentrations of <10 μM. Polyphemusin III caused fast permeabilization of the cytoplasmic membrane of human leukemia cells HL-60, which was measured with trypan blue exclusion assay and lactate dehydrogenase-release assay. Flow cytometry experiments for annexin V-FITC/ propidium iodide double staining revealed that the caspase inhibitor, Z-VAD-FMK, did not abrogate disruption of the plasma membrane by polyphemusin III. Our data suggest that polyphemusin III disrupts the plasma membrane integrity and induces cell death that is apparently not related to apoptosis. In comparison to known polyphemusins and tachyplesins, polyphemusin III demonstrates a similar or lower antimicrobial effect, but significantly higher cytotoxicity against human cancer and transformed cells in vitro.

Keywords: antimicrobial peptide; cytotoxicity; β-hairpin; polyphemusins; tachyplesins; cell death; signaling pathways

1. Introduction

Antimicrobial peptides (AMPs) are important components of the innate host defense in many organisms. AMPs exhibit activity against pathogenic bacteria, fungi, viruses, and protozoans [1–3]. Some antimicrobial peptides are also considered as putative anticancer agents [4–6]. Previous studies demonstrated that β-hairpin cationic antimicrobial peptides, for example, tachyplesin I from horseshoe crab hemocytes, gomesin from spider hemocytes, and protegrin-1 from porcine leukocytes displayed both antibacterial and antitumor activities [7–10].

Polyphemusins are family of β-hairpin cationic antimicrobial peptides that play a role in the innate immunity of horseshoe crabs. They were isolated from hemocytes of the horseshoe crab *Limulus polyphemus* [11]. These peptides are structurally close to another family of horseshoe crab antimicrobial peptides, tachyplesins, isolated from the species *Tachypleus trindentatus, Tachypleus gigas,* and *Carcinoscorpius rotundicauda*. Polyphemusins and tachyplesins polypeptide chains consist of 18 and 17 amino acid residues, respectively, and contain two disulfide bonds. The peptides from both groups have a high net positive charge due to several arginine and lysine residues in their amino acid sequences [11–13]. Polyphemusins and tachyplesins can disrupt both outer and inner membranes of Gram-negative bacteria [14–16]. Cationic and amphipathic properties of polyphemusins and tachyplesins have been implicated as the most essential features for the mode of their action towards microorganisms [14,16,17]. It has been shown that these peptides selectively interact with negatively charged phospholipids of bacterial membranes [14,18].

Similarly to tachyplesins, polyphemusins also exhibit a broad spectrum of biological activities. Naturally occurring and synthetic polyphemusin I, polyphemusin II, and their analogs inhibit growth of both Gram-positive and Gram-negative bacteria, as well as some fungi at submicromolar and micromolar concentrations [11,14,16,19], mammalian tumor cells at micromolar concentrations [8,9], have a high affinity for lipopolysaccharides [11,14], and may cause degradation of *Staphylococcus aureus* biofilms [20].

So far, five β-hairpin peptides (polyphemusin I, polyphemusin II, tachyplesin I, tachyplesin II, tachyplesin III) have been isolated from the four above-mentioned species of horseshoe crabs and only for two of them, tachyplesin I and tachyplesin II, have the precursor nucleotide and amino acid sequences been reported [21]. The complete coding sequences of prepropolyphemusins were obtained by using the preprotachyplesin I sequential blasting in the *Limulus polyphemus* genome database. Interestingly, the gene encoding polyphemusin II was not identified in this database. Instead, we identified the novel isoform named polyphemusin III (PM III). PM III has a molecular mass of 2309.09 Da and the amino acid sequence RRGCFRVCYRGFCFQRCR including six basic arginine residues, providing a net positive charge of +6.

We expressed the recombinant PM III in *Escherichia coli* and investigated cytotoxic properties of polyphemusins against seven bacterial strains, both Gram-positive and Gram-negative, as well as towards four human cancer cell lines and one transformed human cell line. In addition, two types of normal human primary cell cultures were used to determine the peptides' cytotoxicity. We also compared the biological properties of PM III with those of the other two isoforms—polyphemusin I (PM I), polyphemusin II (PM II), and with tachyplesins—tachyplesin I (TP I), tachyplesin II (TP II), and tachyplesin III (TP III).

PM III demonstrated a high cytotoxicity at concentrations of <10 μM. Compared to tachyplesins and other polyphemusins, PM III had higher cytotoxic activities for human cells. In contrast, PM III showed lower antibacterial activity compared to tachyplesins, PM I, and PM II. A cytotoxic effect of PM III was observed after 15 min of incubation without further increase over time. The cell death promoting mechanism presumably was not associated with the caspase-dependent apoptosis, as the disruption of plasma membrane integrity was not abrogated by the caspase inhibitor, Z-VAD-FMK.

2. Results

2.1. Identificantion of Antimicrobial Peptide

Nucleotide sequence alignment of genes encoding polyphemusins PM I and PM III in the genome of the horseshoe crab *Limulus polyphemus* showed that both peptides had the same length, but PM III involved four amino acids substitutions (W3G, Y14F, R15Q, K16R) compared with PM I (Figure 1). Noteworthy, a single nucleotide deletion was detected in the amidation signal GKR site located between the mature polyphemusin III and anionic propiece sequences. The deletion of the guanine nucleotide position appears to cause a shift of the open reading frame, however, the sequencing error by the *Limulus polyphemus* genome sequencing consortium also cannot be excluded. The aim of this study was to investigate the biological activities of a novel polyphemusin.

```
PmI     atgaggaagcttgtagttgctctgtgcctgatgatggtattggctgtgatggtggaagaggccaaggctagg  72
        M   R   K   L   V   V(I) A   L   C   L   M   M   V   L   A   V   M   V   E   E   A   K   A   R
PmIII   atgaggaaactcgtaattgctctatgcctgatgatggtattggctgtgatggtggaagaggccaaggctagg  72
Gap fraction

                                                                              exon      intron
PmI     agatggtgcttagagtgtgttacagggggattttgctatcgcaaatgtcgagggaagagaaagtgagctgat  144
        R   W(G) C   F   R   V   C   Y   R   G   F   C  Y(F) R(Q) K(R) C   R   G   K   R   N
PmIII   aggggtgtttcagagtgtgttacagagggtttttgctttcagagatgtcgagg-aagagaaagtgagttgat  143
Gap fraction

PmI     tttaaaattctgattattttttaaccgtcactataacaagtgattgcgttagtaaagatcaac----atttt  212
PmIII   tttaaaattgtgattatttctaactgtcactatatgaactgatcgcgttagtaaagggtgattgatgacttc  215
Gap fraction

PmI     ggatataaatcaaatccgtctgattctttgaaaaattatatgaatgacgtctgaatctattacatta------  277
PmIII   ggatataaattaagtctgtctgatcctttgaaaaattaagataatgaagtctgaatctgttatcttaatgaagg  287
Gap fraction

PmI     -----------------------------------------------------------------------  277
PmIII   tgtaagaaagattttcgttaaatgtgttgaattattacacttgtacattattctgaagtcatcttgctcctg  359
Gap fraction

PmI     -----------------------------------------------------------------------  277
PmIII   atagggcagtaaactataaatatacgactaatattgttgtatcatccctgttgttaaaggttcaaataaaga  431
Gap fraction

PmI     -------------------aatcttataaaaatcatggtaattttaagtaagaaaacaaccagtctctga  328
PmIII   taagggtttattgtgagtttgaatttataaaagtaaaattgatgtcaattaagaaatcagccagtccctga  503
Gap fraction

PmI     gtcttgaatttaaagattcgtatttggttaaaatttaaaatcaaatacttagcctggccttaacttccgtt  400
PmIII   atcttgaatttgaacaatcatattcgggtaaa-tttaaaaatcaagtacctagtctgatctcgactttttgtt  574
Gap fraction

PmI     cttttgagtggcttgcatatatataaagttaagtttttcgtttttgtatttgcaagctgggccatagtgagggatg  472
PmIII   gtgttgaatgacttgcacatataaaattaaatttttattttgcatttgca----------------gggatt  630
Gap fraction

PmI     ttcacatataaagcttaagctgttgctttttagaacttaagggatatttacagtctcacaactgacatttttat  544
PmIII   ttt-cataaagctaaagctgcggcttttttgtaacttaatgaatatttacagtctcacaaatgtcatttctat  701
Gap fraction

                                                                intron    exon
PmI     gtaaattatcatttcaaaaagatctgtttacgatgcttctgtatagtgaagtacgtgagttccgtgaccgtg  616
                                                              E   V   R   E  F(Y) R(H) D   R
PmIII   attaactatcatgtaaaaaaaatctctttacgatacttctgtatagtgaagtgcgtgagtaccatgatcgtg  773
Gap fraction

PmI     ggtatgatgtaagagccattccagaagaagcgttgtttttcacgacaagacgatatagaagacgacgatgacg  688
        G   Y   D   V   R   A   I   P   E   E   A   L   F   S   R   Q   D   D  I(V) E(D) D  D(E) D   D
PmIII   gatatgatgtaagagccattccagaagaagcgttgtttttcacgacaagacgatgtagatgatgaggataaag  845
Gap fraction

PmI     agtaa   693
        D(E) stop
PmIII   agtaa   850
Gap fraction
```

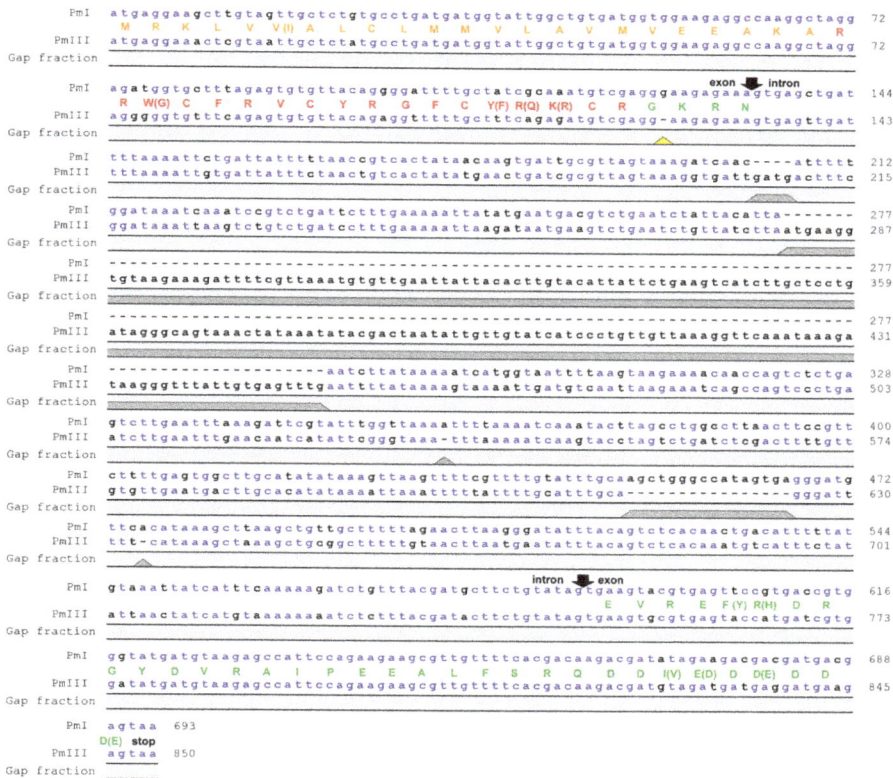

Figure 1. Nucleotide sequence alignment of genes encoding polyphemusins. The genes encoding PM I and PM III were identified in the *Limulus polyphemus* whole genome shotgun sequence (GenBank: AZTN01102408.1 and AZTN01052275.1, respectively). Gaps in the sequences are shown as dashes. Putative exon and intron boundaries are indicated by black arrows. The deduced amino acid sequences of coding region are shown as a colored one-letter code: Signal peptide (orange), mature peptide (red), and anionic propiece (green). The yellow triangle points at the deletion cause a reading frame shift in the sequence of polyphemusin III. Putative prepropolyphemusin III amino acid sequence was translated from corresponding DNA considering that deletion of guanine nucleotide did not occur.

2.2. Expression and Purification of the Recombinant Peptides

To improve the yield of the recombinant polyphemusins and tachyplesins after expression in *E. coli* and to facilitate their purification, the peptides were obtained as a part of the fusion proteins with the N-terminal octahistidine tag and the modified thioredoxin A (M37L). Following cell harvesting, sonication, preparative centrifugation of the cell lysate, affinity chromatography, and specific CNBr cleavage of the fusion proteins, the target peptides were purified by reversed-phase high-performance liquid chromatography (RP-HPLC) in a linear gradient of acetonitrile. MALDI mass spectrometry analysis of the main fractions (Figures S1 and S2) showed that the measured monoisotopic *m/z* matched well with the calculated molecular masses of protonated ions [M+H]$^+$ of corresponding peptides (Table 1).

Table 1. Primary structure and physicochemical characteristics of polyphemusins and tachyplesins.

Peptide	Amino Acid Sequence [1]	Calculated [M+H]+ Monoisotopic Mass, Da [2]	Measured Monoisotopic m/z Value [3]	Net Charge	RP-HPLC Retention Time [4], min	Recombinant Peptide Final Yield, mg/L
PM I	RRWCFRVCYRGFCYRKCR	2454.18	2453.97	+7	35.5	2.4
PM II	RRWCFRVCY**K**GFCYRKCR	2426.18	2426.19	+7	35.4	1.5
PM III	RR**G**CFRVCYRGFC**FQ**RCR	2309.09	2309.01	+6	36.2	5.9
TP I	**KW**CFRVCYRGICYRRCR	2264.10	2264.25	+6	35.5	3.4
TP II	**RW**CFRVCYRGICYRKCR	2264.10	2264.14	+6	35.9	3.0
TP III	**KW**CFRVCYRGICYRKCR	2236.09	2236.07	+6	35.5	3.0

[1] Amino acid substitutions in PM II and PM III (as compared to PM I) and in TP II and TP III (as compared to TP I) are shown in bold. [2] Molecular masses were calculated by considering the presence of four Cys residues forming two disulfide bonds and [3] were determined experimentally using MALDI mass spectrometry. [4] Retention times were measured using semi-preparative reversed-phase high-performance liquid chromatography (RP-HPLC) on a C18 column with a linear gradient from 5 to 80% (v/v) of acetonitrile in water containing 0.1% trifluoroacetic acid (TFA) within 1 h.

2.3. Antimicrobial Activity

The antimicrobial activity of PM III, its isoforms, and tachyplesins was determined by measuring their minimum inhibitory concentrations (MICs) against Gram-positive and Gram-negative bacteria using broth microdilution assay (Table 2). PM III displayed antimicrobial activity in a range of 0.25–2 µM against all strains except *S. aureus* ATCC 29213. However, compared to PM I, TP I, and TP III peptides, PM III demonstrated a 4-fold reduction in activity against the Gram-negative strains *E. coli* ML35p and *K. pneumoniae* (CI 287), and the Gram-positive strain *S. aureus* 209P. PM III had a similar potency against Gram-positive bacteria *B. subtilis* B-886 and *M. luteus* B-1314, and Gram-negative *P. aeruginosa* PAO1 compared to PM I and PM II. Moreover, identical activities were registered against *P. aeruginosa* PAO1 with MIC 0.5 µM among all tested peptides. All the peptides showed markedly reduced activities against *S. aureus* strain ATCC 29213 compared to other strains, with an 8-fold reduction in antimicrobial activity for polyphemusins and at least a 16-fold reduction for tachyplesins compared to *S. aureus* 209P. All tachyplesins demonstrated similar activities, with MICs ranging from 0.06 to 2 µM, except that measured against a low sensitive strain *S. aureus* ATCC 29213. MICs ranges determined for PM I (0.06–0.5 µM) and PM II (0.03–1 µM) were quite similar, with the above exception of that determined for *S. aureus* ATCC 29213. Compared to tachyplesins, PM I and PM II had, overall, higher or identical antibacterial effects.

Table 2. Antimicrobial activities of polyphemusins and tachyplesins.

Strain	Gram	MICs, µM					
		PM I	PM II	PM III	TP I	TP II	TP III
E. coli ML-35p	−	0.062	0.031	0.25	0.062	0.062	0.062
K. pneumoniae (CI 287)	−	0.5	0.5	2	0.5	1	0.5
P. aeruginosa PAO1	−	0.5	0.5	0.5	0.5	0.5	0.5
S. aureus ATCC 29213	+	4	4	16	8	8	16
S. aureus 209P	+	0.5	0.5	2	0.5	0.5	0.5
B. subtilis B-886	+	0.25	0.5	0.5	0.5	0.5	1
M. luteus B-1314	+	0.5	1	0.5	1	1	2

2.4. Cytotoxic Effects on Human Cells

Cytotoxic activities of PM III, its isoforms, and tachyplesins against seven human cell lines were evaluated. Four cancer (HL-60 acute promyelocytic leukemia, HeLa cervix adenocarcinoma, SK-BR-3 breast adenocarcinoma, A549 lung carcinoma), one transformed (HEK 293T transformed human embryonic kidney), and two normal human cell lines (HEF human embryonic fibroblasts and NHA normal human astrocytes) were used for these experiments. Cytotoxicity was measured by incubating the cells with serial dilutions of PM I, PM II, PM III, TP I, TP II, or TP III samples followed by MTT assay after 48 h. The half-maximal inhibitory concentrations (IC_{50}) were measured as the peptide concentration at which cell viability was reduced by 50% in comparison to untreated cells (Table 3).

Table 3. The IC_{50} values measured for polyphemusins and tachyplesins on human cell lines.

Cell Line	IC_{50}, µM					
	PM I	**PM II**	**PM III**	**TP I**	**TP II**	**TP III**
HL-60	7.2 ± 0.5	7.2 ± 0.5	2.5 ± 0.1	4.8 ± 0.3	5.6 ± 0.5	5.0 ± 0.4
HeLa	12.5 ± 0.9	16.4 ± 1.3	6.0 ± 0.2	24.2 ± 1.7	24.4 ± 3.0	13.7 ± 1.3
SK-BR-3	16.0 ± 0.6	17.3 ± 0.6	9.9 ± 0.1	30.1 ± 1.9	34.0 ± 1.3	27.5 ± 0.8
A549	8.8 ± 1.3	10.8 ± 1.9	7.3 ± 0.5	26.5 ± 1.2	28.1 ± 1.7	15.3 ± 1.0
HEK 293T	9.4 ± 1.5	11.3 ± 1.6	7.3 ± 0.4	23.5 ± 1.2	24.6 ± 1.7	19.7 ± 1.9
HEF	8.3 ± 0.7	9.7 ± 0.2	7.0 ± 0.4	13.0 ± 1.5	17.7 ± 1.2	14.1 ± 1.2
NHA	14.5 ± 1.6	18.3 ± 1.4	7.5 ± 0.5	24.7 ± 1.8	29.4 ± 1.7	21.3 ± 1.2

IC_{50} values are represented as the means $\pm$ standard deviations (SD) of at least three independent experiments.

Data analysis revealed that PM III had a potent cytotoxic activity against human cell lines. PM III was the most cytotoxically active among all tested peptides. IC_{50} values determined for PM III on cancer and transformed cell lines were in a range of 2.5–9.9 µM. Compared to PM III, the peptides PM I and PM II showed lower cytotoxic effects, with IC_{50} values ranging from 7.2 to 16.0 µM and from 7.2 to 17.3 µM, respectively. IC_{50} values for PM I or PM II tested against the same cancer, transformed, or normal cells were similar.

Tachyplesins turned out to be less toxic than polyphemusins. Among the investigated tachyplesins, TP III had the strongest cytotoxicity against cancer, transformed, and normal cell lines. The IC_{50} values determined for TP III on cancer and transformed cell lines were in a range of 5.0–27.5 µM, the IC_{50} values determined for the normal cells were of 14.1 µM for HEF and of 21.3 µM for NHA.

The leukemia cell line, HL-60, was the most sensitive to all investigated cytotoxic peptides. Moreover, HL-60 cells were two to three times more sensitive to PM III (IC_{50} = 2.5 µM) than to tachyplesins, PM I, and PM II. In contrast, the lowest sensitivity to cytotoxic peptides was observed for the SK-BR-3 cell line with IC_{50} values for all polyphemusins and tachyplesins ranging from 9.9 to 17.3 µM and from 27.5 to 34.0 µM, respectively.

The normal cell lines showed similar sensitivities to all polyphemusins: PM I (IC_{50} = 8.3 µM for HEF, IC_{50} = 14.5 µM for NHA), PM II (IC_{50} = 9.7 µM for HEF, IC_{50} = 18.3 µM for NHA), and PM III (IC_{50} = 7.0 µM for HEF, IC_{50} = 7.5 µM for NHA). The IC_{50} values determined for HEF and NHA cells were in the same range as for the cancer cell lines. Interestingly, the IC_{50} values of PM III determined for normal cells were several times higher than that for the most sensitive cell line, HL-60.

2.5. Hemolytic Activity

The assay for the hemolytic activity of PM III was performed to determine its effect on the integrity of red blood cells. At a concentration range of 3.125–100 µM, PM III had the highest hemolytic activity among all the peptides tested (Figure 2). The measured half-hemolysis concentration (HC_{50}) value for PM III was of 46 µM. PM I and PM II were less toxic to erythrocytes and caused only ~45% and ~30% hemolysis, respectively, even at the maximal concentration of 100 µM. Tachyplesins also demonstrated low hemolytic effects: TP I, TP II, and TP III lysed 38%, 33%, and 20% of erythrocytes, respectively, at a maximal concentration of 100 µM.

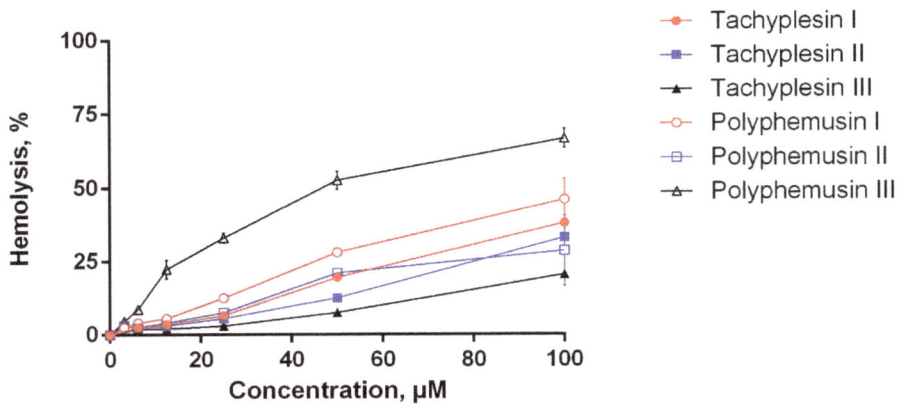

Figure 2. The hemolysis curve showing effects of polyphemusins and tachyplesins on human erythrocytes. The data represent the mean values ± SD for two independent series of triplicated experiments.

2.6. Trypan Blue Assay for Dead Cells

According to the MTT-test, HL-60 was the most sensitive cell culture to PM III. Therefore, to investigate the mechanism of the PM III cytotoxicity, we first assessed a short-time membrane permeabilizing effect of PM III on HL-60 cells at different time points using the trypan blue exclusion assay. PM III was used at two final concentrations: Equal to IC_{50} (2.5 µM) and 2-fold exceeding IC_{50} (5 µM). The experiments were done at 15 min, 1 h, and 4 h following incubation with PM III.

The proportion of dead HL-60 cells was virtually unchanged for all these time points at both concentrations used (Figure 3). In the negative control experiments, the dead cells ratio did not exceed 10%. In contrast, both concentrations of PM III were highly toxic to HL-60 cells, thus giving 42–48% of trypan-stained (dead) cells for 2.5 µM PM III for all incubation times, and 66–71% of dead cells for 5 µM PM III for all incubation times. Thus, the cytotoxic effect of PM III depended on its concentration, but not on the incubation times. We concluded, therefore, that PM III could induce cell death after 15 min of incubation, which is typical for necrotic cell death [22].

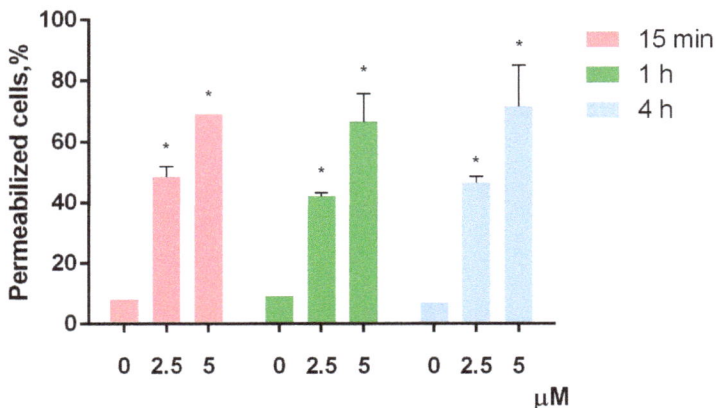

Figure 3. Trypan blue exclusion assay of HL-60 cell death after 15 min (red bars), 1 h (green bars), or 4 h (blue bars) of incubation with PM III (* $p < 0.05$ vs. the control sample of 0 µM for each time interval, respectively).

2.7. Mechanism of Cell Death

To further investigate the effect of PM III on human cells, we performed annexin V-FITC/propidium iodide double staining with subsequent flow cytometric analysis. Annexin V-FITC binds to phosphatidylserine, which is exposed on the outer leaflet of the cellular plasma membrane at the initial stages of apoptosis, whereas propidium iodide (PI) preferentially stains nuclei of dead cells. Therefore, a combination of annexin V-FITC and PI assays allows differentiation between early apoptotic and late apoptotic/necrotic cell populations. PM III was used at two final concentrations of 2.5 and 5 µM. In order to elucidate the predominant mechanism of the PM III action, we applied a widely used caspase inhibitor, Z-VAD-FMK [23].

The results of HL-60 cells double staining, followed by the flow cytometry analysis are shown in Figure 4. The majority of the cells treated with 2.5 or 5 µM PM III were stained with both annexin V-FITC and PI and thus were either late apoptotic or necrotic. This was almost not affected by the presence of the apoptotic inhibitor, Z-VAD-FMK, following 4 h of incubation. In the absence of Z-VAD-FMK, > 40% of double-stained cells were detected for 2.5 µM PM III and >80% for 5 µM PM III. In the presence of Z-VAD-FMK, there were >30% of double-stained cells for 2.5 µM PM III, and > 70% for 5 µM PM III. In contrast, Z-VAD-FMK totally abrogated the effect of the 50 µM apoptotic inducer camptothecin that was used as a positive control.

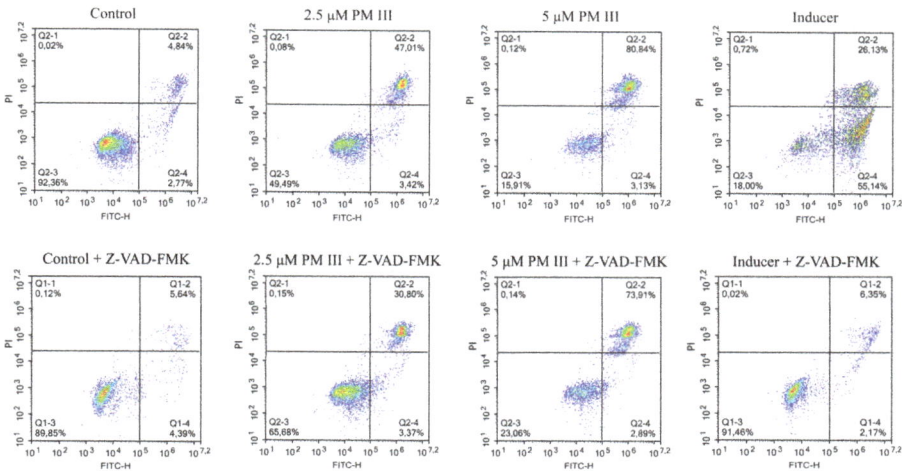

Figure 4. The flow cytometry results of annexin V-FITC/PI double staining of HL-60 cells after 4 h of incubation with PM III (at IC_{50} and $2 \times IC_{50}$) in the presence or absence of the caspase inhibitor, Z-VAD-FMK. Columns, from left to right: Control (untreated cells); 2.5 µM PM III; 5 µM PM III; 50 µM apoptotic inducer, camptothecin. Top row: No Z-VAD-FMK added, bottom row: 50 µM Z-VAD-FMK added. The results are presented as the percentage of viable (AV−PI−), apoptotic (AV+PI−), and late apoptotic/necrotic (AV+PI+) cells.

2.8. Cell Membrane Integrity

The loss of membrane integrity, detected by trypan blue exclusion assay and annexin V-FITC/propidium iodide double staining, was also evaluated by lactate dehydrogenase (LDH)-release. The cytosolic enzyme LDH is released upon cell lysis and therefore can be a marker of cell integrity. The percentage of LDH-leakage from cells enables evaluation of direct cell lysis. The obtained results showed that PM III induced a concentration-dependent lysis in HL-60 cells within 1 h of incubation in a concentration range of 1.56–25 µM (Figure 5).

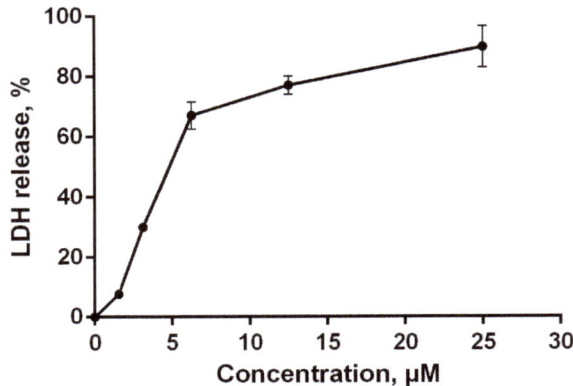

Figure 5. HL-60 cell membrane integrity after treatment with PM III. The data represent the mean values ± SD of two independent series of triplicated experiments.

2.9. Gene Expression Profiling and Oncobox Pathway Analysis

To get a deeper molecular insight into the mechanisms of cell death induced by PM III, we profiled gene expression in the PM III treated (1.25, 2.5, and 5 µM) and intact HL-60 cells. Gene expression profiles were further analyzed using the Oncobox bioinformatical platform to measure activation levels of 376 intracellular signaling pathways. We found a significant inhibition of the Caspase cascade (Figure 6), while the TRAF (tumor necrosis factor receptor (TNF-R)-associated factor) pathway was strongly activated (Figure 7) following the PM III treatment. An additional line of evidence for the non-apoptotic mechanism of the PM III mediated activity was provided by the PTEN pathway. It has been reported that PTEN most frequently had a positive connection to apoptosis [24]. The incubation with PM III strongly downregulated the PTEN signaling. The activation levels of all signaling pathways profiled in this study and case-to-normal ratios for the respective genes are shown in Supplementary Table S1. Taken together, these facts rather argue for a non-apoptotic mode of the PM III action.

We observed a number of molecular pathways promoting survival of the PM III treated cells. For example, the Akt and p38 signaling pathways were sequentially overactivated by increasing concentrations of PM III, thus probably representing the cellular pro-survival response on the PM III cytotoxic activity. Interestingly, we also found a number of immunity-linked pathways, namely Interferon response, Il-2, Il-6, and Il-10 pathways upregulated in most of the PM III-treated cell cultures (Table S1).

Caspase Cascade

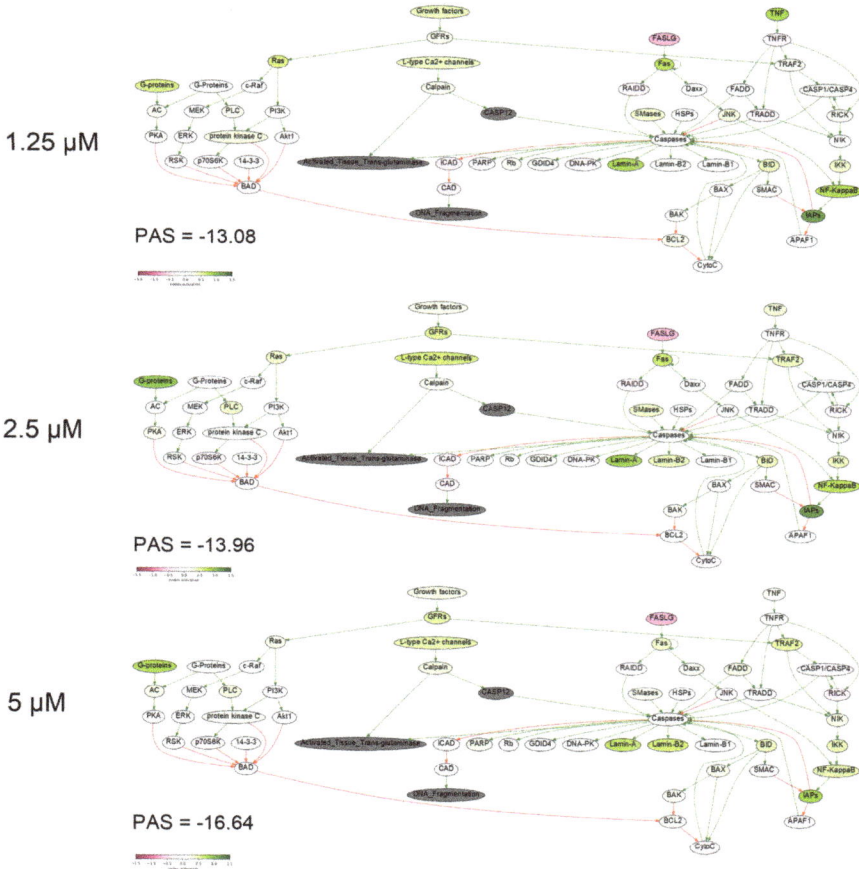

Figure 6. Caspase cascade pathway was inhibited in the PM III treated cells. The pathway was visualized using the Oncobox software (version 1.6.0-dev-1c6b124-modified). The pathway is shown as an interacting network, where green arrows indicate activation, red arrows—inhibition. The color depth of each node of the network corresponds to the logarithms of the case-to-normal (CNR) expression rate for each node, where "normal" is for intact cells, the scale represents an extent of up/downregulation.

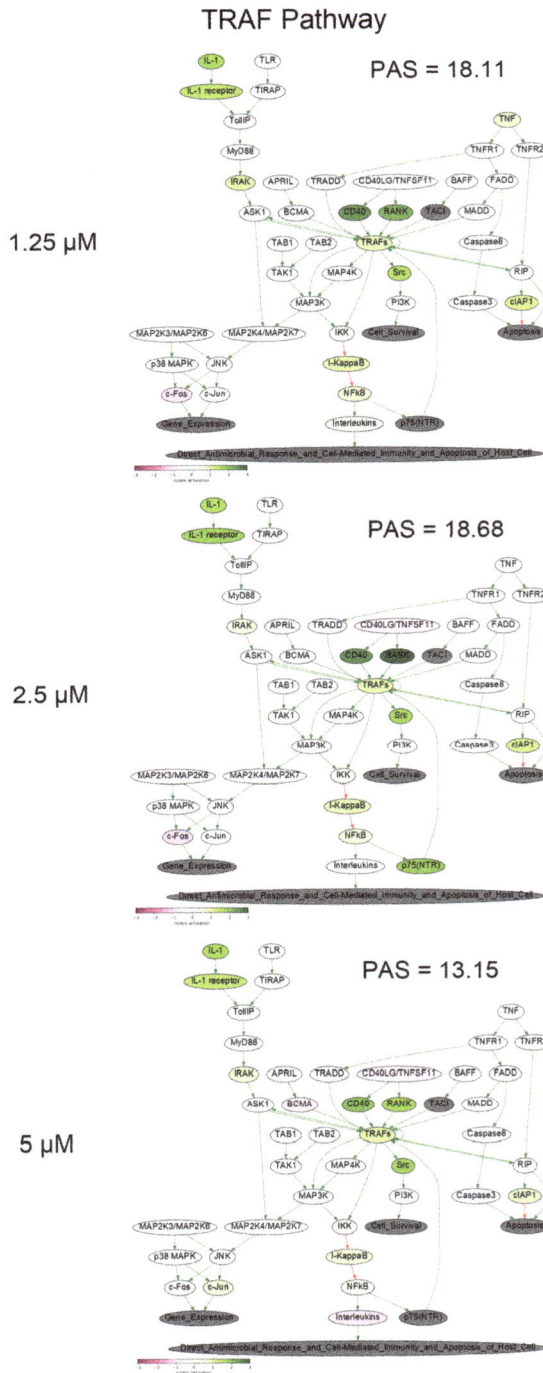

Figure 7. TRAF (tumor necrosis factor receptor (TNF-R)-associated factor) pathway was activated in the PM III treated cells. The pathway was visualized using the Oncobox software (version 1.6.0-dev-1c6b124-modified).

The pathway is shown as an interacting network, where green arrows indicate activation, red arrows—inhibition. The color depth of each node of the network corresponds to the logarithms of the case-to-normal (CNR) expression rate for each node, where "normal" is for intact cells, the scale represents an extent of up/downregulation.

3. Discussion

In this study, for the first time to our knowledge, the antimicrobial peptide PM III was obtained in a bacterial expression system and studied. We examined its cytotoxic potential on bacteria and human cells. We studied PM III activities in comparison with its isoforms: PM I, PM II, and homologous horseshoe crab peptides, tachyplesins. Assessment of the antimicrobial activity of PM III evidenced that its MICs ranged from 0.25 to 2 µM (except that measured against the low sensitive strain, *S. aureus* ATCC 29213). Compared to the antimicrobial activities of PM I and PM II, the activity of PM III was either the same or lower against the bacterial strains tested.

Our experimental data for the obtained recombinant PM I are in line with those obtained earlier for synthetic PM I against Gram-negative and Gram-positive bacteria (with reported MICs not exceeding 1 µM) [14,16,25]. However, several reports on antimicrobial activities of natural and synthetic peptides TP I, TP II, PM I, and PM II demonstrated MICs higher than 1 µM [11,12]. In our study, the MICs of the recombinant tachyplesins did not exceed 2 µM.

PM III also caused half-maximal inhibition of human cell viability in the concentration range of ~2–10 µM. The PM III IC$_{50}$ values were lower than those determined for PM I and PM II. We speculate that the higher cytotoxicity of PM III might be due to its higher hydrophobicity. In comparison to other tested peptides, the retention time of PM III measured during RP-HPLC indicated its higher hydrophobicity (Table 1). These data were congruent with the study results obtained with analogs of the synthetic amphipathic peptide V13K displaying antimicrobial and antitumor activities. Increased hydrophobicity of these analogs caused higher cytotoxic effects [26]. Previously published works showed a correlation between the hydrophobicity of peptides and their affinity to lipid bilayers in general [27–30]. Cell membranes contain different phospholipids, which sustain the amphipathic features due to the formation of hydrophilic and hydrophobic domains in the membrane structure. Well-known differences between the composition of bacterial and mammalian cell membranes provide the evidence for selectivity of the peptides' action. Bacterial membranes predominantly consist of phosphatidylserine, phosphatidylglycerol, and cardiolipin having a net negative charge [31]. Tumor cell bilayers are also enriched in anionic molecules, such as phosphatidylserine, sialylated gangliosides, *O*-glycosylated mucins, and heparin sulfate. In contrast, zwitterionic phospholipids—phosphatidylcholine, phosphatidylethanolamine, and sphingomyelin—are abundant in the cytoplasmic membranes of non-cancer mammalian cells [32]. Electrically neutral normal mammalian membranes prevent their recognition by positively charged antimicrobial peptides, and binding to these membranes is enabled by hydrophobic interactions [33]. Thus, modulation of hydrophobicity of antimicrobial peptides, and also peptoid molecules, may be followed by non-specific interaction with erythrocytes as it was shown in previously published studies [30,34–36]. It was also revealed that antimicrobial peptides require optimal hydrophobicity levels to exhibit antimicrobial activity and retain selectivity [37]. Suboptimal high hydrophobic properties may not only result in increased toxicity to erythrocytes, but even in a reduction of antibacterial activity [37–39]. Several protegrin-1 synthetic analogs with different hydrophobicities were characterized earlier [40]. The analog with substitutions of valine by leucine that was more hydrophobic than naturally occurring protegrin-1 and the analog with substitutions of valine by fluorinated leucine had the most hydrophobic properties than other tested peptides. A highly hydrophobic protegrin-1 analog with fluorinated leucine was shown to be less potent against bacterial strains than naturally occurring protegrin-1. In contrast, the analog with leucine without fluorination exhibited the most pronounced antibacterial activity among all tested peptides. This demonstrates that the susceptibility of bacteria to peptides strongly depends on hydrophobicity levels [40]. These data are in line with the reduced antibacterial and increased hemolytic activities of the PM III peptide as compared to other tested peptides. The hemolytic activity of PM III determined in this study (HC_{50} = 46 µM) was rather high, but the HC_{50} value of PM III was 18-fold higher than its IC_{50} measured for the HL-60 cell line and ~5–7-fold higher than its IC_{50} measured for other cancer cell lines. Therefore, half-hemolysis concentration and IC_{50} effective concentration were in different ranges.

In this study, we obtained and studied the recombinant peptides. Despite the absence of naturally occurring post-translational C-terminal amidation, the recombinant polyphemusins demonstrated both antibacterial and cytotoxic activities. Our data obtained here for PM II matched well with the previously published results [9]. In this study, IC_{50} values for the recombinant PM II measured on human cancer, transformed, and normal cell lines were in a range of 7–18 µM. In the previous report, IC_{50} for synthetic PM II with the amidated C-terminal residue measured against leukemic and normal mononuclear cells ranged from 6 to 13 µM [9]. Furthermore, PM II caused a decrease of tumor cells' viability with an IC_{50} of 6–13 µM, while the IC_{50} determined on mononuclear cells was 13 µM, indicating a general absence of selectivity towards tumor cells [9]. Similarly, we determined the IC_{50} for PM II on tumor cell lines, which ranged from 7 to 17 µM, while the IC_{50} determined for human embryonic fibroblasts and normal human astrocytes was 7 and 18 µM, respectively.

Previous studies revealed that TP I exhibited cytotoxic activity against tumor cells, with IC_{50} values ranging from 6 to 30 µM [9,41]. For example, in the case of glioma stem cells, IC_{50} values for synthetic TP I with the N-terminal acetylation and C-terminal amidation were ~10–20 µM, depending on incubation time [41]. Here, we showed that the recombinant non-amidated TP I had an IC_{50} ranging from 5 to 30 µM for different human tumor cells. The IC_{50} values for human embryonic fibroblasts and normal human astrocytes were 13 and 25 µM, respectively. Comparison with previously published studies indicated similar IC_{50} values for the normal cells. For the synthetic amidated TP I, previously measured IC_{50} for normal mononuclear cells was 15 µM [9]. The IC_{50} value for the naturally occurring TP I on monkey epithelial kidney cells (MA-104) was ~23 µM [42].

Suspension culture properties of HL-60 cells are supposed to be at the bottom of high sensitivity to polyphemusins and tachyplesins. In the previous report, the naturally occurring TP I halved the viability of HL-60 cells at ~10 µM [43]. For the synthetic amidated TP I and PM II peptides, the IC_{50} of 6–16 µM was previously observed on the suspension leukemia cell lines [9].

In this study, using trypan blue exclusion assay at different time points, we showed that the cytotoxic effect of PM III may develop in a relatively short time of 15 min of incubation. Furthermore, based on the data obtained by annexin V-FITC/PI double staining with subsequent flow cytometry, we found that PM III caused the cytotoxic effect most probably without involvement of apoptosis, and that the cytotoxic effect was not affected by the caspase inhibitor Z-VAD-FMK. The previous findings on PM II are in good agreement with our results, as the authors proposed Z-VAD-FMK-independent necrotic-like death of leukemia cells treated with PM II [8,9]. The loss of membrane cell integrity was also demonstrated by LDH-release assay. PM III induced lysis of cells followed by LDH leakage in a concentration-dependent manner within 1 h of incubation. Profiling of the gene expression and analysis of intracellular signaling pathways in human HL-60 cells incubated with PM III also supports the concept that peptide-mediated cell death is implemented likely without induction of apoptosis. In particular, there were no major pro-apoptotic signaling pathways activated by PM III (Table S1). Pathway analysis revealed inactivation of the entire caspase cascade pathway (Figure 6), which means that relative expression levels of most genes involved in this pathway are lower than in the control samples. We did not observe an increased expression for either p53 or its targets, such as TP53AIP1, PMAIP1, BAX, and BCL2. Expressions of these genes were, in most cases, below the normal levels (Table S1. Sheet "CNR"). Thus, we conclude that there were no detected signs of p53 activation linked with the PM III administration.

Summarizing all the above, in this study, PM III revealed the most significant cytotoxic effects against human cell cultures. It had a stronger cytotoxicity towards human leukemia HL-60 cells, as compared with the cytotoxic effect of other peptides tested against HL-60 in this study. Finally, we found that exposure of human leukemia cells to PM III not only caused cytotoxicity, but also mediated an intrinsic immune reaction via enhanced Interferon, Il-2, Il-6, and Il-10 signaling. This immunomodulatory feature of PM III suggests that it may be an attractive target for further biomedical screenings for future drug development.

4. Materials and Methods

4.1. Cell Lines and Culture Conditions

The following tumor and transformed cell lines were used in this study: HL-60 (acute promyelocytic leukemia), HeLa (human cervix adenocarcinoma cells), SK-BR-3 (human breast adenocarcinoma cells), A549 (human lung carcinoma cells), HEK 293T (transformed human embryonic kidney cells), HEF (human embryonic fibroblasts), and NHA (normal human astrocytes) were used as normal cell lines. Tumor and transformed cell lines were obtained from the American Type Culture Collection (ATCC; www.atcc.org). Primary cells HEF (normal human embryonic fibroblasts derived from human embryonic stem cells) and NHA (normal human astrocytes derived from human fetal brain tissue) were obtained and cultured according to the corresponding protocol [44,45]. Briefly, cells were cultured in DMEM/F12 (1:1) or RPMI-1640 medium containing 10% fetal bovine serum (Invitrogen, USA) at 37 °C in the atmosphere containing 5% CO_2 and 95% air according to standard mammalian tissue culture protocols and using a sterile technique. All cell lines were tested by using the LookOut®*Mycoplasma* PCR Detection Kit (Sigma-Aldrich, St. Louis, MO, USA) according to the manufacturer's protocol and found to be free of *Mycoplasma* infection.

4.2. Peptides

All the peptides were obtained by heterologous expression in *E.coli* with subsequent two-step purification as previously described for producing of β-hairpin peptides [46–48]. The recombinant plasmids for expression of the peptides were constructed with the use of pET-based vector as described previously [46]. The peptides were expressed in *E. coli* BL21 (DE3) cells as fusion proteins that included an octahistidine tag, the TrxL carrier protein (*E. coli* thioredoxin A with the Met37Leu mutation), a methionine residue and the mature polyphemusin I (GenBank: 14215.1), polyphemusin II (GenBank: 14216.1), polyphemusin III, tachyplesin I (GenBank: P14213.2), tachyplesin II (GenBank: P14214.2), or tachyplesin III (GenBank: P18252.1). The polyphemusin III primary structure was deduced from the whole genome shotgun sequence of *Limulus polyphemus* (GenBank: AZTN01052275.1). Oligonucleotides were designed based on *E. coli* codon usage bias. *E. coli* BL21 (DE3) cells transformed with the constructed plasmids were grown up to OD_{600} 1.0 and then were induced with 0.2 mM IPTG. The induction was performed at 30 °C for 5 h under stirring with a shaking speed of 220 rpm. The peptides' purification included immobilized metal affinity chromatography (IMAC) of cell lysate, CNBr cleavage of the fusion proteins, and reversed-phase high-performance liquid chromatography (RP-HPLC) as described previously; the peptides had a purity of at least 98% [46]. The RP-HPLC fractions were dried in vacuo, dissolved in water, and analyzed by MALDI-MS (Bruker Daltonics, Bremen, Germany). The obtained non-amidated recombinant analogs of natural polyphemusin I, polyphemusin II, polyphemusin III, tachyplesin I, tachyplesin II, and tachyplesin III were analyzed by automated microsequencing with the use of the Procise cLC 491 Protein Sequencing System (PE Applied Biosystems, Foster City, CA, USA). The peptides' concentrations were estimated based on near-UV absorbance measurement and calculated with the use of extinction coefficients.

4.3. Antimicrobial Assay

Bacterial test cultures were grown in the Mueller-Hinton (MH) medium at 37 °C to mid-log phase and then diluted with the 2 × MH medium supplemented with 1.8% NaCl. 50 µL of the bacterial suspension with a final cell concentration of 10^6 CFU/mL were added to aliquots of 50 µL of the peptide solutions and serially diluted with sterilized 0.1% bovine serum albumin in 96-well flat-bottom polystyrene microplates (Eppendorf, Hamburg, Germany). Bacterial cells were incubated for 24 h at 37 °C and 900 rpm on the plate thermoshaker (Biosan, Riga, Latvia). The minimum inhibitory concentrations (MIC) were determined as the lowest peptide concentration that prevented growth of a test microorganism observed as visible turbidity. The results were expressed as median values of three independent triplicated experiments. Assessment of antimicrobial activities of the recombinant PM III, other polyphemusins, and tachyplesins was conducted against Gram-negative (*Escherichia coli* ML-35p, *Klebsiella pneumoniae* (clinical isolate, CI 287), *Pseudomonas aeruginosa* PAO1) and Gram-positive (*Staphylococcus aureus* ATCC 29213, *Staphylococcus aureus* 209P, *Bacillus subtilis* B-886, *Micrococcus luteus* B-1314) bacteria.

4.4. Cytotoxic Activity Assay

The colorimetric 3-(4,5-dimethylthiazol-2-yl)-2,5-diphenyltetrazolium bromide (MTT) dye reduction assay was used to determine the cytotoxicity of the polyphemusins and tachyplesins. Cells (3×10^3–6×10^3 per well) were placed into 96-well plates in Dulbecco's modified Eagle's medium (DMEM/F12) supplemented with 10% fetal bovine serum (FBS). After incubation in the atmosphere containing 5% CO_2 and 95% air at 37 °C overnight, the media were discarded, and polyphemusins or tachyplesins solutions were added to the cell cultures up to final concentrations of 2.5, 5, 10, 25, and 50 µM in a final volume of 0.1 mL DMEM/F12 with 10% FBS. HL-60 cells (4×10^4 in 50 µL) were added to two-time serial dilutions of polyphemusins solutions at a final concentration of 1.25, 2.5, 5, 10, 25, and 50 µM in 50 µL RPMI-1640 with 10% FBS. 48 hours later, 20 µL of MTT (5 mg/mL) was added into each well and the plates were incubated for 3 h at 37 °C. The plates with HL-60 cells were centrifuged for 10 min at 300 g. The media were discarded and 0.1 mL of dimethyl sulfoxide and isopropanol mixture at a ratio of 1:1 (v/v) was added to each well to dissolve the crystallized formazan. The absorbance at 570 nm was measured by a microplate reader (Eppendorf, Hamburg, Germany).

4.5. Hemolytic Activity Assay

Testing of the hemolytic activity of polyphemusins and tachyplesins was performed using fresh human red blood cells (hBRC). Permeabilization of erythrocyte cytoplasmic membrane results in lysis followed by the release of hemoglobin. hBRC were washed three times with phosphate buffered saline (PBS: 10 mM Na_2HPO_4, 1.76 mM K_2HPO_4, pH 7.4, containing 173 mM NaCl, and 2.7 mM KCl). Two-fold serial dilutions of the peptide solutions were added to 50 µL aliquots of hRBC in the 96-well microplate. The final hBRC concentration was of 4% (v/v) in each well, and the final volume of suspension was 100 µL. After incubation of suspensions for 1.5 h at 37 °C under stirring at 1000 rpm, centrifugation of plates was done at 700 g for 5 min. The supernatant 50 µL aliquots were then transferred into flat-bottomed 96-well microplates. The absorbance at 405 nm was measured in a microplate reader (Eppendorf, Hamburg, Germany), allowing the detection of hemoglobin release. 0.1% Triton X-100 caused a complete lysis of erythrocytes, thus hBRC treated with Triton X-100 were used as a positive control. As PBS did not cause lysis, hBRC in PBS served as a negative control. The percentage of hemolysis was calculated using the following Equation (1):

$$\text{Hemolysis (\%)} = (\text{OD}_{405} \text{ sample} - \text{OD}_{405} \text{ 0\% lysis control})/(\text{OD}_{405} \text{ 100\% lysis control} - \text{OD}_{405} \text{ 0\% lysis control}) \times 100\% \quad (1)$$

The quantitative data resulted from two series of experiments were represented as average means with standard deviations. The experiments were carried out using hBRC obtained from human blood samples of independent donors.

4.6. Trypan Blue Exclusion Assay

Polyphemusin III was diluted in non-supplemented RPMI medium and incubated with 2.5×10^5 HL-60 cells in a volume of 100 µL. After 15 min, 1 h, or 4 h of incubation with 2.5 or 5 µM polyphemusin III, proportions of viable cells were counted in an automated cell counter (Thermo

Fisher Scientific, Waltham, MA, USA) using sterile-filtered 0.4% trypan blue solution. The quantitative data were represented as average means with standard deviations ($\pm$SD) obtained from three independent experiments.

4.7. Annexin V-FITC/Propidium Iodide Double Staining and Flow Cytometry

Cell death analysis with fluorescein isothiocyanate conjugated annexin V (annexin V-FITC)/propidium iodide double staining and dead cells counting with flow cytometry were performed 4 h after addition of polyphemusin III up to a final concentration of 2.5 or 5 μM. The Annexin V-FITC Apoptosis Detection Kit (BD Biosciences, Franklin Lakes, NJ, USA) was used according to the manufacturer's protocol on a NovoCyte flow cytometer (ACEA Biosciences, San Diego, CA, USA). Each experiment was performed in triplicate. The apoptosis inducer camptothecin (Sigma-Aldrich, St. Louis, MO, USA) and the general caspase inhibitor, Z-VAD-FMK (BD Biosciences, Franklin Lakes, NJ, USA), were used. All flow cytometry experiments were performed twice.

4.8. Lactate Dehydrogenase (LDH)-Release Assay

The LDH-release assay (CytoTox 96 Non-Radioactive Cytotoxicity Assay; Promega Corporation, Madison, WI, USA) was performed according to the manufacturer's protocol. Suspension HL-60 cells (4×10^4) were seeded into a 96-well plate in triplicate and incubated for 1 h with various concentrations of polyphemusin III at 100 μL per well in RPMI serum-free medium. Untreated cells served as a control for spontaneous LDH-release and cells treated with 1% Triton X-100 were used as a control for maximal LDH-release. Absorbance was measured at 490 nm using a microplate reader (Eppendorf, Hamburg, Germany). Percent LDH-release was calculated using the following Equation (2):

$$[(\text{experimental LDH-release} - \text{spontaneous LDH-release})/(\text{maximal LDH-release} - \text{spontaneous LDH-release})] \times 100 \quad (2)$$

The dose response curve shown is an average of two independent experiments.

4.9. Statistical Analysis

The GraphPad PRISM 6.0 software (GraphPad Software Inc., San Diego, CA, USA) was used for statistical analysis; the values of $p < 0.05$ were considered statistically significant.

4.10. Gene Expression Profiling and Functional Annotation

RNA extraction was performed immediately before preparation of sequencing libraries using a QIAGEN RNeasy Kit (Qiagen, Venlo, Netherlands) following the manufacturer's protocol. Then, the RNA Integrity Number (RIN) was measured using an Agilent 2100 bio-Analyzer. Agilent RNA 6000 Nano or Qubit RNA Assay Kits were used to measure RNA concentration. A KAPA RNA Hyper with RiboErase (KAPA Biosystems, Wilmington, MA, USA) kit was used for further depletion of ribosomal RNA. For library preparations, we used the Ovation®Universal RNA-Seq System and 1-96 KAPA HyperPrep Kit according to the manufacturer's recommendations. Different adaptors were used for multiplexing samples in one sequencing run. Library concentrations and quality were measured using a Qubit ds DNA HS Assay kit (Life Technologies, Carlsbad, CA, USA) and Agilent Tapestation (Agilent, Santa Clara, CA, USA). RNA sequencing was performed using Illumina HiSeq 3000 equipment for single-end sequencing, 50 bp read length, for approximately 30 million raw reads per each sample. The data quality check was done on an Illumina SAV. De-multiplexing was performed with an Illumina Bcl2fastq2 v 2.17 program.

RNA sequencing FASTQ files were processed with a STAR aligner [49] in the "GeneCounts" mode with the Ensembl human transcriptome annotation (Build version GRCh38 and transcript annotation GRCh38.89). Ensembl gene IDs were converted to HGNC gene symbols using the Complete HGNC dataset (https://www.genenames.org/, database version from 2017 July 13). In total, expression levels were established for 36596 annotated genes with corresponding HGNC identifiers.

The SABiosciences knowledge base was used to determine structures of intracellular molecular pathways as described previously [50,51]. We applied the original Oncobox algorithm [50] for functional annotation and visualization of the primary expression data and for calculating pathway activation strength (PAS) scores and case-to-normal ratios (CNRs). CNRs were calculated as the ratios of expression levels of a gene in the experimental samples to average expression levels in the control samples. PAS values can be both positive and negative, being indicative of up- or downregulation compared to controls.

5. Conclusions

We investigated the properties and mechanism of cytotoxicity of the novel peptide PM III from the horseshoe crab *Limulus polyphemus*. It had the strongest cytotoxicity against human cells among all the peptides interrogated in this study and, despite its high hemolytic activity, may be regarded as a potentially useful object for further studies on cytotoxicity towards tumor cells. We showed here that the cytotoxic activity of PM III is based on fast disruption of the cell membrane.

Supplementary Materials: The following are available online at http://www.mdpi.com/1660-3397/16/12/466/s1. Figure S1: MALDI-MS analysis of the recombinant (**A**) polyphemusin I, (**B**) polyphemusin II and (**C**) polyphemusin III. The experimental $[M+H]^+$ monoisotopic *m/z* is presented in the picture. Figure S2: MALDI-MS analysis of the recombinant (**A**) tachyplesin I, (**B**) tachyplesin II and (**C**) tachyplesin III. The experimental $[M+H]^+$ monoisotopic *m/z* is presented in the picture. Figure S3: Reversed-phase high-performance liquid chromatography (RP-HPLC) of the recombinant (**A**) polyphemusin I, (**B**) polyphemusin II and (**C**) polyphemusin III. RP-HPLC was performed with a linear gradient from 5 to 80% (v/v) of acetonitrile in water containing 0.1% TFA within 1 h. The fractions of the mature recombinant peptides are marked with arrows. Figure S4: Reversed-phase high-performance liquid chromatography (RP-HPLC) of the recombinant (**A**) tachyplesin I, (**B**) tachyplesin II and (**C**) tachyplesin III. RP-HPLC was performed with a linear gradient from 5 to 80% (v/v) of acetonitrile in water containing 0.1% TFA within 1 h. The fractions of the mature recombinant peptides are marked with arrows. Table S1: Pathway activation strength (PAS) and case-to-normal (CNR) values for unaffected and polyphemusin III-treated cells (at the peptide concentration of 1.25, 2.5, and 5 μM).

Author Contributions: M.B.M., P.V.P., A.A.E., I.A.B. performed the experiments; M.B.M., P.V.P., A.A.E., I.A.B., A.A.B., M.I.S., D.V.K., T.V.O. designed the experiments and analyzed data; M.B.M. wrote—prepared the original draft; A.A.E., D.V.K., P.V.P., A.A.B., M.I.S. and T.V.O. wrote—reviewed and edited the paper; T.V.O. contributed to the conception of the work, supervised the whole project, revised the manuscript critically, and prepared it for publication. All authors read and approved the final manuscript.

Funding: This work was supported by Russian Science Foundation (project No. 14-50-00131).

Conflicts of Interest: The authors declare no conflict of interest.

References

1. Brandenburg, L.-O.; Merres, J.; Albrecht, L.-J.; Varoga, D.; Pufe, T. Antimicrobial peptides: Multifunctional drugs for different applications. *Polymers* **2012**, *4*, 539–560. [CrossRef]

2. Mishra, B.; Reiling, S.; Zarena, D.; Wang, G. Host defense antimicrobial peptides as antibiotics: design and application strategies. *Curr. Opin. Chem. Biol.* **2017**, *38*, 87–96. [CrossRef] [PubMed]

3. Zasloff, M. Antimicrobial peptides of multicellular organisms. *Nature* **2002**, *415*, 389–395. [CrossRef] [PubMed]

4. Roudi, R.; Syn, N.L.; Roudbary, M. Antimicrobial peptides as biologic and immunotherapeutic agents against cancer: A comprehensive overview. *Front. Immunol.* **2017**, *8*, 1320. [CrossRef] [PubMed]

5. Deslouches, B.; Di, Y.P. Antimicrobial peptides with selective antitumor mechanisms: prospect for anticancer applications. *Oncotarget* **2017**, *8*, 46635–46651. [CrossRef] [PubMed]

6. Felício, M.R.; Silva, O.N.; Gonçalves, S.; Santos, N.C.; Franco, O.L. Peptides with dual antimicrobial and anticancer activities. *Front. Chem.* **2017**, *5*, 5. [CrossRef] [PubMed]

7. Rodrigues, E.G.; Dobroff, A.S.; Cavarsan, C.F.; Paschoalin, T.; Nimrichter, L.; Mortara, R.A.; Santos, E.L.; Fázio, M.A.; Miranda, A.; Daffre, S.; et al. Effective topical treatment of subcutaneous murine B16F10-Nex2 melanoma by the antimicrobial peptide gomesin. *Neoplasia* **2008**, *10*, 61–68. [CrossRef] [PubMed]

8. Paredes-Gamero, E.J.; Martins, M.N.C.; Cappabianco, F.A.M.; Ide, J.S.; Miranda, A. Characterization of dual effects induced by antimicrobial peptides: Regulated cell death or membrane disruption. *Biochim. Biophys. Acta* **2012**, *1820*, 1062–1072. [CrossRef] [PubMed]

9. Buri, M.V.; Torquato, H.F.V.; Barros, C.C.; Ide, J.S.; Miranda, A.; Paredes-Gamero, E.J. Comparison of cytotoxic activity in leukemic lineages reveals important features of β-hairpin antimicrobial peptides. *J. Cell Biochem.* **2017**, *118*, 1764–1773. [CrossRef] [PubMed]

10. Panteleev, P.V.; Balandin, S.V.; Ivanov, V.T.; Ovchinnikova, T.V. A therapeutic potential of animal β-hairpin antimicrobial peptides. *Curr. Med. Chem.* **2017**, *24*, 1724–1746. [CrossRef] [PubMed]

11. Miyata, T.; Tokunaga, F.; Yoneya, T.; Yoshikawa, K.; Iwanaga, S.; Niwa, M.; Takao, T.; Shimonishi, Y. Antimicrobial peptides, isolated from horseshoe crab hemocytes, tachyplesin II, and polyphemusins I and II: Chemical structures and biological activity. *J. Biochem.* **1989**, *106*, 663–668. [CrossRef] [PubMed]

12. Nakamura, T.; Furunaka, H.; Miyata, T.; Tokunaga, F.; Muta, T.; Iwanaga, S.; Niwa, M.; Takao, T.; Shimonishi, Y. Tachyplesin, a class of antimicrobial peptide from the hemocytes of the horseshoe crab (Tachypleus tridentatus). Isolation and chemical structure. *J. Biol. Chem.* **1988**, *263*, 16709–16713. [PubMed]

13. Muta, T.; Nakamura, T.; Furunaka, H.; Tokunaga, F.; Miyata, T.; Niwa, M.; Iwanaga, S. Primary structures and functions of anti-lipopolysaccharide factor and tachyplesin peptide found in horseshoe crab hemocytes. *Adv. Exp. Med. Biol.* **1990**, *256*, 273–285. [PubMed]

14. Zhang, L.; Scott, M.G.; Yan, H.; Mayer, L.D.; Hancock, R.E. Interaction of polyphemusin I and structural analogs with bacterial membranes, lipopolysaccharide, and lipid monolayers. *Biochemistry* **2000**, *39*, 14504–14514. [CrossRef] [PubMed]

15. Ohta, M.; Ito, H.; Masuda, K.; Tanaka, S.; Arakawa, Y.; Wacharotayankun, R.; Kato, N. Mechanisms of antibacterial action of tachyplesins and polyphemusins, a group of antimicrobial peptides isolated from horseshoe crab hemocytes. *Antimicrob. Agents Chemother.* **1992**, *36*, 1460–1465. [CrossRef] [PubMed]

16. Edwards, I.A.; Elliott, A.G.; Kavanagh, A.M.; Zuegg, J.; Blaskovich, M.A.T.; Cooper, M.A. Contribution of amphipathicity and hydrophobicity to the antimicrobial activity and cytotoxicity of β-hairpin peptides. *ACS Infect. Dis.* **2016**, *2*, 442–450. [CrossRef] [PubMed]

17. Oishi, O.; Yamashita, S.; Nishimoto, E.; Lee, S.; Sugihara, G.; Ohno, M. Conformations and orientations of aromatic amino acid residues of tachyplesin I in phospholipid membranes. *Biochemistry* **1997**, *36*, 4352–4359. [CrossRef] [PubMed]

18. Katsu, T.; Nakao, S.; Iwanaga, S. Mode of action of an antimicrobial peptide, tachyplesin I, on biomembranes. *Biol. Pharm. Bull.* **1993**, *16*, 178–181. [CrossRef] [PubMed]

19. Hong, J.; Hu, J.; Ke, F. Experimental induction of bacterial resistance to the antimicrobial peptide tachyplesin I and investigation of the resistance mechanisms. *Antimicrob. Agents Chemother.* **2016**, *60*, 6067–6075. [CrossRef] [PubMed]

20. Zapotoczna, M.; Forde, É.; Hogan, S.; Humphreys, H.; O'Gara, J.P.; Fitzgerald-Hughes, D.; Devocelle, M.; O'Neill, E. Eradication of staphylococcus aureus biofilm infections using synthetic antimicrobial peptides. *J. Infect. Dis.* **2017**, *215*, 975–983. [CrossRef] [PubMed]

21. Shigenaga, T.; Muta, T.; Toh, Y.; Tokunaga, F.; Iwanaga, S. Antimicrobial tachyplesin peptide precursor. cDNA cloning and cellular localization in the horseshoe crab (Tachypleus tridentatus). *J. Biol. Chem.* **1990**, *265*, 21350–21354. [PubMed]

22. Janko, C.; Munoz, L.; Chaurio, R.; Maueröder, C.; Berens, C.; Lauber, K.; Herrmann, M. Navigation to the graveyard-induction of various pathways of necrosis and their classification by flow cytometry. *Methods Mol. Biol.* **2013**, *1004*, 3–15. [CrossRef] [PubMed]

23. Van Noorden, C.J. The history of Z-VAD-FMK, a tool for understanding the significance of caspase inhibition. *Acta Histochem.* **2001**, *103*, 241–251. [CrossRef] [PubMed]

24. Lu, X.; Cao, L.; Chen, X.; Xiao, J.; Zou, Y.; Chen, Q. PTEN inhibits cell proliferation, promotes cell apoptosis, and induces cell cycle arrest via downregulating the PI3K/AKT/hTERT pathway in lung adenocarcinoma A549 Cells. *Biomed. Res. Int.* **2016**, *2016*, 2476842. [CrossRef] [PubMed]

25. Powers, J.-P.S.; Rozek, A.; Hancock, R.E.W. Structure-activity relationships for the beta-hairpin cationic antimicrobial peptide polyphemusin I. *Biochim. Biophys. Acta* **2004**, *1698*, 239–250. [CrossRef] [PubMed]

26. Huang, Y.-B.; Wang, X.-F.; Wang, H.-Y.; Liu, Y.; Chen, Y. Studies on mechanism of action of anticancer peptides by modulation of hydrophobicity within a defined structural framework. *Mol. Cancer Ther.* **2011**, *10*, 416–426. [CrossRef] [PubMed]

27. Dathe, M.; Wieprecht, T.; Nikolenko, H.; Handel, L.; Maloy, W.L.; MacDonald, D.L.; Beyermann, M.; Bienert, M. Hydrophobicity, hydrophobic moment and angle subtended by charged residues modulate antibacterial and haemolytic activity of amphipathic helical peptides. *FEBS Lett.* **1997**, *403*, 208–212. [CrossRef]

28. Yin, L.M.; Edwards, M.A.; Li, J.; Yip, C.M.; Deber, C.M. Roles of hydrophobicity and charge distribution of cationic antimicrobial peptides in peptide-membrane interactions. *J. Biol. Chem.* **2012**, *287*, 7738–7745. [CrossRef] [PubMed]

29. Tachi, T.; Epand, R.F.; Epand, R.M.; Matsuzaki, K. Position-dependent hydrophobicity of the antimicrobial magainin peptide affects the mode of peptide-lipid interactions and selective toxicity. *Biochemistry* **2002**, *41*, 10723–10731. [CrossRef] [PubMed]

30. Dathe, M.; Meyer, J.; Beyermann, M.; Maul, B.; Hoischen, C.; Bienert, M. General aspects of peptide selectivity towards lipid bilayers and cell membranes studied by variation of the structural parameters of amphipathic helical model peptides. *Biochim. Biophys. Acta* **2002**, *1558*, 171–186. [CrossRef]

31. Yeaman, M.R.; Yount, N.Y. Mechanisms of antimicrobial peptide action and resistance. *Pharmacol. Rev.* **2003**, *55*, 27–55. [CrossRef] [PubMed]

32. Gaspar, D.; Veiga, A.S.; Castanho, M.A.R.B. From antimicrobial to anticancer peptides. A review. *Front. Microbiol.* **2013**, *4*, 294. [CrossRef] [PubMed]

33. Wieprecht, T.; Beyermann, M.; Seelig, J. Binding of antibacterial magainin peptides to electrically neutral membranes: Thermodynamics and structure. *Biochemistry* **1999**, *38*, 10377–10387. [CrossRef] [PubMed]

34. Wieprecht, T.; Dathe, M.; Beyermann, M.; Krause, E.; Maloy, W.L.; MacDonald, D.L.; Bienert, M. Peptide hydrophobicity controls the activity and selectivity of magainin 2 amide in interaction with membranes. *Biochemistry* **1997**, *36*, 6124–6132. [CrossRef] [PubMed]

35. Glukhov, E.; Stark, M.; Burrows, L.L.; Deber, C.M. Basis for selectivity of cationic antimicrobial peptides for bacterial versus mammalian membranes. *J. Biol. Chem.* **2005**, *280*, 33960–33967. [CrossRef] [PubMed]

36. Andreev, K.; Martynowycz, M.W.; Huang, M.L.; Kuzmenko, I.; Bu, W.; Kirshenbaum, K.; Gidalevitz, D. Hydrophobic interactions modulate antimicrobial peptoid selectivity towards anionic lipid membranes. *Biochim. Biophys. Acta Biomembr.* **2018**, *1860*, 1414–1423. [CrossRef] [PubMed]

37. Chen, Y.; Guarnieri, M.T.; Vasil, A.I.; Vasil, M.L.; Mant, C.T.; Hodges, R.S. Role of peptide hydrophobicity in the mechanism of action of alpha-helical antimicrobial peptides. *Antimicrob. Agents Chemother.* **2007**, *51*, 1398–1406. [CrossRef] [PubMed]

38. Glukhov, E.; Burrows, L.L.; Deber, C.M. Membrane interactions of designed cationic antimicrobial peptides: The two thresholds. *Biopolymers* **2008**, *89*, 360–371. [CrossRef] [PubMed]

39. Pasupuleti, M.; Walse, B.; Svensson, B.; Malmsten, M.; Schmidtchen, A. Rational design of antimicrobial C3a analogues with enhanced effects against Staphylococci using an integrated structure and function-based approach. *Biochemistry* **2008**, *47*, 9057–9070. [CrossRef] [PubMed]

40. Gottler, L.M.; de la Salud Bea, R.; Shelburne, C.E.; Ramamoorthy, A.; Marsh, E.N.G. Using fluorous amino acids to probe the effects of changing hydrophobicity on the physical and biological properties of the β-hairpin antimicrobial peptide protegrin-1. *Biochemistry* **2008**, *47*, 9243–9250. [CrossRef] [PubMed]

41. Ding, H.; Jin, G.; Zhang, L.; Dai, J.; Dang, J.; Han, Y. Effects of tachyplesin I on human U251 glioma stem cells. *Mol. Med. Rep.* **2015**, *11*, 2953–2958. [CrossRef] [PubMed]

42. Carriel-Gomes, M.C.; Kratz, J.M.; Barracco, M.A.; Bachére, E.; Barardi, C.R.M.; Simões, C.M.O. In vitro antiviral activity of antimicrobial peptides against herpes simplex virus 1, adenovirus, and rotavirus. *Mem. Inst. Oswaldo Cruz* **2007**, *102*, 469–472. [CrossRef] [PubMed]

43. Zhang, H.; Wu, J.; Zhang, H.; Zhu, Q. Efflux of potassium ion is an important reason of HL-60 cells apoptosis induced by tachyplesin. *Acta Pharmacol. Sin.* **2006**, *27*, 1367–1374. [CrossRef] [PubMed]

44. Xu, C.; Jiang, J.; Sottile, V.; McWhir, J.; Lebkowski, J.; Carpenter, M.K. Immortalized fibroblast-like cells derived from human embryonic stem cells support undifferentiated cell growth. *Stem Cells* **2004**, *22*, 972–980. [CrossRef] [PubMed]

45. Xiong, H.; Gendelman, H.E. Isolation and culture of human neurons, microglia, and astrocytes. In *Current Laboratory Methods in Neuroscience Research*; Xiong, H., Gendelman, H.E., Eds.; Springer: New York, NY, USA, 2014; ISBN 978-1-4614-8793-7.

46. Panteleev, P.V.; Ovchinnikova, T.V. Improved strategy for recombinant production and purification of antimicrobial peptide tachyplesin I and its analogs with high cell selectivity. *Biotechnol. Appl. Biochem.* **2017**, *64*, 35–42. [CrossRef] [PubMed]

47. Panteleev, P.V.; Bolosov, I.A.; Balandin, S.V.; Ovchinnikova, T.V. Design of antimicrobial peptide arenicin analogs with improved therapeutic indices. *J. Pept. Sci.* **2015**, *21*, 105–113. [CrossRef] [PubMed]

48. Panteleev, P.V.; Bolosov, I.A.; Ovchinnikova, T.V. Bioengineering and functional characterization of arenicin shortened analogs with enhanced antibacterial activity and cell selectivity. *J. Pept. Sci.* **2016**, *22*, 82–91. [CrossRef] [PubMed]

49. Dobin, A.; Davis, C.A.; Schlesinger, F.; Drenkow, J.; Zaleski, C.; Jha, S.; Batut, P.; Chaisson, M.; Gingeras, T.R. STAR: Ultrafast universal RNA-seq aligner. *Bioinformatics* **2013**, *29*, 15–21. [CrossRef] [PubMed]

50. Sorokin, M.; Kholodenko, R.; Suntsova, M.; Malakhova, G.; Garazha, A.; Kholodenko, I.; Poddubskaya, E.; Lantsov, D.; Stilidi, I.; Arhiri, P.; et al. Oncobox bioinformatical platform for selecting potentially effective combinations of target cancer drugs using high-throughput gene expression data. *Cancers* **2018**, *10*, 365. [CrossRef] [PubMed]

51. Buzdin, A.; Sorokin, M.; Garazha, A.; Sekacheva, M.; Kim, E.; Zhukov, N.; Wang, Y.; Li, X.; Kar, S.; Hartmann, C.; et al. Molecular pathway activation—New type of biomarkers for tumor morphology and personalized selection of target drugs. *Semin. Cancer Biol.* **2018**. [CrossRef] [PubMed]

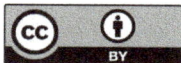

marine drugs

MDPI

Article

Massive Gene Expansion and Sequence Diversification Is Associated with Diverse Tissue Distribution, Regulation and Antimicrobial Properties of Anti-Lipopolysaccharide Factors in Shrimp

Gabriel Machado Matos [1], Paulina Schmitt [2], Cairé Barreto [1], Natanael Dantas Farias [1], Guilherme Toledo-Silva [3], Fanny Guzmán [4], Delphine Destoumieux-Garzón [5], Luciane Maria Perazzolo [1] and Rafael Diego Rosa [1,*]

[1] Laboratory of Immunology Applied to Aquaculture, Department of Cell Biology, Embryology and Genetics, Federal University of Santa Catarina, Florianópolis SC 88040-900, Brazil; gabrielmatos92@gmail.com (G.M.M.); cairebarreto@gmail.com (C.B.); natan.cbio@gmail.com (N.D.F.); l.m.perazzolo@ufsc.br (L.M.P.)
[2] Laboratorio de Genética e Inmunología Molecular, Instituto de Biología, Facultad de Ciencias, Pontificia Universidad Católica de Valparaíso, Valparaíso 2373223, Chile; paulina.schmitt@pucv.cl
[3] Department of Cell Biology, Embryology and Genetics, Federal University of Santa Catarina, Florianópolis SC 88040-900, Brazil; guilherme.toledo@ufsc.br
[4] Núcleo Biotecnología Curauma, Pontificia Universidad Católica de Valparaíso, Valparaíso 2373223, Chile; fanny.guzman@pucv.cl
[5] Interactions Hôtes-Pathogènes-Environnements, Université de Montpellier, CNRS, Ifremer, Université de Perpignan Via Domitia, CEDEX 5, 34090 Montpellier, France; Delphine.Destoumieux.Garzon@ifremer.fr
*   Correspondence: rafael.d.rosa@ufsc.br; Tel.: +55-48-37216163

Received: 15 September 2018; Accepted: 9 October 2018; Published: 11 October 2018

Abstract: Anti-lipopolysaccharide factors (ALFs) are antimicrobial peptides with a central β-hairpin structure able to bind to microbial components. Mining sequence databases for ALFs allowed us to show the remarkable diversity of ALF sequences in shrimp. We found at least seven members of the ALF family (Groups A to G), including two novel Groups (F and G), all of which are encoded by different loci with conserved gene organization. Phylogenetic analyses revealed that gene expansion and subsequent diversification of the ALF family occurred in crustaceans before shrimp speciation occurred. The transcriptional profile of ALFs was compared in terms of tissue distribution, response to two pathogens and during shrimp development in *Litopenaeus vannamei*, the most cultivated species. ALFs were found to be constitutively expressed in hemocytes and to respond differently to tissue damage. While synthetic β-hairpins of Groups E and G displayed both antibacterial and antifungal activities, no activity was recorded for Group F β-hairpins. Altogether, our results showed that ALFs form a family of shrimp AMPs that has been the subject of intense diversification. The different genes differ in terms of tissue expression, regulation and function. These data strongly suggest that multiple selection pressures have led to functional diversification of ALFs in shrimp.

Keywords: host defense peptide; antimicrobial peptide; anti-LPS factor; host-microbe relationship; functional diversity; invertebrate immunity; crustacean; antimicrobial activity

1. Introduction

Anti-lipopolysaccharide factors (ALFs) are multifunctional antimicrobial host defense peptides (AMPs) with the ability to bind to microbial surface molecules. They were initially characterized as potent inhibitors of lipopolysaccharide (LPS)-induced clotting in marine chelicerates, the horseshoe crabs *Tachypleus tridentatus* and *Limulus polyphemus* [1]. In addition to their LPS-binding properties, they were also shown to be highly active against Gram-negative bacteria [2]. In the early 2000s, ALF homologues were identified in hemocyte transcriptomes from two penaeid shrimp, *Litopenaeus setiferus* and *Penaeus monodon* [3,4]. Although ALF sequences have been extensively identified in many species, these AMPs appear to be exclusive of marine chelicerates and crustaceans.

ALFs are genetically encoded as precursor molecules composed of a leader sequence followed by a mature peptide containing two conserved cysteine residues [5]. The three-dimensional structure of both horseshoe crab and shrimp ALFs consists of three α-helices packed against a four-stranded β-sheet [6]. In this structure, the two cysteines flank a central β-hairpin of 20 residues stabilized by a single disulfide bond. This central β-hairpin (also known as "LPS-binding domain" or LPS-BD) is the functional domain of ALFs and holds key charged amino acids involved in the recognition and binding of microbial cell wall components, such as LPS from Gram-negative bacteria, lipoteichoic acid from Gram-positive bacteria and β-glucans from fungi [7]. Indeed, the mechanism of action of ALFs is intimately associated with their ability to bind to those microbial moieties. Notably, ALFs are known to be highly active against a broad range of bacteria, fungi and some enveloped viruses [8].

Different from horseshoe crabs, ALFs form a diverse and multigenic family of AMPs in penaeid shrimp. Shrimp ALFs are composed of five members (Groups A to E), which differ in terms of primary structure and biochemical characteristics [5]. While ALFs from Groups A and D possess anionic properties, Groups B and C are exclusively composed of cationic peptides. Interestingly, while cationic ALFs exhibit potent antimicrobial activities against a broad range of bacterial and fungal strains [9], anionic ALFs from Group D have impaired antimicrobial properties [10]. The limited antibacterial activity of Group D ALFs is likely due to the lack of most residues involved in LPS binding of cationic ALFs from Group B [10]. Group E ALFs were only described in the kuruma prawn *Marsupenaeus japonicus* as cationic (*Mj*ALF-E1) and anionic (*Mj*ALF-E2) peptides, with antimicrobial activity restricted to Gram-negative bacteria [11].

At present, little is known about the evolutionary forces that may have shaped the diversification of ALF sequences in shrimp. To address this question and explore the biological implications of such sequence diversity, we combined a series of molecular, phylogenetic, transcriptional and functional analyses. By using an in silico mapping method, we have identified novel ALF members in different penaeid species. Bayesian phylogenetic reconstructions revealed the existence of seven ALF groups in shrimp: the previously described Groups A to E, and the novel Groups F and G evidenced here. Each ALF group is encoded by a different locus in the shrimp genome. Through a quantitative PCR-based approach, we have assessed the expression of the seven ALF genes in terms of tissue distribution and transcriptional response to two pathogens (*Vibrio harveyi* and WSSV), but also during different shrimp development stages (from fertilized eggs to larval and post-larval stages) in the shrimp *L. vannamei*. Finally, we evaluated the antimicrobial activity of synthetic peptides based on the central β-hairpin of the three novel ALFs identified in *L. vannamei* (Groups E to G) and presented evidence that the sequence diversity of shrimp ALFs can be reflected in their biological properties. Altogether, the tissue distribution, regulation and biological functions of ALF genes reveal that various evolutionary pressures have led to functional diversification of the ALF family in penaeid shrimp.

2. Results

2.1. ALFs from Penaeid Shrimp Comprise a Diverse Family Composed of Seven Members

By using an exhaustive in silico screening approach, we recovered 47 unique ALF sequences (complete CDS) from both publicly available annotated and non-annotated databases for 10 penaeid shrimp species (Decapoda: Penaeidae) (Table S1). With all predicted amino acid sequences in hand, we performed multiple alignments in order to classify the obtained sequences into the five previously described ALF groups (Groups A to E). Surprisingly, from our sequence analysis, shrimp

ALFs clustered into seven distinct groups with specific amino acid sequence signatures (Figure 1A). In addition to already documented ALFs from Groups A to E, we identified here two novel groups that were conveniently named Group F and G (Figure 1A).

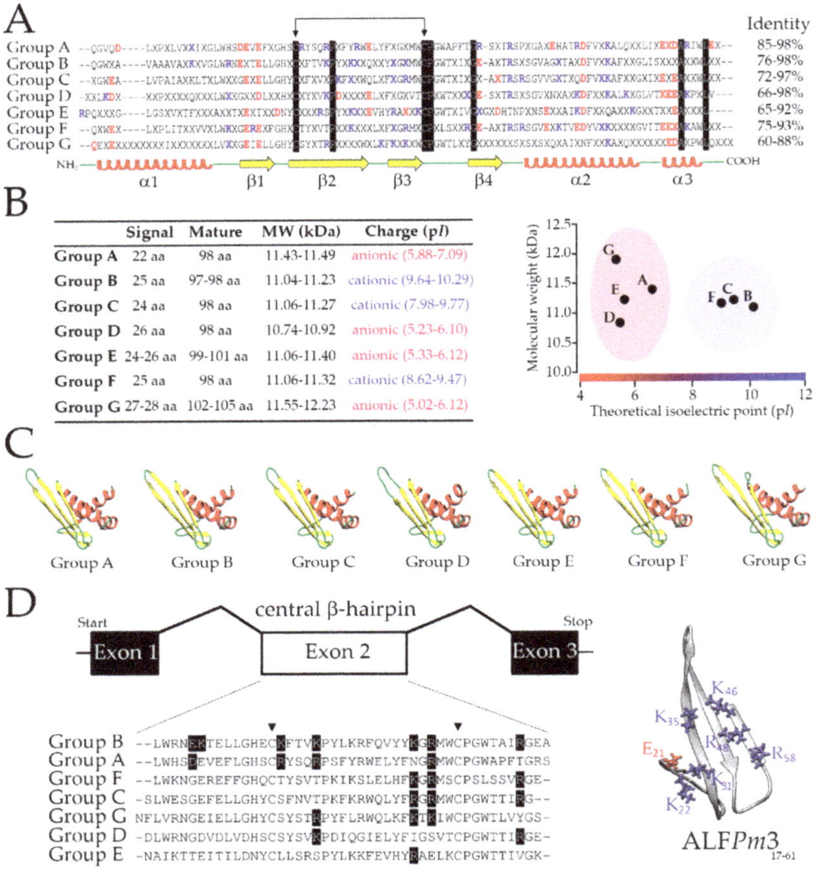

Figure 1. The seven members of the shrimp ALF family. (**A**) Multiple alignments of the consensus amino acid signature of each ALF member (Groups A to G) found in penaeid shrimp. Identical residues are highlighted in black while "X" indicates any amino acid. Positively and negatively charged residues are displayed in blue and red, respectively. The conserved cysteine bond is indicated by the arrows. The position of α-helices (red helices) and β-sheets (yellow arrows) is based on the three-dimensional (3D) structure of ALFPm3 (PDB: 2JOB). Intragroup amino acid identity values are indicated on the right. (**B**) Biochemical properties of shrimp ALFs. MW: molecular weight; pI: theoretical isoelectric point; aa: amino acid residues. (**C**) Predicted 3D structure of *L. vannamei* ALFs. The structural models were built based on the NMR (nuclear magnetic resonance) structure of ALFPm3. (**D**) Not-to-scale schematic representation of ALF genes from *P. monodon*: Group A (*ALFPm2*: EF523561), Group B (*ALFPm3*: EF523562), Group C (*ALFPm6*: JN562340), Group D (*ALFPm8*: NIUS010164210), Group E (*ALFPm9*: NIUS010076396), Group F (*ALFPm10*: NIUS011801312) and Group G (*ALFPm11*: NIUS010749450). Boxes represent the exons, and lines represent the introns. Multiple alignments of the amino acid sequences encoded by the exon 2 (white box). Triangles (▼) indicate the two conserved cysteines. Residues involved in LPS binding of ALFPm3 are highlighted in black.

Across shrimp species, ALFs corresponded to full-length transcripts that encode for precursors composed of a signal peptide (22 to 28 residues), followed by a mature peptide (10.74 to 12.23 kDa) containing two conserved cysteine residues (Figure 1A). Besides their differences in size and molecular weight, shrimp ALFs also displayed contrasting electrostatic characteristics. Notably, while ALFs from Groups B, C and F showed cationic properties, Groups A, D, E and G were composed of anionic ALFs (Figure 1B). However, independently of their differences in primary structure and biochemical properties, the seven ALFs shared a similar three-dimensional architecture: three α-helices packed against a four-stranded β-sheet (Figure 1C). Members of the seven groups were identified in at least four different shrimp species (*Farfantepenaeus aztecus*, *L. vannamei*, *M. japonicus* and *P. monodon*) (Table S1). Remarkably, Group G ALFs were the only members that were not identified in the genus *Fenneropenaeus* (*F chinensis*, *F. indicus* and *F. penicillatus*). On the other hand, two different members from Group C were identified in *F. chinensis* (*FcALF2*: JX853775 and *FcALF3*: JX853776), *M. japonicus* (*MjALF-C1*: AB210110 and *MjALF-C2*: KU160498) and *P. monodon* (*ALFPm6*: JN562340 and *ALFPm7*: KX431031).

Our knowledge of ALF intraspecific sequence diversity was also enriched by the discovery of novel sequences in *F. aztecus* (Groups A to G), *F. penicillatus* (Groups A to F), *L. vannamei* (Groups E to G) and *P. monodon* (Groups D to G). Besides, according to our in silico analyses, some ALFs from *M. japonicus* were classified in a different Group to that previously categorized by Jiang and colleagues [11]. For instance, the sequence *MjALF-A2* [11] is actually a member of Group G and not an ALF from Group A, whereas the cationic *MjALF-D1* (GenBank: KU160499) belongs to Group F and not to Group D (which gathers anionic sequences only). More surprisingly, the sequence *MjALF-E1* (GenBank: KY627760), previously classified as a cationic member of Group E, did not fit in any ALF Group. Indeed, its mature sequence contains an additional cysteine residue (apart of the two cysteines holding the central β-hairpin structure) that is not found in ALFs from either marine chelicerates or crustaceans. Interestingly, coding sequences related to *MjALF-E1* were also found in *P. monodon* and *L. vannamei*. Unlike the three-cysteine-containing sequences from *M. japonicus* and *P. monodon*, the sequences identified in *L. vannamei* contain four cysteines (Figure S1).

2.2. ALF Sequence Diversity Is Gene-Encoded

To gain insights into the origin of the molecular diversity of the shrimp ALF family, we searched for ALF gene sequences in both annotated (GenBank Nucleotide) and non-annotated (Whole-Genome Shotgun Contigs) databases. From our in silico mining analysis, seven unique genomic sequences were identified in *P. monodon*: *ALFPm2* from Group A (GenBank: EF523561), *ALFPm3* from Group B (GenBank: EF523562), *ALFPm6* from Group C (GenBank: JN562340), *ALFPm8* from Group D (GenBank: NIUS010164210), *ALFPm9* from Group E (GenBank: NIUS010076396), *ALFPm10* from Group F (GenBank: NIUS011801312) and *ALFPm11* from Group G (GenBank: NIUS010749450). Each genomic sequence corresponded to a specific ALF member and we found no evidences that ALFs from different Groups could be encoded by a same genomic sequence.

Despite their differences in terms of sequence signatures, all genes shared a similar structural organization: three exons interrupted by two introns (Figure 1D). Every sequence presents a second exon that encodes the four stranded β-sheets, with the two cysteines delimiting the central β-hairpin. This structure holds the seven charged residues involved in LPS binding and is considered as the functional domain of ALFs. As shown in Figure 1D, not all *P. monodon* ALFs contain those conserved residues found in ALFPm3 from Group B [6]. Regarding the other gene regions, the first exon covers the 5′-untranslated region (UTR), the leader sequence and the hydrophobic N-terminal portion of the mature peptide (the first α-helice), and the third exon encodes the two C-terminal α-helices of the mature peptide and the 3′-UTR.

2.3. ALFs Evolved from Gene Duplication Events before Shrimp Speciation

In order to unravel the phylogenetic relationships of the shrimp ALFs, phylogenetic reconstructions were performed with ALF sequences from 38 species of decapod crustaceans (suborders

Dendrobranchiata and Pleocyemata) and three species of marine chelicerates (the horseshoe crabs *Carcinoscorpius rotundicauda*, *L. polyphemus* and *T. tridentatus*) (Table S1). Additionally, we analyzed the ALF-related sequences containing three and four cysteine residues and scygonadins (anionic AMPs from crabs that contain two cysteines flanking 17 amino acid residues [12]). Our Bayesian phylogenetic analysis revealed that ALFs comprise a large and diverse gene family in decapod crustaceans. The first striking piece of information is that the three/four-cysteine-containing peptides (including *Mj*ALF-E1), as well as scygonadins, are not authentic members of the ALF family since they form a separate and distant clade from all other sequences (Figure 2A). Indeed, the ALF clade gathered sequences from both crustaceans and marine chelicerates. Regarding the crustacean group, ALFs were split into two main clades (Figure 2A). The first clade included ALFs from Group A, while the second clade gathered ALFs from six additional groups (B to G). Interestingly, sequences from non-penaeid species (Pleocyemata) were found in all shrimp ALF groups, but they also formed exclusive groups distinct from those found in penaeids (Figure 2A).

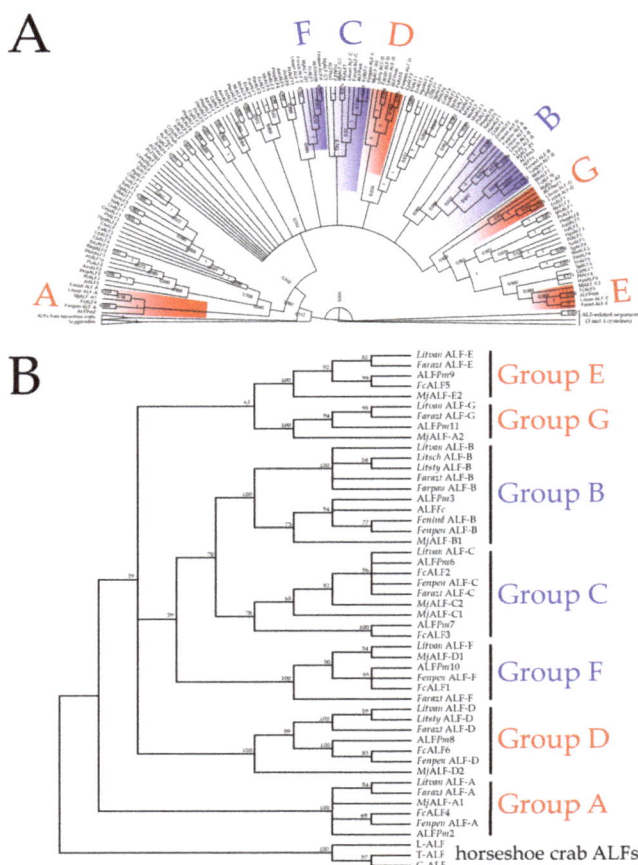

Figure 2. ALFs form a diverse antimicrobial peptide family in decapod crustaceans. (**A**) Bayesian and (**B**) neighbor-joining trees of ALFs from decapod crustaceans and marine chelicerates (horseshoe crabs). Cationic and anionic ALF groups from penaeid shrimp are displayed in blue and red, respectively. Posterior probabilities (Bayesian) and bootstrap values (neighbor-joining) higher than 50% are shown in the nodes. The list of the ALF sequences included in analyses (annotations, sequences and GenBank accession numbers) is provided in Table S1.

Then, an additional phylogenetic tree was constructed to determine the phylogenetic relationships among the seven shrimp ALF groups (A to G) (Figure 2B). In this tree, shrimp ALFs clustered into two main clades: a first clade containing ALFs from Group A and a second clade divided into three branches. Within the second clade, all cationic shrimp ALFs (Groups B, C and F) clustered into one branch, and anionic ALFs from Groups E and G clustered into a second branch (Figure 2B). Group D ALFs clustered in a third branch (Figure 2B). Altogether, our results suggest that the sequence diversity found in the ALF family was likely driven by gene duplication events before the divergence of decapod crustaceans (Dendrobranchiata and Pleocyemata). Notably, the gene expansion and subsequent diversification of the ALF family seems to have occurred in crustaceans and not in marine chelicerates. Actually, in marine chelicerates, only one ALF type was identified (Table S1).

2.4. ALFs Are All Expressed in Individual Shrimps and Differentially Modulated in Response to Tissue Damage

We further focused on the transcriptional profiles of shrimp ALFs in terms of tissue distribution. For gene expression analyses, we considered the seven ALFs from the Pacific white shrimp *L. vannamei* (*Litvan* ALF-A to -G). First, the gene expression distribution of *Litvan* ALFs was assessed in eight different tissues of healthy juveniles by semiquantitative RT-PCR analysis. Overall, *Litvan* ALFs were mainly detected in circulating hemocytes and gills (Figure 3A). Transcripts of *Litvan* ALF-A and *Litvan* ALF-B were detected in foregut, midgut, hemocytes, gills and nerve cord, while the expression of *Litvan* ALF-C was observed in midgut, hemocytes, and gills (Figure 3A). Besides, while the expression of *Litvan* ALF-E and *Litvan* ALF-G was exclusively detected in hemocytes and gills, *Litvan* ALF-F was mainly expressed in the foregut (Figure 3A). Unlike the other ALF groups, the expression of *Litvan* ALF-D was only detected in hemocytes (Figure 3A). For all genes, no signals were observed in hepatopancreas, hindgut and muscle (Figure 3A).

ALF gene expression was then studied in response to infections and wounding. We first asked whether ALF genes were all transcribed in a single animal or whether their diversity reflected inter-individual sequence variability. Transcripts of the seven ALF genes were detected in the circulating hemocytes of every individual shrimp, as determined by RT-qPCR (Figure 3B). However, important variation was observed in the basal transcription of each gene among individuals (Figure 3B). While the basal gene expression of *Litvan* ALF-A to *Litvan* ALF-F varied from 2- to 6-fold among individuals, variations up to 11.3-fold were found for *Litvan* ALF-G gene expression (Figure 3B).

Next, we analyzed the gene expression profile of *Litvan* ALFs in response to microbial challenge and injury. Two unrelated shrimp pathogens were chosen: the Gram-negative *V. harveyi* and the White spot syndrome virus (WSSV). The transcriptional response of *Litvan* ALFs was quantified by RT-qPCR in shrimp hemocytes 48 h after infections. This time point was chosen on the basis of previous studies from our group [13–15]. Anionic ALFs from Groups A, D and E did not respond to pathogens nor to injury (Figure 3C). Conversely, cationic ALFs (Groups B, C and F) and the anionic Group G ALF showed significant changes in expression only in response to tissue injury. Indeed, the expression of *Litvan* ALF-B (2.6-fold), *Litvan* ALF-C (18.7-fold), *Litvan* ALF-F (3.6-fold) and *Litvan* ALF-G (8.3-fold) was significantly induced in circulating hemocytes after the injection of a tissue homogenate prepared from shrimp muscle (Figure 3C). Similarly, the expression of *Litvan* ALF-B (2.7-fold) and *Litvan* ALF-F (4.1-fold) also increased after the injection of sterile seawater. The pathogens (*V. harveyi* and WSSV) did not modulate further ALF expression. Notably, independently of the experimental condition, a high variability in gene expression was observed for all ALFs (Figure 3C).

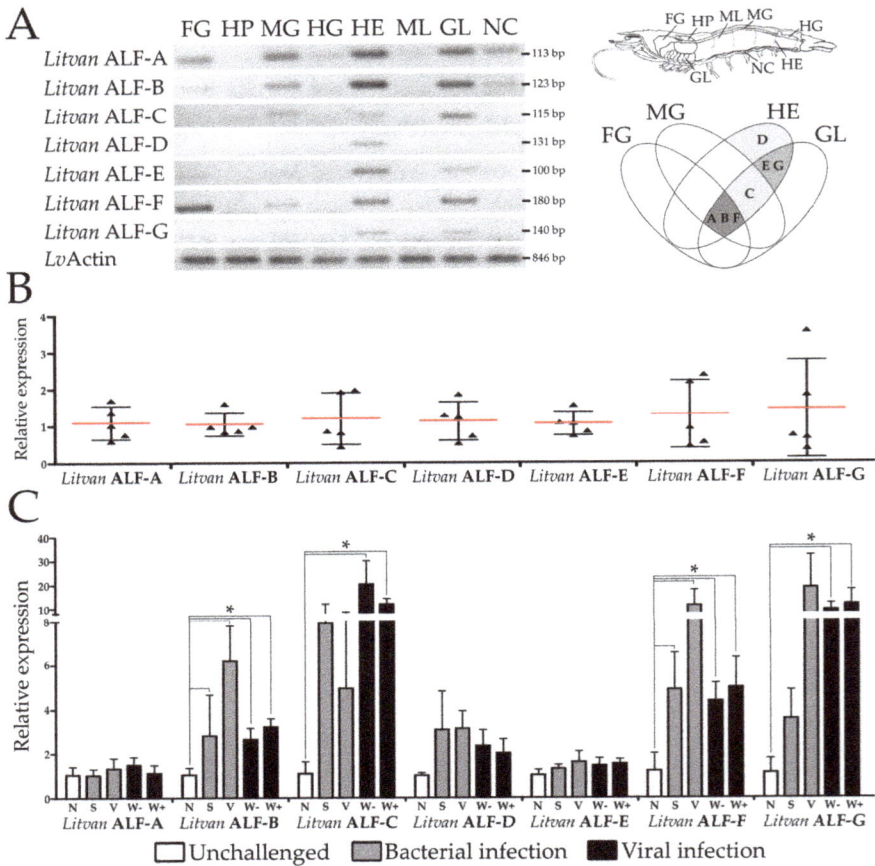

Figure 3. Tissue expression distribution of shrimp ALFS and gene modulation in hemocytes in response to pathogen challenge and tissue damage. (**A**) Semiquantitative RT-PCR analysis of *L. vannamei* ALFs in shrimp tissues: foregut (FG), hepatopancreas (HP), midgut (MG), hindgut (HG), hemocytes (HE), muscle (ML), gills (GL) and nerve cord (NC). The expression of the *Lv*Actin gene was used as endogenous control. The anatomic location of the tissues is indicated in the shrimp image. The Venn diagram summarizes the main sites of expression of *L. vannamei* ALFs. (**B**) mRNA basal levels of *L. vannamei* ALFs in the circulating hemocytes from five individual shrimp. (**C**) Gene expression profile of ALFs in the hemocytes of shrimp at 48 h after experimental infections with *V. harveyi* (grey bars) or WSSV (black bars). Results are presented as mean ± standard deviation of relative expressions (three biological replicates) and statistical differences are indicated by asterisks (*) (one-way ANOVA/Tukey, $p < 0.05$). N: naïve (non-stimulated) shrimp (white bars), S: sterile seawater injury control, V: *V. harveyi* ATCC 14126 (6×10^7 CFU/animal), W−: tissue homogenate inoculum prepared from WSSV-free shrimp, W+: WSSV (3×10^2 viral particles/animal).

2.5. Some ALF Genes Are Transcribed Early in Shrimp Development, while Others Are Mainly Expressed in Juveniles

Finally, we studied the expression of the three new *L. vannamei* ALFs (Groups E, F and G) at different stages of shrimp development: fertilized eggs, nauplii, protozoeae, mysis, postlarvae and juveniles. The expression profile of *Litvan* ALFs from Groups A to D was previously reported [16]. Three distinct patterns of expression were observed for ALF groups E to G over *L. vannamei* development.

ALFs from Groups E and F were detected at all developmental stages, but Group F expression could only be quantified from nauplius stages (Figure 4). Group E expression did not vary significantly over the entire shrimp development, from larvae to juveniles. In contrast, Group F expression was maximum in protozoea III (ZIII) and then decreased significantly in juveniles (PL17) (Figure 4). Finally, Group G ALF was only expressed from protozoea III (ZIII), and its expression increased significantly up to juvenile stages (PL17) (Figure 4).

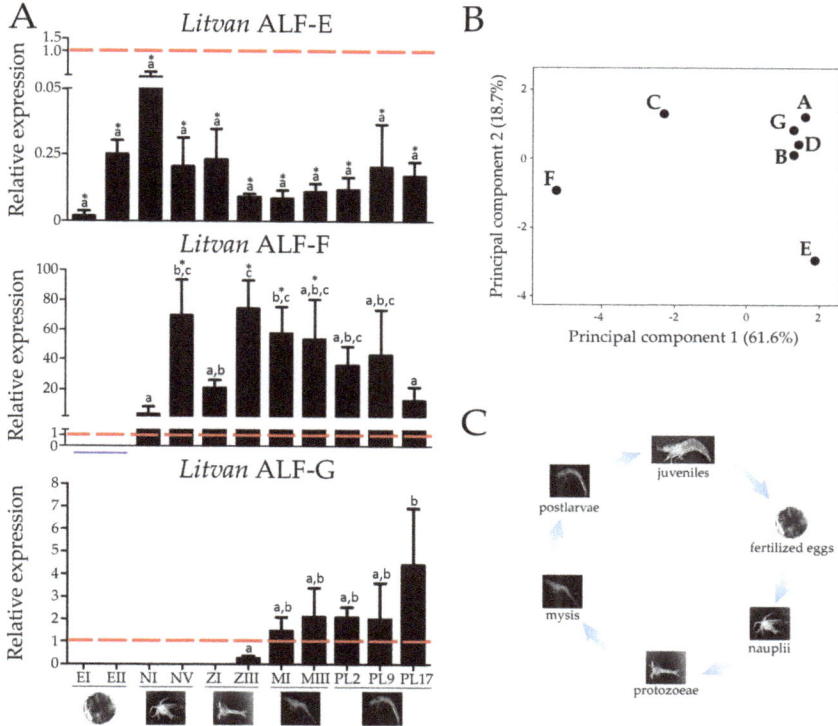

Figure 4. Expression of ALFs during shrimp development. (**A**) Gene expression profile of *Litvan* ALF-E, -F and -G in twelve developmental stages: fertilized eggs at 0–4 h post-spawning (EI), fertilized eggs at 7–11 h post-spawning (EII), nauplius I (NI), nauplius V (NV), protozoea I (ZI), protozoea III (ZIII), mysis I (MI), mysis III (MIII), postlarva 2 (PL2), postlarva 9 (PL9), postlarva 17 (PL17). Representative images of the developmental stages are indicated at the bottom of the graph. Results are present as mean ± standard deviation. The red dotted line indicates the expression in hemocytes from juveniles while the solid blue underline highlights the stages at which the expression was detected (valid dissociation curve) but not quantified (Cq values higher than the limit of quantification). Different letters indicate significant differences among the developmental stages and asterisks (*) shows significant differences between each developmental stage and hemocytes from juveniles (one-way ANOVA/Tukey, $p < 0.05$). (**B**) Results of principal component analysis showing the relationship among the expression profile of *L. vannamei* ALFs during shrimp development. (**C**) The life cycle of the Pacific white shrimp *L. vannamei*.

2.6. Sequence Diversity of Shrimp ALFs Results in Distinct Antimicrobial Properties

The functional domain (central β-hairpin) of the three novel ALF members identified in *L. vannamei* (Groups E, F and G) was generated by chemical synthesis to evaluate their antimicrobial properties. Indeed, this functional domain is considered a good proxy of the full-length ALF antimicrobial properties [9,10,17]. Minimal inhibitory concentration assays were performed against Gram-positive and

Gram-negative bacteria and fungi (yeast and filamentous) (Figure 5). From the three synthetic peptides, *Litvan* ALF-G$_{34-55}$ displayed the broadest range of antimicrobial activity, being effective against all tested Gram-positive bacteria, the Gram-negative *V. nigripulchritudo* and the filamentous fungus *F. oxysporum* (Figure 5). This peptide could also affect the growth of the Gram-negative bacteria *E. coli* and *V. harveyi* at 40 µM (data not shown), but total inhibition was only observed against *V. nigripulchritudo*. Additionally, *Litvan* ALF-G$_{34-55}$ exhibited bactericidal activity against the Gram-positive bacteria *B. cereus*, *B. stationis* and *M. maritypicum*. On the other hand, synthetic β-hairpins of *Litvan* ALF-E$_{32-53}$ could inhibit only the growth of marine Gram-positive bacteria (*B. stationis* and *M. maritypicum*) and *F. oxysporum* (Figure 5). Notably, no antimicrobial activity was observed for *Litvan* ALF-F$_{30-51}$ β-hairpin even at 40 µM. None of the synthetic peptides was able to inhibit the growth of the Gram-negative bacteria *A. salmonicida*, *P. aeruginosa*, *V. alginolyticus* and *V. anguillarum*, and of the yeast *C. albicans*. Thus, according to their synthetic β-hairpin, Group G and to a lower extent Group E ALFs show a broad spectrum of antimicrobial activities, whereas Group F is devoid of antifungal and antibacterial activity. However, in agreement with a very poor conservation of residues involved in LPS binding (Figure 1D), ALFs from Groups E-G were almost inactive against Gram-negative bacteria (Figure 5C).

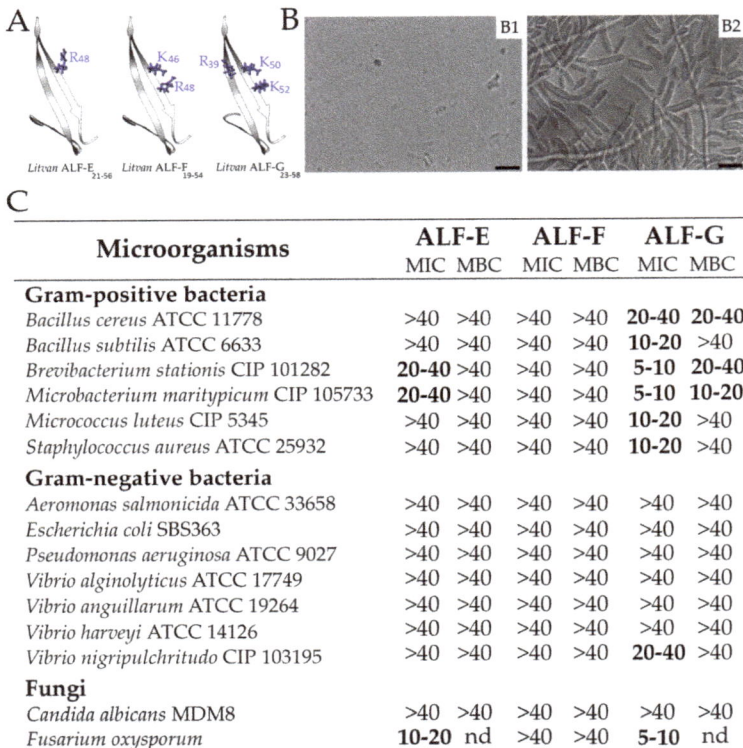

Microorganisms	ALF-E		ALF-F		ALF-G	
	MIC	MBC	MIC	MBC	MIC	MBC
Gram-positive bacteria						
Bacillus cereus ATCC 11778	>40	>40	>40	>40	**20-40**	**20-40**
Bacillus subtilis ATCC 6633	>40	>40	>40	>40	**10-20**	>40
Brevibacterium stationis CIP 101282	**20-40**	>40	>40	>40	**5-10**	**20-40**
Microbacterium maritypicum CIP 105733	**20-40**	>40	>40	>40	**5-10**	**10-20**
Micrococcus luteus CIP 5345	>40	>40	>40	>40	**10-20**	>40
Staphylococcus aureus ATCC 25932	>40	>40	>40	>40	**10-20**	>40
Gram-negative bacteria						
Aeromonas salmonicida ATCC 33658	>40	>40	>40	>40	>40	>40
Escherichia coli SBS363	>40	>40	>40	>40	>40	>40
Pseudomonas aeruginosa ATCC 9027	>40	>40	>40	>40	>40	>40
Vibrio alginolyticus ATCC 17749	>40	>40	>40	>40	>40	>40
Vibrio anguillarum ATCC 19264	>40	>40	>40	>40	>40	>40
Vibrio harveyi ATCC 14126	>40	>40	>40	>40	>40	>40
Vibrio nigripulchritudo CIP 103195	>40	>40	>40	>40	**20-40**	>40
Fungi						
Candida albicans MDM8	>40	>40	>40	>40	>40	>40
Fusarium oxysporum	**10-20**	nd	>40	>40	**5-10**	nd

Figure 5. The antimicrobial spectrum of the novel shrimp ALFs. (**A**) Predicted three-dimensional structure of the central β-hairpin of *Litvan* ALF-E, -F and -G. The structural models were built based on the NMR structure of ALFPm3 (PDB: 2JOB). Conserved residues involved in LPS binding of ALFPm3 are displayed in blue. (**B**) Representative images of the effects of ALFs against *F. oxysporum*: (B1) fugal spore inhibition (antifungal effect); (B2) fungal spore germination (no antifungal activity). Bars = 20 µm. (**C**) Spectrum of antibacterial and antifungal activities of synthetic peptides based on the central β-hairpin of *Litvan* ALF-E, -F and -G. Minimum inhibitory (MIC) and Minimum bactericidal (MBC) concentrations are expressed in µM. nd: non-determined.

3. Discussion

We showed here that shrimp ALFs are composed of seven distinct members (Groups A to G) with contrasting biochemical properties, activities and expression patterns. Particularly, ALF sequences were found to vary from cationic to anionic with important consequences on their antimicrobial activities. Overall, ALFs comprise the most diverse AMPs found in penaeid shrimp. Indeed, such diversity has not been observed in any other gene-encoded AMP families from shrimp, which are exclusively composed of cationic (penaeidins and crustins) or anionic (stylicins) members [8,12]. ALF diversity is encoded by at least seven genes that arose from successive duplications and subsequent mutations (nucleotide substitutions and insertion/deletion events) before decapod crustacean speciation occurred. This indicates that strong evolutionary pressures have driven the functional diversification of ALF genes, giving rise to neo- or sub-functionalization and retention in the shrimp genome.

We found that shrimp ALFs are paralogous genes that evolved before the speciation of the suborder Dendrobranchiata (penaeid shrimp). Indeed, ALF diversity, which is the subject of the present study, goes beyond penaeid shrimp and extends to other decapod species from the suborder Pleocyemata (including crayfish, crabs, lobsters, freshwater prawns, etc.). Some ALF members from non-penaeid decapods fall into the seven groups characterized here for penaeid shrimp. However, the ALF diversity found in the suborder Pleocyemata is different from penaeid shrimp (Dendrobranchiata). It is likely that the remarkable gene expansion and diversification of ALF sequences through gene duplication and subsequent mutation have fueled adaptation to different lifestyles and environments (and their associated pathogens) among crustaceans. Here, we have focused our study on shrimp ALFs, as a good sub-representative of ALF diversity. In order to support our hypothesis, we showed that the biological activities and expression patterns of ALF genes have diverged. In particular, we found that some ALFs are antimicrobial, whereas others are not. Some are expressed early during shrimp development, whereas others are expressed in late developmental stages. Finally, ALFs differ in their tissue distribution and responses to tissue damage. However, much more biological data are still needed on the expression and functions of the different ALF members to understand ALF evolution. This ambitious objective will require the development and use of emerging gene-silencing technologies (such as CRISPR-Cas9 and RNA interference) to achieve specific invalidation of closely-related genes in crustaceans and further phenotyping. Similarly, molecular tools such as in situ hybridization could reveal the tissue specificity of ALFs and thus, they would help in uncovering other biological functions. Finally, a classification of all crustacean ALFs (from both decapod and non-decapod species) based on robust phylogenetic reconstructions may avoid misleading classifications and lead to consensus among researchers.

With the identification of two novel ALF groups, we found that ALFs from Groups E and G share a common ancestor gene. Interestingly, Group G is lacking in species of the genus *Fenneropenaeus* whereas it is found in species of the genera *Farfantepenaeus*, *Litopenaeus*, *Marsupenaeus* and *Penaeus*. Although it cannot be ruled out that data are missing from publicly accessible databases, the absence of Group G in *Fenneropenaeus* could result from a gene loss event within this genus. Alternatively, the duplication event that originated these two genes may not have occurred in the genus *Fenneropenaeus*. Indeed, the evolutionary history of each group traced a particular trajectory in each shrimp species. For instance, while Group C ALFs from *F. chinensis* (FcALF2 and FcALF3 [17]), *M. japonicus* (MjALF-C1 and MjALF-C2 [11]) and *P. monodon* (ALFPm6 and ALFPm7 [18,19]) are composed of two members, in other penaeids this group appears to be composed by a single gene. However, we do not favor this last hypothesis as Group G is found in a diversity of penaeid species. Interestingly, in *L. vannamei*, Group G ALF was shown here to (i) have broader and more potent antimicrobial activity than Group E ALF, according to their β-hairpin activity, and (ii) to be expressed at late developmental stages whereas Group E expression tends to decrease over ontogenesis. Therefore, it is tempting to speculate that Group E confers antimicrobial protection at larval stages when Group G is still not expressed, whereas Group G provides a selective advantage to the *Litopenaeus* genus in facing infections at juvenile and adult stages when they are more exposed to different environmental challenges.

We showed that the expression of the seven ALF genes is simultaneous in the circulating hemocytes of a single shrimp. This result is particularly interesting because it suggests that the different ALF members may act synergistically to improve their antimicrobial properties. However, it is still unknown whether they are produced by the same hemocyte populations. Comparatively, the different penaeidin members of *L. vannamei* (Litvan PEN1/2, -3 and -4) are constitutively expressed by the granular cell populations [20]. Although the expression of ALFs has been detected in hemocytes from juveniles, some members (Groups C, E and F) appeared to be transcribed in larval stages of shrimp development that precede the emergence of these immune cells [21]. Instead, the expression of ALFs from Groups A, B, D and G was quite similar to that observed for other shrimp AMPs that are exclusively produced by hemocytes [16]. On the one hand, the expression of ALFs early in development could be the result of maternal transmission [16,22] but, on the other hand, those transcripts might originate from other shrimp tissues. Interestingly, in different species, including *L. vannamei*, the expression of ALFs from Groups C and F was mainly detected in other tissues (digestive system, gills, eyestalk) than in the circulating hemocytes [17–19]. However, only the expression of ALFs from Group B (ALF*Pm*3 from *P. monodon*) was studied by immune staining [23]. More knowledge about the precise sites of ALF production will contribute to understand the involvement of these AMPs in shrimp epithelial defenses, especially those occurring in gills and intestines [15].

One important finding from this study concerns the differential gene expression pattern of shrimp ALFs in response to various challenges. Indeed, the different ALF genes found across penaeids showed to be responsive to various shrimp pathogens, from viruses to bacteria and filamentous fungi [11,14,15,18]. Moreover, RNA interference (RNAi)-mediated gene silencing assays have confirmed that ALFs are directly involved in shrimp survival to infectious diseases [18,24,25]. Additionally, our results provided new evidences for the role of ALFs in other biological processes. Interestingly, while ALFs from Groups A, D and E were not regulated, the expression of the other ALF genes was induced in response to tissue damage. Particularly, ALFs from Groups C and G were shown to be responsive to a tissue homogenate prepared from shrimp muscle (injury control for the WSSV infection), suggesting that they can be modulated by danger/damage-associated molecular patterns (DAMPs). This nonspecific transcriptional response could be associated with additional biological roles involving the promotion of wound healing and the rapid regeneration of tissues [20]. Additionally, we showed that some ALFs are modulated in the shrimp gut in response to infections, suggesting that ALFs can act as a first line of defense in tissues continuously exposed to microbe-rich environments [15,19]. Therefore, it is possible that those ALF variants have evolved novel functions associated with the control of the intestinal microbiota. The shrimp intestinal microbiota is a complex and dynamic community that is directly influenced by both biotic and abiotic factors [13], but probably it is also by the constitutive expression of immune-related genes. In fact, RNAi experiments revealed that ALFs from Groups B [18] and C [25] play an essential role in the control of the bacterial communities residing in the hemolymph. However, more functional genomic studies are required to understand the role of ALF in shrimp intestinal defenses.

Another relevant conclusion taken is that the antimicrobial activity of the functional domain of ALFs (central β-hairpin) is associated with its primary sequence rather than to its charge. Despite their differences in primary structure and biochemical features, the seven ALF groups shared a similar tertiary structure. However, the residues involved in LPS binding are not conserved among the seven groups, confirming the neo-functionalization hypothesis proposed by Rosa and colleagues [10]. Indeed, LPS binding has been demonstrated for the limulus ALF sequence, which shares a common ancestor with all shrimp ALFs. Taking into account previous studies [9–11,17] and the present results, shrimp ALFs have proved to display a diverse spectrum of antimicrobial activity. While some members exhibited a broad range of antimicrobial activity (Groups B and G), some others displayed limited (Groups A, C and E) or very weak action (Groups D and F). One possible explanation is that the effectiveness of the antimicrobial activity of each ALF group is directly proportional to the amount of positively charged amino acids in its central β-hairpin structure [26]. However, we showed that the highly cationic central β-hairpin structure of *Litvan* ALF-F$_{19-54}$ (p*I* = 9.24) was not active against the microorganisms tested in this study. Likewise, synthetic β-hairpins of the *Fc*ALF1 (Group F) from *F. chinensis* was also poorly active against both Gram-positive and Gram-negative bacteria [17]. Thus, besides their overall net charge, other features may interfere directly on their biological activities. Given these results, the determination of the amino acid residues involved in the interaction with other microbial surface molecules (peptidoglycan, lipoteichoic acid, β-glucans, etc.) may provide valuable information of the mechanism of action of ALFs against other microorganisms beyond Gram-negative bacteria [7].

4. Materials and Methods

4.1. Database Searches and Phylogenetic Reconstructions

ALF sequences were methodically collected from publicly accessible databases and used for the search of homologous sequences in both annotated and non-annotated databases. Only full-length coding sequences were considered. Homology searches were performed using tBLASTx at NCBI. Exon-intron boundaries were defined by alignment of the cDNA and genomic sequences. All nucleotide sequences were manually inspected and analyzed using open-access bioinformatics tools. Three-dimensional models for *L. vannamei* ALFs were built with SWISS-MODEL (https://swissmodel.expasy.org/) using ALF*Pm*3 NMR resolution (PDB: 2JOB1) as a template. Deduced amino acid sequences were aligned using MAFFT multiple alignment program (https://mafft.cbrc.jp/alignment/server/). Bayesian phylogenetic analysis was conducted in MrBayes 3.1.2 (http://mrbayes.sourceforge.net/), using WAG + G as substitution model, with two runs of 10^7 generations, sample rate of 1000 and burn-in of 25%. Neighbor-joining analysis was conducted in MEGA X [27]. Bootstrap sampling was reiterated 1000 times using a 50% bootstrap cutoff. Trees were drawn using FigTree v1.4.2 (http://tree.bio.ed.ac.uk/software/figtree/).

4.2. Animals and Tissue Collection

Litopenaeus vannamei juveniles (10 ± 2 g) and at different development stages were obtained from the Laboratory of Marine Shrimp (Federal University of Santa Catarina, Florianópolis, Brazil). Each developmental stage was identified microscopically and collected as previously described [16] while juveniles were acclimated in controlled conditions for at least one week before any experimentation. Hemolymph was collected from the ventral sinus into a precooled modified Alsever solution (27 mM sodium citrate, 336 mM NaCl, 115 mM glucose, 9 mM EDTA, pH 7.0) and hemocytes were isolated by centrifugation. After hemolymph collection, the following tissues were harvested by dissection: foregut, hepatopancreas, midgut, hindgut, muscle, gills and nerve cord. Tissues were rinsed in Tris-saline solution (10 mM Tris, 330 mM NaCl, pH 7.4), homogenized in TRIzol reagent (Thermo Scientific, Asheville, NC, USA) and processed for semiquantitative RT-PCR analysis.

4.3. Experimental Infections

Two unrelated shrimp pathogens were chosen for experimental infections, the Gram-negative *Vibrio harveyi* and the White spot syndrome virus (WSSV). For the bacterial infection, 6 × 10^7 CFU/animal of *V. harveyi* ATCC 14126 under 100 µL sterile seawater (SSW) or 100 µL SSW (injury control) were injected. For the viral infection, shrimp were injected with 100 µL of a WSSV inoculum containing 3 × 10^2 viral particles. The WSSV inoculum was prepared from muscle tissues of WSSV-infected shrimp as previously described [14]. Animals injected with 100 µL of a tissue homogenate prepared from WSSV-free shrimp were used as injury control for the viral infection. At 48 h post-infections, hemocytes were collected, pooled (three pools of five animals per condition) and processed for gene expression analysis. Naïve (non-stimulated) animals were used as a control for all experimental conditions.

4.4. Semiquantitative RT-PCR Analysis for Tissue Distribution of Gene Expression

Total RNA was extracted using TRIzol reagent (Thermo Scientific, Asheville, NC, USA) according to the manufacturer's protocol. RNA samples were treated with DNase I (Thermo Scientific) at 37 °C for 15 min and precipitated with 0.3 M sodium acetate (pH 5.2) and isopropanol (1:1; *v:v*). RNA amount and quality were assessed by spectrophotometric analysis and the integrity of total RNA was analyzed by 0.8% agarose gel electrophoresis. First strand cDNA was synthesized from 1 μg of total RNA using the RevertAid Reverse Transcription kit (Thermo Scientific, Asheville, NC, USA) and oligo(dT)$_{12\text{-}18}$ primers. PCR reactions were carried out in a 15-μL reaction volume containing 1 μL cDNA, 2 mM MgCl$_2$, 0.4 mM dNTP Mix, 0.4 μM of each primer (Table 1) and 1 U Taq DNA Polymerase (Sinapse, São Paulo, SP, Brazil). PCR conditions were as follows: 1 cycle of denaturation at 95 °C for 10 min followed by 30–35 cycles of 95 °C for 30 s, 60 °C for 30 s and 72 °C for 30 s. PCR products were analyzed by electrophoresis (1.5% agarose gel) and stained by ethidium bromide. The expression of the *Lv*Actin gene was used as endogenous control.

Table 1. Nucleotide sequences of primers used in this study.

Gene	Forward Primer (5′-3′)	Reverse Primer (5′-3′)	Amplicon
*Lv*Actin [1]	TAATCCACATCTGCTGGAAGGTGG	TCACCAACTGGGATGACATGG	846 bp
*Lv*Actin [2]	CCACGAGACCACCTACAAC	AGCGAGGGCAGTGATTTC	142 bp
*Lv*EF1α [2]	TGGCTGTGAACAAGATGGACA	TTGTAGCCCACCTTCTTGACG	103 bp
*Lv*L40 [2]	GAGAATGTGAAGGCCAAGATC	TCAGAGAGAGTGCGACCATC	104 bp
*Lv*RpS6 [2]	AGCAGATACCCTTGGTGAAG	GATGCAACCACGGACTGAC	193 bp
Litvan ALF-A [1,2]	CTGATTGCTCTTGTGCCACG	TGACCCATGAACTCCACCTC	113 bp
Litvan ALF-B [1,2]	GTGTCTCCGTGTTGACAAGC	ACAGCCCAACGATCTTGCTG	123 bp
Litvan ALF-C [1,2]	ATGCGAGTGTCTCGTCCTCAG	TGAGTTTGTTCGCGATGGCC	115 bp
Litvan ALF-D [1,2]	TGTGTTGGTTGTGGCACTGG	CAACGAGGTCAATGTCACCG	131 bp
Litvan ALF-E [1,2]	TGCTACGTGAATCGCAGTCC	CGCTTCCTCTTCCGACAATG	100 bp
Litvan ALF-F [1,2]	AAGCTCTCATTCCTGGTCGG	GGGTGTAACGAAGTACGTGC	180 bp
Litvan ALF-G [1,2]	CCGCTGCATGTCAAGTATCC	TCAGCAGTAGCAGTGTCAGC	140 bp

[1] Primers for semiquantitative analysis of gene expression (RT-PCR); [2] Primers for quantitative analysis of gene expression (RT-qPCR).

4.5. Fluorescence-Based Reverse Transcription Real-Time Quantitative PCR (RT-qPCR)

RT-qPCR amplifications were performed in a final volume of 15 μL containing 0.3 μM of each primer (Table 1), 7.5 μL of reaction mix (Maxima SYBR Green/ROX qPCR Master Mix 2×; Thermo Scientific, Asheville, NC, USA) and 1 μL of cDNA. The RT-qPCR program was 95 °C for 10 min, followed by 40 cycles of 95 °C for 15 s and 60 °C for 1 min. Melt curve analysis was performed to evaluate primer specificity. The eukaryotic translation elongation factor 1-alpha (*Lv*EF1α) and the ribosomal protein *Lv*L40 were used as reference genes of expression data in hemocytes. Relative transcript levels were determined by the comparative standard curve method using a standard curve derived from 2-fold dilution series of a cDNA pool of all samples. Differences we considered significant at $p < 0.05$ (one-way ANOVA and Tukey's multiple comparison test). Gene expression of ALFs during shrimp development was assessed in twelve developmental stages as previously described [16].

4.6. Peptide Synthesis, Oxidation and Characterization

Synthetic peptides based on the central β-hairpin of ALF-E (*Litvan* ALF-E$_{32\text{-}53}$: GCYVNRSPYLKKFEVHYRADVKCG), ALF-F (*Litvan* ALF-F$_{30\text{-}51}$: GCTYFVTPKVKSFELYFKGRMTCG) and ALF-G (*Litvan* ALF-G$_{34\text{-}55}$: GCSYSTRPYFLRWRLKFKSKVWCG) were obtained in a Liberty Blue automated microwave peptide synthesizer (CEM Corp, Matthews, NC, USA) using Fmoc-protected amino acids (Iris Biotech GmBH (Marktredwitz, Germany) and Rink Amide AM resin (loading: 0.6 meq/g). Fmoc deprotection was carried out with 20% *v/v* piperidine in DMF, couplings were performed with DIC/OxymaPure activation (1/1 eq) and additional couplings with TBTU/DIEA/OxymaPure activation (1/2/1 eq). Peptides were cleaved with TFA/TIS/DOT/H$_2$0

(92.5/2.5/2.5/2.5) [trifluoroacetic acid/triisopropylsilane/2,2-(ethylenedioxy)-diethanethiol/ultrapure water] and purified by RP-HPLC (JASCO Corp., Tokyo, Japan) on a XBridge™ BEH C18 column (100 × 4.6 mm, 3.5 μm) (Waters Corp., Milford, MA, USA) with a 0–70% acetonitrile-water mixture gradient over 30 min at a flow rate of 1 mL/min. Peptides were further lyophilized and analyzed by MALDI-TOF mass spectrometry in a LCMS-2020 ESI-MS (Shimadzu Corp., Kyoto, Japan) to confirm their molecular masses.

Then, peptides were oxidized as previously reported [28]. In brief, 5 mg of the crude peptide were first reduced with 10% β-mercaptoethanol (95 °C for 5 min) then dissolved in 50% (v/v) AcOH/H$_2$O and later diluted in 32 mL of oxidation buffer (2 mM guanidinium chloride, 10% isopropyl alcohol and 10% dimethyl sulfoxide). The pH was adjusted to 5.8 with ammonium hydroxide. The peptide solution was subjected to air oxidation at room temperature for 18 h. The peptide solution was then acidified to pH 2.5 and purified using a SPE C18 (Waters Corp., Milford, MA, USA). The peptides were eluted with 5%, 20%, 40%, 60% and 80% acetonitrile in 0.05% TFA ultrapure water at a flow rate of 1 mL/min. The fractions were collected, and the acetonitrile was evaporated on a Savant SPD 1010 SpeedVac Concentrator (Thermo Scientific, Asheville, NC, USA). The fractions were analyzed by MALDI-TOF mass spectrometry.

4.7. Antibacterial and Antifungal Assays

The antimicrobial activity of synthetic peptides was assayed against the Gram-positive bacteria *Bacillus cereus* ATCC 11778, *Bacillus subtilis* ATCC 6633, *Brevibacterium stationis* CIP 101282, *Microbacterium maritypicum* CIP 105733, *Micrococcus luteus* CIP 5345 and *Staphylococcus aureus* ATCC 25932, the Gram-negative bacteria *Aeromonas salmonicida* ATCC 33658, *Escherichia coli* SBS363, *Pseudomonas aeruginosa* ATCC 9027, *Vibrio alginolyticus* ATCC 17749, *Vibrio anguillarum* ATCC 19264, *Vibrio harveyi* ATCC 14126 and *Vibrio nigripulchritudo* CIP103195, the yeast *Candida albicans* MDM8 and the filamentous fungus *Fusarium oxysporum*.

Minimum inhibitory concentrations (MICs) were determined in duplicate by the liquid growth inhibition assay, as previously described [29]. MIC values are expressed as the lowest concentration tested that causes 100% growth inhibition. Poor Broth (PB: 1% peptone, 1% NaCl, pH 7.2) was used for standard bacteria, while PB supplemented with 0.5 M NaCl (PB–NaCl) was used as a culture medium for *Vibrio* strains. For *B. stationis* and *M. maritypicum* cultures, PB–NaCl medium was supplemented with 20 mM KCl, 5 mM MgSO$_4$ and 1.5 mM CaCl$_2$. Potato dextrose broth (Kasvi, São José dos Pinhais, PR, Brazil) at half strength was used for cultures of *F. oxysporum* while Sabouraud medium (1% peptone, 4% glucose, pH 5.6) was used for yeast cultures. The growth of bacteria and yeast was monitored spectrophotometrically ($\lambda = 595$ nm), while *F. oxysporum* hyphae formation was observed in an inverted microscope. After MIC determination, bacterial cultures were plated in nutrient agar for 24–48 h for the determination of the bactericidal activity of the synthetic peptides.

5. Conclusions

In conclusion, the combination of our molecular, transcriptional and functional data revealed that ALFs comprise the most diverse AMP family found in penaeid shrimp. We showed that they are composed of seven members encoded by different genes that follow a diverse pattern of expression. Our results also strongly suggest that the expansion and diversification of shrimp ALFs have shaped novel functions for this AMP family beyond their primary antibacterial properties. Thus, ALFs represent an attractive model to explore the impacts of the molecular diversity of immune-related genes on host-microbe interactions. Finally, ALFs possess the broadest spectrum of antimicrobial activity when compared to other shrimp AMPs. These bioactive peptides undoubtedly show biotechnological potential for the development of novel antibiotics derived from AMPs, as well as for the development of selective breeding programs.

Supplementary Materials: The following are available online at http://www.mdpi.com/1660-3397/16/10/381/s1. Table S1: Sequences and biochemical properties of ALFs from decapod crustaceans and marine chelicerates. Figure S1: Amino acid sequence alignments of ALF-related sequences containing three and four cysteine residues. The predicted signal peptides are in bold and underlined. Asterisks (*) mark the identical amino acid residues while the cysteines are highlighted with a black background. GenBank accession numbers are indicated in brackets.

Author Contributions: Conceptualization, R.D.R., D.D.-G. and L.M.P.; Formal analysis, G.M.M., P.S., C.B., N.D.F., G.T.-S., F.G., D.D.-G., L.M.P. and R.D.R.; Funding acquisition, R.D.R., L.M.P. and P.S.; Investigation, P.S. and R.D.R.; Methodology, G.M.M., P.S., C.B., N.D.F., G.T.-S. and F.G.; Project administration, G.M.M. and R.D.R.; Validation, G.T.-S.; Writing—original draft, G.M.M. and R.D.R.; Writing—review & editing, P.S., G.T.-S., D.D.-G. and L.M.P. All authors commented on the manuscript and discussed the data and implications.

Funding: This research was supported by the Brazilian funding agencies CNPq (MEC/MCTI/CAPES/CNPq/FAPs PVE 401191/2014-1 and MCTI/CNPq Universal 406530/2016-5) and CAPES (CIMAR 1974/2014). P.S. was funded by FONDECYT grant 11150009. G.M.M. and N.D.F. were supported by scholarships provided by FAPESC and C.B. received a scholarship provided by CAPES.

Acknowledgments: The authors are grateful to the Laboratory of Marine Shrimp (Federal University of Santa Catarina, Florianópolis, Brazil) for providing the shrimp used in this study and to Pedro Ismael da Silva Jr. (Butantan Institute, São Paulo, Brazil) for the culture of *Candida albicans* MDM8. We are also in debt to Juan Eberhard for English correction and editing.

Conflicts of Interest: The authors declare no conflict of interest. The funders had no role in the design of the study; in the collection, analyses, or interpretation of data; in the writing of the manuscript, and in the decision to publish the results.

References

1. Tanaka, S.; Nakamura, T.; Morita, T.; Iwanaga, S. Limulus anti-LPS factor: an anticoagulant which inhibits the endotoxin-mediated activation of Limulus coagulation system. *Biochem. Biophys. Res. Commun.* **1982**, *105*, 717–723. [CrossRef]

2. Morita, T.; Ohtsubo, S.; Nakamura, T.; Tanaka, S.; Iwanaga, S.; Ohashi, K.; Niwa, M. Isolation and biological activities of limulus anticoagulant (anti-LPS factor) which interacts with lipopolysaccharide (LPS). *J. Biochem.* **1985**, *97*, 1611–1620. [CrossRef] [PubMed]

3. Gross, P.S.; Bartlett, T.C.; Browdy, C.L.; Chapman, R.W.; Warr, G.W. Immune gene discovery by expressed sequence tag analysis of hemocytes and hepatopancreas in the Pacific White Shrimp, *Litopenaeus vannamei*, and the Atlantic White Shrimp, *L. setiferus*. *Dev. Comp. Immunol.* **2001**, *25*, 565–577. [CrossRef]

4. Supungul, P.; Klinbunga, S.; Pichyangkura, R.; Jitrapakdee, S.; Hirono, I.; Aoki, T.; Tassanakajon, A. Identification of immune-related genes in hemocytes of black tiger shrimp (*Penaeus monodon*). *Mar. Biotechnol.* **2002**, *4*, 487–494. [CrossRef] [PubMed]

5. Tassanakajon, A.; Rimphanitchayakit, V.; Visetnan, S.; Amparyup, P.; Somboonwiwat, K.; Charoensapsri, W.; Tang, S. Shrimp humoral responses against pathogens: antimicrobial peptides and melanization. *Dev. Comp. Immunol.* **2018**, *80*, 81–93. [CrossRef] [PubMed]

6. Yang, Y.; Boze, H.; Chemardin, P.; Padilla, A.; Moulin, G.; Tassanakajon, A.; Pugniere, M.; Roquet, F.; Destoumieux-Garzón, D.; Gueguen, Y.; et al. NMR structure of *r*ALF-*Pm*3, an anti-lipopolysaccharide factor from shrimp: Model of the possible lipid A-binding site. *Biopolymers* **2008**, *91*, 207–220. [CrossRef] [PubMed]

7. Schmitt, P.; Rosa, R.D.; Destoumieux-Garzón, D. An intimate link between antimicrobial peptide sequence diversity and binding to essential components of bacterial membranes. *Biochim. Biophys. Acta Biomembr.* **2016**, *1858*, 958–970. [CrossRef] [PubMed]

8. Destoumieux-Garzón, D.; Rosa, R.D.; Schmitt, P.; Barreto, C.; Vidal-Dupiol, J.; Mitta, G.; Gueguen, Y.; Bachère, E. Antimicrobial peptides in marine invertebrate health and disease. *Philos. Trans. R. Soc. B Biol. Sci.* **2016**, *371*, 20150300. [CrossRef] [PubMed]

9. Somboonwiwat, K.; Marcos, M.; Tassanakajon, A.; Romestand, B.; Gueguen, Y. Recombinant expression and anti-microbial activity of anti-lipopolysaccharide factor (ALF) from the black tiger shrimp *Penaeus monodon*. *Dev. Comp. Immunol.* **2005**, *29*, 841–851. [CrossRef] [PubMed]

10. Rosa, R.D.; Vergnes, A.A.; de Lorgeril, J.; Goncalves, P.; Perazzolo, L.M.; Sauné, L.; Romestand, B.; Fievet, J.; Gueguen, Y.; Bachère, E.; et al. Functional divergence in shrimp anti-lipopolysaccharide factors (ALFs): from recognition of cell wall components to antimicrobial activity. *PLoS ONE* **2013**, *8*, e67937. [CrossRef] [PubMed]

11. Jiang, H.-S.; Zhang, Q.; Zhao, Y.-R.; Jia, W.-M.; Zhao, X.-F.; Wang, J.-X. A new group of anti-lipopolysaccharide factors from Marsupenaeus japonicus functions in antibacterial response. *Dev. Comp. Immunol.* **2015**, *48*, 33–42. [CrossRef] [PubMed]

12. Rosa, R.D.; Barracco, M.A. Antimicrobial peptides in crustaceans. *Invertebr. Surviv. J.* **2010**, *7*, 262–284.

13. Pilotto, M.; Goncalves, A.; Vieira, F.; Seifert, W.; Bachère, E.; Rosa, R.; Perazzolo, L. Exploring the Impact of the Biofloc Rearing System and an Oral WSSV Challenge on the Intestinal Bacteriome of *Litopenaeus vannamei*. *Microorganisms* **2018**, *6*, 83. [CrossRef] [PubMed]

14. Goncalves, P.; Guertler, C.; Bachère, E.; de Souza, C.R.B.; Rosa, R.D.; Perazzolo, L.M. Molecular signatures at imminent death: hemocyte gene expression profiling of shrimp succumbing to viral and fungal infections. *Dev. Comp. Immunol.* **2014**, *42*, 294–301. [CrossRef] [PubMed]

15. Silveira, A.S.; Matos, G.M.; Falchetti, M.; Ribeiro, F.S.; Bressan, A.; Bachère, E.; Perazzolo, L.M.; Rosa, R.D. An immune-related gene expression atlas of the shrimp digestive system in response to two major pathogens brings insights into the involvement of hemocytes in gut immunity. *Dev. Comp. Immunol.* **2018**, *79*, 44–50. [CrossRef] [PubMed]

16. Quispe, R.L.; Justino, E.B.; Vieira, F.N.; Jaramillo, M.L.; Rosa, R.D.; Perazzolo, L.M. Transcriptional profiling of immune-related genes in Pacific white shrimp (*Litopenaeus vannamei*) during ontogenesis. *Fish Shellfish Immunol.* **2016**, *58*, 103–107. [CrossRef] [PubMed]

17. Li, S.; Guo, S.; Li, F.; Xiang, J. Functional Diversity of Anti-Lipopolysaccharide Factor Isoforms in Shrimp and Their Characters Related to Antiviral Activity. *Mar. Drugs* **2015**, *13*, 2602–2616. [CrossRef] [PubMed]

18. Ponprateep, S.; Tharntada, S.; Somboonwiwat, K.; Tassanakajon, A. Gene silencing reveals a crucial role for anti-lipopolysaccharide factors from Penaeus monodon in the protection against microbial infections. *Fish Shellfish Immunol.* **2012**, *32*, 26–34. [CrossRef] [PubMed]

19. Soonthornchai, W.; Chaiyapechara, S.; Klinbunga, S.; Thongda, W.; Tangphatsornruang, S.; Yoocha, T.; Jarayabhand, P.; Jiravanichpaisal, P. Differentially expressed transcripts in stomach of Penaeus monodon in response to AHPND infection. *Dev. Comp. Immunol.* **2016**, *65*, 53–63. [CrossRef] [PubMed]

20. Destoumieux, D.; Muñoz, M.; Cosseau, C.; Rodriguez, J.; Bulet, P.; Comps, M.; Bachère, E. Penaeidins, antimicrobial peptides with chitin-binding activity, are produced and stored in shrimp granulocytes and released after microbial challenge. *J. Cell Sci.* **2000**, *113*, 461–469. [CrossRef] [PubMed]

21. Muñoz, M.; Vandenbulcke, F.; Gueguen, Y.; Bachère, E. Expression of penaeidin antimicrobial peptides in early larval stages of the shrimp *Penaeus vannamei*. *Dev. Comp. Immunol.* **2003**, *27*, 283–289. [CrossRef]

22. Barreto, C.; Coelho, J.R.; Yuan, J.; Xiang, J.; Perazzolo, L.M.; Rosa, R.D. Specific Molecular Signatures for Type II Crustins in Penaeid Shrimp Uncovered by the Identification of Crustin-Like Antimicrobial Peptides in *Litopenaeus vannamei*. *Mar. Drugs* **2018**, *16*, 31. [CrossRef] [PubMed]

23. Somboonwiwat, K.; Bachère, E.; Rimphanitchayakit, V.; Tassanakajon, A. Localization of anti-lipopolysaccharide factor (ALFPm3) in tissues of the black tiger shrimp, *Penaeus monodon*, and characterization of its binding properties. *Dev. Comp. Immunol.* **2008**, *32*, 1170–1176. [CrossRef] [PubMed]

24. De la Vega, E.; O'Leary, N.; Shockey, J.E.; Robalino, J.; Payne, C.; Browdy, C.L.; Warr, G.W.; Gross, P.S.; O'Leary, N.A.; Shockey, J.E.; et al. Anti-lipopolysaccharide factor in *Litopenaeus vannamei* (*Lv*ALF): A broad spectrum antimicrobial peptide essential for shrimp immunity against bacterial and fungal infection. *Mol. Immunol.* **2008**, *45*, 1916–1925. [CrossRef] [PubMed]

25. Wang, X.W.; Xu, J.D.; Zhao, X.F.; Vasta, G.R.; Wang, J.X. A shrimp C-type lectin inhibits proliferation of the hemolymph microbiota by maintaining the expression of antimicrobial peptides. *J. Biol. Chem.* **2014**, *289*, 11779–11790. [CrossRef] [PubMed]

26. Tassanakajon, A.; Somboonwiwat, K.; Amparyup, P. Sequence diversity and evolution of antimicrobial peptides in invertebrates. *Dev. Comp. Immunol.* **2015**, *48*, 324–341. [CrossRef] [PubMed]

27. Kumar, S.; Stecher, G.; Li, M.; Knyaz, C.; Tamura, K. MEGA X: Molecular Evolutionary Genetics Analysis across Computing Platforms. *Mol. Biol. Evol.* **2018**, *35*, 1547–1549. [CrossRef] [PubMed]

28. Alvarez, C.A.; Guzmán, F.; Cárdenas, C.; Marshall, S.H.; Mercado, L. Antimicrobial activity of trout hepcidin. *Fish Shellfish Immunol.* **2014**, *41*, 93–101. [CrossRef] [PubMed]

29. Hetru, C.; Bulet, P. Strategies for the Isolation and Characterization of Antimicrobial Peptides of Invertebrates. *Methods Mol. Biol.* **1997**, *78*, 35–49. [CrossRef] [PubMed]

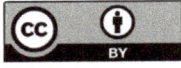

marine drugs

MDPI

Article

In Vitro Vascular-Protective Effects of a Tilapia By-Product Oligopeptide on Angiotensin II-Induced Hypertensive Endothelial Injury in HUVEC by Nrf2/NF-κB Pathways

Jiali Chen [1], Fang Gong [1], Mei-Fang Chen [1], Chengyong Li [2,3], Pengzhi Hong [1], Shengli Sun [2], Chunxia Zhou [1,*] and Zhong-Ji Qian [2,3,*]

[1]   College of Food Science and Technology, Guangdong Ocean University, Zhanjiang 524088, China
[2]   School of Chemistry and Environmental Science, Guangdong Ocean University, Zhanjiang 524088, China
[3]   Shenzhen Institute of Guangdong Ocean University, Shenzhen 518108, China
*   Correspondence: chunxia.zhou@163.com (C.Z.); zjqian78@163.com (Z.-J.Q.);
      Tel.: +86-13828262885 (C.Z.); +86-186-07596590 (Z.-J.Q.)

Received: 3 June 2019; Accepted: 22 July 2019; Published: 23 July 2019

Abstract: Angiotensin II (Ang II) is closely involved in endothelial injury during the development of hypertension. In this study, the protective effects of the tilapia by-product oligopeptide Leu-Ser-Gly-Tyr-Gly-Pro (LSGYGP) on oxidative stress and endothelial injury in Angiotensin II (Ang II)-stimulated human umbilical vein endothelial cells (HUVEC) were evaluated. LSGYGP dose-dependently suppressed the fluorescence intensities of nitric oxide (NO) and reactive oxygen species (ROS), inhibited the nuclear factor-kappa B (NF-κB) pathway, and reduced inducible nitric oxide synthase (iNOS), cyclooxygenase-2 (COX-2), and endothelin-1 (ET-1) expression, as shown by western blot. In addition, it attenuated the expression of gamma-glutamyltransferase (GGT) and heme oxygenase 1 (HO-1), as well as increasing superoxide dismutase (SOD) and glutathione (GSH) expression through the nuclear factor erythroid 2-related factor 2 (Nrf2) pathway. Other experiments revealed that LSGYGP increased the apoptotic inhibition ratio between cleaved-caspase-3/procaspase-3, reduced expressions of pro-apoptotic ratio between Bcl-2/Bax, inhibited phosphorylation of mitogen-activated protein kinases (MAPK), and increased phosphorylation of the serine/threonine kinase (Akt) pathway. Furthermore, LSGYGP significantly decreased Ang II-induced DNA damage in a comet assay, and molecular docking results showed that the steady interaction between LSGYGP with NF-κB may be attributed to hydrogen bonds. These results suggest that this oligopeptide is effective in protecting against Ang II-induced HUVEC injury through the reduction of oxidative stress and alleviating endothelial damage. Thus, it has the potential for the therapeutic treatment of hypertension-associated diseases.

Keywords: tilapia; HUVEC; angiotensin II; NF-κB; Nrf2; endothelial dysfunction

1. Introduction

Endothelial dysfunction is regarded as a predictor of cardiovascular diseases (CVD) and long-term clinical outcomes, such as heart disease, arteriosclerosis, stroke, kidney disease, and hypertension. Hypertension is a CVD which results in high death rates; however, its pathogenesis and precise mechanism, at present, remain unknown. There is a common perception that hypertension is connected with vascular endothelial dysfunction caused by inflammation cytokines and oxidative stress in vascular endothelial cells [1,2]. Research has shown that inflammatory stimulation in endothelial cells could be induced by the extracellular stimulators angiotensin II (Ang II) [3], tumor necrosis factor-alpha (TNF-α) [4], and lipopolysaccharide (LPS) [5] which may cause further vascular endothelial dysfunction.

Ang II is a crucial active peptide produced in the renin–angiotensin system (RAS), which is responsible for regulating downstream cellular factors and physiological responses and, also, directly induces vascular injury through activating inflammation and oxidative stress [6]. Moreover, it has a dominant position in the phase of vascular normal physiology and disease taking part in endothelial damage [7]. It has been reported that other vascular dysfunction-related factors, such as reactive oxygen species (ROS), vasoconstrictor endothelin-1 (ET-1), and nitric oxide (NO), are induced by Ang II [8–10].

ROS is a vital bio-molecular factor, relevantly connected with the damage of endothelial cells and endothelial dysfunction, which participate in the development of CVDs [11]. It promotes the expression levels of anti-oxidant enzymes and inflammatory cytokines, including gamma-glutamyltransferase (GGT), glutathione (GSH), nitric oxide synthase (iNOS), superoxide dismutase (SOD), and cyclooxygenase-2 (COX-2) [12,13], resulting in the activation of the nuclear factor-kappa B (NF-κB) pathway, further activating oxidative stress by the downstream nuclear erythroid 2-related factor 2 (Nrf2) pathway [14,15]. Among these, the Nrf2 pathway, as a key controller of the redox homeostasis gene regulatory network [16], has been shown to be the most critical pathway against oxidative stress [17]. Heme oxygenase 1 (HO-1) functions as a downstream effector of the Nrf2 pathway and as vital antioxidant enzymes to suppress oxidative stress [18]. Moreover, under induction of oxidative stress and nitric oxide, it is mainly regulated by the activation of Nrf-2 and MAPK/ERK pathways in vascular and endothelial cells [19]. Furthermore, oxidative stress and inflammation induced by Ang II causes endothelial damage and even cell death [7], which is relevant to classic apoptotic pathways, including the Bcl-2 family (anti-apoptotic protein Bcl-2 and pro-apoptotic protein Bax) and the serine/threonine kinase (Akt) pathway [20].

Recently, some studies have reported natural compounds which suppress Ang II-induced hypertensive injury [3,6,21,22]; however, little is known about marine fish resources. A review [23] summarized that marine resources broaden chemical space to be explored in the pharmaceutical market. Especially with bioactive peptide, they linked antibody drugs and small molecules due to the advantage that peptides possess the properties of antibodies and small molecules. Tilapia (*Oreochromis niloticus*) plays an important role in aquaculture, expansion of its production in Asia and Africa has increased, which is partially attributable to the high protein content. It's reported that during the process of tilapia filleting, other parts of the fish are wasted, for example, the frame and skin5 may contain approximately 80% protein content, but are underutilized [24]. Gelatin peptides have been widely used in food, cosmetics, and biomedical industries, due to their low molecular weight, high absorption rate, and bioavailability, as well as their antioxidant and anti-hypertensive functional and biological properties [25]. The oligopeptide Leu-Ser-Gly-Tyr-Gly-Pro (LSGYGP) has been purified completely from tilapia skin gelatin hydrolysates, with molecular weight 592.26 Da [26]. According to former studies, this oligopeptide has good antioxidant and anti-photoaging activities [27], but, to our knowledge, the other activities of LSGYGP have not been reported. This study is aimed to investigate whether it is able to protect against cardiovascular injury.

Endothelial cells are directly correlated prominent cells in CVD and, so, it is a good strategy to prevent cardiovascular diseases by inhibiting the stimulation of activated endothelial cells in order to improve excessive inflammatory response in diseases. Therefore, this study focuses on the cytoprotective effects of LSGYGP on Ang II-induced human umbilical vein endothelial cells (HUVEC) injury and the underlying mechanisms, including cytokine expressions of the Nrf2, NF-κB, MAPK, and Akt pathways.

2. Results

2.1. Cytoprotective Effect of LSGYGP on Ang II-Stimulated HUVEC

The cytotoxic concentration (10, 20, 50, and 100 μM) of LSGYGP (Figure 1a) and the evaluation of the protective effects of LSGYGP in Ang II-stimulated HUVEC were determined using an MTT assay. As shown in Figure 1b, at the concentrations tested (10–100 μM), LSGYGP did not affect cell viability, and LSGYGP treatment showed a cytoprotective effect on Ang II-stimulated HUVEC in a dose-dependent manner (Figure 1c).

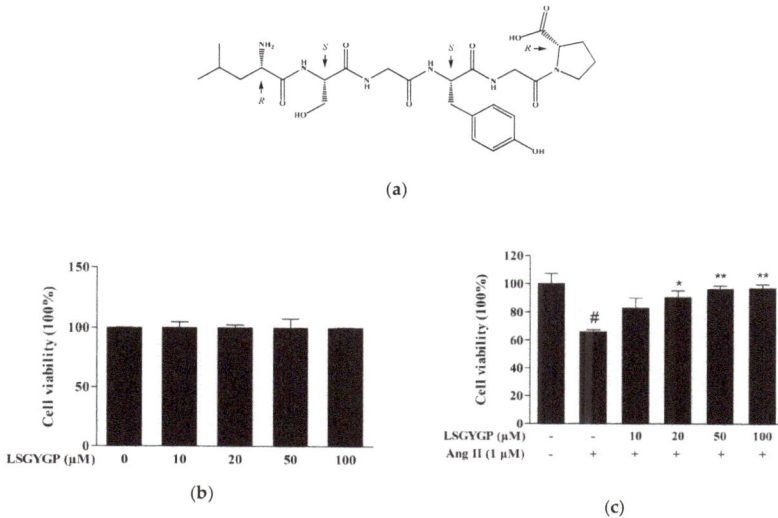

(a)

(b)

(c)

Figure 1. (a) Structure of Leu-Ser-Gly-Tyr-Gly-Pro (LSGYGP). Effect of LSGYGP on the viability of human umbilical vein endothelial cells (HUVEC). (b) and protective effect of LSGYGP on the viability of Ang II-treated HUVEC. (c) Cells were exposed to varying concentrations (10, 20, 50, and 100 µM) of LSGYGP and the cell viability was assessed by MTT assay. # $p < 0.001$, compared with blank group (untreated cells); * $p < 0.05$, ** $p < 0.01$, compared with control group (Ang II-treated cells).

2.2. LSGYGP against NO and ROS Production

As Figure 2a shows, the Ang II group had an obvious effect on NO and ROS levels, as compared to the untreated control. Remarkably, 10 µM treatment with LSGYGP decreased the Ang II-induced increase in NO and ROS generation. LSGYGP significantly attenuates NO and ROS production in a dose-dependent manner.

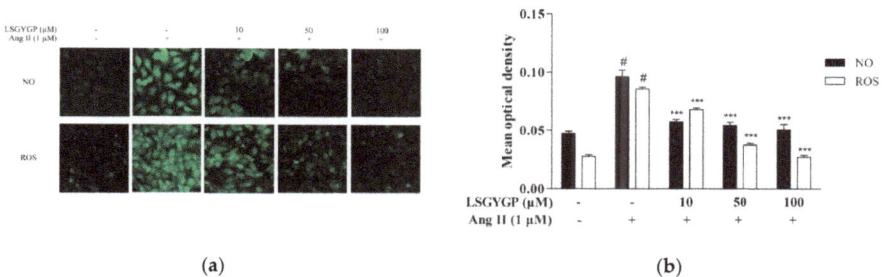

(a)

(b)

Figure 2. (a) Representative 3-amino,4-aminomethyl-2′,7′-difluorescein diacetate (DAF-FM DA) fluorescent images and 2,7-dichlorodihydrofluorescein diacetate (DCFH-DA) fluorescent images of LSGYGP in HUVEC. Mean optical density analysis of cellular DAF-FM DA staining (green fluorescence; an indicator of production of NO) and mean optical density analysis of cellular DCFH-DA staining (green fluorescence; an indicator of production of ROS). (b) Mean optical density analysis of fluorescent images. # $p < 0.001$, compared with blank group (untreated cells); *** $p < 0.001$, compared with control group (Ang II-treated cells).

2.3. Effect of LSGYGP on the Nrf2 Pathway

Nrf2 is a major signaling pathway in oxidative stress reactions. As shown in Figure 3, reduction of SOD, GSH, Nrf2, and HO-1 proteins were discovered in the Ang II-induced HUVEC treatment group; however, a significant restoration was shown when treated with LSGYGP. Compared to the untreated control, Ang II treatment resulted in a significant augmentation of GGT. However, treatment with 50 μM LSGYGP diminished the Ang II-induced increase in GGT expression level. These findings indicate that LSGYGP increased antioxidant enzymes and inhibited the Nrf2 pathway.

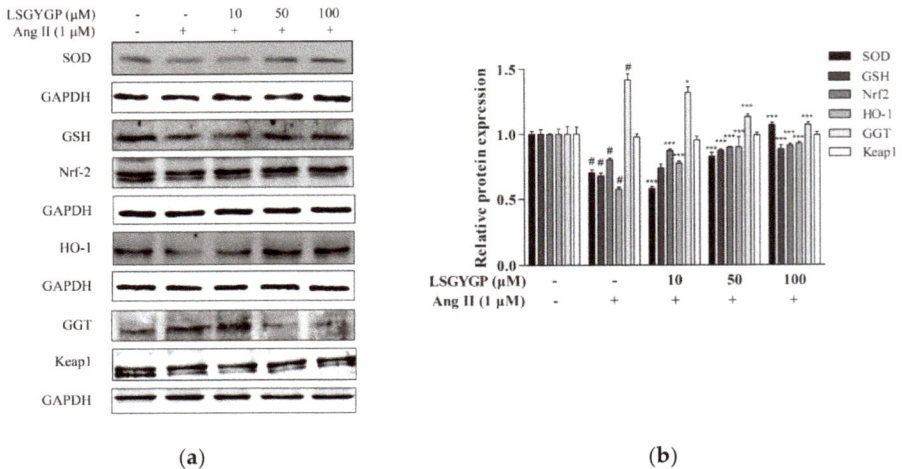

Figure 3. Effects of LSGYGP on the expression of superoxide dismutase (SOD), gamma-glutamyltransferase (GGT), glutathione (GSH), and nuclear erythroid 2-related factor 2 (Nrf2) pathway in HUVEC (**a**,**b**). Protein expression was by western blot, glyceraldehyde-3-phosphate dehydrogenase (GAPDH) was as control. [#] $p < 0.001$, compared with blank group (untreated cells); [*] $p < 0.05$, [***] $p < 0.001$, compared with control group (Ang II-treated cells).

2.4. Effect of LSGYGP on MAPK Pathway

Western blot was used to detect phosphorylation of JNK, ERK, and p38. Moreover, Ang II markedly increased protein expression of phosphorylated p38, JNK, and ERK, as compared to the non-Ang II-treated control. However, the above changes were both markedly reversed by 100 μM treatment with LSGYGP (Figure 4b). The above results indicate that, while Ang II markedly activates endothelial oxidative stress, LSGYGP treatment may attenuate this oxidative damage through MAPK pathways.

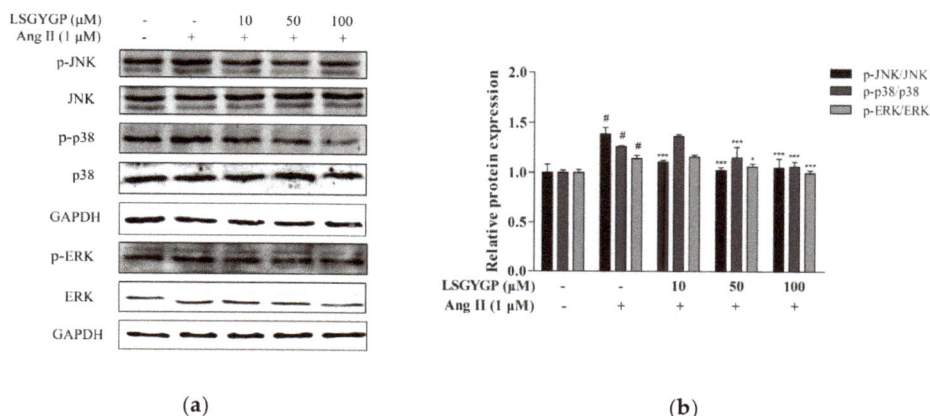

(a)   (b)

Figure 4. (a) HUVEC were exposed to different concentrations (10, 50, and 100 μM) of LSGYGP with 1 μM Ang II to stimulated mitogen-activated protein kinases (MAPK) phosphorylation in cells. (b) Equal amounts of protein were loaded in each lane. # indicate significantly compared with untreated cells; [#] $p < 0.001$, compared with blank group (untreated cells); * $p < 0.05$, *** $p < 0.001$, compared with control group (Ang II-treated cells).

2.5. Effect of LSGYGP on Inflammatory Factor and NF-κB Pathway

As LSGYGP could down-regulate NO production (as per the above summarized results), western blot was used to analyze whether LSGYGP decreased NO expression through iNOS down-regulation (Figure 5a). As shown in Figure 5b, the reduction level of iNOS was consistent with the result of NO production measured in LSGYGP treatment. Furthermore, COX-2 and ET-1 levels were also investigated. As depicted in Figure 5b, expression of COX-2 and ET-1 mainly increased after exposure to Ang II, but treatment of 10 μM LSGYGP markedly blocked the Ang II induced changes. Moreover, the results revealed that LSGYGP may inhibit expression and translocation of NF-κB p65 by suppressing the phosphorylation of IκBα.

Immunocytochemistry and electrophoretic mobility shift assay (EMSA) were applied to further investigate the translocation of NF-κB p65 in Ang II-stimulated HUVEC. Observing images in Figure 5c, the NF-κB p65 sub-unit was transported to the nucleus after Ang II stimulation, as indicated by the NF-κB p65 protein level in the western blot test. Employing image analysis, treatment with Ang II presented a significant increase in the DNA-binding activity of NF-κB, whereas treatment with LSGYGP significantly reduced the Ang II-induced DNA-binding activity of NF-κB (Figure 5d,e), this revealed that p65 might enter the nucleus based on DNA-binding activity.

With the above results, we can identify that Ang II treatment activated endothelial oxidative stress and may cause inflammatory injury, which caused the expression of the relative inflammatory factors and translocation of the NF-κB pathway.

(a)

(b)

(c)

(d)

(e)

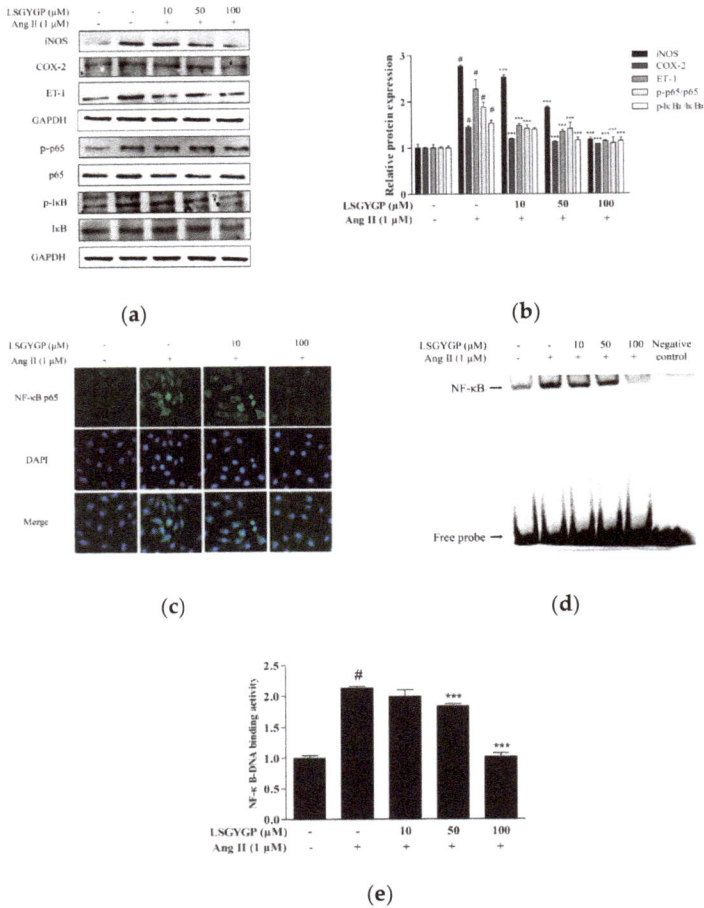

Figure 5. Effects of LSGYGP on the expression of iNOS, COX-2, NF-κB p65, and IκBα in HUVEC (**a**,**b**). Protein expression was by western blot, GAPDH, NF-κB p65, and IκBα were as control, respectively. (**c**) The effect of LSGYGP on translocation of NF-κB p65 in HUVEC. Cells were pre-treated with LSGYGP (10 and 100 μM) and subsequently treated with Ang II (1 μM) for 24 h. Nucleus was stained with DAPI and NF-κB p65 was immunostained with p65 antibody. (**d**,**e**) LSGYGP suppressed the NF-κB activity inside the nucleus of NF-κB in Ang II-stimulated HUVEC. Electrophoretic mobility shift assay (EMSA) was performed to determine the NF-κB activity in nuclear reaction by using DNA probe specific to NF-κB p65. $^{\#}$ $p < 0.001$, compared with blank group (untreated cells); ** $p < 0.01$, *** $p < 0.001$, compared with control group (Ang II-treated cells).

2.6. Effect of LSGYGP on the Akt Pathway

Figure 6 shows a marked augmentation of the expression of Bax and cleaved-caspase-3 (c-caspase-3) and down-regulation of the proliferation-related p-Akt and anti-apoptosis protein Bcl-2 in the Ang II-stimulated group. These results were both reversed by LSGYGP treatment in a dose-dependent manner. The expression of procaspase-3 did not change in any treatment. The effects of LSGYGP on the Bcl-2 family and Akt pathway could explain its vascular-protective effects on endothelial injury.

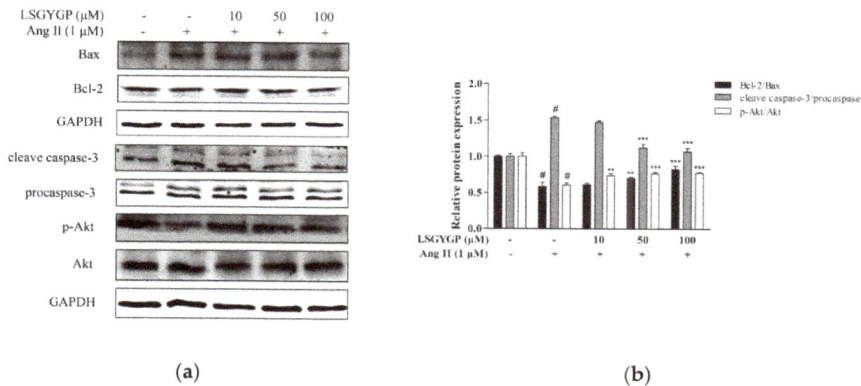

(a)

(b)

Figure 6. (a) The expressions of Bax, Bcl-2, procaspase-3, caspase-3 (p20), and phosphorylation of Akt in HUVEC. GAPDH was used as an internal control. (b) The ratios of Bcl-2/Bax and cleaved-caspase-3/procaspase-3 were calculated. # $p < 0.001$, compared with blank group (untreated cells); ** $p < 0.01$, *** $p < 0.001$, compared with control group (Ang II-treated cells).

2.7. DNA Damage in Comet Assay

In Figure 7a, no visible comets were observed in normal cells. Ang II treatment produced significantly long "comet tails", while 10 μM LSGYGP treatment significantly reduced the comet tail induced by Ang II; the lengths of the comet tails decreased in a dose-dependent manner with LSGYGP treatment (Figure 7b). The above results suggested that Ang II treatment may cause inflammatory injury, which further results in the expression of the relative apoptosis factor and reduction of p-Akt; possibly even DNA damage. LSGYGP reversed these phenomena in a vascular-protective role.

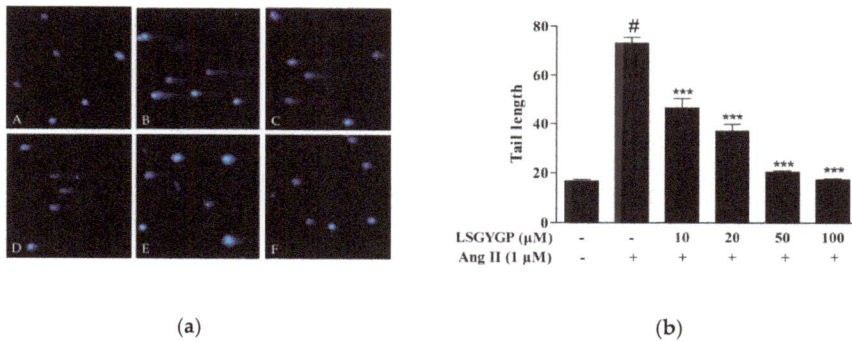

(a)

(b)

Figure 7. (a) Comet assay of HUVEC: (A) cells without treatment (the blank group); (B) cells exposed to 1 μM Ang II (the control group); (C, D, E, and F) cells pretreated with LSGYGP (10, 20, 50, and 100 μM, respectively) prior to treatment with 1 μM Ang II, all both followed by staining with DAPI. Images were obtained using an inverted fluorescence microscope with blue fluorescence (magnification: 10×). (b) Tail lengths of the comets were analyzed. # $p < 0.001$, compared with blank group (untreated cells); *** $p < 0.001$, compared with control group (Ang II-treated cells).

2.8. Docking Results of LSGYGP with NF-κB

Molecular docking results revealed that LSGYGP connected with NF-κB in a steady interaction (Figure 8a). The CDOCKER results of the NF-κB–LSGYGP combination can evaluate the rationality of side-chain backbone interactions (−5.557 kcal/mol), which is shown at 2.0 Å resolution in Figure 8b (as can be seen, the first way is the best). LSGYGP generated 10 hydrogen bonds, with bond lengths of 5.42 Å, 6.41 Å, 4.83 Å, 5.35 Å, 4.74 Å, 4.61 Å, 3.57 Å, 5.24 Å, 5.81 Å, and 5.46 Å with Lys79, Lys79, Gln220, Gln29, Gln29, Met279, Glu282, Lys221, Lys221, and Lys221, respectively, in Table 1.

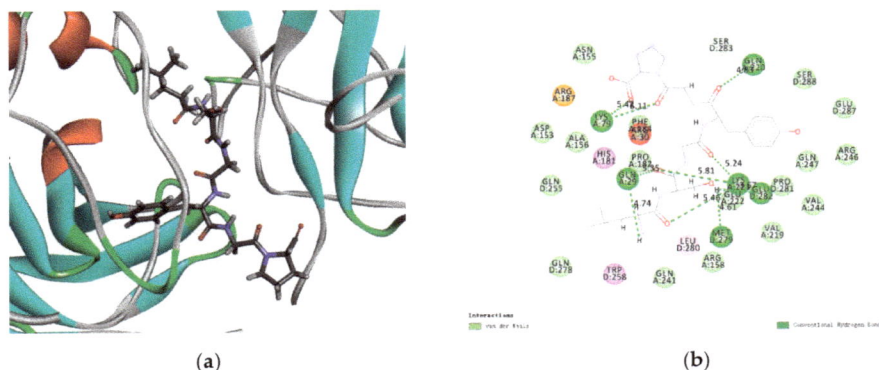

(a)   (b)

Figure 8. General and local overview poses of the best interaction poses after automated docking of peptide-NF-κB p65 active site (**a**), amino acids of LSGYGP involved in hydrogen bonds are represented by thin sticks; (**b**) Bi-dimensional (2D) diagrams of predicted interactions between ligand and NF-κB p65 amino acid residues. LSGYGP is draw by gray lines, and hydrogen bonds of them shown with green dashed lines.

Table 1. LSGYGP contacts with NF-κB (PDB: 1IKN).

Number	Interacting Atoms	Distance (Å)	Interaction Force
1	Lys79	5.42	
2		6.11	
3	Gln220	4.83	
4	Gln29	5.35	
5		4.74	Conventional Hydrogen Bond
6	Met279	4.61	
7	Glu282	3.57	
8		5.24	
9	Lys221	5.81	
10		5.46	

3. Discussion

Recently, the evidence from a great amount of research supports the idea that chronic vascular disease, such as atherosclerosis, hypertension, stroke, and so on, may be attributed to specific endothelial dysfunction for oxidative stress and inflammatory response [28,29]. Endothelial dysfunction of oxidative stress possesses a critical role in CVD, with an increasing amount of evidence [30]. Especially cumulating in the vascular endothelium, Ang II levels are frequently elevated at the initiation and in the progression of hypertension, upon which certain endotheliocytes undergo oxidative stress, which gives rise to endothelial dysfunction [31]. Some studies have provided evidence that endothelial oxidative stress promotes vascular cell apoptosis and increases inflammatory cytokine expression, causing the failure, relaxation, or dilation of arteries, leading to increased tension of the arterial wall [32], which may cause the progression of hypertension. Our study conducted a series of experiments to verify this theory and found that the tilapia by-product peptide LSGYGP can play a protective role and reverse these phenomena.

The ROS we discovered in Ang II-induced HUVEC is a common mediator of endothelial dysfunction and vascular inflammation in the cardiovascular system [33]. According to former studies, Ang II may result in ROS formation by activating nicotinamide adenine dinucleotide/triphosphopyridine nucleotide (NADH/NADPH) oxidases [31,34–36], and the result of ROS fluorescence of our study gave the same result (Figure 2). On one hand, the augmentation of ROS in oxidative stress, with the ability to stimulate the expression of pro-inflammatory factors [37], may further lead to endothelial dysfunction, lipid oxidation, and inflammatory responses [38]. The imbalance between NO with ET-1 is usually regarded as a predictor of hypertension. NO, as a vasoactive substance, might decrease endothelial cell activation through the mechanism of reducing NF-κB activation [39]. From the fluorescence results, it was clearly verified that LSGYGP reduced the Ang II-stimulated levels of NO production. Similarly, the Ang II-stimulated production of ROS was reduced by LSGYGP, as shown by the DCF fluorescence intensity in Figure 2. It has been reported that a great mass of inhibitors of NF-κB activation work by suppressing IκBα phosphorylation and degradation [40]. The results, in terms of the NF-κB pathway, detected phosphorylation of NF-κB in accordance with the above theory. Subsequently, LSGYGP treatment reduced this DNA-binding activity of NF-κB in a dose-dependent manner (Figure 5d).

On the other hand, oxidative stress could activate Nrf2, which is present in low levels under normal conditions, into the cell nucleus. HO-1 expression is regulated by Nrf2 levels, which leads to LSGYGP dose-dependently protecting from oxidative stress injury in vitro. Therefore, further study is needed on the effect of LSGYGP on the Ang II-mediated Nrf2 pathway and observing its relative protein expression. It has been shown that Nrf2, with stimuli, up-regulated the transcription of antioxidant enzymes [41]; the result of SOD in LSGYGP treatment in our study reversed it (Figure 3). Several studies have reported that Ang II activates the family JNK, ERK, and p38 of MAPK, which can result in the activation of NF-κB by phosphorylation and degradation of IκBα [42,43]. We found that LSGYGP had the ability to evidently decrease the pro-inflammatory factors iNOS and COX-2, suppress NF-κB phosphorylation and translocation, suppress MAPK phosphorylation, and suppress the relative protein expression in the Nrf2 pathway in Ang II-mediated HUVEC (Figures 3–5), which presented the same protective effects as Tao's osthole [6]. All in all, these results verify the theory that Ang II-induces ROS production and the NF-κB pathway, and thus activates the subsequent oxidative stress pathways, which both give rise to vascular endothelial injury, leading to endothelial dysfunction and, subsequently, CVD [44].

Yusuke et al. [45] suggested that the Ang II acts in a wide pathway-inhibitive role mechanism, which may be partly traced back to "intra-cellular cross talk" between Ang II and other inflammatory second mediators (NO, ET-1, iNOS, and COX-2) through transcription factor activation (e.g., NF-κB and Nrf2). In our study, LSGYGP suppressed those pathways by mediation of Ang II; we go deeper into the potential mechanisms of this result next. The results of this study suggest the restored expression of the proliferation-associated proteins p-Akt and Bcl-2 after LSGYGP treatment, as well as a marked down-regulation of caspase-3 and Bax (as observed in Figure 6), which is consistent with Shan [46]. The results of investigating the Akt pathway and the comet assay (Figure 7) suggest that oxidative stress further results in endothelial damage, and even cell death, to some degree.

The molecular docking results indicate that LSGYGP could interact with NF-κB, as a stable complex, by hydrogen bonds. A binding energy value of −5.557 kcal/mol in the optimal spatial structure (Figure 8a) was shown by the presence of the hydrogen bond, such that LSGYGP has a strong affinity toward NF-κB. Hydrophobic interactions have been regarded as the most important non-covalent force in the literature, and have been shown to be responsible for multiple phenomena, including the binding of enzymes to substrates, folding of proteins, and structure stabilization of proteins [47]. In the LSGYGP–NF-κB interaction, most of the amino acid interactions are attributed to the hydrophobic amino acids of LSGYGP. It is the amino acids Leu and Pro of LSGYGP that may contribute to the exhibition of inhibitory activity in Figure 8b, with the strong binding effect of hydrophobic interaction improving the binding affinity between NF-κB and LSGYGP. These docking studies imply that LSGYGP alleviates oxidative stress through inhibiting the activation of NF-κB.

This study has firstly reported that LSGYGP acts in a cytoprotective role against Ang II-induced oxidative stress and inflammation. LSGYGP altered the related protein expressions of the NF-κB/Nrf2 signaling pathways and reversed Ang II-induced cell endothelial injury for the first time. The entire signaling pathway of this study is shown in Figure 9. Considering all of the results, we may conclude that LSGYGP effectively attenuated Ang II-stimulated cellular injury by activation of the NF-κB/Nrf2/MAPK/Akt pathways, at both the cellular and molecular levels. This study has also illustrated that Ang II, through oxidative stress, inflammation, and apoptosis pathways, could contribute to injury events in endothelial dysfunction, especially in terms of hypertension and atherosclerosis, but future studies are still necessary to determine the specific receptors involved. Future research should further discuss and confirm that how Ang II to binds the angiotensin type 1-receptor (AT1R) and activates membrane-bound NAD(P)H oxidase for the formation of ROS; how oligopeptide LSGYGP to binds with AT1R through determinate the location for GABARAP. Besides, bioavailability and transport mechanisms of oligopeptide are remains to research for following bioactivity design and application of peptide drugs, these are the key concerns attempted to overcome by using different design strategies in the future.

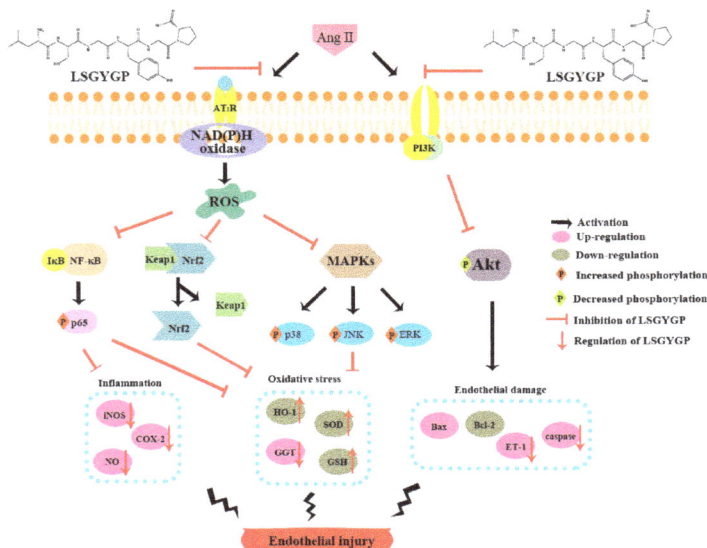

Figure 9. Summary diagram of signaling pathway of this study.

4. Materials and Methods

4.1. Materials

Ang II, 3-(4,5-Dimethylthiazol-2-yl)-2,5-diphenyltetrazolium bromide (MTT), 2,7-dichlorodihydrofluorescein diacetate (DCFH-DA), Dimethyl sulfoxide (DMSO), and 4′,6-diamidino-2-phenylindole (DAPI) were provided by Sigma-Aldrich (St. Louis, MO, USA). LSGYGP was ordered from Hangzhou Dangang Biotechnology Co., Ltd. (Hangzhou, China) with 99.8% purity. The BCA protein assay kit was provided by Thermo Fisher Scientific, Inc. (Waltham, MA, USA). The following antibodies were purchased from Santa Cruz Biotechnology (Santa Cruz, CA, USA): Mouse polyclonal antibodies, including iNOS (sc-7271), COX-2 (sc-19999), SOD (sc-271014), GGT (sc-100746), GSH (sc-71155), Nrf2 (sc-365949), Keap1 (sc-365626), HO-1 (sc-136960), NF-κB p65 (sc-8008), NF-κB p-p65 (sc-136548), IκB-α (sc-1643), p-IκB-α (sc-8404), p-p38 (sc-166182), p-ERK (sc-81492), JNK (sc-7345), p-JNK (sc-6254), and glyceraldehyde-3-phosphate dehydrogenase (GAPDH) (sc-47724); rabbit polyclonal antibodies (ERK, sc-94; p38, sc-535); secondary antibodies, such as goat anti-mouse IgG-HRP (sc-2005) and goat anti-rabbit IgG-HRP (sc-2004). Green fluorescence secondary antibody (Dylight 488, A23220) was acquired from Abbkine (Redlands, CA, USA). 3-amino,4-aminomethyl-2′,7′-difluorescein diacetate (DAF-FM DA) and a chemiluminescent EMSA Kit were purchased from Beyotime Biotechnology (Shanghai, China). All other unmentioned reagents were of analysis grade.

4.2. Cell Culture

Human umbilical vein cells (HUVEC) were obtained from Bena Culture Collection Co., Ltd. (Beijing, China) and grown in Dulbecco's modified Eagle's medium (DMEM): 10% fetal bovine serum (FBS) and 1% penicillin-streptomycin in 5% CO_2 at 37 °C.

4.3. Cell Viability Assay

Cytotoxicity was evaluated by MTT assay. The HUVEC were seeded in 96-well plates (1×10^4 cells/well), pre-treated with LSGYGP (10, 20, 50, and 100 μM; 1 h) and, afterwards, by Ang II (1 μM; 24 h). After removing the cell culture, MTT solution (1 mg/mL; 100 μL) was added to each well for 4 h. Finally, the supernatants were removed and 100 μL DMSO was added to dissolve the formazan crystal. Absorbance at 540 nm was measured with a microplate reader (BioTek, Winooski, VT, USA).

4.4. Determination of NO and ROS

Productions of NO and intracellular ROS were assessed by measuring the fluorescence intensities of DAF-FM DA and DCFH-DA, respectively. Briefly, the cells were seeded in a 24-well plate (1×10^4 cells/well), pre-treated with LSGYGP (10, 50, and 100 μM; 1 h), and then incubated with Ang II (1 μM; 24 h). The cells were washed in phosphate buffered saline (PBS) three times, subsequently being loaded with fluorochrome (5 μM DAF-FM DA, 20 min; 10 μM DCFH-DA, 30 min) at 37 °C in a CO_2 incubator. After being rinsed again, productions of NO and ROS were observed with a fluorescence microscope (Olympus, Tokyo, Japan).

4.5. Western Blot

The HUVEC were cultured in 6-well plates (5×10^6 cells/well). The cells were pre-treated with LSGYGP (10, 50, and 100 μM) for 1 h and subsequently treated with Ang II (1 μM) for 24 h. After treatment, the cells were washed with pre-cooled PBS, harvested by scraping, and lysed using lysis buffer on ice for 30 min. After centrifugation for 10 min at $12,000 \times g$, the supernatants were collected to determine protein concentration using the Pierce BCA Protein Assay Kit. Equal amounts of protein (20–40 μg) were heated with pre-stained markers at 95 °C for 10 min, then were electrophoretically examined using a 10% sodium dodecyl sulfate-polyacrylamide gel electrophoresis (SDS-PAGE), then transferred onto nitrocellulose (NC) filter membranes (Amersham, USA). Non-specific binding sites were blocked with 5% skim milk in Tris-buffered saline Tween-20 (TBST) at room temperature for 3 h, and then incubated overnight at 4 °C with primary antibody (1:500). After being washed with TBST (4 times, 10 min/time), the membranes, following used secondary antibody (1:5000), were treated with horseradish peroxidase (HRP). Blotted antibody signals were detected with an enhanced chemiluminescence (ECL) system (Syngene, Cambridge, UK).

4.6. Immunocytochemistry

The HUVEC were seeded in 24-well plates (5×10^4 cells/well) in advance, treated as described above, and were then harvested. After washing thrice with PBS buffer, the cells were fixed in phosphate buffer solution contained 4% paraformaldehyde (4 °C, 20 min). Then, permeabilization was carried out by using 0.2% Triton X-100 in PBS followed by incubation (4 °C, 10 min). Cells were then blocked with 5% bovine serum albumin (BSA) in PBS, removed and directly incubated overnight at 4 °C with anti-p65 antibody (1:100). After removing the primary antibody, the cells were washed again and incubated, in the dark and at room temperature for 3 h, with the corresponding Goat Anti-Rabbit IgG secondary antibody (1:500; Abbkine, CA, USA). Finally, the nuclei were stained using DAPI (100 ng/mL) for 5 min. The images were then observed under an inverted fluorescence microscope (Olympus, Tokyo, Japan).

4.7. EMSA Assay

The HUVEC were cultured in 6-well plates (1×10^6 cells/well), treated as described above, and were then harvested. Nuclear extracts were collected, according to the manufacturer's instructions of the Nuclear and Cytoplasmic Extraction Kit from Beyotime Biotechnology (Shanghai, China). Protein concentration was determined using the Pierce BCA Protein Assay Kit. The NF-kB probe was 5'-AGT TGA GGG GAC TTT CCC AGG C-3' which reacted with 5 μg nuclear protein. The mixture was then electrophoretically separated on a 6.5% polyacrylamide gel in 0.5X Tris-borate buffer (100 V; 1 h) and transferred onto positive-charge nylon membranes with $0.5 \times$ TBE running buffer for 50 min at 300 mA. The membrane was cross-linked for 15 min under UV light, blocked with blocking solution containing streptavidin-HRP conjugate, and finally visualized using Chemiluminescent EMSA Kit, according to the manufacturer's instructions.

4.8. Comet Assay

The comet assay was performed as described previously [48] to evaluate DNA strand breakdown. Cells were treated as described above and then suspended in PBS (1×10^5 cells/mL). Briefly, 1% low melting point agarose (LMA, 80 μL) was added to the cells (200 cells/μL, 20 μL), which were then put on a slide pre-coated with 0.8% normal agarose (NMA, 100 μL) dissolved in PBS, and covered immediately with a coverslip (4 °C, 15 min). After solidification, the coverslip was cautiously removed. The cells were lysed in a pre-chilled lysis solution containing 2.5 M NaCl, 100 mM Na_2EDTA, 10 mM Tris, 200 mM NaOH, 1% sodium lauroyl sarcosinate, and 1% Triton X-100 at pH 10 (4 °C; 90 min). The slides were placed in an electrophoresis chamber with an alkaline electrophoresis solution (200 mM NaOH and 1 mM Na_2EDTA, pH > 13) for unwinding and expression of alkali-labile sites (30 min) and were subsequently electrophoresed (25 V and 300 mA, 20 min) with aim to draw the negatively charged DNA toward the anode. After neutralization, the cells were stained with DAPI (50 μg/mL, 20 μL) in the dark for 5 min. They were then observed under an invert fluorescence microscope (Olympus, Tokyo, Japan) the DNA damage (average tail length) was quantified using the CASP software to analyze the comet images.

4.9. Molecular Docking

The structure of LSGYGP was drawn using the Chemdraw software (Chemdraw, PerkinElmer Informatics, Boston, MA, USA). The three-dimensional (3D) crystal structure of NF-κB (PDB: 1IKN) was downloaded from the Protein Data Bank (PDB) (http://www.rcsb.org/pdb/). The CDOCKER algorithm in the Discovery Studio (DS) 3.5 software (Accelrys Software Inc., San Diego, CA, USA) was used to simulate the protein–ligand interaction. The high-molecular dynamics method was utilized to randomly search for small molecule (LSGYGP) conformations, and simulated annealing was used to optimize each conformation of the active site of the receptor (NF-κB).

4.10. Statistical Analysis

All analyses were carried out on triplicate samples. The GraphPad Prism 5.0 software (GraphPad Prism Software Inc., La Jolla, CA, USA) was used for the statistical analysis. Multiple-group comparisons were evaluated by one-way ANOVA, accompanied by Dunnett's multiple comparison test for group comparison.

5. Conclusions

In conclusion, Ang II is a well-known powerful inducer of oxidative stress and inflammatory responses in cardiovascular tissues, resulting in atherosclerosis and hypertension. LSGYGP inhibited Ang II-stimulated oxidative stress and vascular endothelial dysfunction; down-regulated iNOS and COX-2 by suppressing the NF-κB pathway; up-regulated SOD and GSH by suppressing the phosphorylation of MAPK; and up-regulated HO-1 by the Nrf2 pathway. Simultaneously, down-regulation of the production of NO and ROS by LSGYGP was involved in the protective process, which could help to protect vascular function. Docking results suggest that LSGYGP may steadily connect with NF-κB by hydrogen bond interactions. This study revealed that LSGYGP has protective effects against the inflammation, oxidant stress, and apoptosis induced by Ang II in HUVEC, which may provide one of the underlying mechanisms for the treatment of Ang II-stimulated endothelial dysfunction and, thus, has potential for application in curing hypertensive disorders.

Author Contributions: J.C. performed the research and wrote the original draft of the manuscripts; Z.-J.Q. conceived and designed the research and edited the manuscripts; F.G. and M.-F.C. analyzed the data; C.L., C.Z., P.H. and S.S. contributed materials and analysis tools. All authors reviewed the final publication.

Funding: The study was supported by the Yangfan Scarce Top Talent Project of Guangdong Province (201433009), Program for Scientific Research Start-Up Funds of Guangdong Ocean University [to Zhong-Ji Qian], Innovation and Strong University Project (2013050204) and the Development Project about Marine Economy Demonstration of Zhanjiang City (2017C8B1).

Conflicts of Interest: The authors declare no conflict of interest.

References

1. Montezano, A.C.; Nguyen Dinh Cat, A.; Rios, F.J.; Touyz, R.M. Angiotensin II and vascular injury. *Curr. Hypertens. Rep.* **2014**, *16*, 431. [CrossRef] [PubMed]
2. Davignon, J. Role of endothelial dysfunction in atherosclerosis. *Circulation* **2004**, *109*, III27–III32. [CrossRef] [PubMed]
3. Zhang, Z.; Wang, M.; Xue, S.J.; Liu, D.H.; Tang, Y.B. Simvastatin ameliorates Angiotensin II-induced endothelial dysfunction through restoration of Rho-BH4-eNOS-NO pathway. *Cardiovasc. Drugs Ther.* **2012**, *26*, 31–40. [CrossRef]
4. Xia, F.; Wang, C.; Jin, Y.; Liu, Q.; Meng, Q.; Liu, K.; Sun, H. Luteolin protects HUVECs from TNF-α-induced oxidative stress and inflammation via its effects on the Nox4/ROS-NF-κB and MAPK pathways. *J. Atheroscler. Thromb.* **2014**, *21*, 768–783. [CrossRef] [PubMed]
5. Xiao, Q.; Qu, Z.; Zhao, Y.; Yang, L.; Gao, P. Orientin ameliorates LPS-induced inflammatory responses through the inhibitory of the NF-κ B pathway and NLRP3 inflammasome. *Evid. Based Complement Altern. Med.* **2017**, *2017*, 1–8. [CrossRef] [PubMed]
6. Tao, L.; Gu, X.; Xu, E.; Ren, S.; Zhang, L.; Liu, W.; Lin, X.; Yang, J.; Chen, C. Osthole protects against Ang II-induced endotheliocyte death by targeting NF-κB pathway and Keap-1/Nrf2 pathway. *Am. J. Transl. Res.* **2019**, *11*, 142–159. [PubMed]
7. Mehta, P.K.; Griendling, K.K. Angiotensin II cell signaling: Physiological and pathological effects in the cardiovascular system. *Am. J. Physiol. Cell Physiol.* **2007**, *292*, C82–C97. [CrossRef] [PubMed]
8. Alonso-Galicia, M.; Maier, K.G.; Greene, A.S.; Cowley, A.W.; Roman, R.J. Role of 20-hydroxyeicosatetraenoic acid in the renal and vasoconstrictor actions of angiotensin II. *Am. J. Physiol. Regul. Integr. Comp. Physiol.* **2002**, *283*, R60–R68. [CrossRef]

9. Gragasin, F.S.; Xu, Y.; Arenas, I.A.; Kainth, N.; Davidge, S.T. Estrogen reduces angiotensin II–induced nitric oxide synthase and NAD(P)H oxidase expression in endothelial cells. *Arterioscler. Thromb. Vasc. Biol.* **2003**, *23*, 38–44. [CrossRef]

10. Hahn, A.W.; Resink, T.J.; Scott-Burden, T.; Powell, J.; Dohi, Y.; Bühler, F.R. Stimulation of endothelin mRNA and secretion in rat vascular smooth muscle cells: A novel autocrine function. *Cell Regul.* **1990**, *1*, 649–659. [CrossRef]

11. Bendall, J.K.; Rinze, R.; Adlam, D.; Tatham, A.L.; de Bono, J.; Channon, K.M. Endothelial Nox2 overexpression potentiates vascular oxidative stress and hemodynamic response to Angiotensin II: Studies in endothelial-targeted Nox2 transgenic mice. *Circ. Res.* **2007**, *100*, 1016–1025. [CrossRef] [PubMed]

12. Sprague, A.H.; Khalil, R.A. Inflammatory cytokines in vascular dysfunction and vascular disease. *Biochem. Pharmacol.* **2009**, *78*, 539–552. [CrossRef] [PubMed]

13. Mueller, C.F.H.; Becher, M.U.; Zimmer, S.; Wassmann, S.; Keuler, B.; Nickenig, G. Angiotensin II triggers release of leukotriene C4 in vascular smooth muscle cells via the multidrug resistance-related protein 1. *Mol. Cell. Biochem.* **2010**, *333*, 261–267. [CrossRef] [PubMed]

14. Cheng, Z.-J.; Vapaatalo, H.; Mervaala, E. Angiotensin II and vascular inflammation. *Med. Sci. Monit.* **2005**, *11*, RA194. [CrossRef] [PubMed]

15. Brasier, A.-R. The nuclear factor-κb-interleukin-6 signalling pathway mediating vascular inflammation. *Cardiovasc. Res.* **2010**, *86*, 211–218. [CrossRef] [PubMed]

16. Xiong, D.; Hu, W.; Ye, S.T.; Tan, Y.S. Isoliquiritigenin alleviated the Ang II-induced hypertensive renal injury through suppressing inflammation cytokines and oxidative stress-induced apoptosis via Nrf2 and NF-κB pathways. *Biochem. Biophys. Res. Commun.* **2018**, *506*, 161–168. [CrossRef]

17. Li, W.; Kong, A.N. Molecular mechanisms of Nrf2-mediated antioxidant response. *Mol. Carcinog.* **2009**, *48*, 91–104. [CrossRef]

18. Kim, Y.M.; Pae, H.O.; Park, J.E.; Lee, Y.C.; Woo, J.M.; Kim, N.-H.; Choi, Y.K.; Lee, B.-S.; Kim, S.R.; Chung, H.-T. Heme oxygenase in the regulation of vascular biology: From molecular mechanisms to therapeutic opportunities. *Antioxid. Redox Signal.* **2011**, *14*, 137–167. [CrossRef]

19. Li, Z.X.; Chen, J.W.; Yuan, F.; Huang, Y.Y.; Zhao, L.Y.; Li, J.; Su, H.X.; Liu, J.; Pang, J.Y.; Lin, Y.C.; et al. Xyloketal B exhibits its antioxidant activity through induction of ho-1 in vascular endothelial cells and zebrafish. *Mar. Drugs* **2013**, *11*, 504–522. [CrossRef]

20. Walensky, L.D. BCL-2 in the crosshairs: Tipping the balance of life and death. *Cell. Death Differ.* **2006**, *13*, 1339–1350. [CrossRef]

21. Li, M.; Liu, X.; He, Y.; Zheng, Q.; Wang, M.; Wu, Y.; Zhang, Y.; Wang, C. Celastrol attenuates angiotensin II mediated human umbilical vein endothelial cells damage through activation of Nrf2/ERK1/2/Nox2 signal pathway. *Eur. J. Pharmacol.* **2017**, *797*, 124–133. [CrossRef] [PubMed]

22. Sivasinprasasn, S.; Pantan, R.; Thummayot, S.; Tocharus, J.; Suksamrarn, A.; Tocharus, C. Cyanidin-3-glucoside attenuates angiotensin II-induced oxidative stress and inflammation in vascular endothelial cells. *Chem. Biol. Interact.* **2016**, *260*, 67–74. [CrossRef] [PubMed]

23. Sable, R.; Parajuli, P.; Jois, S. Peptides, peptidomimetics, and polypeptides from marine sources: A wealth of natural sources for pharmaceutical applications. *Mar. Drugs* **2017**, *15*, 124. [CrossRef] [PubMed]

24. Huang, B.B.; Lin, H.C.; Chang, Y.W. Analysis of proteins and potential bioactive peptides from tilapia (*Oreochromis spp.*) processing co-products using proteomic techniques coupled with BIOPEP database. *J. Funct. Food* **2015**, *19*, 629–640. [CrossRef]

25. Zhuang, Y.; Hou, H.; Zhao, X.; Zhang, Z.; Li, B. Effects of collagen and collagen hydrolysate from jellyfish (*Rhopilema esculentum*) on mice skin photoaging induced by UV irradiation. *J. Food Sci.* **2009**, *74*, H183–H188. [CrossRef] [PubMed]

26. Sun, L.; Zhang, Y.; Zhuang, Y. Antiphotoaging effect and purification of an antioxidant peptide from tilapia (*Oreochromis niloticus*) gelatin peptides. *J. Funct. Food.* **2013**, *5*, 154–162. [CrossRef]

27. Ma, Q.; Liu, Q.; Yuan, L.; Zhuang, Y. Protective EFFECTS of LSGYGP from fish skin gelatin hydrolysates on UVB-Induced MEFs by regulation of oxidative stress and matrix metalloproteinase activity. *Nutrients* **2018**, *10*, 420. [CrossRef]

28. Gu, L.; Bai, W.; Li, S.; Zhang, Y.; Han, Y.; Gu, Y.; Meng, G.; Xie, L.; Wang, J.; Xiao, Y.; et al. Celastrol prevents atherosclerosis via inhibiting LOX-1 and oxidative stress. *PLoS ONE* **2013**, *8*, e65477. [CrossRef]

29. Bermudez, E.A.; Rifai, N.; Buring, J.; Manson, J.E.; Ridker, P.M. Interrelationships among circulating interleukin-6, c-reactive protein, and traditional cardiovascular risk factors in women. *Arterioscler. Thromb. Vasc. Biol.* **2002**, *22*, 1668–1673. [CrossRef]

30. Guzik, T.J.; West, N.E.J.; Black, E.; McDonald, D.; Ratnatunga, C.; Pillai, R.; Channon, K.M. Vascular superoxide production by NAD(P)H oxidase: Association with endothelial dysfunction and clinical risk factors. *Circ. Res.* **2000**, *86*. [CrossRef]

31. Cao, Y.; Zheng, L.; Liu, S.; Peng, Z.; Zhang, S. Total flavonoids from Plumula Nelumbinis suppress angiotensin II-induced fractalkine production by inhibiting the ROS/NF-κB pathway in human umbilical vein endothelial cells. *Exp. Ther. Med.* **2014**, *7*, 1187–1192. [CrossRef] [PubMed]

32. Guzik, T.J.; Hoch, N.E.; Brown, K.A.; McCann, L.A.; Rahman, A.; Dikalov, S.; Goronzy, J.; Weyand, C.; Harrison, D.G. Role of the T cell in the genesis of angiotensin II–induced hypertension and vascular dysfunction. *J. Exp. Med.* **2007**, *204*, 2449–2460. [CrossRef] [PubMed]

33. Griendling, K.K.; Sorescu, D.; Ushio-Fukai, M. NAD(P)H oxidase: Role in cardiovascular biology and disease. *Circ. Res.* **2000**, *86*, 494–501. [CrossRef] [PubMed]

34. Rajagopalan, S.; Kurz, S.; Münzel, T.; Tarpey, M.; Freeman, B.A.; Griendling, K.K.; Harrison, D.G. Angiotensin II-mediated hypertension in the rat increases vascular superoxide production via membrane NADH/NADPH oxidase activation. Contribution to alterations of vasomotor tone. *J. Clin. Investig.* **1996**, *97*, 1916–1923. [CrossRef]

35. Kalinowski, L.; Malinski, T. Endothelial NADH/NADPH-dependent enzymatic sources of superoxide production: Relationship to endothelial dysfunction. *Acta Biochim. Pol.* **2004**, *51*, 459.

36. Harrison, D.; Griendling, K.K.; Landmesser, U.; Hornig, B.; Drexler, H. Role of oxidative stress in atherosclerosis. *Am. J. Cardiol.* **2003**, *91*, 7–11. [CrossRef]

37. Zhao, J.; Liu, J.; Pang, X.; Wang, S.; Wu, D.; Zhang, X.; Feng, L. Angiotensin II induces c-reactive protein expression via AT1-ROS-MAPK-NF-κB signal pathway in hepatocytes. *Cell. Physiol. Biochem.* **2013**, *32*, 569–580. [CrossRef]

38. Murdoch, C.E.; Chaubey, S.; Zeng, L.; Yu, B.; Ivetic, A.; Walker, S.J.; Vanhoutte, D.; Heymans, S.; Grieve, D.J.; Cave, A.C.; et al. Endothelial NADPH Oxidase-2 promotes interstitial cardiac fibrosis and diastolic dysfunction through proinflammatory effects and endothelial-mesenchymal transition. *J. Am. Coll. Cardiol.* **2014**, *63*, 2734–2741. [CrossRef]

39. Bharadwaj, A.S.; Schewitz-Bowers, L.P.; Wei, L.; Lee, R.W.J.; Smith, J.R. Intercellular adhesion molecule 1 mediates migration of Th1 and Th17 cells across human retinal vascular endothelium. *Investig. Ophtalmol. Vis. Sci.* **2013**, *54*, 6917. [CrossRef]

40. Gyeong-Jin, Y.; Il-Whan, C.; Gi-Young, K.; Byung-Woo, K.; Cheol, P.; Su-Hyun, H.; Sung-Kwon, M.; Hee-Jae, C.; Young-Chae, C.; Kee Yoeup, P.; et al. Anti-inflammatory potential of saponins derived from cultured wild ginseng roots in lipopolysaccharide-stimulated RAW 264.7 macrophages. *Int. J. Mol. Med.* **2015**, *35*, 1690–1698. [CrossRef]

41. Peng, S.; Hou, Y.; Yao, J.; Fang, J. Activation of Nrf2-driven antioxidant enzymes by cardamonin confers neuroprotection of PC12 cells against oxidative damage. *Food Funct.* **2017**, *8*, 997–1007. [CrossRef] [PubMed]

42. Daniels, D.; Yee, D.K.; Faulconbridge, L.F.; Fluharty, S.J. Divergent behavioral roles of angiotensin receptor intracellular signaling cascades. *Endocrinology* **2005**, *146*, 5552–5560. [CrossRef] [PubMed]

43. Wang, W.; Huang, X.R.; Canlas, E.; Oka, K.; Truong, L.D.; Deng, C.; Bhowmick, N.A.; Ju, W.; Bottinger, E.P.; Lan, H.Y. Essential role of Smad3 in angiotensin II–induced vascular fibrosis. *Circ. Res.* **2006**, *98*, 1032–1039. [CrossRef] [PubMed]

44. Hansson, G.K.; Hermansson, A. The immune system in atherosclerosis. *Nat. Immunol.* **2011**, *12*, 204–212. [CrossRef] [PubMed]

45. Suzuki, Y.; Ruiz-Ortega, M.; Lorenzo, O.; Ruperez, M.; Esteban, V.; Egido, J. Inflammation and angiotensin II. *Int. J. Biochem. Cell Biol.* **2003**, *35*, 881–900. [CrossRef]

46. Shan, H.; Zhang, S.; Wei, X.; Li, X.; Qi, H.; He, Y.; Liu, A.; Luo, D.; Yu, X. Protection of endothelial cells against Ang II-induced impairment: Involvement of both PPARα and PPARγ via PI3K/Akt pathway. *Clin. Exp. Hypertens.* **2016**, *38*, 571–577. [CrossRef] [PubMed]

47. Manimaran, D.; Ghanendra, S.; Sridhar, M.; Kaliaperumal, J.; Muniyaraj, S.; Mohankumar, T.; Vijayakumar, R.; Manigandan, K.; Balakrishnan, R.; Elangovan, N. Molecular insights of newly identified potential peptide inhibitors of hypoxia inducible factor 1α causing breast cancer. *J. Mol. Struct.* **2019**, *1177*, 558–563. [CrossRef]
48. Lu, Y.; Liu, Y.; Yang, C. Evaluating in vitro DNA damage using comet assay. *Jove-J. Vis. Exp.* **2017**, *128*, e56450. [CrossRef]

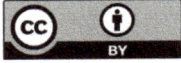

marine drugs

MDPI

Article

Antihypertensive Effect in Vivo of QAGLSPVR and Its Transepithelial Transport Through the Caco-2 Cell Monolayer

Liping Sun [1], Beiyi Wu [1], Mingyan Yan [2], Hu Hou [3] and Yongliang Zhuang [1,*]

[1] Yunnan Institute of Food Safety, Kunming University of Science and Technology, No. 727 South Jingming Road, Kunming 650500, China; kmlpsun@163.com (L.S.); wubeiyi1994@163.com (B.W.)
[2] Shandong Provincial Key Laboratory of Biochemical Engineering, College of Marine Science and Biological Engineering, Qingdao University of Science and Technology, Qingdao 266042, China; yanmingyan@qust.edu.cn
[3] Food Science and Technology, Ocean University of China, No 5, Yushan Road, Qingdao 266005, China; houhu@ouc.edu.cn
* Correspondence: ylzhuang@kmust.edu.cn; Tel./Fax: +86-871-6592-0216

Received: 23 March 2019; Accepted: 25 April 2019; Published: 13 May 2019

Abstract: The peptide QAGLSPVR, which features high angiotensin-I-converting enzyme (ACE) inhibitory activity, was identified in our previous study. In this study, the in vivo antihypertensive effect of QAGLSPVR was evaluated. Results showed that QAGLSPVR exerts a clear antihypertensive effect on spontaneously hypertensive rats (SHRs), and the systolic and diastolic blood pressures of the rats remarkably decreased by 41.86 and 40.40 mm Hg, respectively, 3 h after peptide administration. The serum ACE activities of SHRs were determined at different times, and QAGLSPVR was found to decrease ACE activities in serum; specifically, minimal ACE activity was found 3 h after administration. QAGLSPVR could be completely absorbed by the Caco-2 cell monolayer, and its transport percentage was 3.5% after 2 h. The transport route results of QAGLSPVR showed that Gly-Sar and wortmannin exert minimal effects on the transport percentage of the peptide ($p > 0.05$), thus indicating that QAGLSPVR transport through the Caco-2 cell monolayer is not mediated by peptide transporter 1 or transcytosis. By contrast, cytochalasin D significantly increased QAGLSPVR transport ($p < 0.05$); thus, QAGLSPVR may be transported through the Caco-2 cell monolayer via the paracellular pathway.

Keywords: QAGLSPVR; antihypertensive effect; Caco-2 cell monolayer; transport routes

1. Introduction

Hypertension is considered a public cardiovascular disease and an important risk factor of myocardial infarction, cerebral infarction, and renal failure. Angiotensin I-converting enzyme (ACE) plays a key role in controlling hypertension. ACE inhibition is an important method often used to treat high blood pressure [1]. Previous studies show that many peptides from food materials have ACE inhibitory (ACEI) activity and decrease blood pressure [2,3]. This function of peptides has received considerable research attention.

Previous studies showed some bioactive peptides existed good antihypertensive activity in vivo [4,5]. Bioactive peptides with high ACEI activities in vitro can exert antihypertensive activity in vivo when they are absorbed intact in the target organ through the intestinal tract [6]. Although some peptides have in vitro ACEI activity, no antihypertensive activity in spontaneously hypertensive rats (SHRs) has yet been observed after oral administration in vivo. Thus, theACEI activities of peptides may be affected by the absorption and metabolismin vivo [7]. Caco-2 cells are human colon adenocarcinoma cell clones. The structures and functions of Caco-2 cells are similar to those of differentiated intestinal epithelial cells [8]. Therefore, a Caco-2 cell monolayer model is often used in simulated intestinal transport experiments in vitro. Previous studies have studied the transepithelial transports of antihypertensive peptides by Caco-2 cell monolayer model [8,9].

In our previous studies, enzymatic hydrolysates of tilapia skin gelatin were obtained using simulated gastrointestinal digestion. The hydrolysates were isolated and purified, and QAGLSPVR was obtained by successive chromatography of the gelatin hydrolysates [10]. The molecular weight of QAGLSPVR is 826.4661 Da, and its IC_{50} of ACEI activity is 68.35 µM [10]. The present study aims to confirm the in vivo antihypertensive effect of QAGLSPVR by using the SHR model. The transepithelial transport of QAGLSPVR was evaluated according to the Caco-2 cell monolayer model via an ultra-performance liquid chromatograph coupled to a Q Exactive hybrid quadrupole-orbitrap mass spectrometer (UPLC-Q-Orbitrap-MS^2). Finally, the transport routes of QAGLSPVR in the Caco-2 cell monolayer were analyzed.

2. Results

2.1. Changes in Blood Pressure over Time

As shown in Figure 1A,B, the systolic (SBP) and diastolic (DBP) blood pressure of SHRs obviously decreased after a single treatment of oral QAGLSPVR. The SBP and DBP obtained were lowest 3 h after QAGLSPVR administration. Compared with those of the control group, the SBP and DBP of the QAGLSPVR- treated group significantly decreased by 41.86 and 40.40 mm Hg (p <0.05), respectively, 3 h after administration. Similar results were found in the group of SHRs receiving 10 mg/kg body weight (BW) captopril serving as positive control.

ACE activities in the serum of SHRs were determined after a single oral administration of 20 mg/kg BW QAGLSPVR. As shown in Figure 1C, serum ACE activities in the QAGLSPVR group significantly decreased3 h after administration ($p < 0.05$) compared with those of the control group. Thereafter, serum ACE activities increased with time. This trend is consistent with the change in blood pressure of SHRs.

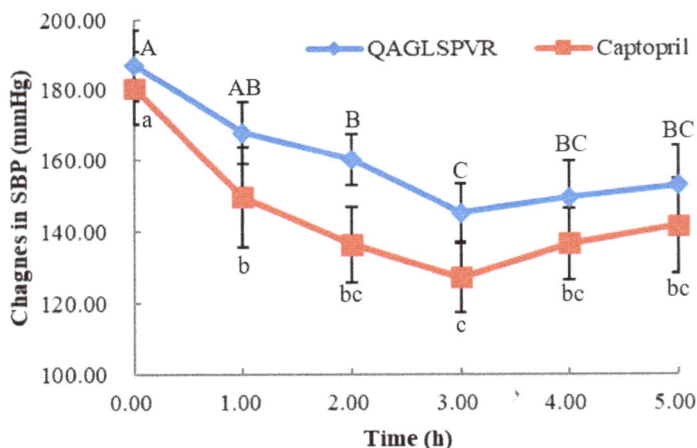

(A)

Figure 1. *Cont.*

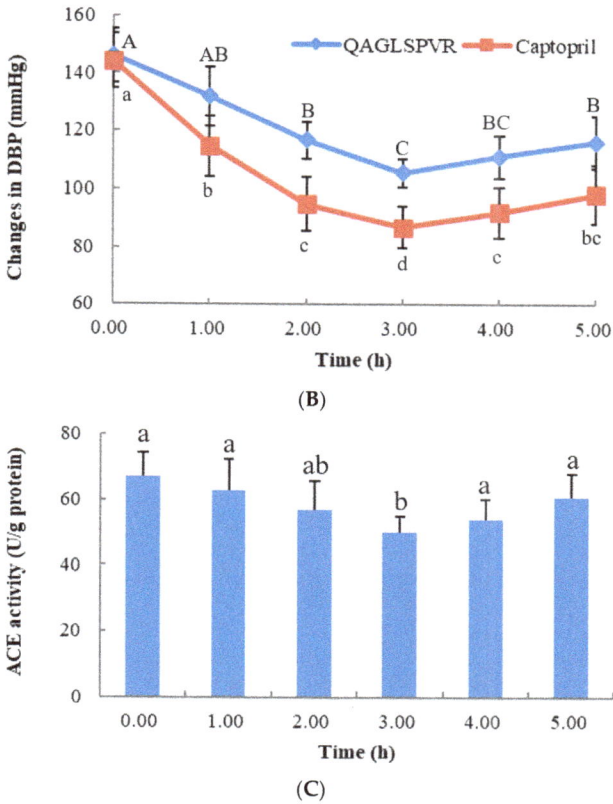

Figure 1. In vivo effects of 20 mg/kg BW QAGLSPVR and 10 mg/kg BW captopril on spontaneously hypertensive rats, (**A**): systolic blood pressure (SBP), different capital letters indicated significant differences for QAGLSPVR with different times and different lowercase letters indicated significant differences for captopril with different times; (**B**): diastolic blood pressure (DBP), different capital letters indicated significant differences for QAGLSPVR with different times and different lowercase letters indicated significant differences for captopril with different times; (**C**): ACE activity in serum, different letters indicated significant differences for QAGLSPVR with different times ($p < 0.05$).

2.2. Transport through the Caco-2 Cell Monolayer

QAGLSPVR transport was analyzed using the Caco-2 cell monolayer model. Qualitative and quantitative analyses of QAGLSPVR were performed using UPLC-Q-Orbitrap-MS^2. Figure 2A,B respectively show the total and extract ion chromatograms of QAGLSPVR in the apical chamber (AP) of the Caco-2 cell monolayer. Figure 2C,D respectively show the total and extract ion chromatograms of QAGLSPVR in the basal chamber (BL). QAGLSPVR identification was conducted using *De Novo*™ software (Peak Studio 7.5, Bioinformatics Solutions, Inc., Waterloo, ON. Canada) (Figure 2E).

As shown in Figure 3A, QAGLSPVR transport was determined at different times. QAGLSPVR could be transported intact by the Caco-2 cell monolayer, and the transport percentage increased over time. The QAGLSPVR transport percentage was 3.5% 2 h after administration.

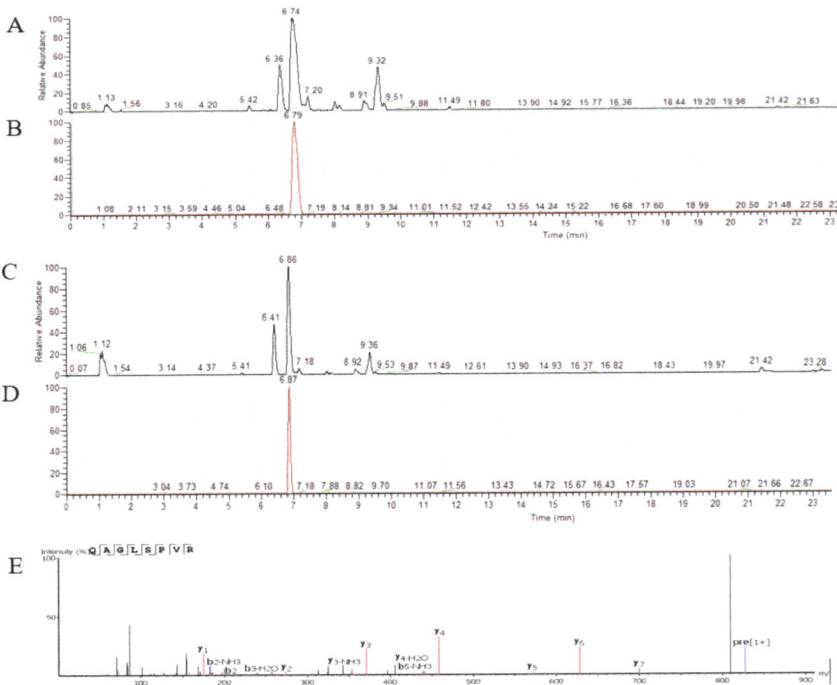

Figure 2. The chromatograms of QAGLSPVR as detected by UPLC-Q-Orbitrap-MS^2, (**A**): Total ion chromatograms of apical chamber; (**B**): Extract ion chromatograms of QAGLSPVR in apical chamber; (**C**): Total ion chromatograms of basal chamber, (**D**): Extract ion chromatograms of QAGLSPVR in basal chamberand; (**E**): Identification of QAGLSPVR by *De Novo*™ software.

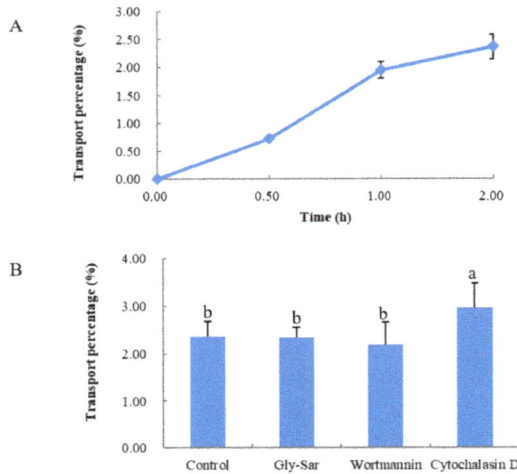

Figure 3. Transepithelial transport of QAGLSPVR in presence of inhibitory/disruptors for different transportation routes by Caco-2 cell monolayer, (**A**): Transport percentage of QAGLSPVR at different times, (**B**): Transport percentage of QAGLSPVR in different routes. Different letters indicated significant differences ($p < 0.05$).

Figure 3B shows the transport routes of QAGLSPVR in the Caco-2 cell monolayer. Gly-Sar had no significant effect on QAGLSPVR transport ($p > 0.05$), which means QAGLSPVR transport through the Caco-2 cell monolayer is not mediated by peptide transporter 1 (PepT1). Wortmannin did not significantly affect QAGLSPVR transport ($p > 0.05$), which means QAGLSPVR transport through the Caco-2 cell monolayer is not mediated by transcytosis. Finally, cytochalasin D significantly increased QAGLSPVR transport ($p < 0.05$) through the cell monolayer, thus indicating that QAGLSPVR may be transported via the paracellular pathway.

3. Discussion

In our previous study, QAGLSPVR was separated and identified from tilapia skin gelatin hydrolysates, and its IC_{50} for ACEI activity in vitro was found to be 68.35 μM [10]. Bioactive peptides are exposed through systemic circulation in human tissues [11]. Unfortunately, bioactive peptides may be hydrolyzed before they reach the target tissues during passage through and absorption by the small intestine. While some bioactive peptides show in vitro ACEI activity, they do not exhibit antihypertensive effects in vivo after oral administration to SHRs. For example, FKGRYYP was identified from chicken muscle hydrolysates, and its IC_{50} for ACEI activity in vitro was found to be 0.55 mM [12]; however, no antihypertensive activity of this peptide was observed after oral administration to SHRs. Therefore, bioactive peptides must resist systemic peptidase degradation prior to reaching their target sites to exert their function in vivo. The application of antihypertensive peptides is limited when they have no ACEI activity after oral administration. In this study, we confirmed the antihypertensive effect of QAGLSPVR on the SBP and DBP of SHRs after a single oral administration of the peptide. Results showed that QAGLSPVR effectively reduces the SBP and DBP of SHRs. SBP and DBP reached maximum effect 3 h after QAGLSPVR administration. This outcome is similar to the results of a number of antihypertensive peptides, such as YASGR [13] and MEGAQEAQGD [5]. The experimental results showed that the antihypertensive effect of QAGLSPVR on SHRs is consistent with its in vitro ACEI activity.

Different ACEI peptides have different metabolic pathways and tissue distributions due to their different molecular structures [14]. Serum ACEI activity plays an important role in regulating blood pressurein vivo. Therefore, ACE activities in the serum of SHRs were evaluated after QAGLSPVR administration. The results indicated that QAGLSPVR could decrease the serum ACE activities of SHRs and regulate their blood pressures. Boonla et al. reported that rice bran protein hydrolysate can regulate plasma ACE levels to decrease the blood pressures of the 2k-1c renovascular hypertensive rats [15]. The results of this previous study are similar to those of the current work.

QAGLSPVR was proven to produce a clear antihypertensive effect on SHRs in this study. To validate whether QAGLSPVR could be completely absorbed to regulate blood pressure, the transport percentage of QAGLSPVR was evaluated via the Caco-2 cell monolayer model. Caco-2 cells can be used as an in vitro model of the human intestinal epithelium due to the various brush border membrane enzymes characterizing these cells [16]. At least eight membrane enzymes are expressed by Caco-2 cells. The brush border membrane enzymes are membrane peptidases and can hydrolyze peptides into short fragments prior to absorption of peptides [9,17]. As shown in Figure 3A, QAGLSPVR could be transported intact by the Caco-2 cell monolayer, and the QAGLSPVR transport percentage was 3.5% after 2 h. Previous studies have shown that many food-derived bioactive peptides, such as QIGLF [8], TNGIIR [18], RKQLQGVN [19], and YLGYLEQ [20], could be absorbed intact through the Caco-2 cell monolayer. This finding is similar to our results.

The characteristics of peptides, including their amino acid compositions and sequences, molecular weights, hydrogen-bond capacity, charge, and hydrophobicity, play key roles in transport over the intestinal epithelium [21]. Many studies have indicated that the transport and mechanism of peptides are highly associated with their chain length [22,23]. Some peptides with low molecular weights can cross the intestinal epithelium easily. In general, di- and tri-peptides can be absorbed by H^+-coupled PepT1.Peptides with a range of four to nine amino acid residues can be successfully transported by the paracellular pathway. Some peptides with 10 amino acid residues and higher are generally believed to be transported by transcytosis.

Several transport enhancers or inhibitors were selected to study the transport mechanisms of QAGLSPVR through the Caco-2 cell monolayer. Gly-Sar is a good substrate for PepT1 and used to evaluate the transport mechanisms of QAGLSPVR. As shown in Figure 3B, Gly-Sar had no significant effect on QAGLSPVR transport ($p > 0.05$), which means QAGLSPVR transport through the Caco-2 cell monolayer is not mediated by PepT1. A previous study indicated that PepT1 is mainly responsible for the transport of di-peptides and tri-peptides but not peptides containing three amino acids and higher [24]. This finding was in accordance with our results. Wortmannin, a transcytos inhibitor, had no significant effect on QAGLSPVR transport ($p > 0.05$), which means QAGLSPVR transport through the Caco-2 cell monolayer is not mediated by transcytosis. In contrast to these substances, cytochalasin D, a disruptor of tight junctions (TJs), significantly increased QAGLSPVR transport ($p < 0.05$), thus revealing that QAGLSPVR could be transported through the Caco-2 cell monolayer via the paracellular pathway. Our results are consistent with those of some food-derived peptides, such as RVPSL [25], QIGLF [8], TNGIIR [18], and GGYR [26].

Quirós et al. found that LHLPLP is degraded to HLPLP, which shows high antihypertensive effects in animal models [27]. Guo et al. reported that intact RLSFNP and its breakdown fragments F, FNP, SFNP, and RLSF could be detected in the RLSFNP transport solution through the Caco-2 cell monolayer and that RLSFNP fragments, such as FNP, SFNP, and RLSF, contribute to ACEI activities [28]. Therefore, the potential structural changes of QAGLSPVR through the Caco-2 cell monolayer should be evaluated in future studies.

4. Materials and Methods

4.1. Materials and Reagents

QAGLSPVR was synthesized by Shanghai Synpeptide Co., Ltd. (Shanghai, China). Captopril was purchased from Sinopharm Shantou Jinshi Pharmaceutical Co., Ltd. (Guangdong, China).Caco-2 cells were provided by the Kunming Institute of Zoology (Kunming, China). The ACE activity determination kit used in this work was provided by Shanghai Tongwei Biological Technology Co., Ltd. (Shanghai, China).

4.2. Animal Treatment

4.2.1. Animals

Forty-five rats (male, SHRs, SPF; body weight (BW), 240–280 g) were provided by Beijing Vital River Laboratory Animal Technology Co., Ltd. (Beijing, China). The rats were maintained under normal conditions and fed ad libitum under temperature (22 ± 3 °C), humidity (60 ± 5%), and light (12 h light/dark cycle) control. During all animal experiments, strong adherence to International Code of Ethics and National Institutes of Health guidelines for the care and use of laboratory animals was ensured. All rats were divided into three groups (n = 15 per group) after 1 week of feeding; these groups were (1) the control group (normal saline), (2) the positive group (captopril, 10 mg/kg BW dose), and (3) the QAGLSPVR group (QAGLSPVR, 20 mg/kg BW dose).

4.2.2. Measurement of Blood Pressure

The SBP and DBP of the SHRs were measured using the tail-cuff method (IITC Life Science, Woodland, CA., USA) 0, 1, 2, 3, 4, and 5 h after QAGLSPVR administration.

4.2.3. Determination of Serum ACE Activities

Serum was collected from SHRs at 0, 1, 2, 3, 4, and 5 h after intervention, and ACE activities were measured using a kit (Shanghai Tongwei Biological Technology Co., Ltd., Shanghai, China). The determination method strictly complied with the kit instructions.

4.3. Transepithelial Transport of QAGLSPVR

Caco-2 cells (1×10^5 cells/well) were routinely cultured in Dublecco's modified Eagle's medium with 15% FBS, 100 mg/mL streptomycin and 100 U/mL penicillin. Caco-2 cell monolayer was cultured in six-well Transwell plastic plates in a humidified incubator with 5% CO_2 at 37 °C and Caco-2 cell monolayer can be used to perform transport experiments when the transepithelial resistance is higher than 400 Ω/cm^2 [29]. The Caco-2 cell culture medium was substituted with Hank's balanced salt solution (HBSS) buffer (preheated at 37 °C for 30 min) prior to the transport experiment. The cell monolayer was cultured in HBSS buffer and maintained at 37 °C for 2 h. QAGLSPVR (2 mg/mL, 1.5 mL, dissolved in HBSS) was added to the AP of the cell monolayer, while HBSS buffer (2.5 mL) was added to the BL. The Caco-2 cell monolayer was cultured for 0.5, 1, or 2 h in an incubator at 37 °C. The AP and BL fractions were collected at different times. QAGLSPVR concentrations in the BL were detected by UPLC-Q-Orbitrap-MS^2 analysis according to our previous method [9], and the transport percentages of QAGLSPVR at different times were calculated.

The transport patterns of QAGLSPVR through the Caco-2 cell monolayer were studied using different transport inhibitors and enhancers [15]. In brief, Gly-Sar, wortmannin, and cytochalasin D were dissolved in DMSO (final concentration of DMSO in HBSS = 0.05%) and final concentrations of 25 mM, 500 nM, and 0.5 µg/mL, respectively. The Caco-2 cell monolayer was pre-incubated with Gly-Sar (a peptide transporter PepT1 substrate), wortmannin (a transcytosis inhibitor), or cytochalasin D (a TJ disruptor) for 30 min followed by addition of 1.5 mL of 2 mg/mL QAGLSPVR to the AP and 2.5 mL of fresh HBSS to the BL. After 2 h of incubation, the QAGLSPVR content in the BL was determined via UPLC-Q-Orbitrap-MS^2 analysis according to our previous method [9], and transport percentages were calculated.

4.4. Statistical Analysis

The data were expressed as mean ± standard deviation. Statistical analysis was performed using SPSS software (version 19.0, IBM Inc., Chicago, IL., USA). Differences were considered significant at p value < 0.05.

5. Conclusions

The antihypertensive effect in vivo of QAGLSPVR derived from tilapia skin gelatin hydrolysates was determined, and the peptide revealed a clear antihypertensive effect on SHRs. The ability of the peptide to inhibit ACE activity in serum was considered a key factor of the antihypertensive effect of QAGLSPVR in vivo. QAGLSPVR could be transported intact by the Caco-2 cell monolayer and may be transported through this layer via the paracellular pathway. Therefore, QAGLSPVR could be effectively absorbed and regulate hypertension in vivo.

Author Contributions: L.S. and Y.Z.: Project Design and Writing; B.W.: Sample Collection and Data Collection; M.Y.: Animal Experiment Analysis; L.S. and H.H.: Cell Experiment Analysis.

Funding: This research was funded by the National Natural Science Foundation of China, grant number: 31360381.

Conflicts of Interest: The authors declare no conflict of interest.

References

1. Abdelhedi, O.; Nasri, R.; Mora, L.; Jridi, M.; Toldra, F.; Nasri, M. In silico analysis and molecular docking study of angiotensin I-converting enzyme inhibitory peptides from smooth-hound viscera protein hydrolysates fractionated by ultrafiltration. *Food Chem.* **2018**, *239*, 453–463. [CrossRef]
2. Ngo, D.H.; Vo, T.S.; Ryu, B.M.; Kim, S.K. Angiotensin-I-converting enzyme (ACE) inhibitory peptides from Pacific cod skin gelatin using ultrafiltration membranes. *Process Biochem.* **2016**, *51*, 1622–1628.
3. Zhuang, Y.; Sun, L.; Li, B. Production of the angiotensin-I-converting enzyme (ACE)-inhibitory peptide from hydrolysates of jellyfish (*Rhopilema esculentum*) collagen. *Food Bio. Technol.* **2012**, *5*, 1622–1629. [CrossRef]

4. Zhuang, Y.; Sun, L.; Zhang, Y.; Liu, G. Antihypertensive effect of long-term oral administration of jellyfish (*Rhopilemaesculentum*) collagen peptides on renovascular hypertension. *Mar. Drugs* **2012**, *10*, 417–426. [CrossRef] [PubMed]

5. Guo, M.; Chen, X.; Wu, Y.; Zhang, L.; Huang, W.; Yuan, Y.; Fang, M.; Xie, J.; Wei, D. Angiotensin I-converting enzyme inhibitory peptides from Sipuncula (*Phascolosoma esculenta*): Purification, identification, molecular docking and antihypertensive effects on spontaneously hypertensive rats. *Process Biochem.* **2017**, *63*, 84–95. [CrossRef]

6. Foltz, M.; van der Pijl, P.C.; Duchateau, G.S. Current in vitro testing of bioactive peptides is not valuable. *J. Nutr.* **2010**, *140*, 117–118. [CrossRef] [PubMed]

7. García-Mora, P.; Martín-Martínez, M.; Bonache, M.A.; González-Múniz, R.; Peñas, E.; Frias, J.; Martinez-Villaluenga, C. Identification, functional gastrointestinal stability and molecular docking studies of lentil peptides with dual antioxidant and angiotensin I converting enzyme inhibitory activities. *Food Chem.* **2017**, *221*, 464–472. [CrossRef] [PubMed]

8. Ding, L.; Zhang, Y.; Jiang, Y.; Wang, L.; Liu, B.; Liu, J. Transport of egg white ACE-inhibitory peptide, Gln-Ile-Gly-Leu-Phe, in human intestinal Caco-2 cell monolayers with cytoprotective effect. *J. Agric. Food Chem.* **2014**, *62*, 3177–3182. [CrossRef] [PubMed]

9. Aiello, G.; Ferruzza, S.; Ranaldi, G.; Sambuy, Y.; Arnoldi, A.; Vistoli, G.; Lammi, C. Behavior of three hypocholesterolemic peptides from soy protein in an intestinal model based on differentiated Caco-2 cell. *J. Func. Food.* **2018**, *45*, 363–370. [CrossRef]

10. Yuan, L.; Sun, L.; Zhuang, Y. Preparation and identification of novel inhibitory angiotensin-I-converting enzyme peptides from tilapia skin gelatin hydrolysates: Inhibition kinetics and molecular docking. *Food Func.* **2018**, *9*, 5251–5259.

11. Balti, R.; Bougatef, A.; Sila, A.; Guillochon, D.; Dhulster, P.; Nedjar-Arroume, N. Nine novel angiotensin I-converting enzyme (ACE) inhibitory peptides from cuttlefish (*Sepia officinalis*) muscle protein hydrolysates and antihypertensive effect of the potent active peptide in spontaneously hypertensive rats. *Food Chem.* **2015**, *170*, 519–525. [CrossRef]

12. Fujita, H.; Yokoyama, K.; Yoshikawa, M. Classification and antihypertensive activity of angiotensin I-converting enzyme inhibitory peptides derived from food proteins. *J. Food Sci.* **2000**, *65*, 564–569.

13. Zhao, Y.; Li, B.; Dong, S.; Liu, Z.; Zhao, X.; Wang, J.; Zeng, M. A novelACE inhibitory peptide isolated from Acaudina molpadioidea hydrolysate. *Peptides* **2009**, *30*, 1028–1033. [CrossRef] [PubMed]

14. Albaladejo, P.; Bouaziz, H.; Duriez, M.; Gohlke, P.; Levy, B.I.; Safar, M.E.; Benetos, A. Angiotensin converting enzyme inhibition prevents the increase in aortic collagen in rats. *Hypertension* **1994**, *23*, 74. [CrossRef] [PubMed]

15. Boonla, O.; Kukongviriyapan, U.; Pakdeechote, P.; Kukongviriyapan, V.; Pannangpetch, P.; Thawornchinsombut, S. Peptides-derived from thai rice bran improves endothelial function in 2K-1C renovascular hypertensive rats. *Nutrients* **2015**, *7*, 5783–5799. [CrossRef]

16. Ding, L.; Wang, L.; Zhang, T.; Yu, Z.; Liu, J. Hydrolysis and transepithelial transport of two corn gluten derived bioactive peptides in human Caco-2 cell monolayers. *Food Res. Int.* **2018**, *106*, 475–480. [CrossRef] [PubMed]

17. Howell, S.; Kenny, A.J.; Turner, A.J. A survey of membrane peptidases in two human colonic cell lines, Caco-2 and HT-29. *Biochem. J.* **1992**, *284*, 595–601. [CrossRef]

18. Ding, L.; Wang, L.; Yu, Z.; Zhang, T.; Liu, J. Digestion and absorption of an egg white ACE-inhibitory peptide in human intestinal Caco-2 cell monolayers. *Int. J. Food Sci. Nut.* **2016**, *67*, 111–116. [CrossRef]

19. Fernández-Tomé, S.; Sanchón, J.; Recio, I.; Hernández-Ledesma, B. Transepithelial transport of lunasin and derived peptides: Inhibitory effects on the gastrointestinal cancer cells viability. *J. Food Comp. Ana.* **2018**, *68*, 101–110. [CrossRef]

20. Cakir-Kiefer, C.; Miclo, L.; Balandras, F.; Dary, A.; Soligot, C.; Le Roux, Y. Transport across Caco-2 cell monolayer and sensitivity to hydrolysis of two anxiolytic peptides from alpha(s1)-casein, alpha-casozepine, and alpha(s1)-casein-(f91−97): Effect of bile salts. *J. Agric. Food Chem.* **2011**, *59*, 11956–11965. [CrossRef]

21. Martínez-Maqueda, D.; Miralles, B.; Recio, I.; Hernández-Ledesma, B. Antihypertensive peptides from food proteins: A review. *Food Func.* **2012**, *3*, 350–361. [CrossRef]

22. Chen, M.; Li, B. The effect of molecular weights on the survivability of caseinderived antioxidant peptides after the simulated gastrointestinal digestion. *Innov. Food Sci. Emer. Technol.* **2012**, *16*, 341–348. [CrossRef]

23. Miner-Williams, W.M.; Stevens, B.R.; Moughan, P.J. Are intact peptides absorbed from the healthy gut in the adult human. *Nutr. Res. Rev.* **2014**, *27*, 308–329. [CrossRef]

24. Terada, T.; Inui, K.I. (Section A: Molecular, structural, and cellular biology of drug transporters) Peptide transporters: Structure, function, regulation and application for drug delivery. *Curr. Drug Metab.* **2004**, *5*, 85–94. [CrossRef]

25. Ding, L.; Wang, L.; Zhang, Y.; Liu, J. Transport of antihypertensive peptide RVPSL, ovotransferrin 328–332, in human intestinal Caco-2 cell monolayers. *J. Agric. Food Chem.* **2015**, *63*, 8143–8150. [CrossRef]

26. Shimizu, K.; Sato, M.; Zhang, Y.; Kouguchi, T.; Takahata, Y.; Morimatsu, F.; Shimizu, M. Molecular size of collagen peptide reverses the permeability of Caco-2 cells. *Biosci. Biotechnol. Biochem.* **2010**, *74*, 1123–1125. [CrossRef] [PubMed]

27. Quirós, A.; Contreras, M.D.M.; Ramos, M.; Amigo, L.; Recio, I. Stability to gastrointestinal enzymes and structure–activity relationship of b-casein peptides with antihypertensive properties. *Peptides* **2009**, *30*, 1848–1853. [CrossRef]

28. Guo, Y.; Gan, J.; Zhu, Q.; Zeng, X.; Sun, Y.; Wu, Z.; Pan, D. Transepithelial transport of milk-derived angiotensin I-converting enzyme inhibitory peptide with the RLSFNP sequence. *J. Sci. Food Agric.* **2017**, *98*, 976–983. [CrossRef]

29. Sun, L.; Liu, Q.; Fan, J.; Li, X.; Zhuang, Y. Purification and characterization of peptides inhibiting MMP-1 activity with C-terminate of Gly-Leu from simulated gastrointestinal digestion hydrolysates of tilapia (*Oreochromis niloticus*) skin gelatin. *J. Agric. Food Chemi.* **2018**, *66*, 593–601.

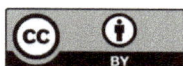

marine drugs

MDPI

Article

Preparation, Identification, and Activity Evaluation of Eight Antioxidant Peptides from Protein Hydrolysate of Hairtail (*Trichiurus japonicas*) Muscle

Xiu-Rong Yang [1], Lun Zhang [1], Dong-Ge Ding [1], Chang-Feng Chi [2,*], Bin Wang [1,*] and Jian-Cong Huo [1]

[1]   Zhejiang Provincial Engineering Technology Research Center of Marine Biomedical Products, School of Food and Pharmacy, Zhejiang Ocean University, 1st Haidanan Road, Zhoushan 316022, China; yxr1948008999@163.com (X.-R.Y.); Zl15525864652@163.com (L.Z.); 9001000@163.com (D.-G.D.); yujia0112@sina.com (J.-C.H.)

[2]   National and Provincial Joint Laboratory of Exploration and Utilization of Marine Aquatic Genetic Resources, National Engineering Research Center of Marine Facilities Aquaculture, School of Marine Science and Technology, Zhejiang Ocean University, 1st Haidanan Road, Zhoushan 316022, China

*   Correspondence: chichangfeng@hotmail.com (C.-F.C.); wangbin4159@hotmail.com (B.W.); Tel./Fax: +86-580-255-4818 (C.-F.C.); Tel./Fax: +86-580-255-4781 (B.W.)

Received: 12 November 2018; Accepted: 26 December 2018; Published: 2 January 2019

Abstract: In this report, protein of hairtail (*Trichiurus japonicas*) muscle was separately hydrolyzed using five kinds of proteases (alcalase, trypsin, neutrase, pepsin, and papain), and the papain- and alcalase-hydrolysates showed higher 2,2-diphenyl-1-picrylhydrazyl radicals (DPPH•) and hydroxyl radical (HO•) scavenging activity than other three protease hydrolysates. Therefore, the protein hydrolysate of hairtail muscle (HTP) was prepared using binary-enzymes hydrolysis process (papain + alcalase). Subsequently, eight antioxidant peptides were purified from HTP using membrane ultrafiltration and chromatography technology, and their amino acid sequences were identified as Gln-Asn-Asp-Glu-Arg (TJP1), Lys-Ser (TJP2), Lys-Ala (TJP3), Ala-Lys-Gly (TJP4), Thr-Lys-Ala (TJP5), Val-Lys (TJP6), Met-Lys (TJP7), and Ile-Tyr-Gly (TJP8) with molecular weights of 660.3, 233.0, 217.1, 274.1, 318.0, 245.1, 277.0, and 351.0 Da, respectively. TJP3, TJP4, and TJP8 exhibited strong scavenging activities on DPPH• (EC$_{50}$ 0.902, 0.626, and 0.663 mg/mL, respectively), HO• (EC$_{50}$ 1.740, 2.378, and 2.498 mg/mL, respectively), superoxide anion radical (EC$_{50}$ 2.082, 2.538, and 1.355 mg/mL, respectively), and 2,2′-azino-bis-3-ethylbenzothiazoline-6-sulfonic acid (ABTS) radical (EC$_{50}$ 1.652, 0.831, and 0.586 mg/mL, respectively). Moreover, TJP3, TJP4, and TJP8 showed higher reducing power and inhibiting ability on lipid peroxidation in a linoleic acid model system. These results suggested that eight isolated peptides (TJP1 to TJP8), especially TJP3, TJP4, and TJP8 might serve as potential antioxidants applied in the pharmaceutical and health food industries.

Keywords: hairtail (*Trichiurus japonicas*); muscle; peptide; antioxidant activity

1. Introduction

Reactive oxygen species (ROS) such as superoxide anion radical (O$_2^-$•), hydrogen peroxide (H$_2$O$_2$), hydroxyl radical (HO•), and singlet oxygen (^{1}O$_2$), are formed in aerobic organisms as a natural by-product of oxygen metabolism and play vital roles in the physiological processes involved in signal transduction and homeostasis [1,2]. Under normal conditions, superfluous ROS are effectively eliminated by antioxidant enzymes and non-enzymatic factors in organisms [3]. An imbalance in pro-oxidant/antioxidant can induce oxidative stress, trigger accumulated ROS production, and result in cell damage and many health disorders, such as diabetes mellitus, coronary heart diseases, cancer, hepatic diseases, and inflammatory diseases [4,5]. Additionally, oxidation is believed to the major course of food deterioration because ROS-mediated oxidation can react with lipids, proteins, amino acids, vitamins, and cholesterol to produce undesirable off-flavors, and potentially toxicity during food processing, transportation, and storage [3,6]. Therefore, it is very important for pharmaceutical, health food, and food processing and preservation industries to develop efficient antioxidants [7]. At present, some artificial antioxidants including butylated hydroxytoluene (BHT), butylated hydroxyanisole (BHA), and tertiary butylhydroquinone (TBHQ) show stronger antioxidant activities and have been widely used in medicine and food industry for retarding oxidation in organisms and food [4,7]. However, the side effects of synthetic antioxidants such as liver damage and carcinogenesis causes consumer anxiety and significantly affect their application [7,8]. Therefore, there has been a major interest in searching for efficient antioxidants from natural sources as alternatives to synthetic antioxidants for countering these adverse effects.

At present, dietary antioxidant ingredients including vitamins, carotenoids, flavonoids, phenols, saccharides, and peptides, have been continually investigated for their health benefits in terms of their scavenging potential of free radicals and low toxicity [9]. Among them, bioactive peptides released from food proteins under controlled proteolysis have aroused wide public concern not only in their possibilities as natural alternatives to synthetic antioxidants, but also for their beneficial effects, lack of residual side effects, and functionality in food systems [10].

Antioxidant peptides from food resources are inactive in the amino acid sequence of their parent proteins and are produced by in vitro enzymatic hydrolysis [7]. These peptides with 2 to 20 amino acid residues are considered to be easy absorption and no hazardous immunoreactions. More importantly, antioxidant peptides can exert their activity as free radical scavengers, peroxide decomposers, metal inactivators and oxygen inhibitors to protect food and organisms from ROS [11–13]. In recent years, antioxidant peptides derived from seafood were more attractive and have been isolated and identified from diverse marine organisms, such as swim bladders of miiuy croaker (*Miichthys miiuy*) [6], bluefin leatherjacket (*Navodon septentrionalis*) heads and skin [8,14], thornback ray skins [15], *Palmaria palmate* [16], viscera and carcass of Nile tilapia [17], *Pinctada fucata* [18], pectoral fin of salmon [19], and jellyfish gonad [20]. Zhao et al. isolated ten antioxidant peptides from swim bladders of miiuy croaker, and PYLRH and GIEWA exhibited stronger scavenging activities on 2,2-diphenyl-1-picrylhydrazyl radicals (DPPH•), hydroxyl radical (HO•), and superoxide anion radical (O_2^- •) than other eight peptides. Furthermore, FPYLRH and GIEWA could effectively inhibit lipid peroxidation in the β-carotene linoleic acid and in the linoleic acid emulsion system [6]. Harnedy et al. prepared and identified 17 peptides from the macroalgal species *Palmaria palmata*, and SDITRPGGNM showed the highest oxygen radical absorbance capacity and ferric reducing antioxidant power activity with values of 152.43 ± 2.73 and 21.23 ± 0.90 nmol TE/μmol peptide, respectively [16]. MCLDSCLL (P1) and HPLDSLCL (P2) showed potent antioxidant activities against DPPH• and 2,2'-azinobis-(3-ethylbenzothiazoline-6-sulfonic acid) (ABTS) radical (ABTS⁺•) and inhibiting copper-catalyzed human low-density lipoprotein (LDL) oxidation [21]. GAERP, GEREANVM, and AEVG from cartilage protein hydrolysate of spotless smoothhound exhibited good scavenging activities on DPPH•, HO•, ABTS⁺•, and O_2^- •. Furthermore, GAERP, GEREANVM, and AEVG could protect H_2O_2-induced HepG2 cells from oxidative stress by decreasing the content of malonaldehyde (MDA) and increasing the levels of superoxide dismutase (SOD), catalase (CAT), glutathione peroxidase (GSH-Px), and glutathione reductase (GSH-Rx) [12]. These studies indicated that seafood-derived peptides had strong antioxidant activity and could be served as ingredients in functional food and food systems to protect food quality by reducing oxidative stress.

Hairtail (*Trichiurus japonicas*) belongs to cutlassfish family of Trichiuridae and is found throughout tropical and temperate waters worldwide. In China, hairtail is one of the four major aquatic products and wildly distributed in the Yellow Sea, the Bo Hai Sea, and the East China Sea. In our previous research, hairtail hydrolysates chelation with iron (Fe-FPH chelate) had higher hemoglobin regeneration efficiency (HRE), longer exhaustive swimming time, and higher SOD activity.

Additionally, Fe-FPH chelate was found to significantly decrease levels the MDA content, visibly enhance the GSH-Px activity in liver and reduce blood lactic acid of rats [22,23]. Therefore, the aim of this work was to (i) optimize the two-step sequential enzymolysis technology; (ii) isolate and identify the antioxidant peptides; and (iii) evaluate the activities of isolated peptides form protein hydrolysate of hairtail muscle in vitro.

2. Results and Discussion

2.1. Preparation of Protein Hydrolysate from Hairtail (T. japonicas) Muscle (HTP)

2.1.1. Effect of Different Proteases on Protein Hydrolysates from Hairtail (*T. japonicas*) Muscle (HTP)

HO• is a highly reactive radical and can destroy all types of macromolecules such as nucleic acids (mutations), carbohydrates, lipids (lipid peroxidation), proteins and amino acids [24]. DPPH is the traditional and perhaps the most popular standard of the position (g-marker) and intensity of electron paramagnetic resonance (EPR) signals [25]. Therefore, DPPH• and HO• has been widely applied to evaluate the antioxidant ability of compounds to act as free radical scavengers or hydrogen donors [7,25,26].

Chemical treatment, enzymatic hydrolysis, and microbial fermentation of food proteins can be used for bioactive peptides production. However, the enzymatic hydrolysis method is preferred in the food and pharmaceutical industries because the other methods may leave residual organic solvents or toxic chemicals in the final products [7]. Treatment of protein substrate with different proteases will produce several types of protein hydrolysates, which exhibit various extents of antioxidant activities against various antioxidant systems [7,14]. Therefore, the specificity of the enzyme used for the proteolysis is one of the most important factors for the production of bioactive peptides.

In the experiment, defatted proteins of hairtail muscle were separately hydrolyzed with alcalase, trypsin, neutrase, pepsin, and papain at designed conditions and the antioxidant capacities of the resulted hydrolysates at the concentration of 6.0 mg protein/mL were shown in Figure 1. The data indicated that HO• scavenging capacities of the protein hydrolysates were significantly influenced by the type of protease ($p < 0.05$). The DPPH• scavenging activities of alcalase and papain hydrolysates were 53.45 ± 1.05% and 47.75 ± 2.34%, respectively, which were significantly higher than those of trypsin (37.05 ± 0.97%), neutrase (35.05 ± 0.97%), and pepsin (39.85 ± 1.28%) hydrolysates ($p < 0.05$) (Figure 1A). The HO• scavenging activities of neutrase, alcalase, and papain hydrolysates were 50.61 ± 1.16%, 48.76 ± 1.64%, and 48.89 ± 1.58%, respectively, which were significantly higher than those of trypsin (35.21 ± 0.67%) and pepsin (33.29 ± 1.01%) hydrolysates ($p < 0.05$) (Figure 1B). However, there were no significant differences on the HO• scavenging activities of neutrase, alcalase, and papain hydrolysates at the concentration of 6.0 mg protein/mL ($p > 0.05$). In addition, the active sites of papain were lie in basic amino acids, particularly Arg- and Lys-; and the active sites of alcalase were lie in Ala-, Leu-, Val-, Tyr-, Phe-, and Try-. The active sites are significantly different between alcalase and papain, which will help to shorten the hydrolysis time and improve the hydrolysis degree (DH) of protein hydrolysates [7,27,28].

Under the designed conditions, the protein hydrolysate of hairtail (*T. japonicas*) muscle was prepared using binary-enzymes hydrolysis process (papain + alcalase) and referred to as HTP, and the antioxidant activity of protein hydrolysates was presented in Figure 2. At the concentration of 6.0 mg protein/mL, DPPH• and HO• scavenging activities of HTP were 60.72 ± 1.05% and 58.17 ± 1.53%, respectively, which was significantly higher than those of the hydrolysates prepared separately using papain and alcalase ($p < 0.05$). Therefore, papain and alcalase were selected for the preparation of protein hydrolysate of hairtail muscle.

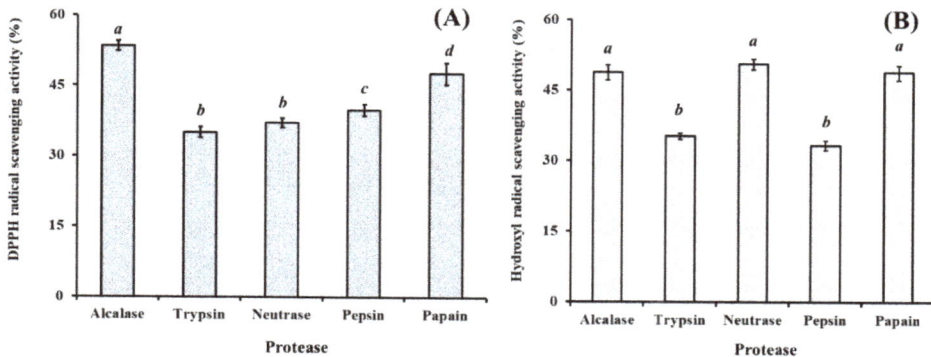

Figure 1. DPPH• (**A**) and HO• (**B**) scavenging activities of different enzymatic hydrolysates from hairtail (*T. japonicas*) muscle at the concentration of 6.0 mg protein/mL. All data are presented as the mean ± SD of triplicate results. [a–d] Values with same letters indicate no significant difference of different sample at same concentrations ($p > 0.05$).

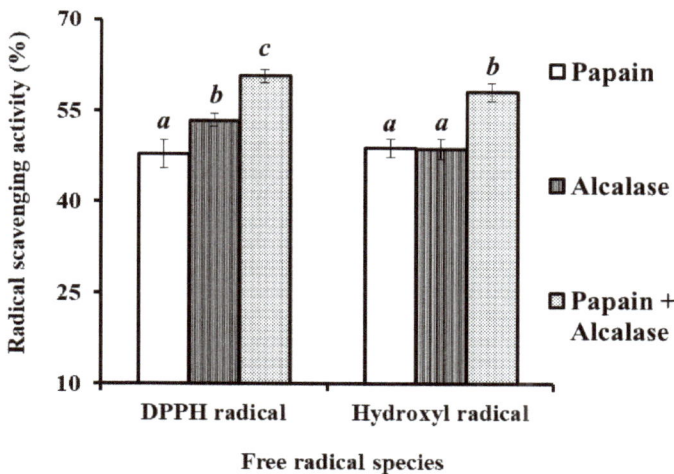

Figure 2. Effect of Papain, Alcalase, and Papain + Alcalase on DPPH• and HO• scavenging activities of protein hydrolysates from hairtail (*T. japonicas*) muscle at the concentration of 6.0 mg protein/mL. All data are presented as the mean ± SD of triplicate results. [a–c] Values with same letters indicate no significant difference of different sample at same concentrations ($p > 0.05$).

2.2. Purification of Antioxidant Peptides from Protein Hydrolysate from Hairtail (T. japonicas) Muscle (HTP)

2.2.1. Fractionation of HTP Using Membrane Ultrafiltration

Membrane ultrafiltration is usually used to enrich the particle sizes of functional molecules and is widely applied in food and beverage processing, biotechnological applications, and pharmaceutical industry [6,7]. Consequently, HTP was divided into four fractions including HTP-I (<1 kDA), HTP-II (1–3 kDa), HTP-III (3–5 kDa), and HTP-IV (>5 kDa) by ultrafiltration with a molecular weight (MW) Cut Off (MWCO) membrane of 1, 3, and 5 kDa. At the concentration of 6.0 mg protein/mL, DPPH• and HO• scavenging activities of HTP-I were 62.13 ± 1.97% and 78.6 ± 1.74%, respectively, which were significantly stronger than those of HTP, HTP-II, HTP-III, and HTP-IV ($p < 0.05$) (Figure 3). The activities of protein hydrolysates and their fractions were affected by the multiple peptides with different chain length and amino acid composition. Sila et al. [7] and Chi et al. [29] reported that MWs of hydrolysates play an important factor in their bioactivities, and hydrolysate fractions with smaller MW showed stronger antioxidant activity than those of larger MW hydrolysates. In the report, HTP-I with short chain peptides showed stronger radical scavenging activity, and this finding was in line with previous reports that the antioxidant abilities of protein hydrolysates were negatively correlated with their average MW [29,30]. Therefore, HTP-I was selected for the subsequent chromatographic separation.

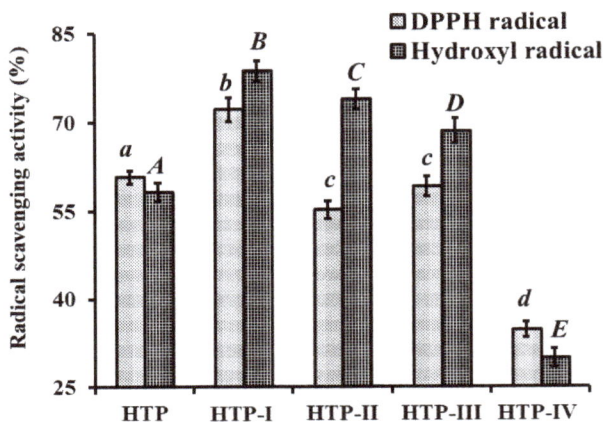

Figure 3. DPPH• and HO• scavenging activity of HTP and its fractions by membrane ultrafiltration at the concentration of 6.0 mg protein/mL. All data are presented as the mean ± SD of triplicate results. $^{a-c}$ or $^{A-E}$ Column wise values with same superscripts of this type indicate no significant difference ($p > 0.05$).

2.2.2. Anion-Exchange Chromatography of HTP-I

Peptides contain acidic and/or hydrophobic amino acid residues such as glutamic acid (Glu), tyrosine (Tyr), methionine (Met), and leucine (Leu), and can be sticks to the anion-exchange resins [31,32]. In addition, acidic and/or hydrophobic amino acid residues in amino acid sequences of peptides will enhance their bioactivities [7,33]. Therefore, anion exchange resins including DEAE-52 cellulose and Q Sepharose FF are usually applied to purified bioactive peptides from protein hydrolysates [8,34,35].

As shown in Figure 4A, five fractions (DE-1 to DE-5) were separated from HTP-I using a DEAE-52 cellulose column. Amongst them, DE-1 and DE-2 were eluted using deionized water, DE-3 was eluted using 0.1 M NaCl, DE-4 was eluted using 0.5 M NaCl, and DE-5 was eluted using 1.0 M NaCl. DPPH• and HO• scavenging activities of HTP-I and five eluted fractions were showed in Figure 4B, and the results indicated that DPPH• (58.91 ± 1.89%) and HO• (69.74 ± 2.61%) scavenging abilities of DE-3 were significantly stronger than those of HTP-I (DPPH•: 40.13 ± 1.16%; HO•: 45.6 ± 1.35%), DE-1 (DPPH•: 24.51 ± 1.06%; HO•: 37.9 ± 2.33%), DE-2 (DPPH•: 47.7 ± 1.51%; HO•: 35.29 ± 1.18%), DE-4 (DPPH•: 30.64 ± 1.25%; HO•: 29.39 ± 1.63%), and DE-5 (DPPH•: 7.29 ± 1.67%; HO•: 13.51 ± 0.99%) at the concentration of 5.0 mg protein/mL ($p < 0.05$). The results indicated that the highest antioxidant activity of the peptides obtained in DE-3 might be due to the acidic amino acid residues in their peptide sequences. Therefore, DE-3 was selected for the following experiment.

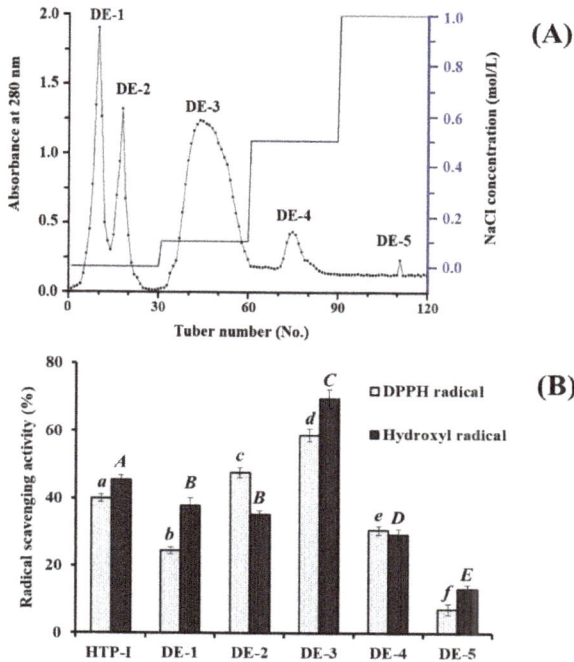

Figure 4. Elution profile of HTP-I in DEAE-52 cellulose anion-exchange chromatography (**A**) and radical scavenging activity of HTP-I and its four subfractions at the concentration of 5.0 mg protein/mL (**B**). All data are presented as the mean ± SD of triplicate results. $^{a-f}$ or $^{A-E}$ Values with same superscripts of this type indicate no significant difference ($p > 0.05$).

2.2.3. Gel Filtration Chromatography (GFC) of DE-3

GFC is a well-accepted separated technique on the basis of molecular size and usually applied to either fractionate molecules and complexes in a sample into fractions with a particular size range, or remove salt from a preparation of macromolecules [3,36]. Therefore, GFC is often used to separate peptides from protein hydrolysates and their fractions [6,7].

As shown in Figure 5A, DE-3 was separated into two fractions of DE-3-1 and DE-3-2 using a Sephadex G-15 column, and each fraction was collected, lyophilized, and then evaluated for DPPH• and HO• scavenging activity. Figure 5B indicated that DPPH• and HO• scavenging activities of DE-3-2 were 69.21 ± 0.91% and 84.16 ± 1.26% at the concentration of 5.0 mg protein/mL, which were significantly higher than those of DE-3 (DPPH• 58.91 ± 1.89%; HO• 69.74 ± 2.61%) and DE-3-1 (DPPH• 36.27 ± 0.79%; HO• 41.38 ± 1.49%) ($p < 0.05$). Therefore, fraction DE-3-2 was selected for the following isolation process.

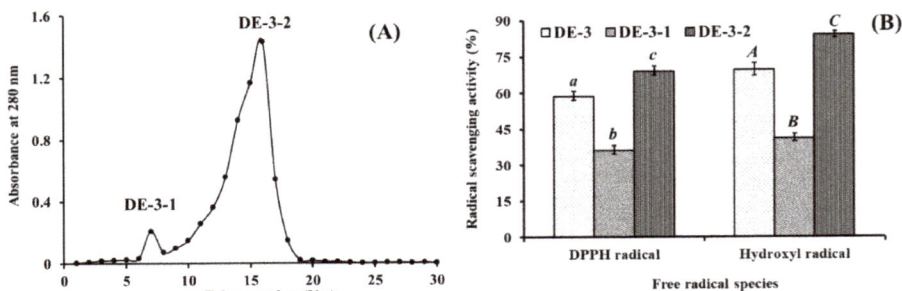

Figure 5. Elution profile of DE-3 in Sephadex G-15 chromatography (**A**) and radical scavenging activities of DE-3 and its fractions at 5.0 mg protein/mL concentration (**B**). All data are presented as the mean ± SD of triplicate results. [a-c] or [A-C] Column wise values with same superscripts of this type indicate no significant difference ($p > 0.05$).

2.2.4. Isolation of Peptides from DE-3-2 by Reverse-Phase High Performance Liquid Chromatography (RP-HPLC)

RP-HPLC is an effective technique applied to purify and quantify peptides in a mixture solution on their hydrophobic character [37]. The retention time (RT) can qualitatively analyze the isolated peptide and adjusted by changing the ratio of methanol or acetonitrile in mobile phase, and the peak area can be used for quantitative analysis of the isolated peptide [3,38]. As shown in Figure 6, DE-3-2 was finally purified using RP-HPLC system on an Agilent 1260 HPLC system with a Zorbax C-18 column, and the eluted peptides were gathered separately in accordance with chromatographic peaks. Among all chromatographic fractions, eight peptides with RT of 8.919 min (TJP1), 9.189 min (TJP2), 12.112 min (TJP3), 13.829 min (TJP4), 14.209 min (TJP5), 17.237 min (TJP6), 19.772 min (TJP7), and 20.436 min (TJP8) showed high radical scavenging activities. Therefore, TJP1-TJP8 were collected and lyophilized for amino acid sequence identification and activity evaluation.

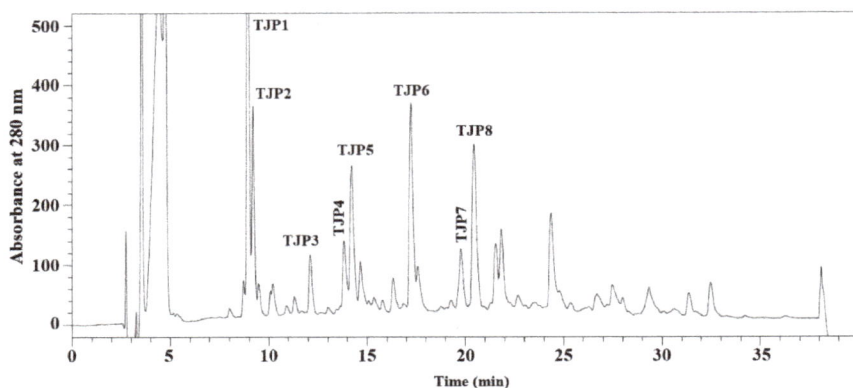

Figure 6. Elution profile of DE-3-2 separated by RP-HPLC system on a Zorbax, SB C-18 column (4.6 × 250 mm) from 0 to 40 min.

2.3. *Amino Acid Sequence Analysis and Mass Spectrometry of Peptides from Protein Hydrolysates of Hairtail Muscle*

For more detailed discussion on the structure-function relationship, the amino acid composition, sequences, and molecular mass of eight isolated peptides (TJP1-TJP8) were determined using protein sequencer and ESI-MS, and the results were shown in Figure 7 and Table 1. The amino acid sequences of eight isolated peptides (TJP1-TJP8) were identified as Gln-Asn-Asp-Glu-Arg (TJP1), Lys-Ser (TJP2), Lys-Ala (TJP3), Ala-Lys-Gly (TJP4), Thr-Lys-Ala (TJP5), Val-Lys (TJP6), Met-Lys (TJP7), and Ile-Tyr-Gly (TJP8) with molecular weights of 660.3, 233.0, 217.1, 274.1, 318.0, 245.1, 277.0, and 351.0 Da, respectively, which were agreed well with their theoretical masses of 660.6, 233.3, 217.3, 274.3, 318.4, 245.3, 277.4, and 351.4 Da.

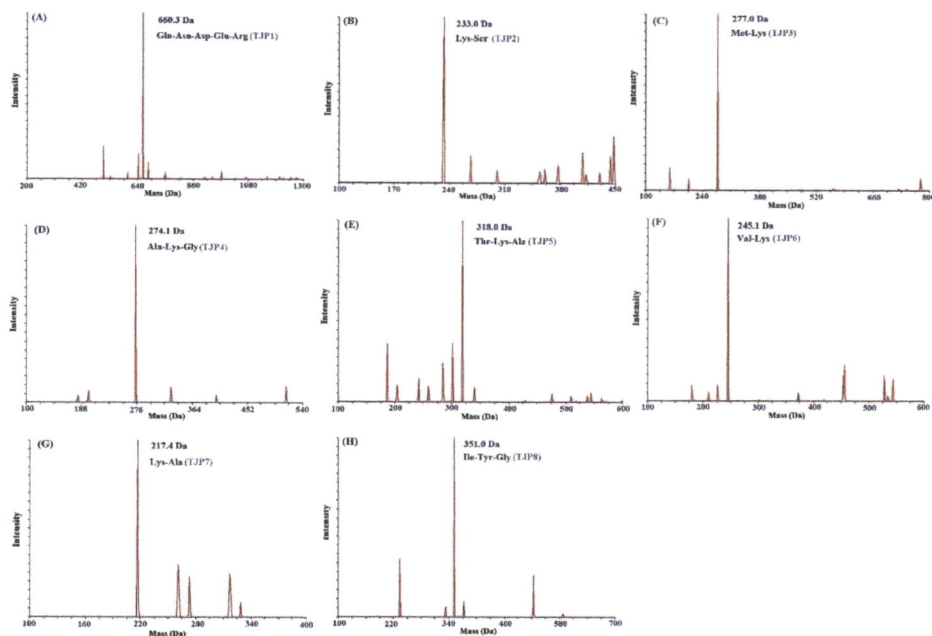

Figure 7. Mass spectra of TJP1 (A), TJP2 (B), TJP3 (C), TJP4 (D), TJP5 (E), TJP6 (F), TJP7 (G), and TJP8 (H) from protein hydrolysate of hairtail (*T. japonicas*) muscle.

Table 1. Retention time, amino acid sequences, and molecular mass of eight isolated peptides (TJP1 to TJP8) from protein hydrolysate of hairtail (*T. japonicas*) muscle.

	Retention time (min)	Amino acid sequence	Theoretical mass/observed mass (Da)
TJP1	8.919	Gln-Asn-Asp-Glu-Arg	660.3/660.6
TJP2	9.189	Lys-Ser	233.0/233.3
TJP3	12.112	Lys-Ala	217.1/217.3
TJP4	13.829	Ala-Lys-Gly	274.1/274.3
TJP5	14.209	Thr-Lys-Ala	318.0/318.4
TJP6	17.237	Val-Lys	245.1/245.3
TJP7	19.772	Met-Lys	277.0/277.4
TJP8	20.436	Ile-Tyr-Gly	351.0/351.4

2.4. Antioxidant Activity

To better evaluate the antioxidant activity of eight isolated peptides (TJP1 to TJP8) from protein hydrolysate of hairtail (*T. japonicas*) muscle, four kinds of radical (DPPH•, HO•, O_2^- •, and ABTS$^+$•) scavenging assays, reducing power, and lipid peroxidation inhibition assay were tested, and the results were presented in Table 2 and Figures 8–10.

Table 2. Radical scavenging activity of eight isolated peptides (TJP1 to TJP8) from protein hydrolysate of hairtail (*T. japonicas*) muscle.

	EC$_{50}$ (mg/mL)			
	DPPH•	**HO•**	**O$_2^-$ •**	**ABTS$^+$•**
TJP1	4.95	6.865	2.753	1.925
TJP2	7.68	5.634	4.296	2.496
TJP3	0.902	1.740	2.082	1.652
TJP4	0.626	2.378	2.538	0.831
TJP5	1.425	5.261	4.911	3.527
TJP6	1.262	3.845	>10.000	2.835
TJP7	3.150	4.993	4.427	8.752
TJP8	0.663	2.498	1.835	0.586
Glutathione (GSH)	0.251	0.758	0.456	0.078

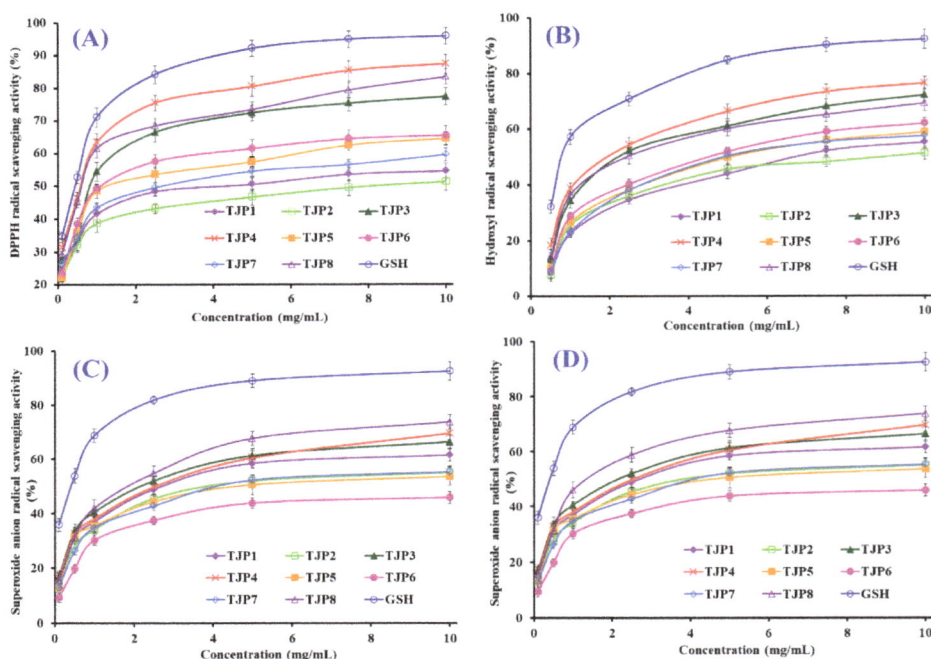

Figure 8. DPPH• (**A**); HO• (**B**); O$_2^-$ • (**C**); and ABTS$^+$• (**D**) scavenging activities of eight isolated peptides (TJP1 to TJP8) from protein hydrolysate of hairtail (*T. japonicas*) muscle. All data are presented as the mean ± SD of triplicate results.

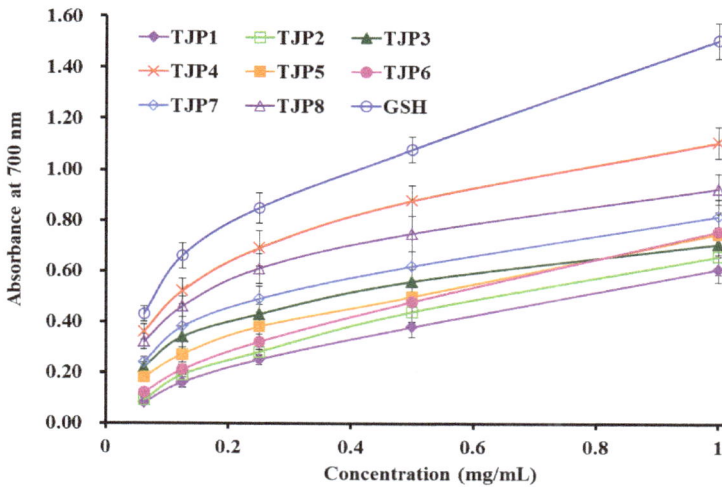

Figure 9. Reducing power of eight isolated peptides (TJP1 to TJP8) from protein hydrolysate of hairtail (*T. japonicas*) muscle. All data are presented as the mean ± SD of triplicate results.

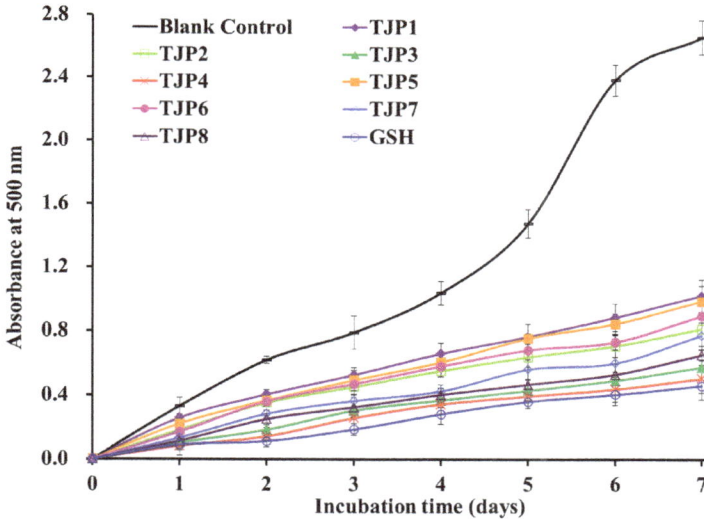

Figure 10. Lipid peroxidation inhibition assays of eight isolated peptides (TJP1 to TJP8) from protein hydrolysate of hairtail (*T. japonicas*) muscle. All data are presented as the mean ± SD of triplicate results.

2.4.1. Radical Scavenging Activity

DPPH• Scavenging Activity

DPPH• shows maximal absorbance at 517 nm in its oxidized form, and the absorbance wears off with the free radical accepting an electron [3]. As shown in Figure 8A, eight isolated peptides (TJP1 to TJP8) showed strong DPPH• scavenging activities and there was also a positive correlation between the concentration and the radical-scavenging activity. The half elimination ratio (EC_{50}) values of TJP3, TJP4, and TJP8 were 0.902, 0.626, and 0.663 mg/mL, respectively, and TJP4 exhibited the highest

DPPH• scavenging ability among eight isolated peptides, but its activity was still lower than that of the positive control of glutathione (GSH) at the same concentration. The EC_{50} value of TJP4 was lower than those of most antioxidant peptides from protein hydrolysates of loach (PSYV: 17.0 mg/mL) [39], miiuy croaker (GIEWA: 0.78 mg/mL) [6], scalloped hammerhead cartilage (GPE: 2.43 mg/mL; GARGPQ: 2.66 mg/mL; GFTGPPGFNG: 1.99 mg/mL) [12], blue mussel (YPPAK: 2.62 mg/mL) [26], bluefin leatherjacket (GPP: 1.927 mg/mL; WEGPK: 4.438 mg/mL; GVPLT: 4.541 mg/mL) [8,14], skate cartilages (FIMGPY: 2.60 mg/mL; GPAGDY: 3.48 mg/mL; IVAGPQ: 3.93 mg/mL) [24], grass carp skin (GFGPL: 2.249 mg/mL; VGGRP: 2.937 mg/mL) [40], and salmon pectoral fin (TTANIEDRR: 2.503 mg/mL) [41]. However, the EC_{50} value of TJP4 was higher than those of peptides from protein hydrolysates of Chinese leek (GSQ: 0.61 mg/mL) [42], miiuy croaker (FPYLRH: 0.51 mg/mL) [6], grass carp skin (HFGBPFH: 0.20 mg/mL) [40], and skate muscle (APPTAYAQS: 0.614 mg/mL; NWDMEKIWD 0.289 mg/mL) [10]. Therefore, these data indicated that eight isolated peptides (TJP1 to TJP8), especially TJP3, TJP4, and TJP8 had the strong capacity to contribute an electron or hydrogen radical for suppressing the DPPH• reaction.

HO• Scavenging Activity

HO• is a highly reactive radical to the organism and only can be eliminated by endogenous and dietary antioxidants. Therefore, it is the ideal assay for searching the radical scavenging agent of organism. The abilities of eight isolated peptides (TJP1 to TJP8) were investigated, and the dose-related effects were observed at different peptide concentrations ranging from 0 to 10.0 mg/mL (Figure 8B). EC_{50} values of TJP3, TJP4, and TJP8 were 1.740, 2.378, and 2.498 mg/mL, respectively, and TJP3 exhibited the highest HO• scavenging ability among all isolated peptides at the same concentration. EC_{50} value of TJP3 was lower than those of peptides from protein hydrolysates of bluefin leatherjacket heads (WEGPK: 5.567 mg/mL; GPP: 2.385 mg/mL; GVPLT: 4.149 mg/mL) [8], weatherfish loach (PSYV: 2.64 mg/mL) [39], skate cartilages (FIMGPY: 3.04 mg/mL; GPAGDY: 3.92 mg/mL; IVAGPQ: 5.03 mg/mL) [24], and grass carp skin (PYSFK: 2.283mg/mL; VGGRP: 2.055 mg/mL) [40]. However, the EC_{50} value of TJP3 was higher than those of antioxidant peptides from protein hydrolysates of miiuy croaker (FPYLRH: 0.68 mg/mL; GIEWA: 0.71 mg/mL) [6], spotless smoothhound cartilage (GAERP: 0.25 mg/mL; GEREANVM: 0.34 mg/mL; AEVG: 0.06 mg/mL) [3], blue mussel (YPPAK: 0.228 mg/mL) [26], giant squid (NGLEGLK: 0.313 mg/mL; NADFGLNGLEGLA: 0.612 mg/mL) [43], conger eel (LGLNGDDVN: 0.687 mg/mL) [44], and skate muscle (APPTAYAQS: 0.390 mg/mL; NWDMEKIWD 0.176 mg/mL) [10]. TJP3, TJP4, and TJP8 showed strong HO• scavenging ability, which indicated that it could serve as a HO• scavenger for decreasing or eliminating the damage caused by HO• in food industries and biological systems.

O_2^-• Scavenging Assay

O_2^-• is the most common free radical generated in vivo, and can promote oxidative reaction to generate peroxy and hydroxyl radicals. Superoxide dismutase protects the cell from the deleterious effects of superoxides in living organisms. Therefore, it is important to search safe and efficient antioxidants for scavenging O_2^-•. Figure 8C indicated the O_2^-• scavenging ratios of eight isolated peptides (TJP1 to TJP8) drastically increased with increasing concentration ranging from 0.1 to 10 mg/mL, but their activities were still lower than that of glutathione (GSH) at the same concentration. EC_{50} values of TJP3, TJP4, and TJP8 were 2.082, 2.538, and 1.355 mg/mL, respectively. Therefore, TJP8 played a significant role in O_2^-• scavenging. EC_{50} value of TJP8 was lower than those of peptides from protein hydrolysates of miiuy croaker swim bladders (FYKWP:1.92 mg/mL; FTGMD:3.04 mg/mL; YLPYA:3.61 mg/mL; GFYAA:3.03 mg/mL; FSGLR:3.35 mg/mL; VPDDD:4.11 mg/mL) [6], bluefin leatherjacket heads (WEGPK: 3.223 mg/mL; GPP: 4.668 mg/mL; GVPLT: 2.8819 mg/mL) [8], and skate cartilage (FIMGPY: 1.61 mg/mL; GPAGDY: 1.66 mg/mL; IVAGPQ: 1.82 mg/mL) [24]. However, EC_{50} value of TJP8 was higher than those of protein hydrolysates of croceine croaker muscle (YLMR: 0.450 mg/mL; VLYEE: 0.693 mg/mL; MILMR: 0.993 mg/mL) [32], skate muscle

(APPTAYAQS: 0.215 mg/mL; NWDMEKIWD 0.132 mg/mL) [10], *Mytilus coruscus* (SLPIGLMIAM: 0.3168 mg/mL) [45], miiuy croaker swim bladders (GFEPY: 0.87 mg/mL; FPPYERRQ: 0.68 mg/mL; FPYLRH: 0.34 mg/mL; GIEWA: 0.30 mg/mL) [6], round scad (HDHPVC: 0.265 mg/mL; HEKVC: 0.235 mg/mL) [46], monkfish muscle (EWPAQ: 0.624 mg/mL; FLHRP: 0.101 mg/mL; LMGQW: 0.042 mg/mL) [47], and croceine croaker scales (GFRGTIGLVG: 0.463 0.151 mg/mL; GPAGPAG: 0.099 mg/mL; GFPSG: 0.151 mg/mL) [48]. $O_2^- \bullet$ is catalyzed into hydrogen peroxide and oxygen by superoxide dismutases (SOD) in organism. Therefore, TJP3, TJP4, and TJP8 can be applied to eliminate $O_2^- \bullet$ damage together with SOD in biological systems.

ABTS$^+\bullet$ Scavenging Assay

The ABTS$^+\bullet$ is reactive towards most antioxidants and the blue ABTS$^+\bullet$ with an absorption maximum of 734 nm is converted back to its colorless neutral form during this reaction [3]. Therefore, ABTS$^+\bullet$ scavenging assay is one of the most widely assay used to screen anti-radical peptides. As shown in Figure 8D, eight isolated peptides (TJP1 to TJP8) showed strong ABTS$^+\bullet$ scavenging activities in a dose-effect manner with EC_{50} values of 1.925, 2.496, 1.652, 0.831, 3.527, 2.835, 8.752, and 0.586 mg/mL, respectively. TJP4 and TJP8 showed the strongest ABTS$^+\bullet$ scavenging activity among eight isolated peptides, but still weaker than glutathione (GSH) did at the same concentration. The EC_{50} values of TJP4 and TJP8 were significantly lower than those of peptides from protein hydrolysates of salmon (FLNEFLHV: 1.548 mg/mL) [41], skate cartilages (FIMGPY: 1.04 mg/mL; IVAGPQ: 1.29 mg/mL) [24], bluefin leatherjacket heads (WEGPK: 5.407 mg/mL; GPP: 2.472 mg/mL; GVPLT: 3.124 mg/mL) [8], and corn gluten meal (FLPF: 1.497 mg/mL; LPF: 1.013 mg/mL; LLPF: 1.031 mg/mL) [49]. However, The EC_{50} values of TJP4 and TJP8 were significantly higher than those of peptides from protein hydrolysates of skate cartilages (GPAGDY: 0.77 mg/mL) [24], grass carp skin (GFGPL: 0.328 mg/mL; VGGRP: 0.465 mg/mL) [40], scalloped hammerhead cartilage (GPE: 0.24 mg/mL; GARGPQ: 0.18 mg/mL; GFTGPPGFNG: 0.29 mg/mL) [12], and *Sphyrna lewini* muscle (WDR:0.34 mg/mL; PYFNK: 0.12 mg/mL) [33]. These results indicated that eight isolated peptides (TJP1 to TJP8), especially TJP4 and TJP8, have the strong ability to convert ABTS$^+\bullet$ to its colorless neutral form and hold back the radical chain reaction.

2.4.2. Reducing Power

The reducing power is an important indicator for evaluating the activities of antioxidant peptides [30]. As shown in Figure 9, eight isolated peptides (TJP1 to TJP8) exhibited dose-dependent reducing power at the concentrations ranged from 0.5 mg/mL to 10 mg/mL, and TJP4 showed the higher capacity to reduce ferric ions (Fe^{3+}) to ferrous ions (Fe^{2+}) than other seven antioxidant peptides. However, the reducing power of eight isolated peptides (TJP1 to TJP8) was lower that of the positive control of GPS.

2.4.3. Lipid Peroxidation Inhibition Assay

In the experiment, DPPH$\bullet$, HO$\bullet$, $O_2^- \bullet$, and ABTS$^+\bullet$ scavenging assays have been used to assess the antioxidant activities of eight isolated peptides (TJP1 to TJP8), but oxidative process in biological systems or food products is complicated and embroiled in different kinds of reactions for propagation of lipid radicals and lipid hydroperoxides in the presence of oxygen [3,37]. The radical scavenging assays only measured an antioxidant property, which cannot reflect its role as an antioxidant to protect organism and/or food systems from lipid oxidation [3,32]. As a consequence, we investigated the abilities of eight isolated peptides (TJP1 to TJP8) to control lipid peroxidation in a linoleic acid model system, and the result was presented in Figure 10. The absorbance at 500 nm of sample solutions with eight isolated peptides (TJP1 to TJP8), respectively, was significantly lower than that of the negative control (without antioxidant), and TJP3, TJP4, and TJP8 revealed similar abilities on lipid oxidation inhibition to that of positive control of GSH. The presented results demonstrated that eight isolated peptides (TJP1 to TJP8) could effectively hold back lipid peroxidation in the tested system during seven days of incubation. Furthermore, eight isolated peptides (TJP1 to TJP8) were isolated from the food resource of hairtail (*T. japonicas*) muscl and considered safer than chemical antioxidants. Therefore, we can increase the using dose of isolated peptides (TJP1 to TJP8) to compensate the flaw that their antioxidant activity is lower than that of chemical antioxidants.

3. Discussion

At present, hundreds of antioxidant peptides have been isolated from different resources. However, there is still insufficient evidence to elucidate the structure-activity relationship of antioxidant peptides. Generally, molecular size, hydrophobicity, and amino acid composition and sequence are deemed to play key roles in their antioxidant capacities [7,50].

Bioactivities of antioxidant peptides are highly dependent on their molecular size because small antioxidants have the higher possibility to interact with free radicals to prevent the lipid peroxidation [3,33]. Furthermore, smaller peptides are more likely to pass through the blood-brain barrier to perform their physiological functions in the body and have the high possibility to develop into new drugs [30,51]. Therefore, shorter size peptides especially peptides with 2–10 amino acid residues are deemed to obtain stronger radical scavenging and lipid peroxidation inhibition activities than long-chain peptides [6,7]. In the study, eight isolated peptides (TJP1 to TJP8) from protein hydrolysate of hairtail muscle are dipeptides (TJP2, TJP3, TJP6, and TJP7), tripeptides (TJP4, TJP5, and TJP8), or pentapeptide (TJP1), which help them to contact the target more easily to exert their bioactive properties.

More importantly, amino acids play a critical role in the antioxidant of peptides. Sila and Bougatef reported that hydrophobic amino acids, such as Leu, Ile, Ala, Val, and Met, had high reactivity to hydrophobic PUFAs and exert their significant effects on radical scavenging in lipid-rich foods [7,33]. Zhao et al. presented that the Ile and Ala residues contribute to the lipid peroxidation inhibitory and radical-scavenging and activities of GIEWA [6]. Therefore, Ala in the sequence of TJP4 and Ile residues in the sequence of TJP8 should positively influence its antioxidant activity. Dávalos et al. [52] and Xing et al. [53] confirmed that Met residue showed the highest antioxidant activity among all the amino acids because its large hydrophobic group can help peptides to facilitate the contacts with hydrophobic radical species. Wu et al. further reported that Met residue in PMRGGGGYHY might work as a reactive site, where the peptide could scavenge oxidants through the formation of a sulfoxide structure after oxidation to stop free-radical chain reactions [54]. Moreover, aromatic residues of aromatic amino acids—including Phe, Trp, and Ty—can keep radical stable during the scavenging process through contributing protons to electron deficient radicals [38]. Tyr residues could turn free radicals into more stable phenoxy radicals to stop the peroxidizing chain reaction [55]. Therefore, Met residues in the sequences of TJP3 and Tyr residues in the sequences TJP8 should be the important contributors for the antioxidant activity of TJP3 and TJP8.

Polar amino acids is reported to play a critical role in HO• scavenging and metal ion chelating activities because of their carboxyl and amino groups in the side chains [56,57]. Zhu et al. reported that peptides consisted of Lys, Glu, and Asp were identified to have strong abilities to chelate metal ions as well as scavenge HO• [57]. Ren et al. have reported that basic peptides had greater capacity to scavenge HO• than acidic or neutral peptides [58]. Hu et al. reported that the presence of basic amino acid of Lys was one of the main reasons for the antioxidant activity of NWDMEKIWD [10]. Gly residue is found to contribute significantly to antioxidant activity since the single hydrogen atom in its side chain can provide a high flexibility to the peptide backbone, serving as proton-donors and neutralizing active free radical species [59,60]. Therefore, polar amino acids including Lys and Gly residues could play a critical role in the radical scavenging activities of TJP3, TJP4, and TJP8.

4. Experimental Section

4.1. Materials

Hairtail (*T. japonicas*) muscle was purchased from Fengmao Market in Zhoushan city of China. Bovine serum albumin (BSA), DEAE-52 cellulose and Sephadex G-15 were purchased from Shanghai Source Poly Biological Technology Co., Ltd. (Shanghai, China). Acetonitrile (ACN) of LC grade and trifluoroacetic acid (TFA) were purchased from Thermo Fisher Scientific Co., Ltd. (Shanghai, China). Phosphate buffered saline (PBS, pH 7.2), DPPH, and ABTS were purchased from Sigma Chemicals Co. (USA). QNDER(TJP1), KS(TJP2), KA(TJP3), AKG(TJP4), TKA(TJP5), VK(TJP6), MK(TJP7), and IYG(TJP8) with purity higher than 98% were synthesized in China Peptides Co. (Suzhou, China). All other reagents were analytical grade and purchased from Sinopharm Chemical Reagent Co., Ltd. (Shanghai, China).

4.2. Preparation of Protein Hydrolysate from Hairtail (*T. japonicas*) Muscle

The hairtail (*T. japonicas*) muscle was homogenized and blended with isopropanol at a ratio of 1:4 (w/v) and stand at 30 ± 2 °C for 1 h. The supernatant was drained and the residue was defatted using isopropanol at a ratio of 1:4 (w/v) at 75 ± 2 °C for 90 min. Finally, the supernatant was then removed and the solid precipitate was air-dried at 35 ± 2 °C.

The resulted precipitate was dispersed in distilled water (DW) at a ratio of 1:10 (w/v), and hydrolyzed separately using trypsin at pH 7.8, 37.5 °C, alcalase at pH 8.5, 50 °C, neutrase at pH 7.0, 50 °C, papain at pH 7.0, 50 °C and pepsin at pH 2.0, 37.5 °C with total enzyme dose 2% (w/w, 2 g enzyme/100 g defatted precipitate powder). In 4 h, the protein hydrolysates were heated to 95 °C for 10 min and centrifuged at 12,000 g for 15 min, and the five supernatants were lyophilized. Protein hydrolysates prepared separately using alcalase and papain exhibited the highest HO• scavenging activity among five protein hydrolysates. Therefore, defatted precipitate of hairtail muscle was scattered in DW at a ratio of 1:5 (w/v), and hydrolyzed using papain and alcalase for 5 and 6 h successively on above hydrolysis conditions. The resulted hydrolysate was treated in the same manner as the above method and referred to as HTP.

The concentrations of protein hydrolysate and its fractions were expressed as mg protein/mL and measured by the dye binding method of Bradford (1976) with BSA as the standard protein.

4.3. Isolation of Peptides from HTP

4.3.1. Fractionation of HTP by Ultrafiltration

HTP was fractionated using ultrafiltration (8400, Millipore, Hangzhou, China) with 1, 3, and 5 kDa MWCO membranes (Millipore, Hangzhou, China), and four fractions termed HTP-I (MW < 1 kDa), HTP-II (MW 1–3 kDa), HTP-III (MW 3–5 kDa), and HTP-IV (MW > 5 kDa) were collected and lyophilized.

4.3.2. Anion-Exchange Chromatography

HTP-I solution (5 mL, 40.0 mg/mL) was injected into a DEAE-52 cellulose column (1.6 × 80 cm) pre-equilibrated with DW, and stepwise eluted with 150 ml DW, 0.1 M NaCl, 0.5 M NaCl, and 1.0 M NaCl solution at a flow rate of 1.0 mL/min, respectively. Each eluate (5 mL) was monitored at 280 nm. Finally, five fractions (DE-1 to DE-5) were pooled and lyophilized on the chromatographic peaks.

4.3.3. Gel Filtration Chromatography

DE-3 solution (5 mL, 10.0 mg/mL) was separated on a Sephadex G-15 column (2.6 × 160 cm) eluted with DW at a flow rate of 0.6 mL/min. Each eluate (3 mL) was collected and monitored at 280 nm, and fraction of DE-3-2 with higher activity than others were collected and lyophilized.

4.3.4. RP-HPLC

DE-3-2 was further purified on an Agilent 1260 HPLC system (Agilent Ltd., Santa Rosa, California, USA) with a Zorbax, SB C-18 column (4.6 × 250 mm). The sample was eluated with a linear gradient of acetonitrile (0–50% in 0–40 min) in 0.1% TFA at a flow rate of 0.8 mL/min. Eight peptides (TJP1 to TJP8) were isolated on the absorbance at 280 nm and lyophilized.

4.4. Determination of Amino Acid Sequence and Molecular Mass

The amino acid sequences and molecular masses of eight isolated peptides (TJP1 to TJP8) was measured on an Applied Biosystems 494 protein sequencer (Perkin Elmer/Applied Biosystems Inc., Foster City, CA, USA) and a Q-TOF mass spectrometer coupled with an electrospray ionization source (ESI), respectively.

4.5. Antioxidant Activity

The DPPH•, HO•, O_2^-•, and ABTS$^+$• scavenging activities of eight isolated peptides (TJP1 to TJP8) were measured on the previous method [52], and the EC_{50} was defined as the concentration where a sample caused a 50% decrease of the initial concentration of radical. The reducing power assay of eight isolated peptides (TJP1 to TJP8) was determined by the description of a literature report [30]. The lipid peroxidation inhibition assay of eight isolated peptides (TJP1 to TJP8) were determined in a linoleic acid model system on the method of Wang et al. [33].

4.6. Statistical Analysis

The data are reported as the mean ± standard deviation (SD) with three determinations. A one-way analysis of variance (ANOVA) test for differences between means of each group was applied to analyzed data using SPSS 19.0 (Statistical Program for Social Sciences, SPSS Corporation, Chicago, IL, USA). A p-value of less than 0.05 was considered statistically significant.

5. Conclusions

In the experiment, eight isolated peptides (TJP1 to TJP8) from protein hydrolysate of hairtail (*T. japonicas*) muscle prepared with alcalase + papain were isolated and identified as QNDER (TJP1), KS (TJP2), KA (TJP3), AKG (TJP4), TKA (TJP5), VK (TJP6), MK (TJP7), and IYG (TJP8), respectively, which exhibited high antioxidant activities through radical scavenging, reducing power, and lipid peroxidation inhibition assays. On the present results, the peptide fractions and isolated peptides (TJP1 to TJP8) from protein hydrolysate of hairtail (*T. japonicas*) muscle may be applied as an ingredient in new functional foods, and detailed studies will be done to illustrate the relationship between the activities and structures of eight isolated peptides. In addition, animal feeding experiments on isolated peptides (TJP1 to TJP8) will be conducted to evaluate their in vivo antioxidant effects.

Author Contributions: B.W. and J.-C.H. conceived and designed the experiments. X.-R.Y., D.-G.D., and L.Z. performed the experiments and analyzed the data. C.-F.C. and B.W. contributed the reagents, materials, and analytical tools and wrote the paper.

Funding: This work was funded by the National Natural Science Foundation of China (NSFC) (no. 81673349), International S&T Cooperation Program of China (2012DFA30600), Zhejiang Province Public Technology Research Project (LGN18D060002), and Natural Science Foundation of Zhejiang Province of China (LY17C200011).

Acknowledgments: The authors thank Zhao-Hui Li at Beijing agricultural biological testing center for his technical support on the isolation and amino acid sequence identification of peptides from hairtail (*T. japonicas*) muscle.

Conflicts of Interest: The authors declare no conflict of interest.

References

1. Rahman, M.S.; Choi, Y.H.; Choi, Y.S.; Alam, M.B.; Lee, S.H.; Yoo, J.C. A novel antioxidant peptide, purified from Bacillus amyloliquefaciens, showed strong antioxidant potential via Nrf-2 mediated heme oxygenase-1 expression. *Food Chem.* **2018**, *239*, 502–510. [CrossRef] [PubMed]
2. Zheng, Z.; Si, D.; Ahmad, B.; Li, Z.; Zhang, R. A novel antioxidative peptide derived from chicken blood corpuscle hydrolysate. *Food Res. Int.* **2018**, *106*, 410–419. [CrossRef] [PubMed]
3. Tao, J.; Zhao, Y.Q.; Chi, C.F.; Wang, B. Bioactive peptides from cartilage protein hydrolysate of spotless smoothhound and their antioxidant activity In vitro. *Mar. Drugs* **2018**, *16*, 100. [CrossRef] [PubMed]
4. Gogineni, V.; Hamann, M.T. Marine natural product peptides with therapeutic potential: Chemistry, biosynthesis, and pharmacology. *BBA—Gen. Subj.* **2018**, *1862*, 81–196. [CrossRef] [PubMed]
5. Carocho, M.; Morales, P.; Ferreira, I.C.F.R. Antioxidants: Reviewing the chemistry, food applications, legislation and role as preservatives. *Trends Food Sci. Technol.* **2018**, *71*, 107–120. [CrossRef]
6. Zhao, W.H.; Luo, Q.B.; Pan, X.; Chi, C.F.; Sun, K.L.; Wang, B. Preparation, identification, and activity evaluation of ten antioxidant peptides from protein hydrolysate of swim bladders of miiuy croaker (*Miichthys miiuy*). *J. Funct. Foods* **2018**, *47*, 503–511. [CrossRef]
7. Sila, A.; Bougatef, A. Antioxidant peptides from marine by-products: Isolation, identification and application in food systems. A review. *J. Funct. Foods* **2016**, *21*, 10–26. [CrossRef]
8. Chi, C.F.; Wang, B.; Wang, Y.M.; Zhang, B.; Deng, S.G. Isolation and characterization of three antioxidant peptides from protein hydrolysate of bluefin leatherjacket (*Navodon septentrionalis*) heads. *J. Funct. Foods* **2015**, *12*, 1–10. [CrossRef]
9. Cömert, E.D.; Gökmen, V. Evolution of food antioxidants as a core topic of food science for a century. *Food Res. Int.* **2018**, *105*, 76–93. [CrossRef]
10. Hu, F.Y.; Chi, C.F.; Wang, B.; Deng, S.G. Two novel antioxidant nonapeptides from protein hydrolysate of skate (*Raja porosa*). Muscle. *Mar. Drugs* **2015**, *13*, 1993–2009. [CrossRef]
11. Shahidi, F.; Janitha, P.K.; Wanasundara, P.D. Phenolic antioxidants. *Crit. Rev. Food Sci.* **1992**, *32*, 67–103. [CrossRef] [PubMed]
12. Li, X.R.; Chi, C.F.; Li, L.; Wang, B. Purification and identification of antioxidant peptides from protein hydrolysate of scalloped hammerhead (*Sphyrna lewini*) cartilage. *Mar. Drugs* **2017**, *15*, 61. [CrossRef] [PubMed]
13. Wang, B.; Gong, Y.D.; Li, Z.R.; Yu, D.; Chi, C.F.; Ma, J.Y. Isolation and characterisation of five novel antioxidant peptides from ethanol-soluble proteins hydrolysate of spotless smoothhound (*Mustelus griseus*) muscle. *J. Funct. Foods* **2014**, *6*, 176–185. [CrossRef]
14. Chi, C.F.; Wang, B.; Hu, F.Y.; Wang, Y.M.; Zhang, B.; Deng, S.G.; Wu, C.W. Purification and identification of three novel antioxidant peptides from protein hydrolysate of bluefin leatherjacket (*Navodon septentrionalis*) skin. *Food Res. Int.* **2015**, *73*, 124–139. [CrossRef]
15. Lassoued, I.; Mora, L.; Nasri, R.; Jridi, M.; Toldrá, F.; Aristoy, M.C.; Barkia, A.; Nasri, M. Characterization and comparative assessment of antioxidant and ACE inhibitory activities of thornback ray gelatin hydrolysates. *J. Funct. Foods* **2015**, *13*, 225–238. [CrossRef]
16. Harnedy, P.A.; O'Keeffe, M.B.; FitzGerald, R.J. Fractionation and identification of antioxidant peptides from an enzymatically hydrolysed Palmaria palmata protein isolate. *Food Res. Int.* **2017**, *100 (Pt 1)*, 416–422. [CrossRef]
17. Silva, J.F.X.; Ribeiro, K.; Silva, J.F.; Cahú, T.B.; Bezerra, R.S. Utilization of tilapia processing waste for the production of fish protein hydrolysate. *Anim. Feed Sci. Technol.* **2014**, *196*, 96–106. [CrossRef]
18. Ma, Y.; Wu, Y.; Li, L. Relationship between primary structure or spatial conformation and functional activity of antioxidant peptides from Pinctada fucata. *Food Chem.* **2018**, *264*, 108–117. [CrossRef]
19. Ahn, C.B.; Kim, J.G.; Je, J.Y. Purification and antioxidant properties of octapeptide from salmon byproduct protein hydrolysate by gastrointestinal digestion. *Food Chem.* **2014**, *147*, 78–83. [CrossRef]
20. Zhang, Q.; Song, C.; Zhao, J.; Shi, X.; Sun, M.; Liu, J.; Fu, Y.; Jin, W.; Zhu, B. Separation and characterization of antioxidative and angiotensin converting enzyme inhibitory peptide from jellyfish gonad hydrolysate. *Molecules* **2018**, *23*, E94. [CrossRef]
21. Jin, J.E.; Ahn, C.B.; Je, J.Y. Purification and characterization of antioxidant peptides from enzymatically hydrolyzed ark shell (Scapharca subcrenata). *Process Biochem.* **2018**, *72*, 170–176. [CrossRef]

22. Huang, S.; Lin, H.; Deng, S.G. Study of anti-fatigue effect in rats of ferrous chelates including hairtail protein hydrolysates. *Nutrients* **2015**, *7*, 9860–9871. [CrossRef]
23. Lin, H.M.; Deng, S.G.; Huang, S.B.; Li, Y.J.; Song, R. The effect of ferrous-chelating hairtail peptides on iron deficiency and intestinal flora in rats. *J. Sci. Food Agric.* **2016**, *96*, 2839–2844. [CrossRef] [PubMed]
24. Pan, X.; Zhao, Y.Q.; Hu, F.Y.; Wang, B. Preparation and identification of antioxidant peptides from protein hydrolysate of skate (*Raja porosa*) cartilage. *J. Funct. Foods* **2016**, *25*, 220–230. [CrossRef]
25. Hamlaoui, I.; Bencheraiet, R.; Bensegueni, R.; Bencharif, M. Experimental and theoretical study on DPPH radical scavenging mechanism of some chalcone quinoline derivatives. *J. Mol. Struct.* **2018**, *1156*, 385–389. [CrossRef]
26. Wang, B.; Li, L.; Chi, C.F.; Ma, J.H.; Luo, H.Y.; Xu, Y.F. Purification and characterisation of a novel antioxidant peptide derived from blue mussel (*Mytilus edulis*) protein hydrolysate. *Food Chem.* **2013**, *138*, 1713–1719. [CrossRef] [PubMed]
27. Bougatef, A.; Balti, R.; Haddar, A.; Jellouli, K.; Souissi, N.; Nasri, M. Antioxidant and functional properties of protein hydrolysates of bluefin tuna (*Thunnus thynnus*) heads as influenced by the extent of enzymatic hydrolysis. *Biotechnol. Bioprocess Eng.* **2012**, *17*, 841–852. [CrossRef]
28. Luo, H.Y.; Wang, B.; Li, Z.R.; Chi, C.F.; Zhang, Q.H.; He, G.Y. Preparation and evaluation of antioxidant peptide from papain hydrolysate of Sphyrna lewini muscle protein. *LWT-Food Sci. Technol.* **2013**, *51*, 281–288. [CrossRef]
29. Chi, C.F.; Cao, Z.H.; Wang, B.; Hu, F.Y.; Li, Z.R.; Zhang, B. Antioxidant and functional properties of collagen hydrolysates from spanish mackerel skin as influenced by average molecular weight. *Molecules* **2014**, *19*, 11211–11230. [CrossRef] [PubMed]
30. Li, Z.; Wang, B.; Chi, C.; Gong, Y.; Luo, H.; Ding, G. Influence of average molecular weight on antioxidant and functional properties of cartilage collagen hydrolysates from *Sphyrna lewini*, *Dasyatis akjei* and *Raja porosa*. *Food Res. Int.* **2013**, *51*, 283–293. [CrossRef]
31. Chi, C.F.; Hu, F.Y.; Wang, B.; Li, Z.R.; Luo, H.Y. Influence of amino acid compositions and peptide profiles on antioxidant capacities of two protein hydrolysates from skipjack tuna (*Katsuwonus pelamis*) dark muscle. *Mar. Drugs* **2015**, *13*, 2580–2601. [CrossRef] [PubMed]
32. Chi, C.F.; Hu, F.Y.; Wang, B.; Ren, X.J.; Deng, S.G.; Wu, C.W. Purification and characterization of three antioxidant peptides from protein hydrolyzate of croceine croaker (*Pseudosciaena crocea*) muscle. *Food Chem.* **2015**, *168*, 662–667. [CrossRef] [PubMed]
33. Wang, B.; Li, Z.R.; Chi, C.F.; Zhang, Q.H.; Luo, H.Y. Preparation and evaluation of antioxidant peptides from ethanol-soluble proteins hydrolysate of *Sphyrna lewini* muscle. *Peptides* **2012**, *36*, 240–250. [CrossRef] [PubMed]
34. Wiriyaphan, C.; Chitsomboon, B.; Yongsawadigul, J. Antioxidant activity of protein hydrolysates derived from threadfin bream surimi byproducts. *Food Chem.* **2012**, *132*, 104–111. [CrossRef]
35. Sudhakar, S.; Nazeer, R.A. Preparation of potent antioxidant peptide from edible part of shortclub cuttlefish against radical mediated lipid and DNA damage. *LWT—Food Sci. Technol.* **2015**, *64*, 593–601. [CrossRef]
36. Lafarga, T.; Hayes, M. Bioactive peptides from meat muscle and by-products: Generation, functionality and application as functional ingredients. *Meat Sci.* **2014**, *98*, 227–239. [CrossRef]
37. Agrawal, H.; Joshi, R.; Gupta, M. Isolation, purification and characterization of antioxidative peptide of pearl millet (*Pennisetum glaucum*) protein hydrolysate. *Food Chem.* **2016**, *204*, 365–372. [CrossRef] [PubMed]
38. Orsini Delgado, M.C.; Nardo, A.; Pavlovic, M.; Rogniaux, H.; Añón, M.C.; Tironi, V.A. Identification and characterization of antioxidant peptides obtained by gastrointestinal digestion of amaranth proteins. *Food Chem.* **2016**, *197*, 1160–1167. [CrossRef]
39. You, L.; Zhao, M.; Regenstein, J.M.; Ren, J. Purification and identification of antioxidative peptides from loach (*Misgurnus anguillicaudatus*) protein hydrolysate by consecutive chromatography and electrospray ionizationmass spectrometry. *Food Res. Int.* **2010**, *43*, 1167–1173. [CrossRef]
40. Cai, L.; Wu, X.; Zhang, Y.; Li, X.; Ma, S.; Li, J. Purification and characterization of three antioxidant peptides from protein hydrolysate of grass carp (*Ctenopharyngodon idella*) skin. *J. Funct. Foods* **2015**, *16*, 234–242. [CrossRef]
41. Ahn, C.B.; Cho, Y.S.; Je, J.Y. Purification and anti-inflammatory action of tripeptide from salmon pectoral fin byproduct protein hydrolysate. *Food Chem.* **2015**, *168*, 151–156. [CrossRef] [PubMed]

42. Hong, J.; Chen, T.T.; Hu, P.; Yang, J.; Wang, S.Y. Purification and characterization of an antioxidant peptide (GSQ) from Chinese leek (*Allium tuberosum* Rottler) seeds. *J. Funct. Foods* **2014**, *10*, 1–10. [CrossRef]

43. Rajapakse, N.; Mendis, E.; Byun, H.G.; Kim, S.K. Purification and in vitro antioxidative effects of giant squid muscle peptides on free radical-mediated oxidative systems. *J. Nutr. Biochem.* **2005**, *9*, 562–569. [CrossRef] [PubMed]

44. Ranathunga, S.; Rajapakse, N.; Kim, S.K. Purification and characterization of antioxidantative peptide derived from muscle of conger eel (*Conger myriaster*). *Eur. Food Res. Technol.* **2006**, *222*, 310–315. [CrossRef]

45. Kim, E.K.; Oh, H.J.; Kim, Y.S.; Hwang, J.W.; Ahn, C.B.; Lee, J.S.; Jeon, Y.J.; Moon, S.H.; Sung, S.H.; Jeon, B.T.; et al. Purification of a novel peptide derived from *Mytilus coruscus* and in vitro/in vivo evaluation of its bioactive properties. *Fish Shellfish Immunol.* **2013**, *34*, 1078–1084. [CrossRef] [PubMed]

46. Jiang, H.; Tong, T.; Sun, J.; Xu, Y.; Zhao, Z.; Liao, D. Purification and characterization of antioxidative peptides from round scad (*Decapterus maruadsi*) muscle protein hydrolysate. *Food Chem.* **2014**, *154*, 158–163. [CrossRef] [PubMed]

47. Chi, C.F.; Wang, B.; Wang, Y.M.; Deng, S.G.; Ma, J.H. Isolation and characterization of three antioxidant pentapeptides from protein hydrolysate of monkfish (*Lophius litulon*) muscle. *Food Res. Int.* **2014**, *55*, 222–228. [CrossRef]

48. Wang, B.; Wang, Y.; Chi, C.; Hu, F.; Deng, S.; Ma, J. Isolation and characterization of collagen and antioxidant collagen peptides from scales of croceine croaker (*Pseudosciaena crocea*). *Mar. Drugs* **2013**, *11*, 4641–4661. [CrossRef] [PubMed]

49. Zhuang, H.; Tang, N.; Yuan, Y. Purification and identification of antioxidant peptides from corn gluten meal. *J. Funct. Foods* **2013**, *5*, 1810–1821. [CrossRef]

50. Agyei, D.; Ongkudon, C.M.; Wei, C.Y.; Chan, A.S.; Danquah, M.K. Bioprocess challenges to the isolation and purification of bioactive peptides. *Food Bioprod. Process.* **2016**, *98*, 244–256. [CrossRef]

51. Deane, R.; Du Yan, S.; Submamaryan, R.K.; LaRue, B.; Jovanovic, S.; Hogg, E.; Welch, D.; Manness, L.; Lin, C.; Yu, J.; et al. RAGE mediates amyloid-beta peptide transport across the blood-brain barrier and accumulation in brain. *Nat. Med.* **2003**, *9*, 907–913. [CrossRef] [PubMed]

52. Dávalos, A.; Miguel, M.; Bartolomé, B.; López-Fandiño, R. Antioxidant activity of peptides derived from egg white proteins by enzymatic hydrolysis. *J. Food Protect.* **2004**, *67*, 1939–1944. [CrossRef]

53. Xing, L.; Hu, Y.; Hu, H.; Ge, Q.; Zhou, G.; Zhang, W. Purification and identification of antioxidative peptides from dry-cured Xuanwei ham. *Food Chem.* **2016**, *194*, 951–958. [CrossRef] [PubMed]

54. Wu, R.; Wu, C.; Liu, D.; Yang, X.; Huang, J.; Zhang, J.; Liao, B.; He, H. Antioxidant and anti-freezing peptides from salmon collagen hydrolysate prepared by bacterial extracellular protease. *Food Chem.* **2018**, *248*, 346–352. [CrossRef] [PubMed]

55. Sheih, I.C.; Wu, T.K.; Fang, T.J. Antioxidant properties of a new antioxidative peptide from algae protein waste hydrolysate in different oxidation systems. *Bioresource Technol.* **2009**, *100*, 3419–3425. [CrossRef] [PubMed]

56. Gimenez, B.; Aleman, A.; Montero, P.; Gomez-Guillen, M.C. Antioxidant and functional properties of gelatin hydrolysates obtained from skin of sole and squid. *Food Chem.* **2009**, *114*, 976–983. [CrossRef]

57. Zhu, C.Z.; Zhang, W.G.; Zhou, G.H.; Xu, X.L.; Kang, Z.L.; Yin, Y. Isolation and identification of antioxidant peptides from Jinhua ham. *J. Agric. Food Chem.* **2013**, *61*, 1265–1271. [CrossRef]

58. Ren, J.Y.; Zhao, M.M.; Shi, J.; Wang, J.S.; Jiang, Y.M.; Cui, C.; Kakuda, Y.; Xue, S.J. Purification and identification of antioxidant peptides from grass carp muscle hydrolysates by consecutive chromatography and electrospray ionization-mass spectrometry. *Food Chem.* **2008**, *108*, 727–736. [CrossRef]

59. Chen, C.; Chi, Y.J.; Zhao, M.Y.; Lv, L. Purification and identification of antioxidant peptides from egg white protein hydrolysate. *Amino Acids* **2012**, *43*, 457–466. [CrossRef]

60. Nimalaratne, C.; Bandara, N.; Wu, J. Purification and characterization of antioxidant peptides from enzymatically hydrolyzed chicken egg white. *Food Chem.* **2015**, *188*, 467–472. [CrossRef]

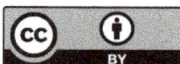

![marine drugs logo] *marine drugs*

MDPI

Article

Novel Antibacterial Peptides Isolated from the Maillard Reaction Products of Half-Fin Anchovy (*Setipinna taty*) Hydrolysates/Glucose and Their Mode of Action in *Escherichia Coli*

Jiaxing Wang [1], Rongbian Wei [2] and Ru Song [1,*]

[1] Key Laboratory of Health Risk Factors for Seafood of Zhejiang Province, School of Food Science and Pharmacy, Zhejiang Ocean University, Zhoushan 316000, China; 18868005756@163.com

[2] School of Marine Science and Technology, Zhejiang Ocean University, Zhoushan 316000, China; rbwei@zjou.edu.cn

*   Correspondence: rusong656@163.com; Tel.: +86-580-255-4781

Received: 19 November 2018; Accepted: 8 January 2019; Published: 10 January 2019

Abstract: The Maillard reaction products (MRPs) of half-fin anchovy hydrolysates and glucose, named as HAHp(9.0)-G MRPs, were fractionated by size exclusion chromatography into three major fractions (F1–F3). F2, which demonstrated the strongest antibacterial activity against *Escherichia coli* (*E. coli*) and showed self-production of hydrogen peroxide (H_2O_2), was extracted by solid phase extraction. The hydrophobic extract of F2 was further isolated by reverse phase-high performance liquid chromatography into sub-fractions HE-F2-1 and HE-F2-2. Nine peptides were identified from HE-F2-1, and two peptides from HE-F2-2 using liquid chromatography-electrospray ionization/multi-stage mass spectrometry. Three peptides, FEDQLR (HGM-Hp1), ALERTF (HGM-Hp2), and RHPEYAVSVLLR (HGM-Hp3), with net charges of −1, 0, and +1, respectively, were synthesized. The minimal inhibitory concentration of these synthetic peptides was 2 mg/mL against *E. coli*. Once incubated with logarithmic growth phase of *E. coli*, HGM-Hp1 and HGM-Hp2 induced significant increases of both extracellular and intracellular H_2O_2 formation. However, HGM-Hp3 only dramatically enhanced intracellular H_2O_2 production in *E. coli*. The increased potassium ions in *E. coli* suspension after addition of HGM-Hp1 or HGM-Hp2 indicated the destruction of cell integrity via irreversible membrane damage. It is the first report of hydrolysates MRPs-derived peptides that might perform the antibacterial activity via inducing intracellular H_2O_2 production.

Keywords: half-fin anchovy hydrolysates; Maillard reaction products; antibacterial peptide; identification; self-production of hydrogen peroxide; membrane damage

1. Introduction

Antibiotics play crucial roles in saving lives and improving human and animal health. However, bacterial pathogens commonly develop antimicrobial resistance due to the extensive use of the antibiotics [1]. As an effective first line of defense against invading pathogens, antimicrobial peptides (AMPs) play a crucial role on the innate immune systems of organisms. The significant advantage of AMPs is their strong antibacterial activity against a very broad spectrum of microorganisms and low rates of bacterial resistance [2]. Natural AMPs can be isolated and characterized from practically all-living organisms [3]. Marine organisms are a good source of AMPs. Recently, an increasing number of AMPs have been isolated from various protein hydrolysates of marine organism sources. For instance, a peptide, CgPep33, rich in cysteine residue was isolated from oyster muscle hydrolysates [4]. Series of short peptides were derived from *Barbel* muscle protein hydrolysates and *Sardinella* (*Sardinella aurita*) hydrolysates [5,6]. One decapeptide GLSRLFTALK was separated from protein hydrolysates of anchovy cooking wastewater [7]. The antibacterial activity of AMPs is related with many factors, such as molecular weight, net charges, hydrophobic domains, and specific amino acid residues in sequences [8].

Maillard reaction (MR), also defined as a non-enzymatic browning reaction, usually occurs in thermal food processing or food storage between amino (amino acid, peptide or protein) and carbonyl groups (e.g. reducing sugar) [9]. The antibacterial activities of some Maillard reaction products (MRPs) or MRP-rich foods, such as chitosan-glucosamine MRPs [10], ε-polylysine-chitosan MRPs [11], xylan-chitosan MRPs [12], roast bread [13], and coffee [14], have attracted great attention in recent years. However, the antibacterial mechanism of MRPs is not yet fully understood. Rufian-Henares and Cueva (2009) reported that coffee melanoidins could exhibit antibacterial activity through metal-chelating of membrane [15]. The bacteriostatic or bactericidal effects of coffee melanoidins were observed at low and high concentrations [16]. Recently, Mueller et al. (2011) identified hydrogen peroxide (H_2O_2) generated in coffee brew as a major antibacterial component of coffee [17]. In our previous study, we reported the broad spectrum of half-fin anchovy hydrolysates (HAHp) against food spoilage bacteria [18]. In addition, we found a dramatic increase of extracellular or intracellular H_2O_2 formation in *Escherichia coli* (*E. coli*) cells after incubation with the HAHp-derived MRPs (HAHp(9.0)-G MRPs) [19].

H_2O_2 is an example of a reactive oxygen species [20]. The generated H_2O_2 from MRPs can oxidize almost every compound in the cell, resulting in internal damage associated with increase of membrane permeability [21]. However, to our best knowledge, few studies are focused on the antibacterial activity of peptides isolated from protein hydrolysates MRPs. In addition, the contribution of H_2O_2 formation induced by MRP-derived peptides to the antibacterial activity is still not fully understood. For this reason, in this study, HAHp(9.0)-G MRPs were isolated to identify peptides with antibacterial activity and the capacity of H_2O_2 self-production. Furthermore, the effects of identified peptides on intracellular and extracellular H_2O_2 accumulation on logarithmic phase of *E. coli* cells were investigated to reveal the contribution of H_2O_2 formation to the antibacterial effect, inducing by addition of antibacterial peptides.

2. Results and Discussion

2.1. Purification of Antibacterial and H_2O_2 Self-Produced Peptidic Fraction

HAHp(9.0)-G MRPs were separated into three fractions (F1–F3) by HPLC system (Figure 1A). At the actual peptide concentration of 0.18 mg/mL, the antibacterial activity of F2 reached 57.29% against the growth of *E. coli* cells, significantly stronger than the other two fractions (33.22% for F1 and 2.50% for F3) ($p < 0.05$) (Figure 1B). The most bioactive fraction F2 also had the strongest H_2O_2 self-production capacity among these fractions (Figure 1C). In recent years, much more attention has been paid to the antibacterial activity of H_2O_2 in MRPs. For example, Hauser et al. [21] reported the generated H_2O_2 (about 100 μM) in a polyethylene film coated with an active fraction derived from the ribose-lysine MRPs resulted in a log-reduction of >5 log-cycles against *E. coli*. In the present study, the fraction of F2 was collected for further purification.

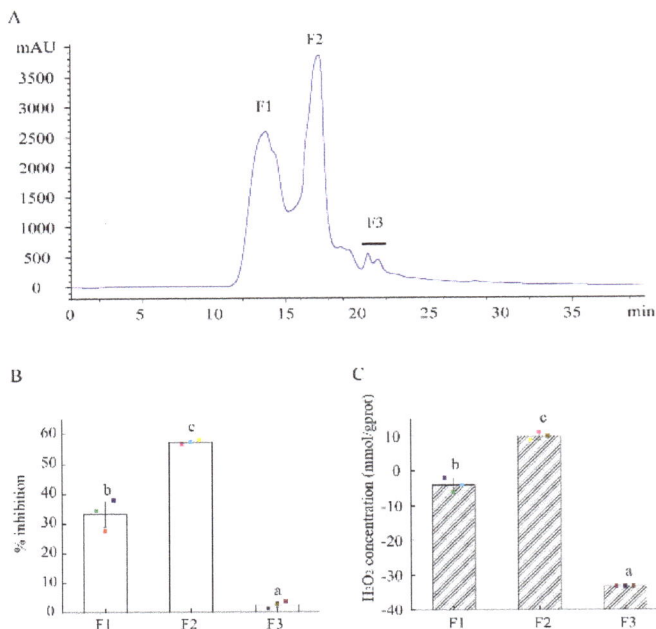

Figure 1. Isolation of HAHp(9.0)-G MRPs and activity of separated fractions. (**A**) The size exclusion chromatography (SEC) of MRPs isolated by high performance liquid chromatography (HPLC) method, detected at 220 nm. (**B**) The percentage inhibition of isolated fractions against *E. coli* cells. (**C**) H_2O_2 self-produced concentration of isolated fractions. The actual peptide concentration of isolated fractions was 0.18 mg/mL in the percentage inhibition and H_2O_2 production assays. Spots in (**B**,**C**) represent the raw data. The results are expressed as the mean $\pm$ standard deviation ($n = 3$). Different letters (a–c) in (**B**,**C**) represent significant differences among isolated fractions ($p < 0.05$).

Through Cleanert® S C18-N solid phase extraction, the active fraction F2 was further isolated into hydrophilic and hydrophobic extracts. At the actual peptide concentration of 0.15 mg/mL, the percentage inhibition of hydrophobic extract of F2 against *E. coli* was 20.98 $\pm$ 1.39%, remarkably higher than that of the hydrophilic counterpart (11.61 $\pm$ 2.27%) ($p < 0.05$) (Figure 2A). Therefore, the hydrophobic extract of F2 (HE-F2) was selected for further purification using a C_{18} column (4.6 $\times$ 250 mm, 5 µm) based on the hydrophobic property of peptides. As shown in Figure 2B, HE-F2 was separated into two major peaks, HE-F2-1 and HE-F2-2. HE-F2-1 demonstrated stronger antibacterial activity than HE-F2-2 ($p < 0.01$) (Figure 2C). A similar result was found for the self-produced H_2O_2 concentrations in HE-F2-1 and HE-F2-2 ($p < 0.05$) (Figure 2D). The results in Figure 1; Figure 2 suggest that the self-production of H_2O_2 could be an important contributor for the observed antibacterial activity of active peptidic fractions derived from HAHp(9.0)-G MRPs.

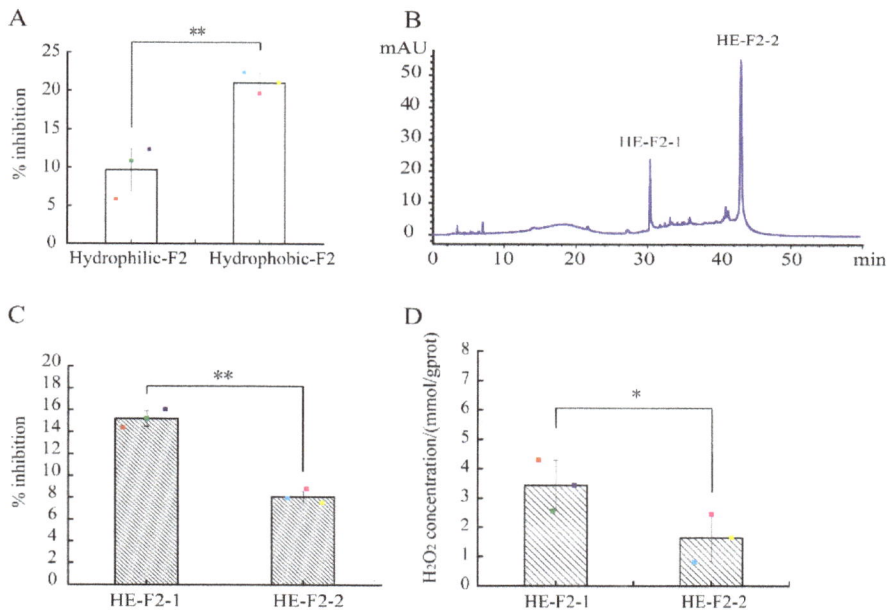

Figure 2. Purification of active fraction F2 using reverse phase high performance liquid chromatography (RP-HPLC) and the activities of sub-fractions assay: (**A**) percentage inhibition of hydrophilic and hydrophobic extracts of F2; (**B**) chromatogram of active fraction F2 by RP-HPLC, measured at 280 nm; (**C**) percentage inhibition of F2-1 and F2-2; and (D) H_2O_2 production capacity of F2-1 and F2-2. Spots in (**A,C,D**) represent the raw data. The results are expressed as the mean ± standard deviation ($n = 3$). The symbol of "******" and "*****" in (**A,C,D**) represent significant differences of $p < 0.01$ and $p < 0.05$, respectively.

2.2. Identification of Peptide by Liquid Chromatography–Electrospray Ionization/Multi-Stage Mass Spectrometry (LC-ESI-Q-TOF-MS/MS)

HE-F2-1 and HE-F2-2 were subjected to LC-ESI-Q-TOF-MS/MS analysis to identify all potential peptides. The molecular mass of peptide was identified according to its proton charged [M + H]H⁺ precursor ion. A few peptides were matched with actin cytoplasmic 1 (*Clupea harengus*) in the protein database of *Clupeoidei* after searching in NCBI; however, the −10lgP scores of these peptides were below 35 (data not shown), suggesting low confidence for these matched peptides. Therefore, in this study, we used de novo analysis to identify potential peptides. After collapses of the precursor ion into series fragments, a single peptide fragment could be auto-matched by de novo peptides sequencing [22]. Peptides with average local confidence scores (ALC) ≥ 95% and local confidence of each residue in peptide sequence ≥ 90% in HE-F2-1 and HE-F2-2 through de novo peptide automated spectrum processing are listed in Table 1.

The mass of identified peptides in HE-F2-1 and HE-F2-2 ranged from 700 Da to 1700 Da. Peptide sequences analysis in the antimicrobial peptide database (APD) database (http://aps.unmc.edu/AP/main.html) and NCBI non-redundant peptide database (http://www.ncbi.nlm.nih.gov/blast) indicated that no AMPs or peptides had the identical sequences with these identified peptides herein. In this study, these identified peptides had different sequences. Nevertheless, nine peptides, namely K̲GTAVPTAAEATAQR̲, FEDQLR̲, SVVMLR̲, LDVLADK̲, EGDALDELR̲, EAGAEFDKAAEEVKR̲, MEVLLLER̲, VATVSLPR̲, and R̲HPEYAVSVLLR̲, had common cationic arginine (R) or lysine (K) residues at the N- or C-terminus of sequences. In addition, the other peptides, ALER̲TF and

LLDRLPRPL, had R residues within sequences. The cationic R or K residues in the sequences of identified peptides were consistent with some published studies, such as peptides RKSGDPLGR and AKPGDGAGSGPR derived from protamex hydrolysates of Atlantic mackerel byproducts [23], and a synthetic peptide VRRFPWWWPFLRR with a wide antibacterial spectrum [24]. The presence of positively charged residues at the N- or C-terminus could contribute to the interaction with negatively charged phospholipids present on *E. coli* membrane surface [8]. Similarly, we identified seven peptides (RVAPEEHPTL, WLPVVR, FFTQATDLLSR, VLLLWR, VLLVLLR, VLLALWR, and LLSWYDNEFGYSNR) from HAHp(9.0)-G MRPs that had R residues at the N- or C-terminus [25]. In consideration of the characteristics of peptide sequences in Table 1, it was quite apparent that the presence of R residue, especially at C- or N- terminus, could be a typical property for the peptides derived from HAHp(9.0)-G MRPs.

Table 1. Identification of peptides in HE-F2-1 and HE-F2-2 using LC-ESI-Q-TOF-MS/MS.

No.	Peptide Sequence	RT [a]/min	Tag Length	ALC [b]/%	m/z	z	Mass	Intensity	Local Confidence/%
HE-F2-1	KGTAVPTAAEATAQR	11.31	15	97	491.2670	3	1470.7790	1.44×10^6	96 91 95 90 95 100 100 100 100 100 100 100 100 100 100
	FEDQLR	15.66	6	99	404.2030	2	806.3922	1.32×10^7	100 100 100 98 100 100
	ALERTF	16.13	6	98	368.7024	2	735.3915	2.70×10^6	100 100 100 99 97 96
	SVVMLR	17.11	6	98	352.7097	2	703.4051	2.97×10^5	94 97 100 100 100 100
	LDVLADK	19.64	7	99	387.2238	2	772.4330	1.58×10^6	99 100 100 100 100 100 100
	LLDRLPRPL	22.97	9	98	364.9008	3	1091.6810	5.02×10^6	100 100 100 99 99 98 99 97 98
	EGDALDELR	25.25	9	98	509.2465	2	1016.4770	1.49×10^6	93 95 100 100 100 100 100 100 100
	EAGAEFDKAAEEVKR	28.22	15	97	550.6095	3	1648.8060	3.47×10^6	98 94 95 90 95 99 100 100 100 100 100 100 99 100 100
	MEVLLLER	35.99	8	99	501.7868	2	1001.5580	4.58×10^6	100 100 100 100 100 100 100 100
HE-F2-2	VATVSLPR	23.43	8	98	421.7583	2	841.5021	5.85×10^6	100 100 99 98 99 98 96 98
	RHPEYAVSVLLR	26.20	12	99	720.4086	2	1438.8044	2.39×10^8	99 100 100 100 100 100 99 99 99 100 100 100

[a] RT is the retention time in LC system connected to ESI-Q-TOF-MS. [b] ALC is the average local confidence scores.

2.3. Physicochemical Property of Synthetic Peptides

Considering the presence of R residue in peptide sequences related with antibacterial activity, F or Y residue in peptide sequence consistent with the specific absorbance of HE-F2-1 or HE-F2-2 at 280 nm, and the intensity of identified peptides, we selected peptide FEDQLR derived from HE-F2-1 (named as HGM-Hp1), and peptide RHPEYAVSVLLR from HE-F2-2 (named as HGM-Hp3) for synthesis. Besides R and F residues in sequence, peptide ALERTF was the only one in Table 1 with net charge of 0 (see Table 2), therefore peptide ALERTF was also synthesized (named as HGM-Hp2). The purity (>98%) of the peptides was verified by RP-HPLC. The properties of ESI-MS and helical wheel projection of the three synthetic peptides are shown in Figure 3.

Table 2. Physiochemical property of synthetic peptides.

Peptides	Measured/Theoretical Weight/Da	pI [a]	Net Charge	Hydrophobicity/ (Kcal/mol)	GRAVY [b]	Instability Index	Secondary Structure
FEDQLR (HGM-Hp1)	807.07/806.3910	4.00	−1	+14.79	−1.400	72.53	Random coil (100%)
ALERTF (HGM-Hp2)	735.85/735.3903	6.65	0	+11.13	−0.050	28.90	Random coil (100%)
RHPEYAVSVLLR (HGM-Hp3)	1438.42/1438.8021	9.53	+1	+14.45	−0.133	73.08	Random coil (100%)

[a] pI represents isoelectric point. [b] GRAVY means the grand average of hydropathicity. The PepDraw Tool was used to estimate the molecular weight, pI, net charge and hydrophobicity of the peptides, available at http://www.tulane.edu/~{}biochem/WW/PepDraw/. GRAVY and instability index of peptides were predicted using ProtParam Tool (http://web.expasy.org/protparam/). The secondary structure of peptides HGM-Hp1, HGM-Hp2, and HGM-Hp3 were predicted using the program SOPMA available at Network Protein Sequence (NPS)® (https://npsa-prabi.ibcp.fr).

Based on the precursor ion of $[M + H]H^+$, the measured molecular weights of HGM-Hp1, HGM-Hp2 and HGM-Hp3 were calculated as 807.07 Da, 735.85 Da, and 1438.42 Da, respectively, which were in very good agreement with their theoretical values (see Table 1). The ESI-MS results in Figure 3 suggest that the peptides were successfully synthesized. The property of α-helices in protein or peptide can be observed in the plot of wheel projection [26]. Usually, hydrophobic amino acids are concentrated on one side of the helix, and polar or hydrophilic amino acids are located on the other side [27]. According to the wheel projection, HGM-Hp1 possessed hydrophobic F_1 and L_5 residues on the hydrophobic side, while the charged residues E_2D_3 and R_6 were observed on the opposite side (diagram in Figure 3A). In the projection diagram of HGM-Hp2, the hydrophobic L_2 and F_6 residues were concentrated on the hydrophobic side, and the negatively charged E_3 and positively charged R_4 residues were located on the opposite side (diagram in Figure 3B). In contrast, HGM-Hp3 might form α-helices in the wheel projection due to more hydrophobic and hydrophilic residues concentrated on the opposite sides (diagram in Figure 3C).

To further reveal the characteristics of these synthetic peptides, their physicochemical properties were compared, as summarized in Table 2.

HGM-Hp3 had larger molecular weight than the other two peptides. The pI value of 4.00 and net charge of −1 for peptide HGM-Hp1 indicated its acidic characteristics. By comparison, the positively charged property was predicted in peptide HGM-Hp3 according to its pI value of 9.53 and net charge of +1. GRAVY is associated with the hydrophobicity of peptide or protein, which is calculated by the sum of hydropathy values of all amino acids divided by the peptide or protein length [28]. The negative and positive values of GRAVY suggest corresponding hydrophilic and hydrophobic properties of peptides [25]. In this sense, the negative GRAVY values of HGM-Hp1 (−1.400), HGM-Hp2 (−0.050), and HGM-Hp3 (−0.133) indicated potential hydrophilic property of these peptides. Furthermore, the hydrophobicity, as measured by an experimentally determined Wimley–White scale and associated with the free energy transitioning a peptide from aqueous environment to a hydrophobic environment, was similar for HGM-Hp1 (+14.79 Kcal/mol) and HGM-Hp3 (+14.45 Kcal/mol). The ProtParam Tool predicted the instability indexes of HGM-Hp1 and HGM-Hp3 were 72.53 and 73.08, which belong to the unstable peptide category. The secondary structures of the three synthetic peptides were predicted to form 100% random-coil structures obtained from the NPS@SOPMA secondary structure prediction.

Compared with the traditional AMPs with > 50 amino acid residues, all of the synthetic peptides in this study are small (<1.5 kDa) and have a substantial portion of hydrophobic residues. The random coil structures were predicted for the three synthetic peptides (Table 2), although the helical wheel projection of these peptides are observed in Figure 3. Generally, peptides without disulfides are often in disorder when dissolved in aqueous solutions [29,30]. However, the AMPs with a random coil structure can be structured in aqueous solution once contacted with biological membrane or dissolved in hydrophobic environment, which could contribute to the binding with membrane, or occurrence of self-aggregation [31].

The actual secondary structures of these synthetic peptides under membrane mimic solvents were analyzed using circular dichroism (CD) measurements, as shown in Figure 4.

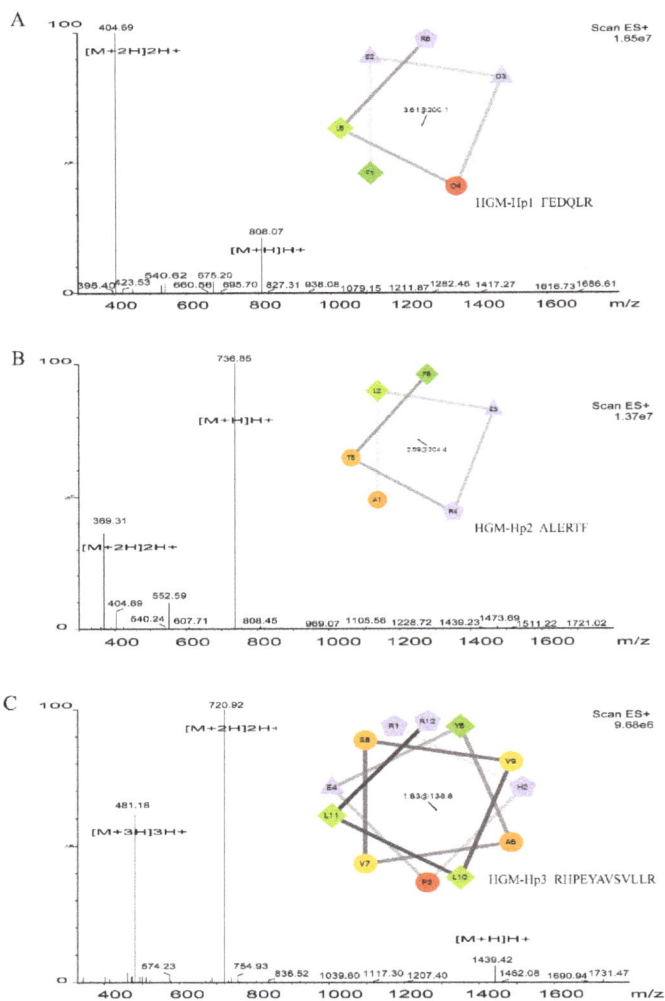

Figure 3. ESI-MS and helical wheel projection of synthetic peptides: (**A**) HGM-Hp1, FEDQLR; (**B**) HGM-Hp2, ALERTF; and (**C**) HGM-Hp3, RHPEYAVSVLLR. The helical wheel projection of HGM-Hp1, HGM-Hp2, and HGM-Hp3 (insert diagrams in Figures (**A–C**)) were performed using the online website tool (http://rzlab.ucr.edu/scripts/wheel/wheel.cgi). In helical wheel projection, circles and diamonds represent hydrophilic and hydrophobic residues, respectively. The green color, whose intensity decreases proportionally to the hydrophobicity, represents the most hydrophobic residue. Non-hydrophobic portions are encoded in yellow. The red color is used to encode hydrophilic residues, whose intensity represents the extent of hydrophilicity. The charged residues are encoded in light blue. Negatively charged and positively charged residues are displayed as triangles and pentagons, respectively. The hydrophobic moment is denoted in the center.

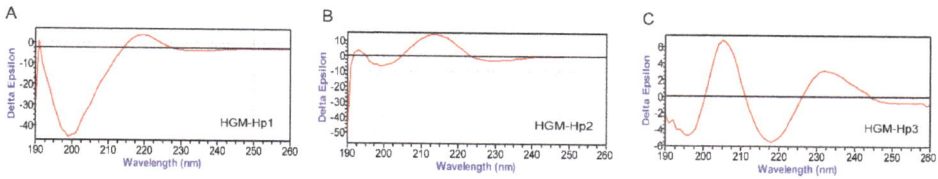

Figure 4. CD spectra of synthetic peptides in membrane-mimicking solution (1.6 mmol/L sodium dodecyl sulfate (SDS), dissolved in 10 mmol/L PBS, pH 7.4): (**A**) HGM-Hp1; (**B**) HGM-Hp2; and (**C**) HGM-Hp3. The peptide concentration was 0.5 mg/mL.

The negative band at 200 nm, due to random coil structure [32], was observed in HGM-Hp1 and HGM-Hp2. However, besides the negative band at 200 nm, other positive CD signals, such as a weak peak at 191 nm and a broad band at 219 nm, were noticed in the CD spectrum of HGMp1. Similarly, two positive bands at 193 nm and 214 nm were found in the CD spectrum of HGMp2. The results in Figure 4A,B suggest that peptides HGM-Hp1 and HGM-Hp2 could form random coil and other structures upon interaction with membrane-mimicking solvents. By comparison, the peptide HGM-Hp3 may tend to form type I β-turn structure in the membrane-mimicking solvents, with a negative band at 196 nm, and a positive band at 205 nm [33]. Protein or peptide with a maximum at 202 nm and a minimum at 216 nm in the CD spectrum could adopt a β-sheet conformation [34]. As shown in the CD spectrum of HGMp3 (Figure 4C), a positive band at 205 nm and a negative band at 218 nm may indicate some kind of β-sheet structure formation.

2.4. Antibacterial Activity and H_2O_2 Self-Production of Synthetic Peptides

The antibacterial activity and self-production of H_2O_2 of the three synthetic peptides were compared, as shown in Figure 5.

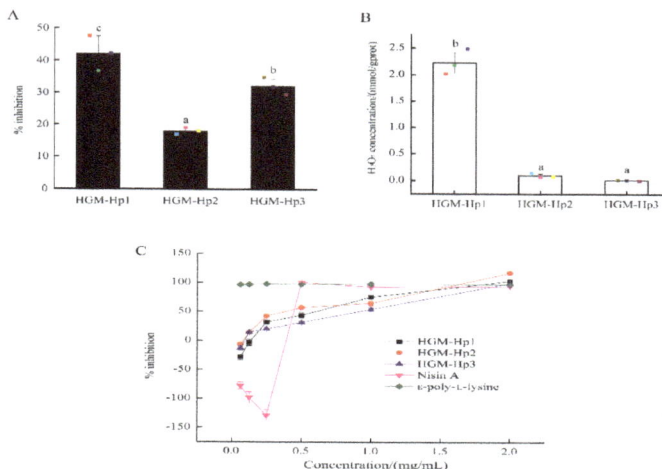

Figure 5. Antibacterial activity and H_2O_2 self-production of synthetic peptides: (**A**) percentage inhibition against *E. coli* cells; (**B**) H_2O_2 self-production of synthetic peptides at the actual peptide concentration of 0.25 mg/mL; and (**C**) percentage inhibition of synthetic peptides, nisin A and ε-poly-lysine against *E. coli* at different concentrations. Raw data in (**A**,**B**) are displayed as spots. The results are expressed as the mean ± standard deviation (*n* = 3). Different letters (a–c) in (**A**,**B**) indicate significant differences among samples (*p* < 0.05).

At the actual peptide concentration of 0.25 mg/mL, HGM-Hp1 demonstrated the highest percentage inhibition ($42.10 \pm 5.36\%$), in contrast to HGM-Hp2 ($17.93 \pm 1.03\%$) and HGM-Hp3 ($32.14 \pm 2.19\%$) ($p < 0.05$) (Figure 5A). In addition, the peptide HGM-Hp1 exhibited the highest H_2O_2 self-production capacity among the three synthetic peptides ($p < 0.05$) (Figure 5B). All synthetic peptides showed concentration-dependent inhibition of the growth of *E. coli* cells, as shown in Figure 5C. In addition, no growth of *E. coli* cells was observed after treatment with the synthetic peptides at the actual peptide concentration of 2 mg/mL. Therefore, the MIC was 2 mg/mL for peptides HGM-Hp1, HGM-Hp2, and HGM-Hp3 against the growth of *E. coli*. By comparison, nisin A, an AMP from *Lactococcus lactis*, had negative inhibition effects on *E. coli* cells at the concentration below 0.5 mg/mL. The antibacterial effect of nisin A reached a plateau (100% inhibition) when its concentration was increased to 0.5 mg/mL. Similar to our results, Tong et al. [1] reported the MIC of nisin against *Enterococcus faecalis* was 1 g/L (actual concentration of 0.5 mg/mL). Natural ε-poly-lysine has a broad antimicrobial activity against Gram-negative and Gram-positive bacteria [35]. In this study, the percentage inhibition on *E. coli* was 95.99% after treatment with 62.5 µg/mL of ε-poly-lysine. This result was in agreement with the MIC of ε-poly-lysine solution, which was less than 100 µg/mL against *E. coli* [36]. ε-poly-lysine consists of 25–30 positively charged L-lysine residues, which are responsible for its strong antibacterial activity [35].

As an anionic peptide, HGM-Hp1 (FEDQL**R**), with the positively charged residue R at the C-terminus, may not contribute to the interaction with the negatively charged bacterial membrane surface. We speculated specific residues in HGM-Hp1 could be associated with its antibacterial activity. By searching the AMPs in APD database, we found HGM-Hp1 (F**ED**QLR) had the same two residues (ED) in the sequence as some reported anionic peptides, such as peptides D**ED**LDE (net charge: −5) and D**ED**DD (net charge: −5) isolated from *Xenopus laevis* skin [37,38], and the surface-tethered peptide GATP**ED**LNQKLS (net charge: −1) [38]. The more amphiphilic and smaller is the peptide, the more it diffuses through the membrane to exert bacteriostatic effect [39]. The smallest molecule size of HGM-Hp2 might be a significant contributor to its inhibitory effect against *E. coli*.

HGM-Hp3 had a relatively higher molecular weight than HGM-Hp1 or HGM-Hp2 (see Table 2), which might be an inconvenient factor for its quick diffusion in biomembrane. Nonetheless, the sequence property of HGM-Hp3 (**RH**PEYA**VS**VL**LR**), such as the cationic net charge, the presence of positively charged residues R at the C- and RH at the N- terminus, and the hydrophobic regions (AV, VLL) in sequence, were consistent with some cationic antibacterial peptides in APD database. For example, Hilpert et al. (2009) [38] reported a surface-tethered cationic peptide **R**RAAVVLIVI**RR** (net charge: +4) with R residues at C- and N- terminus, and hydrophobic regions (AAVVLIVI). Kim et al. (2016) [40] identified a cationic peptide L**RHK**VYGYCVLGP (net charge: +2) from American cockroach *Periplaneta americana* (*Linnaeus*) with positively charged residues (RHK) close to the N-terminus, and hydrophobic regions (VL) in sequence. Obviously, the sequence characteristics of HGM-Hp3 could be responsible for its inhibitory effect on the growth of *E. coli*.

2.5. Antibacterial Activity of Synthetic Peptides on the Logarithmic Growth Phase of E. coli and Intracellular and Extracellular H_2O_2 Formation

The logarithmic growth phase of *E. coli* cells suspended in saline were added to the synthetic peptide solution. In that case, peptides could easily contact with the newly formed *E. coli* cell membrane. After incubation at 37 °C for 3 h, the percentage inhibition of synthetic peptides on logarithmic phase of *E. coli* was measured, and the induced production of intracellular and extracellular H_2O_2 in *E. coli* cells by addition of synthetic peptides were investigated as well.

As shown in Figure 6A, HGM-Hp1 still demonstrated the strongest inhibitory activity on the growth of logarithmic phase *E. coli* cells among the three synthetic peptides. However, the percentage inhibitions of HGM-Hp2 and HGM-Hp3 on logarithmic phase *E. coli* cells were not in accordance with the result of Figure 5A. It was noticed that HGM-Hp2 showed higher percentage inhibition ($25.54 \pm 0.57\%$) than HGM-Hp3 ($18.15 \pm 1.30\%$) ($p < 0.05$) after incubated with logarithmic phase of *E.*

coli cells. Interestingly, after incubation of 3 h at 37 °C, the H_2O_2 concentrations of bare HGM-Hp1 and HGM-Hp2 (peptide controls) (Figure 6B) were obviously higher than their H_2O_2 self-productions in Figure 5B. Although the incubation of bare peptide at 37 °C contributed to produce more H_2O_2, the concentration of extracellular H_2O_2 in *E. coli* cells after treatment with HGM-Hp1 or HGM-Hp2 at 37 °C for 3 h was significantly higher than those observed in the bare bacteria or their peptide controls ($p < 0.05$) (Figure 6B).

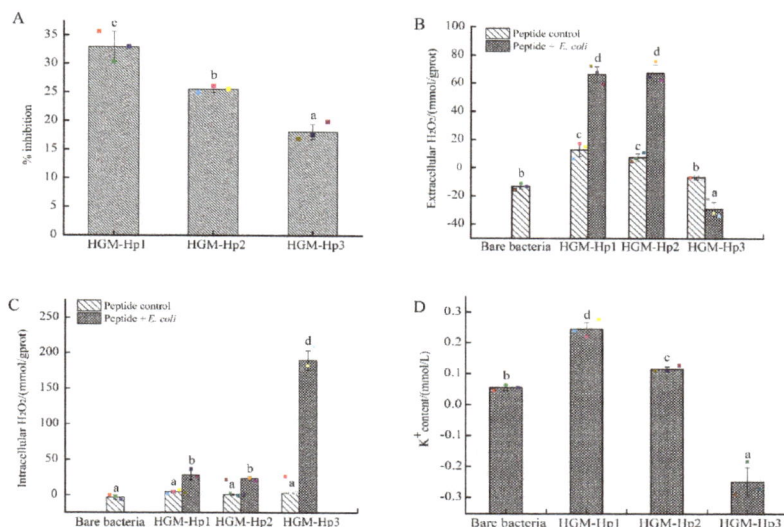

Figure 6. Antibacterial activity of synthetic peptides on the logarithmic growth phase of *E. coli* cells: (**A**) percentage inhibition; (**B**) extracellular H_2O_2 concentration; (**C**) intracellular H_2O_2 concentration; and (**D**) extracellular potassium ion (K^+) content. Raw data are displayed as spots. *E. coli* cells and peptides treated under the same conditions were used as the bare bacteria and peptide control, respectively. The results are represented as the mean ± standard deviation (*n* = 3). Different letters (a–d) indicate significant differences among samples ($p < 0.05$).

Likewise, the intracellular H_2O_2 concentration in *E. coli* cells after incubation with HGM-Hp1 or HGM-Hp2 were significantly higher than those in the bare bacteria or their peptide controls ($p < 0.05$) (Figure 6C). In contrast, the increase of extracellular H_2O_2 production was not observed in the logarithmic phase of *E. coli* cells after treatment of HGM-Hp3 (Figure 6B). Nevertheless, the highest intracellular H_2O_2 concentration in *E. coli* cells was induced by HGM-Hp3 addition (189.74 mmol/gprot), which was dramatically increased than those in HGM-Hp1 (28.16 mmol/gprot) or HGM-Hp2 (23.35 mmol/gprot) treatment ($p < 0.05$) (Figure 6C). The results in Figure 6 suggest that peptides HGM-Hp1, HGM-Hp2, and HGM-Hp3 induced intracellular H_2O_2 production in logarithmic phase of *E. coli* cells. This result is similar to our previous study of HAHp(9.0)-G MRPs, which induced H_2O_2 production in *E. coli* cells after 3 h of incubation at 37 °C [19]. In a recent study, Bucekova et al. (2018) [41] reported the antibacterial activity of honey samples incubated at 45 °C was enhanced by 25% when compared to untreated honeys, and significantly increased H_2O_2 accumulation and glucose oxidase activity were detected as well in the honey samples exposed to 45 °C. This means the H_2O_2 formation in samples or treated cells could play a crucial role for the antibacterial activity of mild thermal products or MRPs.

However, the H_2O_2 production in *E. coli* cells induced by HGM-Hp1 and HGM-Hp2 addition were different from the case of HGM-Hp3. Apparently, the treatments of HGM-Hp1 and HGM-Hp2 quickly resulted in extracellular H_2O_2 accumulation in the logarithmic phase of *E. coli* cells, while

HGM-Hp3 caused dramatic increases of intracellular H_2O_2 accumulation. The aqueous solution of logarithmic phase *E. coli* cells could provide enough cell membranes for interaction with peptides, which could contribute to the rapid permeation of smaller peptides HGM-Hp1 (807.07 Da) and HGM-Hp2 (735.85 Da) into the biomembrane as compared with the relatively large peptide of HGM-Hp3 (1438.42 Da). Furthermore, the dramatic increases of intracellular H_2O_2 accumulation in logarithmic phase of *E. coli* cells after addition of synthetic peptides also suggested the undergone oxidative stress induced by these synthetic peptides.

High ROS level in cells can lead to oxidative damage to cell membranes, and finally result in morphological and physiological changes [42,43]. In this context, measuring the efflux of K^+ from bacterial cells, a classical method to assess the membrane damage caused by antimicrobial agents [44–46], was a priority to determine after addition of synthetic peptides. As shown in Figure 6D, the amount of extracellular K^+ ions in HGM-Hp1 or HGM-Hp2 treatment was significantly higher than that in the bare bacteria (without synthetic peptide addition) ($p < 0.05$). The trend of K^+ content variations of peptide treatments was consistent with the change of their percentage inhibitions (Figure 6A). The higher the K^+ content was in the cell suspension after treatment, the more serious was the observed membrane damage. In addition, the results in Figure 6D suggest that the destruction of membrane integrity could contribute to dramatic increase of extracellular H_2O_2 in HGM-Hp1 and HGM-Hp2 treatments, due to accumulated intracellular H_2O_2 leakage. Based on the result of Figure 6, we supposed that the intracellular H_2O_2 accumulation might play an important role on the antibacterial action of synthetic peptides via ROS trigger pathway, especially for shorter peptides such as HGM-Hp1 and HGM-Hp2. To the best of our knowledge, it is the first report of antibacterial peptide derived from the MRPs of marine protein hydrolysates could perform the antibacterial activity via inducing intracellular H_2O_2 production.

3. Materials and Methods

3.1. Materials

Half-fin anchovy (*Setipinna taty*), were bought from the local aquatic market in Zhoushan City, China. The strain of *E. coli* CGMCC 1.1100 used as the indicative bacterium was provided by School of Food Science and Pharmacy, Zhejiang Ocean University. H_2O_2 and K^+ assay kits were purchased from Jiancheng Bioengineering Institute (Nanjing, China). Reagents used in HPLC or RP-HPLC, and MS were chromatographic and mass spectrometric grade, respectively. Other reagents were analytical grade and were commercially available.

3.2. Preparation of HAHp(9.0)-G MRPs

HAHp was prepared according to our previous method [18]. In brief, the minced half-fin anchovy was blended with deionized water at a ratio of 1:4 (w/v). The pH of the mixture was adjusted to 2.0 using 6 mol/L HCl, then preincubated at 37 °C for 30 min. Pepsin was added at a ratio of 1100 U/g and incubated at 37 °C for 2.4 h. The hydrolysis was terminated by heating at 95 °C for 10 min to inactive pepsin. Then, the hydrolysates were adjusted to pH of 5.0 using 6 mol/L NaOH, and centrifuged at 10,000× *g* for 20 min at 4 °C (Himae CF 16 RX versatile compact centrifuge, Tokyo, Japan) to remove insoluble material (including upper layer of fat and sediments). The soluble hydrolysates, namely HAHp, were filtered and adjusted to pH of 9.0. After centrifugation of 10 min at 6000× *g*, the supernatant was blended with glucose at a ratio of 100:3 (v/m), followed by thermal treatment at 120 °C for 100 min. The generated dark brown products, designated as HAHp(9.0)-G MRPs, were kept at −20 °C until use. The mass of peptide in HAHp(9.0)-G MRPs was 6.71 mg/mL. The production rate of peptide in HAHp(9.0)-G MRPs per 100 g content of half-fin anchovy (wet weight) was 2.68%.

3.3. Peptide Concentration Determination

Peptide concentration was determined using the method of O-phthalaldehyde (OPA) described by Bougherra et al. (2017) [47] with slight modifications. Briefly, 25 µL of sample were mixed with 1 mL of OPA solution. After completely blending, 600 µL of the mixture solution were added into a micro cuvette. The absorbance was determined at 340 nm with a UV-vis 1200 spectrophotometer (Hitachi, Tokyo, Japan). Glutathione was used as a standard peptide to make standard curve.

3.4. Antibacterial Assay

The antibacterial activity of isolated fractions was determined using the method of 96-well micro-plate [18]. Briefly, 100 µL of *E. coli* cells at the logarithmic phase were pipetted into 10 mL of sterilized nutrient broth to prepare the *E. coli* suspension. Then, 50 µL of samples were added with 50 µL of *E. coli* suspension and incubated at 37 °C for 24 h. The absorbance of sample (A_S) was measured at 630 nm by a SM-800 micro-plate reader (Shanghai Utrao Medical Instrument Co., Ltd, China). The antibacterial activity, indicated as the percentage inhibition, was calculated according to the following equation:

$$\text{Percentage inhibition (\%)} = [A_C - (A_S - A_{SB})]/(A_C - A_B)] \times 100 \tag{1}$$

where A_C is the absorbance of control, with the same volume of distilled water instead of sample solution; A_S is the absorbance of the sample; A_{SB} is the absorbance of sample blank, with same volume of distilled water in substitute of *E. coli* suspensions; and A_B is the absorbance of distilled water.

3.5. H_2O_2 Assay

The amount of H_2O_2 self-production in isolated fractions or peptides was determined using the H_2O_2 assay kit. Briefly, 250 µL of Reagent 1 (incubated at 37 °C) were added with 25 µL of sample, and 250 µL of Reagent 2. After complete blending, the absorbance of sample tube (A_S) was measured at 405 nm using a micro-cuvette. The amount of H_2O_2 was calculated according to the following equation:

$$H_2O_2 \text{ content (mmol/gprot)} = [(A_S - A_B)/(A_C - A_B)] \times 163/P_C \tag{2}$$

where A_B is the absorbance of blank tube, using the same volume of double-distilled water instead of the sample; A_C is the absorbance of standard tube, using the same volume of 163 mmol/L H_2O_2 instead of the sample; 163 is the concentration of standard H_2O_2 solution (mmol/L); and P_C is the protein concentration (mg/mL).

3.6. Purification of H_2O_2 Self-Production Peptides from HAHp(9.0)-G MRPs

3.6.1. SEC

After being filtered through a 0.22 µm micro-filter, the filtration of HAHp(9.0)-G MRPs was used for purification. The isolation of peptidic components was carried out by employing a 1260 Agilent HPLC system equipped with a PL aquagel-OH 30 column (75 × 300 mm, 8 µm, Agilent Technologies, Inc., Santa Clara, CA, USA), with separation mass ranging from 100 to 30,000 Dalton. The injection volume of HAHp(9.0)-G MRPs was 20 µL. The isolation process was firstly eluted with 30% acetonitrile at a flow rate of 0.5 mL/min under temperature of 25 °C and the UV absorption was measured at 220 nm. The purification was repeated 20 times at the same elution conditions to collect enough isolated fractions for further assay. The freeze-dried isolated fractions were dissolved in distilled water. The antibacterial activity (measured as percentage inhibition) and H_2O_2 self-production capacity (represented as mmol/gprot) of isolated fractions were assayed. The active peptic fraction was then selected for further purification.

3.6.2. Solid Phase Extraction (SPE) and Purification by RP-HPLC

The active fraction F2 isolated from SEC was separated using a small SPE cartridge (Cleanert® S C18-N, 500 mg/3mL, Agela Technologies, Tianjin, China). Prior to elution with 3 mL of 30% methanol (containing 0.1% formic acid), the SPE cartridge was pre-activated with 6 mL methanol and then rinsed with 12 mL water. The filtrate or eluent were collected and designated as the hydrophilic extract. The absorbed hydrophobic compounds were washed off with 3 mL of 70% acetonitrile. The hydrophilic and hydrophobic components of the extract were lyophilized separately. After being re-dissolved in distilled water, the percentage inhibitions of hydrophilic and hydrophobic components of F2 on the growth of *E. coli* cells were measured by utilizing the 96-well micro-plate method (described in the Section 2.3).

The hydrophobic extract of F2, which showed the largest percentage inhibition, was loaded onto a RP-HPLC system equipped with a C_{18} column (4.6 × 250 mm, 5 μm, Sunfire™, Waters, MA, USA) for further separation. Solvent A, 0.1% (v/v) trifluoroacetic acid (TFA) in water, and solvent B, 100% acetonitrile with 0.1% (v/v) TFA, were used for elution. A gradient elution was carried out as follows: 0–25 min, 5–45% solvent B; 25–30 min, 45–85% solvent B; 30–40 min, 85–95% solvent B; 40–50 min, 95–5% solvent B; 50–60 min, 95–5% solvent B, at a constant flow rate of 1.0 mL/min, and measured at 280 nm. Major separated peaks of F2 were collected, then freeze-dried. The percentage inhibitions of major peaks in F2 against *E. coli* cells, as well as the H_2O_2 self-production capacity were measured and compared.

3.6.3. Identification of Peptide by LC-ESI-Q-TOF-MS/MS

The bioactive peak derived from RP-HPLC was subjected to LC-ESI-Q-TOF-MS/MS analysis, aiming to identify all potential peptides. The separation was performed on a Nano Aquity UPLC system (Waters Corporation, Milford, MA, USA), coupled with a quadrupole-Orbitrap mass spectrometer (Q-Exactive) (Thermo Fisher Scientific, Bremen, Germany) and equipped with an online nano-electrospray ion source. Elution was carried out by applying the UPLC system, according to the following procedures: 4 μL of sample were loaded on a C_{18} column (75 μm × 250 mm, 3 μm, Eksigent, Livermore, CA, USA). Solvent A (0.1% formic acid in water) and solvent B (acetonitrile with 0.1% formic acid) were used for the gradient elution, 0–45 min, 5–30% solvent B; 45–50 min, 30–80% solvent B; 50–52 min, 80% solvent B; 53 min, 5% solvent B; 53–60 min, 5% solvent B, at a flow rate of 300 nL/min. First order MS detection was performed in a positive MS-mode with resolution of 70,000, and the automatic gain control (AGC) was set at 1×10^6, mass-to-charge ratio scanning from 350 to 1600 m/z. At each elution time, ten strongest ions were automatically selected for MS/MS analysis using a higher energy collisional dissociation (HCD). The resolution of MS/MS was 17,500, and AGC was set at 2×10^5. Raw data files of peptides acquired on the Q-TOF from the samples were searched against the protein database of *Clupeoidei* in NCBI. Through homology analysis in *Clupeoidei*, peptide was considered a match if its −10lgP score was greater than 80. Furthermore, de novo peptide automated spectrum processing was performed using the PEAKS Studio software (7.0) (Bioinformatics Solutions Inc., Waterloo, Canada) (http://www.bioinfor.com). PEAKS Studio awards confidence scores for the entire range of amino acid sequences studied [48]. In de novo peptide, the ALC and local confidence scores indicate that the probability of peptide sequence is correct [48]. In this study, de novo sequences of peptides with ALC ≥ 95%, and local confidence of each amino acid residue ≥ 90% were set for validation of predicted peptides.

3.7. Peptide Synthesis

Three peptides were synthesized by Synpeptide Co., Ltd. (Shanghai, China) based on their sequences. The purity of synthetic peptide was determined (>98%) using HPLC analysis. Furthermore, the molecular mass of synthetic peptides was also measured using MS analysis under ESI positive mode. The helical wheel projection of peptide was performed using an online tool (http://rzlab.ucr. edu/scripts/wheel/wheel.cgi).

3.8. CD Spectroscopy of Synthetic Peptides

The secondary structure of synthetic peptides in membrane mimic solution (1.6 mM SDS, dissolved in 10 mM PBS, pH 7.4) was evaluated as in our previous method [25] using a Chirscan circular dichroism spectrometer (Applied Photophysics Ltd., Surrey, UK) at 25 °C according to the following parameters: scanning wavelength from 190 to 260 nm in 1 mm quartz cuvette, scanning speed of 100 nm/min, step size of 1 nm, and 0.5 nm bandwidth. Spectra were corrected for background contributions by subtraction of appropriate blanks. The delta epsilon in degrees was displayed as a function of the wavelength in nanometers.

3.9. Physicochemical Property of Synthetic Peptides

The molecular weight (Da), pI, net charge and hydrophobicity of peptides were estimated using the PepDraw Tool (http://www.tulane.edu/~{}biochem/WW/PepDraw/). The GRAVY and instability index of peptides were predicted by ProtParam Tool (http://web.expasy.org/protparam/). Homology searches of peptides were performed using the APD (http://aps.unmc.edu/AP/main.html) and BLAST program in NCBI non-redundant peptide database (http://www.ncbi.nlm.nih.gov/blast). The secondary structure of synthetic peptides was predicted by the protein sequence analysis tool of Hierarchial Neural Network in NPS@ analysis (https://npsa-prabi.ibcp.fr) with SOPMA method [49].

3.10. MIC Determination of Synthetic Peptides

The MIC of synthetic peptides against *E. coli* was determined using a twofold microdilution method described in our previous study [18] with slight modifications. In brief, various concentrations of synthetic peptides (50 μL, stock peptide concentration of 4 mg/mL dissolved in distilled water) were added to a sterile 96-well microplate. Then, 50 μL of *E. coli* suspension at logarithmic phase in broth medium were added to every well. After incubation of 24 h at 37 °C, the MIC is defined as the lowest concentration of peptide at which no visible bacterial growth is observed. Furthermore, the growth of *E. coli* cells was measured by the optical density at 630 nm using a SM-800 micro-plate reader (Shanghai Utrao Medical Instrument Co., Ltd., China) after incubation of different concentrations of synthetic peptides. The same volume of distilled water instead of peptide was used in positive control, and no bacteria with peptide was used in negative control. The percentage inhibition of synthetic peptides was calculated according to the Equation (1) described in Section 3.4. The antibacterial effects of nisin A and ε-poly-L-lysine, two commercial peptides used in food preservatives, were compared in the same conditions. Four replicas were performed in each concentration.

3.11. Intracellular and Extracellular H_2O_2 Formation in Logarithmic Phase of E. coli Induced by Synthetic Peptides

The capacity of synthetic peptide, which induced intracellular and extracellular H_2O_2 production in the logarithmic growth phase of *E. coli* cells after treatment of 3 h at 37 °C, was investigated, referring to the method of our previous studies [19]. Briefly, after incubation of 3 h at 37 °C, the mixture was centrifuged at 4000× *g* for 5 min; the supernatants were collected for detection of extracellular H_2O_2 content. The remaining pellets were blended with 300 μL of icy saline and ultrasonically treated in ice bath (5 of pulses, 2 min of each pulse) to destroy the cell membrane completely. After centrifugation at 4000× *g* for 5 min, the supernatants were collected and utilized for the assay of intracellular H_2O_2 concentration. An equivalent volume of distilled water instead of the synthetic peptide solution incubated with *E. coli* cells at the same conditions was designated as the bare bacteria group. Before and after ultrasonic treatment, the supernatants of the bare bacteria group were collected. In addition, the H_2O_2 self-production of synthetic peptides after addition of saline with a ratio of 1:1 (*v/v*) treated under the same conditions was measured as the control. The H_2O_2 concentrations of all groups were determined using the H_2O_2 assay kit. The efflux of K^+ from *E. coli* cells (the supernatants without ultrasonic treatment) after incubation of synthetic peptides was determined using the K^+ assay kit and expressed as mmol/L. All determinations were performed in triplicate for each group.

3.12. Statistical Analysis

Data are presented as mean $\pm$ standard deviation ($n = 3$). Statistical analysis was performed using the SPSS® software (SPSS Statistical Software 19.0, Inc., Chicago, IL, USA). The independent sample *t*-test was used to evaluate the significant differences between two samples ($p < 0.05$ or $p < 0.01$).

4. Conclusions

Several short peptides were identified from the active peptidic fractions derived from HAHp(9.0)-G MRPs. The synthesized peptides HGM-Hp1 (FEDQLR), HGM-Hp2 (ALERTF), and HGM-Hp3 (RHPEYAVSVLLR) had different net charges. However, they possessed positive R residue, and a portion of hydrophobic residues in their sequences. After incubation of 3 h at 37 °C with logarithmic growth phase of *E. coli* cells, the synthetic peptides induced dramatic increases of extracellular and/or intracellular H_2O_2 accumulation. Significant increases of K^+ were also detected in HGM-Hp1 and HGM-Hp2 treatments. Our results suggest that HAHp(9.0)-G MRPs are a good source of antibacterial peptides. These identified peptides could have potential use to treat Gram-negative infections in general. Furthermore, H_2O_2 production might be a potential cause of the antibacterial activity for these synthetic peptides.

Author Contributions: J.W. performed the experiments; R.W. contributed to discussion and revision of the paper; and R.S. performed the experiments, analyzed the data, and wrote the paper.

Funding: This work was funded by grants from the National Natural Science Foundation of China (31671959) and Zhejiang Provincial Natural Science Foundation of China (LY15C200018).

Conflicts of Interest: The authors declare no conflict of interest.

References

1. Tong, Z.; Zhang, Y.; Ling, J.; Ma, J.; Huang, L.; Zhang, L. An in vitro study on the effects of nisin on the antibacterial activities of 18 antibiotics against *Enterococcus faecalis*. *PLoS ONE* **2014**, *9*, e89209. [CrossRef] [PubMed]
2. Aoki, W.; Kuroda, K.; Ueda, M. Next generation of antimicrobial peptides as molecular targeted medicines. *J. Biosci. Bioeng.* **2012**, *114*, 365–370. [CrossRef] [PubMed]
3. Patel, S.; Akhtar, N. Antimicrobial peptides (AMPs): The quintessential 'offense and defense' molecules are more than antimicrobials. *Biomed. Pharmacother.* **2017**, *95*, 1276–1283. [CrossRef] [PubMed]
4. Liu, Z.; Dong, S.; Xu, J.; Zeng, M.; Song, H.; Zhao, Y. Production of cysteine-rich antimicrobial peptide by digestion of oyster (*Crassostrea gigas*) with alcalase and bromelin. *Food Control* **2008**, *19*, 231–235. [CrossRef]
5. Sila, A.; Nedjar-Arroume, N.; Hedhili, K.; Chataigne, G.; Balti, R.; Nasri, M.; Dhulster, P.; Bougatef, A. Antibacterial peptides from barbel muscle protein hydrolysates: Activity against some pathogenic bacteria. *LWT-Food Sci. Technol.* **2014**, *55*, 183–188. [CrossRef]
6. Jemil, I.; Abdelhedi, O.; Nasri, R.; Mora, L.; Jridi, M.; Aristoy, M.C.; Toldrá, F.; Nasri, M. Novel bioactive peptides from enzymatic hydrolysate of Sardinelle (*Sardinella aurita*) muscle proteins hydrolysed by *Bacillus subtilis* A26 proteases. *Food Res. Int.* **2017**, *100*, 121–133. [CrossRef] [PubMed]
7. Tang, W.; Zhang, H.; Wang, L.; Qian, H.; Qi, X. Targeted separation of antibacterial peptide from protein hydrolysate of anchovy cooking wastewater by equilibrium dialysis. *Food Chem.* **2015**, *168*, 115–123. [CrossRef]
8. Dashper, S.G.; Liu, S.W.; Reynolds, E.C. Antimicrobial peptides and their potential as oral therapeutic agents. *Int. J. Pept. Res. Ther.* **2007**, *13*, 505–516. [CrossRef]
9. Hodge, J.E. Dehydrated foods, chemistry of browning reactions in model systems. *J. Agric. Food Chem.* **1953**, *1*, 928–943. [CrossRef]

10. Chung, Y.C.; Kuo, C.L.; Chen, C.C. Preparation and important functional properties of water-soluble chitosan produced through Maillard reaction. *Bioresour. Technol.* **2005**, *96*, 1473–1482. [CrossRef] [PubMed]

11. Liang, C.X.; Yuan, F.; Liu, F.G.; Wang, Y.Y.; Gao, Y.X. Structure and antimicrobial mechanism of ε-polylysine–chitosan conjugates through Maillard reaction. *Int. J. Biol. Macromol.* **2014**, *70*, 427–434. [CrossRef] [PubMed]

12. Wu, S.; Hu, J.; Wei, L.; Du, Y.; Shi, X.; Zhang, L. Antioxidant and antimicrobial activity of Maillard reaction products from xylan with chitosan/chitooligomer/glucosamine hydrochloride/taurine model systems. *Food Chem.* **2014**, *148*, 196–203. [CrossRef] [PubMed]

13. Lindenmeier, M.; Faist, V.; Hofmann, T. Structural and functional characterization of pronyl-lysine, a novel protein modification in bread crust melanoidins showing in vitro, antioxidative and phase I/II enzyme modulating activity. *J. Agric. Food Chem.* **2002**, *50*, 6997–7006. [CrossRef] [PubMed]

14. Monente, C.; Bravo, J.; Vitas, A.I.; Arbillaga, L.; Peña, M.P.D.; Cid, C. Coffee and spent coffee extracts protect against cell mutagens and inhibit growth of food-borne pathogen microorganisms. *J. Funct. Foods* **2015**, *12*, 365–374. [CrossRef]

15. Rufian-Henares, J.A.; Morales, F.J. Antimicrobial activity of melanoidins against *Escherichia Coli*, is mediated by a membrane-damage mechanism. *J. Agric. Food Chem.* **2008**, *56*, 2357–2362. [CrossRef] [PubMed]

16. Rufian-Henares, J.A.; Cueva, S.P. Antimicrobial activity of coffee melanoidins-a study of their metal-chelating properties. *J. Agric. Food Chem.* **2009**, *57*, 432–438. [CrossRef] [PubMed]

17. Mueller, U.; Sauer, T.; Weigel, I.; Pichner, R.; Pischetsrieder, M. Identification of H_2O_2 as a major antimicrobial component in coffee. *Food Funct.* **2011**, *2*, 265–272. [CrossRef]

18. Song, R.; Wei, R.B.; Zhang, B.; Wang, D.F. Optimization of the antibacterial activity of half-fin anchovy (*Setipinna taty*) hydrolysates. *Food Bioprocess Technol.* **2012**, *5*, 1979–1989. [CrossRef]

19. Song, R.; Shi, Q.; Yang, P.; Wei, R. In vitro membrane damage induced by half-fin anchovy hydrolysates/glucose Maillard reaction products and the effects on oxidative status in vivo. *Food Funct.* **2018**, *9*, 785–796. [CrossRef]

20. Tong, G.; Du, F.; Wu, W.; Wu, R.; Liu, F.; Liang, Y. Enhanced reactive oxygen species (ROS) yields and antibacterial activity of spongy $ZnO/ZnFe_2O_4$ hybrid micro-hexahedra selectively synthesized through a versatile glucose-engineered co-precipitation/annealing process. *J. Mater. Chem. B* **2013**, *1*, 2647–2657. [CrossRef]

21. Hauser, C.; Müller, U.; Sauer, T.; Augner, K.; Pischetsrieder, M. Maillard reaction products as antimicrobial components for packaging films. *Food Chem.* **2014**, *145*, 608–613. [CrossRef] [PubMed]

22. Lin, L.; Li, B.F. Radical scavenging properties of protein hydrolysates from Jumbo flying squid (*Dosidicus eschrichitii Steenstrup*) skin gelatin. *J. Sci. Food Agric.* **2006**, *86*, 2290–2295. [CrossRef]

23. Ennaas, N.; Hammami, R.; Beaulieu, L.; Fliss, I. Purification and characterization of four antibacterial peptides from protamex hydrolysate of Atlantic mackerel (*Scomber scombrus*) by-products. *Biochem. Biophys. Res. Commun.* **2015**, *462*, 195–200. [CrossRef] [PubMed]

24. Lawyer, C.; Pai, S.; Watabe, M.; Borgia, P.; Mashimo, T.; Eagleton, L.; Watabe, K. Antimicrobial activity of a 13 amino acid tryptophan-rich peptide derived from a putative porcine precursor protein of a novel family of antibacterial peptides. *FEBS Lett.* **1996**, *390*, 95–98. [CrossRef]

25. Song, R.; Shi, Q.Q.; Yang, P.Y.; Wei, R.B. Identification of antibacterial peptides from Maillard reaction products of half-fin anchovy hydrolysates/glucose via LC-ESI-QTOF-MS analysis. *J. Funct. Foods* **2017**, *36*, 387–395. [CrossRef]

26. Zhu, X.; Zhang, L.; Wang, J.; Ma, Z.; Xu, W.; Li, J.; Shan, A. Characterization of antimicrobial activity and mechanisms of low amphipathic peptides with different α-helical propensity. *Acta Biomater.* **2015**, *18*, 155–167. [CrossRef]

27. Zhang, J.; Movahedi, A.; Wang, X.; Wu, X.; Yin, T.; Zhuge, Q. Molecular structure, chemical synthesis, and antibacterial activity of ABP-dHC-cecropin A from drury (*Hyphantria cunea*). *Peptides* **2015**, *68*, 197–204. [CrossRef]

28. Kyte, J.; Doolittle, R.F. A simple method for displaying the hydropathic character of a protein. *J. Mol. Biol.* **1982**, *157*, 105–132. [CrossRef]

29. Falla, T.J.; Karunaratne, D.N.; Hancock, R.E.W. Mode of action of the antimicrobial peptide indolicidin. *J. Biol. Chem.* **1996**, *271*, 19298–19303. [CrossRef]

30. Genaro, R.; Zanetti, M. Structural features and biological activities of the cathelicidin-derived antimicrobial peptide. *Biopolymers* **2000**, *55*, 31–49. [CrossRef]

31. Powers, J.P.S.; Hancock, R.E.W. The relationship between peptide structure and bacterial activity. *Peptides* **2003**, *24*, 1681–1691. [CrossRef] [PubMed]

32. Kelly, S.M.; Price, N.C. The use of circular dichroism in the investigation of protein structure and function. *Curr. Protein Pept. Sci.* **2000**, *1*, 1349–1384. [CrossRef]

33. Kelly, S.M.; Jess, T.J.; Price, N.C. How to study proteins by circular dichroism. *Biochim. Biophys. Acta (BBA)-Proteins Proteom.* **2005**, *1751*, 119–139. [CrossRef] [PubMed]

34. Wall, J.S.; Williams, A.; Wooliver, C.; Martin, E.B.; Cheng, X.L.; Heidel, R.E.; Kennel, S.J. Secondary structure propensity and chirality of the amyloidophilic peptide p5 and its analogues impacts ligand binding—In vitro characterization. *Biochem. Biophys. Rep.* **2016**, *8*, 89–99. [CrossRef] [PubMed]

35. Yu, H.; Huang, Y.; Huang, Q. Synthesis and characterization of novel antimicrobial emulsifiers from ε-Polylysine. *J. Agric. Food Chem.* **2009**, *58*, 1290–1295. [CrossRef] [PubMed]

36. Zhou, C.; Li, X.; Sharif, A.R.M.; Poon, Y.F.; Cao, Y.; Chang, M.W.; Leong, S.S.; Chan-Park, M.B. A photopolymerized antimicrobial hydrogel coating derived from epsilon-poly-L-lysine. *Biomaterials* **2011**, *32*, 2704–2712. [CrossRef] [PubMed]

37. Li, S.; Hao, L.; Bao, W.; Zhang, P.; Su, D.; Cheng, Y.; Nie, L.; Wang, G.; Hou, F.; Yang, Y. A novel short anionic antibacterial peptide isolated from the skin of Xenopus laevis with broad antibacterial activity and inhibitory activity against breast cancer cell. *Arch. Microbiol.* **2016**, *198*, 473–482. [CrossRef]

38. Hilpert, K.; Elliott, M.; Jenssen, H.; Kindrachuk, J.; Fjell, C.D.; Körner, J.; Winkler, D.F.; Weaver, L.L.; Henklein, P.; Ulrich, A.S.; et al. Screening and characterization of surface-tethered cationic peptides for antimicrobial activity. *Chem. Biol.* **2009**, *16*, 58–69. [CrossRef]

39. Teixeira, V.; Feio, M.J.; Bastos, M. Role of lipids in the interaction of antimicrobial peptides with membranes. *Prog. Lipid Res.* **2012**, *2*, 149–177. [CrossRef]

40. Kim, I.W.; Lee, J.H.; Subramaniyam, S.; Yun, E.Y.; Kim, I.; Park, J.; Hwang, J.S. De novo transcriptome analysis and detection of antimicrobial peptides of the American Cockroach Periplaneta americana (*Linnaeus*). *PLoS ONE* **2016**, *11*, e0155304. [CrossRef]

41. Bucekova, M.; Juricova, V.; Marco, G.D.; Gismondi, A.; Leonardi, D.; Canini, A.; Majtan, J. Effect of thermal liquefying of crystallised honeys on their antibacterial activities. *Food Chem.* **2018**, *269*, 335–341. [CrossRef] [PubMed]

42. Ning, C.; Wang, X.; Li, L.; Zhu, Y.; Li, M.; Yu, P.; Zhou, L.; Zhou, Z.; Chen, J.; Tan, G.; et al. Concentration ranges of antibacterial cations for showing the highest antibacterial efficacy but the least cytotoxicity against mammalian cells: Implications for a new antibacterial mechanism. *Chem. Res. Toxicol.* **2015**, *28*, 1815–1822. [CrossRef] [PubMed]

43. Liao, W.; Lai, T.; Chen, L.; Fu, J.; Sreenivasan, S.T.; Yu, Z.; Ren, J. Synthesis and characterization of a walnut peptides-zinc complex and its antiproliferative activity against human beast Carcinoma cells through the induction of apoptosis. *J. Agric. Food Chem.* **2016**, *104*, 849–859.

44. Lee, H.; Hwang, J.S.; Lee, J.; Kim, J.; Lee, D.G. Scolopendin 2, a cationic antimicrobial peptide from centipede, and its membrane-active mechanism. *Biochim. Biophys. Acta (BBA)-Biomembr.* **2015**, *1848*, 634–642. [CrossRef] [PubMed]

45. Miao, J.; Liu, G.; Ke, C.; Fan, W.; Li, C.; Chen, Y.; Dixon, W.; Song, M.; Cao, Y.; Xiao, H. Inhibitory effects of a novel antimicrobial peptide from kefir against *Escherichia coli*. *Food Control* **2016**, *65*, 63–72. [CrossRef]

46. Riazi, S.; Dover, S.E.; Chikindas, M.L. Mode of action and safety of lactosporin, a novel antimicrobial protein produced by *Bacillus coagulans* ATCC7050. *J. Appl. Microbiol.* **2012**, *113*, 714–722. [CrossRef] [PubMed]

47. Bougherra, F.; Dilmi-Bouras, A.; Balti, R.; Przybylski, R.; Adoui, F.; Elhameur, H.; Chevalier, M.; Flahaut, C.; Dhulster, P.; Naima, N. Antibacterial activity of new peptide from bovine casein hydrolyzed by a serine metalloprotease of Lactococcus lactis subsp lactis BR16. *J. Funct. Foods* **2017**, *32*, 112–122. [CrossRef]

48. Ma, B.; Zhang, K.Z.; Hendrie, C.; Liang, C.Z.; Li, M.; Doherty-Kirty, A.; Lajoie, G. PEAKS: Powerful software for peptide de novo sequencing by tandem massspectrometry. *Rapid Commun. Mass Spectrom.* **2003**, *17*, 2337–2342. [CrossRef]

49. Combet, C.; Blanchet, C.; Geourjon, C.; Deléage, G. NPS@: Network protein sequence analysis. *Trends Biochem. Sci.* **2000**, *25*, 147–150. [CrossRef]

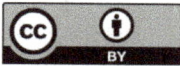

marine drugs

MDPI

Article

A Novel Natural Influenza A H1N1 Virus Neuraminidase Inhibitory Peptide Derived from Cod Skin Hydrolysates and Its Antiviral Mechanism

Jianpeng Li [1], Yiping Chen [1], Ning Yuan [1], Mingyong Zeng [1,*], Yuanhui Zhao [1,*], Rilei Yu [2], Zunying Liu [1], Haohao Wu [1] and Shiyuan Dong [1]

[1]   College of Food Science and Engineering, Ocean University of China, Qingdao 266003, China; changjing@stu.ouc.edu.cn (J.L.); chenyiping@stu.ouc.edu.cn (Y.C.); ningy1@126.com (N.Y.); liuzunying@ouc.edu.cn (Z.L.); wuhaohao@ouc.edu.cn (H.W.) dongshiyuan@ouc.edu.cn (S.D.)
[2]   School of Medicine and Pharmacy, Ocean University of China, Qingdao 266003, China; ryu@ouc.edu.cn
*   Correspondence: mingyz@ouc.edu.cn (M.Z.); zhaoyuanhui@ouc.edu.cn (Y.Z.);
    Tel./Fax: +86-532-6678-2427 (M.Z.); +86-532-8203-2400 (Y.Z.)

Received: 13 September 2018; Accepted: 6 October 2018; Published: 10 October 2018

Abstract: In this paper, a novel natural influenza A H1N1 virus neuraminidase (NA) inhibitory peptide derived from cod skin hydrolysates was purified and its antiviral mechanism was explored. From the hydrolysates, novel efficient NA-inhibitory peptides were purified by a sequential approach utilizing an ultrafiltration membrane (5000 Da), sephadex G-15 gel column and reverse-phase high-performance liquid chromatography (RP-HPLC). The amino acid sequence of the pure peptide was determined by electrospray ionization Fourier transform ion cyclotron resonance mass spectrometry (ESI-FTICR-MS) was PGEKGPSGEAGTAGPPGTPGPQGL, with a molecular weight of 2163 Da. The analysis of the Lineweacer–Burk model indicated that the peptide was a competitive NA inhibitor with Ki of 0.29 mM and could directly bind free enzymes. In addition, docking studies suggested that hydrogen binding might be the driving force for the binding affinity of PGEKGPSGEAGTAGPPGTPGPQGL to NA. The cytopathic effect reduction assay showed that the peptide PGEKGPSGEAGTAGPPGTPGPQGL protected Madin–Darby canine kidney (MDCK) cells from viral infection and reduced the viral production in a dose-dependent manner. The EC_{50} value was 471 ± 12 µg/mL against H1N1. Time-course analysis showed that PGEKGPSGEAGTAGPPGTPGPQGL inhibited influenza virus in the early stage of the infectious cycle. The virus titers assay indicated that the NA-inhibitory peptide PGEKGPSGEAGTAGPPGTPGPQGL could directly affect the virus toxicity and adsorption by host cells, further proving that the peptide had an anti-viral effect with multiple target sites. The activity of NA-inhibitory peptide was almost inactivated during the simulated in vitro gastrointestinal digestion, suggesting that oral administration is not recommended. The peptide PGEKGPSGEAGTAGPPGTPGPQGL acts as a neuraminidase blocker to inhibit influenza A virus in MDCK cells. Thus, the peptide PGEKGPSGEAGTAGPPGTPGPQGL has potential utility in the treatment of the influenza virus infection.

Keywords: cod skin; NA-inhibitory peptide; influenza virus; neuraminidase; molecular docking; adsorption

1. Introduction

   The influenza virus remains a highly contagious pathogen that causes high morbidity and mortality [1]. In 2009, the influenza A (H1N1) virus first emerged and resulted in more than 8000 deaths worldwide [2]. Furthermore, the number of patients suffering from influenza continues to grow.

Neuraminidase (NA), a surface glycoprotein, is a major structural component of the virion and plays an important role in virus replication [3]. Therefore, it is essential to explore the inhibition of NA in order to control the influenza virus.

NA inhibitors can bind to the active site of the viral NA to interfere with the virus replication [1] and are a promising target for screening anti-influenza drugs. Current NA inhibitor drugs, such as zanamivir and oseltamivir [4,5], significantly affect the duration of infection and clinical diseases [6]. However, the pharmaceutical drug efficacy, resistance and cost remain to be solved [7]. In addition, the NA inhibitor drugs may lead to some side effects, such as potential neurotoxicity, digestive discomfort and respiratory diseases [8]. Hence, it is necessary to develop alternative and natural NA inhibitors. Recently, many NA-inhibitory peptides have been found to show potential as antiviral drugs. For example, Amri et al. [9] found that some cyclic peptides, RRR and RRP, showed high NA-inhibitory activity. In addition, Upadhyay et al. [10] found that the mimosine tetrapeptide (M-FFY) also showed high NA-inhibitory activity. However, natural NA-inhibitory peptide was seldom reported.

Cod is an important fish species in China. Lots of scraps are generated during the processing and utilization of cod, which can lead to the waste of resources and environmental pollution. Thus, it is necessary to make full use of the cod scraps. More than 80% of the dry matter of cod skin [11] is collagen, which is rich in proline and L-hydroxyproline [12]. Both proline and L-hydroxyproline contain a pyrrolidine structure [13] and this group can act as hydrogen bond donors or receptors to exert anti-influenza effects by binding to neuraminidase, thus allowing the formation of proline-containing polypeptide inhibitors. A number of studies have showed that synthetic pyrrolidine-containing compounds exhibited high NA-inhibitory activity [14,15], which suggested that natural pyrrolidine-containing substances (proline and L-hydroxyproline) might also play an important role in the inhibition of NA. Recently, cod skins were widely applied in the preparation of ACE-inhibitory peptides [16,17]. However, the preparation of natural NA-inhibitory peptides from cod skin hydrolysates was not reported. Therefore, the peptide derived from cod skin hydrolysates might have the high potential in the inhibition of NA. In addition, it has been reported that the influenza-infection cycle involves several distinct steps [5,18]. Hemagglutinin (HA), a significant surface glycoprotein, also plays an important role in viral infection by mediating viral entry and fusion [19–21]. Thus, it is significant to further investigate the potential mechanisms of peptides against the influenza A virus.

To the best of our knowledge, the preparation of natural influenza A H1N1 virus neuraminidase inhibitory peptide from cod skin hydrolysates has seldom been reported. The study aims to prepare efficient NA-inhibitory peptides from cod skin hydrolysates. We identified the NA-inhibitory peptides with high activities by electrospray ionization Fourier transform ion cyclotron resonance mass spectrometry (ESI-FTICR-MS). In addition, molecular docking simulations were conducted to investigate the interactions between the peptides and NA. Moreover, the mechanism of the peptide against the influenza virus was also discussed. This study can provide previously unknown information about the effect of the novel NA-inhibitory peptides on influenza A H1N1 virus and alternative approach for antiviral therapy.

2. Results and Discussion

2.1. Isolation and Purification of Neuraminidase (NA)-Inhibitory Peptide

The enzymatic hydrolysates of cod skins were firstly ultrafiltered with an 5 K membrane to obtain the components whose molecular weight were less than 5000 Da. The IC_{50} value of the ultrafiltrate was 6.4 mg/mL (Table 1). The NA-inhibitory peptides were then fractionated using a Sephadex G-15 gel column and Fractions A–F were obtained at 220 nm (Figure 1A). The NA inhibition assays of these fractions showed that Fraction D exhibited high NA-inhibitory activity ($IC_{50} = 3.50 \pm 0.11$ mg/mL). The fractions with the same molecular weight peaked simultaneously in the Sephadex G-15 gel column [22]. Therefore, Fraction D may be a mixture and needs to be further fractionated by reverse-phase high-performance liquid chromatography (RP-HPLC).

Table 1. Purification procedure of NA-inhibitory peptides.

Components	Purification	IC_{50} (mg/mL)	Purification Fold
Hydrolysates (<5000 Da)	Ultrafiltration	6.40 ± 0.13 [a]	1.00
D	Sephadex G-15	3.50 ± 0.11 [b]	1.83
D1	RP-HPLC	0.89 ± 0.07 [c]	7.19

Mean $\pm$ standard deviation (SD) ($n = 3$). Values with different superscript letters are significantly different ($p < 0.05$).

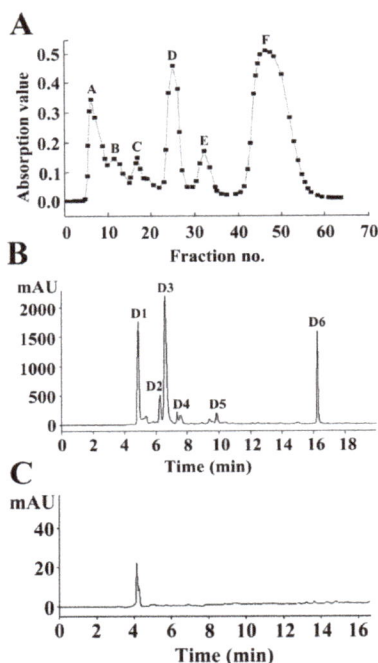

Figure 1. Isolation and purification of NA-inhibitory peptides using a Sephadex G-15 gel column (**A**) and reverse-phase high-performance liquid chromatography (RP-HPLC) (**B**). Purity identification of neuraminidase (NA)-inhibitory peptide D1 (**C**).

RP-HPLC is a common tool for isolating and purifying the polypeptides [22]. After 5 min of elution, six major peaks were detected at 220 nm, among which the peak corresponding to Fraction D1 exhibited a relatively high intensity (Figure 1B). Fraction D1 exhibited the high activity ($IC_{50} = 0.89 \pm 0.07$ mg/mL). After a two-step purification process, Fraction D1 was purified by 7.19 times (Table 1), suggesting that the NA-inhibitory activity of cod skin peptides can be significantly improved by fractionation and purification. In addition, Fraction D1 exhibited a single peak in an analytical C_{18} HPLC column (Figure 1C), suggesting that the purity of D1 had met the requirement for sequencing.

2.2. Identification of the NA-Inhibitory Peptide

ESI-FTICR-MS can simultaneously dissociate multiple precursor ions and has a wide detection range, high resolution, and high precision [23]. To determine the matching degree of the identification sequence, the sequence results were matched by using the Swiss Prot database. The matching result showed that the determined sequence was PGEKGPSGEAGTAGPPGTPGPQGL with a molecular mass of 2163 Da (Figure 2). The peptide consisted of 24 amino acid residues and proline accounted for a quarter.

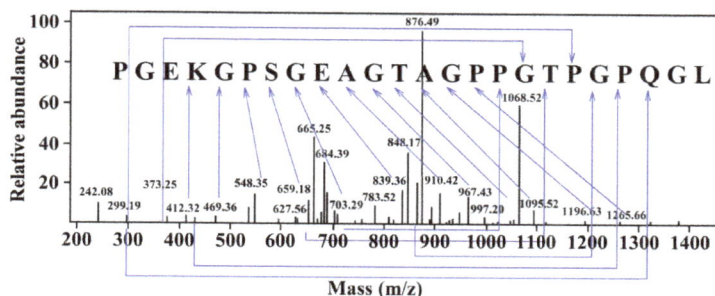

Figure 2. Electrospray ionization Fourier transform ion cyclotron resonance mass spectrometry (ESI-FTICR-MS) spectra of the amino acid sequences of Fraction D1.

2.3. Mode of Action and Molecular Docking of PGEKGPSGEAGTAGPPGTPGPQGL

To determine the mode of action of the NA-inhibitory peptide, a Lineweaver–Burk kinetic model was used to explore the relationship between the reaction rate and the substrate concentration. As shown in Figure 3, PGEKGPSGEAGTAGPPGTPGPQGL (peptide P) is a competitive NA inhibitor (Ki = 0.29 mM), suggesting that the peptide P can directly bind free enzyme. Such a binding results in a decrease in substrate affinity at the active site [24]. The binding of NA to a substrate or competitive inhibitor of amino acid residues is the highly specific binding [25]. A number of studies have shown that modes of action of NA inhibitors include competitive, non-competitive, uncompetitive and mixed modes. For example, Park et al. [26] obtained 2-hydroxy-3-methyl-3-butenyl alkyl (HMB) from *Angelica keiskei* and HMB was a non-competitive inhibitor with Ki of 14.0 ± 1.5 μM (IC$_{50}$ = 12.3 μM). Nguyen et al. [27] isolated eight oligostilbenes from *Vitis amurensis*, which were all non-competitive inhibitors with Ki of 8–25 μM (IC$_{50}$ = 8.94–234.61 μM). Jiang et al. [28] isolated indole alkaloid from *Streptomyces* sp. FIM090041, which was a competitive inhibitor with Ki of 13.5 μM (IC$_{50}$ = 67.8 μM). In addition, oseltamivir was a competitive inhibitor of chemically synthesized drugs. Compared with those NA inhibitors, the NA-inhibitory intensity of the peptide P was relatively low. Thus, the synergistic combination with other inhibitors should be further explored based on this study.

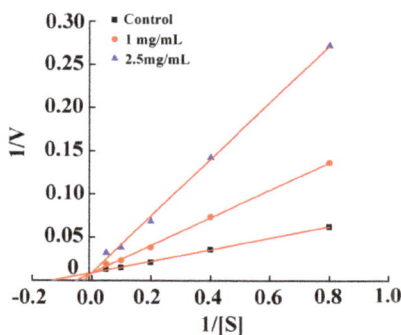

Figure 3. Kinetic study of the NA inhibition profile of PGEKGPSGEAGTAGPPGTPGPQGL.

For the purpose of understanding the interaction mechanism between peptide P and NA, molecular docking was performed. Prior to docking, the conformation of the peptide P was determined using molecular dynamics (MD). Peptide P has several conformations in the solution. Two main clusters were identified. Two minimum-energy conformations of peptide P from the two main clusters were selected for binding modes determination. As shown in Figure 4, Conformation A forms 6 hydrogen bonds with the residues Asn347, Asp151 and Lys150, whereas Conformation B only forms 3 hydrogen bonds with the residues Lys150, Asn347 and Ser369. In addition, Pro21 of Conformation A is important in the formation of hydrogen bonds. Thus, Conformation A is probably more energetically favorable to bind to the NA. Our docking studies suggested that hydrogen binding might be the driving force for the binding affinity of peptide P to NA. Li et al. [22] also reported that the hydrogen binding was the main driving force for the binding affinity of PNVA to angiotensin converting enzyme (ACE). The binding site of the NA is filled with charged residues and properly introducing charged residues to the NA can be a way to increase the binding affinity of peptide P analogues.

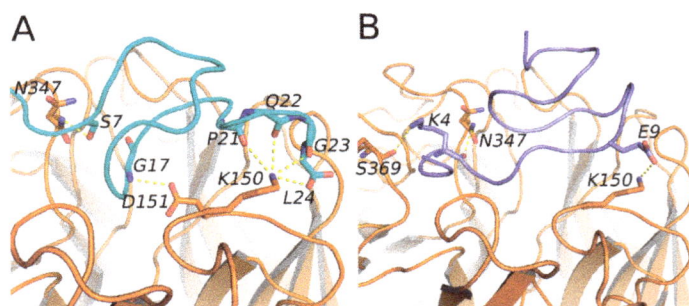

Figure 4. Probable binding mode of peptide PGEKGPSGEAGTAGPPGTPGPQGL at H1N1 NA. Conformation of the peptide was determined by MD simulations. Conformation of the peptide was clustered from the last 50 ns MD. (**A**,**B**) show the binding modes of the two minimum-energy conformations (Conformation **A** and Conformation **B**) of the peptide extracted from the two largest clusters at the binding site of NA. The dashed lines show the hydrogen bonds formed between residues from the peptide and residues of the NA.

2.4. Cytotoxicity and Antiviral Activity of Peptide PGEKGPSGEAGTAGPPGTPGPQGL on Madin–Darby Canine Kidney (MDCK) Cells

The peptide P exhibited no significant cytotoxicity in Madin–Darby canine kidney (MDCK) cells at a concentration of 250 μg/mL or less ($p > 0.05$), while peptide P significantly reduced the viability of MDCK cells at concentrations over 250 μg/mL ($p < 0.05$) (Figure 5B). The inhibitory effect of the peptide P on the H1N1 virus was examined in vitro. MDCK cells treated with H1N1 (Figure 5A) exhibited cytoplasmic shrinkage, loss of cell-cell contract, and reduction in cell numbers. After co-treatment with peptide P, MDCK cell morphology was changed slightly and appeared healthy with a regular shape compared with the control cells. The treatment with 62.5~1000 μg/mL peptide P significantly reduced the cytopathic effect (CPE) and peptide P increased the viability of virus-infected cells dose-dependently (Figure 5C). The peptide P at a concentration of 250 μg/mL inhibited H1N1 by 42%, which showed a lower antiviral effect than ribavirin ($p < 0.05$). The EC_{50} value of peptide P against H1N1 was 471 ± 12 μg/mL. Test results indicated that peptide P could protect MDCK cells from viral infection and reduced the viral production in a dose-dependent manner.

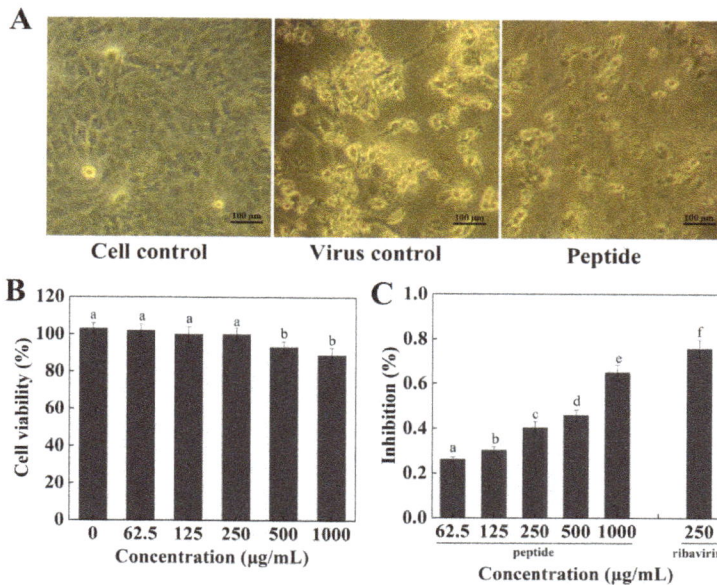

Figure 5. (**A**) Morphological changes in H1N1-infected MDCK cells; (**B**) Cell viability of Madin–Darby canine kidney (MDCK) cells after being incubated with the peptide at different concentrations for 48 h; (**C**) Inhibitory effects of the peptide on influenza virus H1N1 infection in MDCK cells. Values of three replicates are expressed as mean ± standard deviation. Different lowercase letters indicate significantly different values ($p < 0.05$).

2.5. Inhibitory Effects of Peptide PGEKGPSGEAGTAGPPGTPGPQGL on Different Stages of Viral Replication

To determine the stages in which the peptide P plays a role in the influenza virus life cycle, a time-of-addition experiment was conducted. MDCK cells treated with H1N1 exhibited the shrinkage of cytoplasm, loss of cell–cell contract, and apoptosis (Figure 6A). The MDCK-cell morphology was different in three stages and the pretreatment group appeared healthier than adsorption and after-adsorption groups, with regular shapes. A significant protection effect was observed when the peptide P was added before viral adsorption and the inhibition ratio was 73%, which was slightly lower than the positive control of ribavirin (75%) (Figure 6B), suggesting that the possible target of peptide P was located in the cell surface and could reduce viral virulence. In addition, the viability of the infected cells was partly recovered by the peptide P during viral adsorption, and the inhibition ratio was 58%, which was significantly lower than positive control of ribavirin (75%) (Figure 6B), indicating that peptide P could effectively prevent the attachment of virus and cells. Moreover, peptide P showed less inhibition rates by approximately 31.5% against H1N1 when it was added after the infection (Figure 6B), indicating that peptide P could inhibit an after-adsorption step of the influenza virus life cycle. In addition, the IC$_{50}$ values in three different stages of viral replication were increased according to the following order: pretreatment < adsorption < after-adsorption (Figure 6B). The result was consistent with the results of inhibition assays. Overall, the time-course analysis showed that the peptide P mainly inhibited influenza virus in the early stage of the infectious cycle.

Previous studies reported the protein-enriched fraction (PEF) that isolated from the larvae of housefly had strong antiviral activity against influenza virus at a very early stage of the interaction with virus particles or their entry into the cells [29]. The extract of *Ginkgo biloba* (EGB) could directly interact with influenza virus and markedly reduce the infectivity of the virus by preventing the adsorption to host cells [30]. The theaflavin derivatives had a direct effect on viral particle infectivity [31]. Similar to the results in the study, these studies also indicated that the inhibition of influenza virus occurred in the early stage of the infectious cycle. Ding et al. [32] reported that chlorogenic acid (CHA) inhibited influenza virus in the late stage of the infectious cycle.

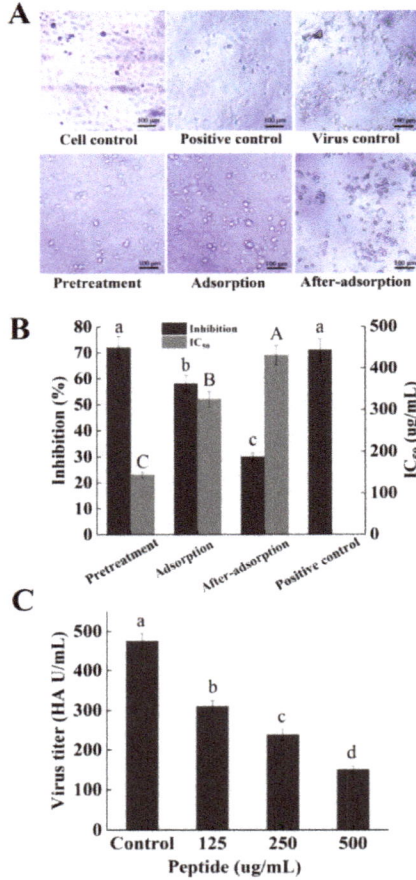

Figure 6. (**A**) Morphological changes of H1N1-infected MDCK cells under different treatment conditions. (i) Pretreatment, (ii) adsorption, (iii) after-adsorption; (**B**) MDCK cells were infected with the peptide under three different treatment conditions; (**C**) hemagglutination (HA) titers of influenza virus H1N1 treated with different concentrations of peptide. Values of three replicates are expressed as mean ± standard deviation. Different letters indicate significantly different values (*p* < 0.05).

2.6. Hemagglutination (HA) Assay

To explore whether the inhibitory effect of the peptide P on H1N1 was cell-specific or not, the virus titers in MDCK cell supernatants were measured by hemagglutination (HA) assay. The virus particles contain hemagglutinin protein, which binds to receptors on the surface of erythrocytes and causes hemagglutination (HA) [33]. The maximum dilution ratio of red blood cell agglutination can be set as the HA titer in HA experiments with different dilutions of virus. Some active substances can bind to the surface of the virus and block the hemagglutinin, thereby preventing the combination of red blood cells and inhibiting hemagglutination. As shown in Figure 6C, the HA titer of the virus was inhibited by the peptide P dose-dependently and the peptide P could significantly reduce the virus titer at the concentration over 125 μg/mL ($p < 0.05$). The NA-inhibitory peptide P could affect the virus toxicity and adsorption by host cells, further proving that the peptide had an anti-viral effect with multiple target sites. Wang et al. [29] also reported that PEF could decrease the infectious capacity in HA titer and prevent the attachment of virus and cells. In addition, Haruyama et al. [30] reported that EGB contained an anti-influenza virus substance that directly affected influenza virus particles and disrupted the function of hemagglutinin in the adsorption to host cells.

2.7. Simulated Digestion Test on NA-Inhibitory Peptide

The NA-inhibitory peptides need to resist digestive enzymes in vivo to maintain the stability of the peptides. In the simulated environment of the digestive tract, the activity the NA-inhibitory peptides before and after digestion were measured. To explore the behaviors of the peptide in the digestive tract in vitro, the peptide P was treated with digestive enzymes. After the simulated digestion, the activity of the NA-inhibitory peptide was significantly decreased ($p < 0.05$), indicating the instability of the NA-inhibitory peptide during the simulated in vitro gastrointestinal digestion (Figure 7). Kuba et al. [34] extracted ACE inhibitory peptide Trp-Leu from Tofuyo (fermented soybean food) and suggested that the inhibitory activity of Trp-Leu was completely preserved after the simulated digestion. Different peptides have different tolerances to gastrointestinal proteases. The activities of some functional peptides were increased after digestion and could be taken orally as a prodrug through sustained release or direct digestion. However, the activity of NA-inhibitory peptide in cod skin hydrolyzates after digestion was not ideal, so oral administration is not recommended. There are many ways to uptake the NA-inhibitory peptides, including adsorption, injection, oral administration and other ways. Therefore, it is necessary to further explore other routes of entry.

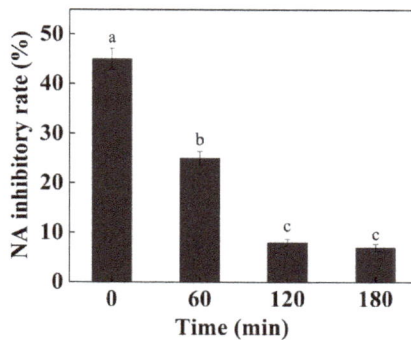

Figure 7. NA-inhibitory rate of the peptide PGEKGPSGEAGTAGPPGTPGPQGL during the simulated in vitro gastrointestinal digestion. Values of three replicates are expressed as mean ± standard deviation. Different lowercase letters indicate significantly different values ($p < 0.05$).

3. Materials and Methods

3.1. Reagents

Cod skins were purchased from Shandong Meijia Group Co., Ltd. (Rizhao, China). Ribavirin (50 mg/mL) was purchased from Cisen Pharmaceutical Co., Ltd. (Jining, China). Zorbax SB-C18 column (9.4 mm × 250 mm) was obtained from Agilent Technologies (Santa Clara, CA, USA). RPM1640 medium, fetal bovine serum (FBS), penicillin and streptomycin were obtained from Gibco (Grand Island, NY, USA). 4-Methylumbelliferyl-N-acetyl-α-D-neuralminic acid (MUNANA) and 2-(N-morpholino) ethanesulphonic acid (MES) were bought from Sigma (St. Louis, MO, USA). Influenza virus H1N1 neuraminidase (NA) was kindly made by the School of Medicine and Pharmacy,

Ocean University of China (Qingdao, China). All other chemicals were bought from local commercial sources and were of the highest purity available.

3.2. Cells and Viruses

MDCK cells were purchased from Shanghai Institute of Biochemistry and Cell Biology (Shanghai, China), and maintained in RPM1640 medium included 10% of FBS, 100 U/mL of penicillin and 100 µg/mL of streptomycin. The influenza virus A/Puerto Rico/8/1934 (H1N1) was obtained from Wuhan Institute of Virology (Wuhan, China), and grown in 10-day-old embryonated eggs at 36.5 °C for 72 h. As for infection, virus propagation solution was diluted in phosphate buffered saline (PBS) containing 0.2% bovine serum albumin (BSA) and then added into the cells at the indicated multiplicity of infection (MOI). Viruses were allowed to be adsorbed 60 min at 37 °C. After removing the virus inoculum, cells were maintained in infecting media (RPM1640, 4 µg/mL trypsin) at 37 °C in 5% CO_2.

3.3. Protein Extraction of Cod Skins

The protein of cod skins was prepared according to the method described by Zhao et al. [35]. Briefly, 100 g of cod skins were firstly cut up and homogenized in 600 mL of distilled water. Then, protein of cod skins was extracted from the homogenates in a water bath at 85 °C for 6 h and centrifuged (5000× g, 30 min) to obtain the solutions. The solutions were freeze-dried with a lyophilizer (Ningbo Scientz Biotechnology Co., Ltd., Ningbo, China).

3.4. Preparation of Cod Skin Protein Hydrolysates

The freeze-dried cod skin protein was initially dissolved in water and its substrate concentration was adjusted to 22 mg/mL. After that, pepsin (1.6 kU/g protein) was added into the solution and hydrolyzed in a water bath at 37 °C for 6.8 h. Afterward, the pepsin was inactivated at 100 °C for 10 min. After centrifugation at 5000× g for 30 min, the ultrafiltration precipitation was carried out with 5 K membrane (Millipore Isopore, Billerica, MA, USA). The precipitate obtained was freeze-dried and stored for use.

3.5. Purification of NA-Inhibitory Peptide

The Sephadex G-15 column (2.6 cm × 65 cm) was used to purify the NA-inhibitory peptides. The flow rate was 1.2 mL/min and double distilled water was used for elution. After that, the Zorbax SB-C18 column (9.4 mm × 250 mm, Agilent, CA, USA) equipped with an Agilent 1260 infinity HPLC system (Agilent Technology, Mississauga, ON, Canada) was used to analyze the peptides in the hydrolysates at a flow rate of 1.5 mL/min. An acetonitrile gradient from 5% to 40% was adopted for 20-min elution to separate groups of peptides. Chromatographic separation was carried out at 35 °C. The components were collected at the absorbance of 220 nm and freeze-dried for further analysis.

3.6. NA-Inhibitory Activity Assay

The NA activity assay was performed according to the previous method with slight modifications [36]. Briefly, the sample (10 µL) and NA solution (30 µL) were added to a 96-well plate. After the incubation at 37 °C for 30 min, 60 µL of reaction buffer (33 mM MES buffer, pH = 3.5; 4 mM $CaCl_2$; 10 µL MUNANA) was added. After the incubation under the same conditions, 100 µL of stop solution (83% ethanol; 14 mM NaOH) was added to each well. The fluorescence intensity was measured with a SpectraMax M5 plate reader (Molecular Decices, Sunnyvale, CA, USA) with the excitation and emission wavelengths of 355 and 460 nm, respectively; 10 µL of PBS and 30 µL of NA were used as the positive control, and 10 µL of PBS and 30 µL of PBS were used as the negative control.

The hydrolysates (10 µL) and NA (30 µL) were used as the samples and 10 µL of hydrolysates and 30 µL of PBS were used as the negative control of the sample. The inhibition activity is calculated as:

$$\text{Inhibition activity}(\%) = \frac{(A_{PC} - A_{NC}) - \left(A_{Sample} - A_{SNC}\right)}{A_{PC} - A_{NC}} \times 100\% \tag{1}$$

PC: positive control, NC: negative control, SNC: negative control of the sample.

3.7. Amino Acid Sequence Analysis

The peptides were sequenced using ESI-FTICR-MS. The sequencing was completed in the Beijing Proteome Research Center (Beijing, China).

3.8. NA Inhibition Mode

The mode of NA inhibition was determined according to the previous method with slight modifications [37]. Various concentrations of MUNANA (1.25, 2.5, 5, 10 and 20 µM) were incubated with NA in the absence or presence (0–2.5 mg/mL) of the peptide P at 37 °C. The inhibition kinetics of NA in the presence of peptide P was determined based on the Lineweaver–Burk plot. The inhibitor constant Ki was calculated by plotting $1/V_{max}$ versus the concentrations of peptide P.

3.9. Molecular Dynamics Simulation

The initial conformation of the peptide P was produced with the xleap module in AMBER 16. The protonation states of the peptide P residues were predicted with the PropKa 3.1 method [38]. The initial model was minimized and refined through molecular dynamics (MD) simulations with the Amber 16 package and ff14SB force field [39]. The system was minimized and equilibrated according the previous method [40]. The SHAKE algorithm was used for the MD simulations [41]. The long-range electrostatic interactions were modeled using the particle-mesh ewald (PME) method [42]. MD trajectories were analyzed with VMD [43] and molecules were drawn with PyMol (Schrödinger LLC, Portland, OR, USA).

3.10. Docking

Docking the MD refined structures of peptide P to H1N1 (PDB Code: 1RUZ) [44] was performed in AutoDock 4.2 [45]. Gasteiger charges were used and nonpolar hydrogens of the macromolecule and ligand were merged. A grid box with the dimensions of 60 Å × 60 Å × 60 Å and a grid spacing of 0.375 Å was set up and centered at the geometric center of the binding box defined with the bound ligand in the crystal structure. Docking was performed by using a Lamarckian genetic algorithm (LGA), with the receptor treated as a rigid body. The docking results were analyzed by AutoDock Tools. The produced conformations were selected based the docking score and manual analysis.

3.11. Cytotoxicity Test by MTT Assay

The MTT assay was used to determine the effect of the peptide on the viability of MDCK cells [5,46]. The 96-well plates were used to culture the MDCK cells. After adding 10 µL of PBS containing MTT (0.5 mg/mL) into each well, the solution was incubated at 37 °C for 4 h. After removing the supernatant, 200 µL of DMSO was added into each well. The optical density (OD) for each well was determined at 570 nm. The IC_{50} was calculated as the concentration of the sample at which the number of viable cells was decreased to 50% of that in the cell control.

3.12. Cytopathic Effect (CPE) Reduction Assay

The cytopathic effect (CPE) reduction assay was performed according to the previous method [5,47]. MDCK cells were firstly infected with influenza A H1N1 virus (IAV) (MOI = 0.1) and then treated with different concentrations of peptide in triplicate after removing the virus inoculum. After 48-h incubation, 4% formaldehyde was used to fix the cells for 20 min. After removing formaldehyde, 0.1% crystal violet was used to stain the cells for 30 min. After elution of the dye with methanol, the intensity of crystal violet staining for each well was measured at 570 nm.

3.13. Acting Mode of Inhibitory Peptide

In order to investigate the inhibitory effects of the peptide on the influenza at different stages of replication, time course analysis was determined according to the previous method [5]. In the pretreatment assay, influenza A virus (IAV, MOI = 3.0) was pretreated with 250 µg/mL of the peptide at 37 °C for 1 h before infection. Then, the virus/peptide mixture was added to MDCK cells for 1 h at 4 °C, and the culture solutions were removed and replaced by sample-free solutions. In the adsorption assay, MDCK cells were infected in solutions containing 250 µg/mL of the peptide at 4 °C after 1-h adsorption and then the culture solutions were removed and replaced by sample-free solutions. In the post-adsorption assay, the virus suspension was added into each well containing a confluent MDCK cell monolayer and then the cells were treated with 250 µg/mL of the peptide after removing the virus inoculums. At 24 h, the antiviral activity was detected by the CPE inhibition assay as described above.

3.14. HA Assay

The hemagglutination (HA) assay was performed as previously reported [48]. The virus solutions (10^5 PFU/mL) were serially diluted in 96-well plates, followed by adding different dilutions of NA-inhibitory peptides. The same volume of 1% standardized chicken red blood cells (cRBCs) prepared according to the World Health Organization (WHO) manuals were added to each well. After 60-min incubation at 4 °C, RBCs in negative wells were sedimented to form red buttons, whereas positive wells had an opaque appearance without sedimentation. HA titers were given as hemagglutination units/50 µL (HAU/50 µL).

3.15. Simulated Digestion Assay

Simulated digestion assay was performed according to the previous method with slight modifications [49]. The NA-inhibitory peptide was dissolved in deionized water to prepare 10 mg/mL solution. The pH was adjusted to 2.0 with 1 mol/L HCl and then pepsin (2.86% of the substrate, dry basis) was added. Digestion was performed at 37 °C for 2 h, followed by boiling for 10 min to stop the enzyme activation. Subsequently, the pH was adjusted to 7.5 with 0.2 mol/L NaOH. After adding chymotrypsin (4.00% of substrate, dry basis), the reaction was carried out at 37 °C for 1 h. The sample was submerged in a 95 °C water bath for 10 min to terminate the enzymatic digestion and cooled on ice to room temperature. Then, trypsin (4.00% of substrate, dry basis) was added, and the above steps were repeated. Afterwards, the digested mixtures were centrifuged at 10,000× *g* for 10 min to obtain the digestive juices. The NA inhibition assay in digestive juices was detected as described above.

3.16. Statistical Analysis

The data were expressed as mean ± standard deviation (SD). The results were validated by one-way analysis of variance (ANOVA). Duncan's multiple range tests were performed to determine the differences between means (significance level was set at 5%) using SPSS 20.0 (SPSS Inc., Chicago, IL, USA).

4. Conclusions

The novel NA-inhibitory peptide PGEKGPSGEAGTAGPPGTPGPQGL was first prepared from cod skin hydrolysates. Docking studies suggested that hydrogen binding might be the driving force for the binding affinity of the peptide to NA. Time-course analysis showed that the peptide inhibited influenza virus in the early stage of the infectious cycle. The assay of virus titers indicated that the

NA-inhibitory peptide could directly affect the virus toxicity and the adsorption by host cells, further proving that the peptide had an anti-viral effect with multiple target sites. The activity of NA-inhibitory peptide was almost inactivated during the simulated in vitro gastrointestinal digestion, suggesting that oral administration was not recommended and the need to further explore other routes of entry. Furthermore, the antiviral activities of peptide against H1N1 in vivo need to be further investigated in order to facilitate the development of peptide in preventing influenza virus infection. The peptide exhibits potential utility in the control of influenza virus infections. This study provides a theoretical basis for guiding the discovery of new natural anti-influenza drugs.

Author Contributions: Data curation, J.L. and N.Y.; Project administration, Y.Z.; Software, R.Y.; Validation, Y.C., Z.L., H.W. and S.D.; Visualization, Z.L.; Writing—original draft, J.L.; Writing—review and editing, M.Z. and Y.Z.

Funding: This project was supported by Ningbo Agricultural Science and Technology Key Projects (2017C110006), Qingdao Science and Technology Development Project (No. 17-3-3-46-nsh) and Natural Science Foundation of Shandong Province (No. ZR2015CM011).

Conflicts of Interest: The authors declare no conflict of interest.

References

1. Baron, Y.; Glasner, A.; Meningher, T.; Achdout, H.; Gur, C.; Lankry, D.; Vitenshtein, A.; Meyers, A.F.A.; Mandelboim, M.; Mandelboim, O. Neuraminidase-mediated, NKp46-dependent immune-evasion mechanism of influenza viruses. *Cell Rep.* **2013**, *3*, 1044–1050. [CrossRef] [PubMed]

2. Li, Y.; Lin, Z.; Guo, M.; Xia, Y.; Zhao, M.; Wang, C.; Xu, T.; Chen, T.; Zhu, B. Inhibitory activity of selenium nanoparticles functionalized with oseltamivir on H1N1 influenza virus. *Int. J. Nanomed.* **2017**, *12*, 5733–5743. [CrossRef] [PubMed]

3. Matrosovich, M.N.; Matrosovich, T.Y.; Gray, T.; Roberts, N.A.; Klenk, H.D. Neuraminidase is important for the initiation of influenza virus infection in human airway epithelium. *J. Virol.* **2004**, *78*, 12665–12667. [CrossRef] [PubMed]

4. Lee, M.Y.; Yen, H.L. Targeting the host or the virus: Current and novel concepts for antiviral approaches against influenza virus infection. *Antivir. Res.* **2012**, *96*, 391–404. [CrossRef] [PubMed]

5. Wang, W.; Cui, Z.Q.; Zhang, P.; Hao, C.; Zhang, X.E.; Guan, H.S. In vitro inhibitory effect of carrageenan oligosaccharide on influenza A H1N1 virus. *Antivir. Res.* **2011**, *92*, 237–246. [CrossRef] [PubMed]

6. Jiang, L.; Fantoni, G.; Couzens, L.; Gao, J.; Plant, E.; Ye, Z.; Eichelberger, M.C.; Wan, H. Comparative efficacy of monoclonal antibodies that bind to different epitopes of the 2009 pandemic H1N1 influenza virus neuraminidase. *J. Virol.* **2016**, *90*, 117–128. [CrossRef] [PubMed]

7. Hayden, F.G.; Pavia, A.T. Antiviral management of seasonal and pandemic influenza. *J. Infect. Dis.* **2006**, *194*, 119–126. [CrossRef] [PubMed]

8. Yen, H.L.; Mckimm-Breschkin, J.L.; Choy, K.T.; Wong, D.D.Y.; Cheung, P.P.H.; Zhou, J.; Ng, I.H.; Zhu, H.; Webby, R.J.; Guan, Y.; et al. Resistance to neuraminidase inhibitors conferred by an R292K mutation in a human influenza virus H7N9 isolate can be masked by a mixed R/K viral population. *MBio* **2013**, *4*, e00396-13. [CrossRef] [PubMed]

9. Amri, N.; Parikesit, A.A.; Tambunan, U.S.F. In silico design of cyclic peptides as influenza virus, a subtype H1N1 neuraminidase inhibitor. *Afr. J. Biotechnol.* **2013**, *11*, 11474–11491.

10. Upadhyay, A.; Chompoo, J.; Taira, N.; Fukuta, M.; Gima, S.; Tawata, S. Solid-phase synthesis of mimosine tetrapeptides and their inhibitory activities on neuraminidase and tyrosinase. *J. Agric. Food Chem.* **2011**, *59*, 12858–12863. [CrossRef] [PubMed]

11. Yuan, N.; Zeng, M.Y.; Gao, F.Z.; Guo, X.M.; Wang, H.T.; Zhao, Y.H.; Wang, W. Preparation of active peptide from cod skins with inhibitory activity on influenza virus neuraminidase. *Chin. J. Mar. Drugs* **2012**, *31*, 1–7.

12. Nagai, T.; Suzuki, N. Preparation and partial characterization of collagen from paper nautilus (*Argonauta argo, Linnaeus*) outer skin. *Food Chem.* **2002**, *76*, 149–153. [CrossRef]

13. Mattice, W.L.; Mandelkern, L. Ordered structures in sequential copolypeptides containing L-proline or 4-hydroxy-L-proline. *J. Am. Chem. Soc.* **1970**, *92*, 5285–5287. [CrossRef] [PubMed]

14. Wang, G.T.; Chen, Y.; Wang, S.; Gentles, R.; Sowin, T.; Kati, W.; Muchmore, S.; Giranda, V.; Stewart, K.; Sham, H.; et al. Design, synthesis, and structural analysis of influenza neuraminidase inhibitors containing pyrrolidine cores. *J. Med. Chem.* **2001**, *44*, 1192–1201. [CrossRef] [PubMed]

15. Hanessian, S.; Bayrakdarian, M.; Luo, X. Total synthesis of A-315675: A potent inhibitor of influenza neuraminidase. *J. Am. Chem. Soc.* **2002**, *124*, 4716–4721. [CrossRef] [PubMed]

16. Himaya, S.W.A.; Ngo, D.H.; Ryu, B.M.; Kim, S.K. An active peptide purified from gastrointestinal enzyme hydrolysate of Pacific cod skin gelatin attenuates angiotensin-1 converting enzyme (ACE) activity and cellular oxidative stress. *Food Chem.* **2012**, *132*, 1872–1882. [CrossRef]

17. Ngo, D.H.; Vo, T.S.; Ryu, B.M.; Kim, S.K. Angiotensin-I-converting enzyme (ACE) inhibitory peptides from Pacific cod skin gelatin using ultrafiltration membranes. *Process Biochem.* **2016**, *51*, 1622–1628. [CrossRef]

18. Madrahimov, A.; Helikar, T.; Kowal, B.; Lu, G.; Rogers, J. Dynamics of influenza virus and human host interactions during infection and replication cycle. *Bull. Math. Biol.* **2013**, *75*, 988–1011. [CrossRef] [PubMed]

19. Lin, Z.; Li, Y.; Guo, M.; Xu, T.; Wang, C.; Zhao, M.; Wang, H.; Chen, T.; Zhu, B. The inhibition of H1N1 influenza virus-induced apoptosis by silver nanoparticles functionalized with zanamivir. *RSC Adv.* **2017**, *7*, 742–750. [CrossRef]

20. Lauster, D.; Glanz, M.; Bardua, M.; Ludwig, K.; Hellmund, M.; Hoffmann, U.; Hamann, A.; Böttcher, C.; Haag, R.; Hackenberger, C.P.R.; et al. Multivalent peptide-nanoparticle conjugates for influenza-virus inhibition. *Angew. Chem. Int. Ed.* **2017**, *56*, 5931–5936. [CrossRef] [PubMed]

21. Xiao, S.; Si, L.; Tian, Z.; Jiao, P.; Fan, Z.; Meng, K.; Zhou, X.; Wang, H.; Xu, R.; Han, X.; et al. Pentacyclic triterpenes grafted on CD cores to interfere with influenza virus entry: A dramatic multivalent effect. *Biomaterials* **2016**, *78*, 74–85. [CrossRef] [PubMed]

22. Li, J.; Liu, Z.; Zhao, Y.; Zhu, X.; Yu, R.; Dong, S.; Wu, H. Novel natural angiotensin converting enzyme (ACE)-inhibitory peptides derived from sea cucumber-modified hydrolysates by adding exogenous proline and a study of their structure–activity relationship. *Mar. Drugs* **2018**, *16*, 271. [CrossRef] [PubMed]

23. Irungu, J.; Go, E.P.; Zhang, Y.; Dalpathado, D.S.; Liao, H.X.; Haynes, B.F.; Desaire, H. Comparison of HPLC/ESI-FTICR MS versus MALDI-TOF/TOF MS for glycopeptide analysis of a highly glycosylated HIV envelope glycoprotein. *J. Am. Soc. Mass Spectr.* **2008**, *19*, 1209–1220. [CrossRef] [PubMed]

24. Sangsawad, P.; Roytrakul, S.; Choowongkomon, K.; Kitts, D.D.; Chen, X.M.; Meng, G.; Lichan, E.; Yongsawatdigul, J. Transepithelial transport across Caco-2 cell monolayers of angiotensin converting enzyme (ACE) inhibitory peptides derived from simulated in vitro gastrointestinal digestion of cooked chicken muscles. *Food Chem.* **2018**, *251*, 77–85. [CrossRef] [PubMed]

25. Sun, H.; Li, T.J.; Zhao, X.H. Ace inhibition and enzymatic resistance in vitro of a casein hydrolysate subjected to plastein reaction in the presence of extrinsic proline and ethanol- or methanol-water fractionation. *Int. J. Food Prop.* **2014**, *17*, 386–398. [CrossRef]

26. Park, J.Y.; Jeong, H.J.; Kim, Y.M.; Park, S.J.; Rho, M.C.; Park, K.H.; Ryu, Y.B.; Lee, W.S. Characteristic of alkylated chalcones from Angelica keiskei on influenza virus neuraminidase inhibition. *Bioorg. Med. Chem. Lett.* **2011**, *21*, 5602–5604. [CrossRef] [PubMed]

27. Nguyen, T.N.A.; Dao, T.T.; Tung, B.T.; Hwanwon, C.; Eunhee, K.; Junsoo, P.; Seongil, L.; Wonkeun, O. Influenza A (H1N1) neuraminidase inhibitors from Vitis amurensis. *Food Chem.* **2011**, *124*, 437–443. [CrossRef]

28. Jiang, H.L.; Wang, C.X.; Jiang, N.Y.; Chen, M.H.; Peng, F.; Xie, Y.; Jiang, H. Neuraminidase inhibitors produced by the marine derived *Streptomyces* sp. FIM090041. *Chin. J. Antibiot.* **2012**, *37*, 265–268.

29. Wang, F.; Ai, H.; Lei, C. In vitro anti-influenza activity of a protein-enriched fraction from larvae of the housefly (*Musca domestica*). *Pharm. Biol.* **2013**, *51*, 405–410. [CrossRef] [PubMed]

30. Haruyama, T.; Nagata, K. Anti-influenza virus activity of Ginkgo biloba leaf extracts. *J. Nat. Med.* **2013**, *67*, 636–642. [CrossRef] [PubMed]

31. Zu, M.; Yang, F.; Zhou, W.; Liu, A.; Du, G.; Zheng, L. In vitro anti-influenza virus and anti-inflammatory activities of theaflavin derivatives. *Antivir. Res.* **2012**, *94*, 217–224. [CrossRef] [PubMed]

32. Ding, Y.; Cao, Z.; Cao, L.; Ding, G.; Wang, Z.; Xiao, W. Antiviral activity of chlorogenic acid against influenza A (H1N1/H3N2) virus and its inhibition of neuraminidase. *Sci. Rep.* **2017**, *7*, 45723. [CrossRef] [PubMed]

33. Wang, L.B.; Chen, Q.Y.; Wu, X.M.; Che, Y.L.; Wang, C.Y.; Chen, R.J.; Zhou, L.J. Isolation of a reassortant H1N2 swine Flu strain of type "Swine-Human-Avian" and its genetic variability analysis. *BioMed Res. Int.* **2018**, 2018. [CrossRef] [PubMed]

34. Kuba, M.; Tanaka, K.; Tawata, S.; Takeda, Y.; Yasuda, M. Angiotensin I-converting enzyme inhibitory peptides isolated from tofuyo fermented soybean food. *Biosci. Biotechnol. Biochem.* **2003**, *67*, 1278–1283. [CrossRef] [PubMed]

35. Zhao, H.Y.; Liang, C.C.; Miao, J.L.; Li, G.Y. Preparation and composition analysis of cod skin collagen protein. *Chin. J. Mar. Drugs* **2005**, *24*, 30–32.

36. Cao, H.P.; Tao, P.Z.; Du, G.H. Establishment and application of high throughput screening model for influenza virus neuraminidase inhibitors in vitro. *Acta Pharm. Sin.* **2002**, *37*, 930–933.

37. Jag, R.; Ramos, M.; Recio, I. Angiotensin converting enzyme-inhibitory activity of peptides isolated from Manchego cheese. Stability under simulated gastrointestinal digestion. *Int. Dairy J.* **2004**, *14*, 1075–1080.

38. Olsson, M.H.M.; Søndergaard, C.R.; Rostkowski, M.; Jensen, J.H. PROPKA3: Consistent treatment of internal and surface residues in empirical pK_a predictions. *J. Chem. Theory Comput.* **2011**, *7*, 525–537. [CrossRef] [PubMed]

39. Hornak, V.; Abel, R.; Okur, A.; Strockbine, B.; Roitberg, A.; Simmerling, C. Comparison of multiple AMBER force fields and development of improved protein backbone parameters. *Proteins* **2010**, *65*, 712–725. [CrossRef] [PubMed]

40. Tabassum, N.; Tae, H.S.; Jia, X.; Kaas, Q.; Jiang, T.; Adams, D.J.; Yu, R. Role of Cys I-Cys III disulfide bond on the structure and activity of α-conotoxins at human neuronal nicotinic acetylcholine receptors. *ACS Omega* **2017**, *2*, 4621–4631. [CrossRef] [PubMed]

41. Miyamoto, S.; Kollman, P.A. Settle: An analytical version of the SHAKE and RATTLE algorithm for rigid water models. *J. Comp. Chem.* **1992**, *13*, 952–962. [CrossRef]

42. Darden, T.; York, D.; Pedersen, L. Particle mesh Ewald: An $N \cdot \log(N)$ method for Ewald sums in large systems. *J. Chem. Phys.* **1993**, *98*, 10089–10092. [CrossRef]

43. Humphrey, W.F.; Dalke, A.; Schulten, K. VMD: visual molecular dynamics. *J. Mol. Graph.* **1996**, *14*, 33–38. [CrossRef]

44. Xu, X.; Zhu, X.; Dwek, R.A.; Stevens, J.; Wilson, I.A. Structural characterization of the 1918 influenza virus H1N1 neuraminidase. *J. Virol.* **2008**, *82*, 10493–10501. [CrossRef] [PubMed]

45. Morris, G.M.; Huey, R.; Lindstrom, W.; Sanner, M.F.; Belew, R.K.; Goodsell, D.S.; Olson, A.J. AutoDock4 and AutoDockTools4: Automated docking with selective receptor flexibility. *J. Comput. Chem.* **2010**, *30*, 2785–2791. [CrossRef] [PubMed]

46. Talarico, L.B.; Damonte, E.B. Interference in dengue virus adsorption and uncoating by carrageenans. *Virology* **2007**, *363*, 473–485. [CrossRef] [PubMed]

47. Wang, W.; Zhang, P.; Yu, G.L.; Li, C.X.; Hao, C.; Qi, X.; Zhang, L.J.; Guan, H.S. Preparation and anti-influenza A virus activity of k-carrageenan oligosaccharide and its sulphated derivatives. *Food Chem.* **2012**, *133*, 880–888. [CrossRef]

48. Sriwilaijaroen, N.; Kadowaki, A.; Onishi, Y.; Gato, N.; Ujike, M.; Odagiri, T.; Tashiro, M.; Suzuki, Y. Mumefural and related HMF derivatives from Japanese apricot fruit juice concentrate show multiple inhibitory effects on pandemic influenza A (H1N1) virus. *Food Chem.* **2011**, *127*, 1–9. [CrossRef]

49. Sangsawad, P.; Roytrakul, S.; Yongsawatdigul, J. Angiotensin converting enzyme (ACE) inhibitory peptides derived from the simulated in vitro gastrointestinal digestion of cooked chicken breast. *J. Funct. Foods* **2017**, *29*, 77–83. [CrossRef]

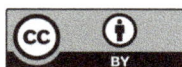

MDPI

St. Alban-Anlage 66

4052 Basel

Switzerland

Tel. +41 61 683 77 34

Fax +41 61 302 89 18

www.mdpi.com

Marine Drugs Editorial Office

E-mail: marinedrugs@mdpi.com

www.mdpi.com/journal/marinedrugs

www.ingramcontent.com/pod-product-compliance
Lightning Source LLC
Chambersburg PA
CBHW051704210326
41597CB00032B/5366